FIRST AID FOR THE®

USMLE STEP 1 2018

TAO LE, MD, MHS
Associate Clinical Professor
Chief, Section of Allergy and Immunology
Department of Medicine
University of Louisville School of Medicine

VIKAS BHUSHAN, MD
Boracay

MATTHEW SOCHAT, MD
Fellow, Department of Hematology/Oncology
St. Louis University School of Medicine

KIMBERLY KALLIANOS, MD
Assistant Professor, Department of Radiology and Biomedical Imaging
University of California, San Francisco

YASH CHAVDA, DO
Resident, Department of Emergency Medicine
St. Barnabas Hospital, Bronx

ANDREW ZUREICK
University of Michigan Medical School
Class of 2018

MEHBOOB KALANI, MD
Resident, Department of Internal Medicine
Allegheny Health Network Medical Education Consortium

Mc
Graw
Hill
Education

New York / Chicago / San Francisco / Athens / London / Madrid / Mexico City
Milan / New Delhi / Singapore / Sydney / Toronto

First Aid for the® USMLE Step 1 2018: A Student-to-Student Guide

Photo and line art credits for this book begin on page 707 and are considered an extension of this copyright page. Portions of this book identified with the symbol ℞ are copyright © USMLE-Rx.com (MedIQ Learning, LLC). Portions of this book identified with the symbol ℞ are copyright © Dr. Richard Usatine. Portions of this book identified with the symbol ✶ are under license from other third parties. Please refer to page 707 for a complete list of those image source attribution notices.

First Aid for the® is a registered trademark of McGraw-Hill Education.

1 2 3 4 5 6 7 8 9 0   LMN   22 21 20 19 18

ISBN 978-1-26-011612-0
MHID 1-26-011612-3
ISSN 1532-6020

Notice

Medicine is an ever-changing science. As new research and clinical experience broaden our knowledge, changes in treatment and drug therapy are required. The authors and the publisher of this work have checked with sources believed to be reliable in their efforts to provide information that is complete and generally in accord with the standards accepted at the time of publication. However, in view of the possibility of human error or changes in medical sciences, neither the authors nor the publisher nor any other party who has been involved in the preparation or publication of this work warrants that the information contained herein is in every respect accurate or complete, and they disclaim all responsibility for any errors or omissions or for the results obtained from use of the information contained in this work. Readers are encouraged to confirm the information contained herein with other sources. For example and in particular, readers are advised to check the product information sheet included in the package of each drug they plan to administer to be certain that the information contained in this work is accurate and that changes have not been made in the recommended dose or in the contraindications for administration. This recommendation is of particular importance in connection with new or infrequently used drugs.

This book was set in Electra LT Std by Rainbow Graphics.
The editors were Bob Boehringer and Christina M. Thomas.
Project management was provided by Rainbow Graphics.
The production supervisor was Jeffrey Herzich.
LSC Communications was printer and binder.

This book is printed on acid-free paper.

International Edition ISBN 978-12-6028815-5, MHID 1-26-028815-3.
Copyright © 2018. Exclusive rights by McGraw-Hill Education for manufacture and export. This book cannot be re-exported from the country to which it is consigned by McGraw-Hill Education. The International Edition is not available in North America.

McGraw-Hill Education books are available at special quantity discounts to use as premiums and sales promotions, or for use in corporate training programs. To contact a representative please visit the Contact Us pages at www.mhprofessional.com.

Dedication

To the contributors to this and past editions, who took time to share their knowledge, insight, and humor for the benefit of students and physicians everywhere.

Contents

▶ SECTION I	GUIDE TO EFFICIENT EXAM PREPARATION	1

▶ SECTION I SUPPLEMENT	SPECIAL SITUATIONS	27

▶ SECTION II	HIGH-YIELD GENERAL PRINCIPLES	29

Contributing Authors

MAJED H. ALGHAMDI, MBBS
King Abdulaziz University College of Medicine

VIJAY BALAKRISHNAN
Emory University School of Medicine
Class of 2018

BRIAN BALLARD
Michigan State University School of Osteopathic Medicine
Class of 2018

HUMOOD BOQAMBAR
Royal College of Surgeons in Ireland
Class of 2018

TARUNPREET DHALIWAL
St. George's University School of Medicine
Class of 2018

RACHEL L. KUSHNER, MSc
Mercer University School of Medicine
Class of 2018

LAUREN N. LESSOR
St. George's University School of Medicine
MD/PhD Candidate, Class of 2018

JONATHAN LI
University of Michigan Medical School
Class of 2018

SCOTT MOORE, DO
Assistant Professor of Medical Laboratory Sciences
Weber State University

JUN YEN NG, MBBS
Princess Alexandra Hospital

CONNIE QIU
Lewis Katz School of Medicine at Temple University
MD/PhD Candidate, Class of 2021

KALLI A. SARIGIANNIS
Oakland University William Beaumont School of Medicine
Class of 2018

SARAH SCHIMANSKY, MB BCh BAO
Resident, Department of Ophthalmology
Gloucestershire Hospitals NHS Foundation Trust

JESSE D. SENGILLO
SUNY Downstate College of Medicine
Class of 2018

ISABELLA T. WU
Tulane University School of Medicine
Class of 2019

VAISHNAVI VAIDYANATHAN
University of Missouri-Kansas City School of Medicine
Class of 2018

IMAGE AND ILLUSTRATION TEAM

ARTEMISA GOGOLLARI, MD
PhD Candidate
University for Health Sciences, Medical Informatics, and Technology, Austria

MATTHEW HO ZHI GUANG
University College Dublin (MD), Dana Farber Cancer Institute (PhD)
MD/PhD Candidate

VICTOR JOSE MARTINEZ LEON, MD
Central University of Venezuela

AIDA K. SARCON
St. George's University School of Medicine
Class of 2018

RENATA VELAPATIÑO, MD
San Martin de Porres University School of Medicine
Hospitalist, Clinica Internacional

Associate Authors

ANUP CHALISE, MBBS
Nepal Medical College and Teaching Hospital
Class of 2017

CATHY CHEN
University of Mississippi School of Medicine
Class of 2019

MATTHEW S. DELFINER
Resident, Internal Medicine
Temple University Hospital

RICHARD A. GIOVANE, MD
University of Alabama
Department of Family Medicine

JOSEPH G. MONIR
University of Florida College of Medicine
Class of 2018

ALEX MULLEN
University of Mississippi School of Medicine
Class of 2019

VASILY OVECHKO
Pirogov Russian National Research Medical University
Class of 2019

ERIKA J. PARISI
Frank H. Netter MD School of Medicine at Quinnipiac University
Class of 2018

JOHN POWER
Icahn School of Medicine at Mount Sinai
Class of 2018

MIGUEL ROVIRA
University of Michigan Medical School
Class of 2018

IMAGE AND ILLUSTRATION TEAM

BENJAMIN F. COMORA
Alabama College of Osteopathic Medicine
DO/MBA Candidate

NAKEYA KHOZEMA DEWASWALA, MBBS
Lokmanya Tilak Muncipal Medical College
Class of 2016

ANTONIO N. YAGHY, MD
University of Balamand School of Medicine

Faculty Advisors

MEESHA AHUJA, MD
Psychiatrist
Rhode Island Hospital

DIANA ALBA, MD
Clinical Instructor
University of California, San Francisco

MARK A.W. ANDREWS, PhD
Lake Erie College of Osteopathic Medicine at Seton Hill
Greensburg, Pennsylvania

MARIA ANTONELLI, MD
Assistant Professor, Division of Rheumatology
MetroHealth Medical Center, Case Western Reserve University

HERMAN SINGH BAGGA, MD
Urologist, Allegheny Health Network
University of Pittsburgh Medical Center, Passavant

SHIN C. BEH, MD
Assistant Professor, Department of Neurology & Neurotherapeutics
UT Southwestern Medical Center at Dallas

PAULETTE BERND, PhD
Professor, Department of Pathology and Cell Biology
Columbia University College of Physicians and Surgeons

ANISH BHATT, MD
Clinical Fellow
University of California, San Francisco

SHELDON CAMPBELL, MD, PhD
Professor of Laboratory Medicine
Yale School of Medicine

BROOKS D. CASH, MD
Professor of Medicine, Division of Gastroenterology
University of South Alabama School of Medicine

SHIVANI VERMA CHMURA, MD
Adjunct Clinical Faculty, Department of Psychiatry
Stanford University School of Medicine

JAIMINI CHAUHAN-JAMES, MD
Psychiatrist
NYC Health + Hospitals

PETER V. CHIN-HONG, MD
Professor, Department of Medicine
University of California, San Francisco School of Medicine

BRADLEY COLE, MD
Assistant Professor
Loma Linda University School of Medicine

LINDA S. COSTANZO, PhD
Professor, Physiology & Biophysics
Virginia Commonwealth University School of Medicine

ANTHONY L. DeFRANCO, PhD
Professor, Department of Microbiology and Immunology
University of California, San Francisco School of Medicine

CHARLES S. DELA CRUZ, MD, PhD
Associate Professor, Department of Pulmonary and Critical Care Medicine
Yale School of Medicine

CONRAD FISCHER, MD
Associate Professor, Medicine, Physiology, and Pharmacology
Touro College of Medicine

JEFFREY J. GOLD, MD
Associate Professor, Department of Neurology
Assistant Professor, University of California, San Diego School of Medicine

RAYUDU GOPALAKRISHNA, PhD
Associate Professor, Department of Integrative Anatomical Sciences
Keck School of Medicine of University of Southern California

RYAN C.W. HALL, MD
Assistant Professor, Department of Psychiatry
University of South Florida

LOUISE HAWLEY, PhD
Immediate Past Professor and Chair, Department of Microbiology
Ross University School of Medicine

JEFFREY W. HOFMANN, MD, PhD
Resident, Department of Pathology
University of California, San Francisco School of Medicine

BRIAN C. JENSEN, MD
Assistant Professor of Medicine and Pharmacology
University of North Carolina Health Care

CLARK KEBODEAUX, PharmD

Clinical Assistant Professor, Pharmacy Practice and Science
University of Kentucky College of Pharmacy

MICHAEL R. KING, MD

Instructor, Department of Pediatric Anesthesiology
Northwestern University Feinberg School of Medicine

THOMAS KOSZTOWSKI, MD

Spine Instructor
The Warren Alpert Medical School of Brown University

KRISTINE KRAFTS, MD

Assistant Professor, Department of Basic Sciences
University of Minnesota School of Medicine

GERALD LEE, MD

Assistant Professor, Departments of Pediatrics and Medicine
Emory University School of Medicine

KACHIU C. LEE, MD, MPH

Assistant Clinical Professor, Department of Dermatology
Brown University, Providence, Rhode Island

WARREN LEVINSON, MD, PhD

Professor, Department of Microbiology and Immunology
University of California, San Francisco School of Medicine

PETER MARKS, MD, PhD

Center for Biologics Evaluation and Research
US Food and Drug Administration

J. RYAN MARTIN, MD

Assistant Professor of Obstetrics, Gynecology, and Reproductive Sciences
Yale School of Medicine

DOUGLAS A. MATA, MD, MPH

Brigham Education Institute and Brigham and Women's Hospital
Harvard Medical School

SOROUSH RAIS-BAHRAMI, MD

Assistant Professor, Departments of Urology and Radiology
University of Alabama at Birmingham School of Medicine

SASAN SAKIANI, MD

Fellow, Transplant Hepatology
Cleveland Clinic

ROBERT A. SASSO, MD

Professor of Clinical Medicine
Ross University School of Medicine

MELANIE SCHORR, MD

Assistant in Medicine
Massachusetts General Hospital

NATHAN W. SKELLEY, MD

Assistant Professor, Department of Orthopaedic Surgery
University of Missouri, The Missouri Orthopaedic Institute

SHEENA STANARD, MD, MHS

Assistant Professor, Department of Obstetrics and Gynecology
University of Rochester School of Medicine and Dentistry

HOWARD M. STEINMAN, PhD

Assistant Dean, Biomedical Science Education
Albert Einstein College of Medicine

MARY STEINMANN, MD

Assistant Professor, Department of Psychiatry
University of Utah School of Medicine

RICHARD P. USATINE, MD

Professor, Dermatology and Cutaneous Surgery
University of Texas Health Science Center San Antonio

PRASHANT VAISHNAVA, MD

Assistant Professor, Department of Medicine
Mount Sinai Hospital and Icahn School of Medicine

J. MATTHEW VELKEY, PhD

Assistant Dean, Basic Science Education
Duke University School of Medicine

BRIAN WALCOTT, MD

Clinical Instructor, Department of Neurological Surgery
University of California, San Francisco

TISHA WANG, MD

Associate Clinical Professor, Department of Medicine
David Geffen School of Medicine at UCLA

SYLVIA WASSERTHEIL-SMOLLER, PhD

Professor Emerita, Department of Epidemiology and Population Health
Albert Einstein College of Medicine

ADAM WEINSTEIN, MD

Assistant Professor, Pediatric Nephrology and Medical Education
Geisel School of Medicine at Dartmouth

ABHISHEK YADAV, MBBS, MSc

Associate Professor of Anatomy
Geisinger Commonwealth School of Medicine

KRISTAL YOUNG, MD

Clinical Instructor, Department of Cardiology
Huntington Hospital, Pasadena, California

Preface

With the 28th edition of *First Aid for the USMLE Step 1*, we continue our commitment to providing students with the most useful and up-to-date preparation guide for the USMLE Step 1. This edition represents an outstanding revision in many ways, including:

- 35 entirely new high-yield topics reflecting evolving trends in the USMLE Step 1.

- Extensive text revisions, new mnemonics, clarifications, and corrections curated by a team of more than 40 medical student and resident physician authors who excelled on their Step 1 examinations and verified by a team of expert faculty advisors and nationally recognized USMLE instructors.

- A new section on learning and memory science in Section I, Guide to Efficient Exam Preparation.

- Updated with 35+ new full-color photos to help visualize various disorders, descriptive findings, and basic science concepts. Additionally, revised imaging photos have been labeled and optimized to show both normal anatomy and pathologic findings.

- Updated study tips on the opening page of each chapter.

- Improved integration of clinical images and illustrations to better reinforce and learn key anatomic concepts.

- Improved organization of text, figures, and tables throughout for quick review of high-yield topics.

- Updated with 50+ new and revised diagrams and illustrations as part of our ongoing collaboration with USMLE-Rx (MedIQ Learning, LLC).

- Reorganized Rapid Review section to present high-yield concepts by topic and with page numbers to the corresponding text.

- Revitalized coverage of current, high-yield print and digital resources in Section IV with clearer explanations of their relevance to USMLE Step 1 review.

- Real-time Step 1 updates and corrections can be found exclusively on our blog, www.firstaidteam.com.

We invite students and faculty to share their thoughts and ideas to help us continually improve *First Aid for the USMLE Step 1* through our blog and collaborative editorial platform. (See How to Contribute, p. xvii.)

Louisville	Tao Le
Boracay	Vikas Bhushan
St. Louis	Matthew Sochat
New York City	Yash Chavda
Ann Arbor	Andrew Zureick
Pittsburgh	Mehboob Kalani
San Francisco	Kimberly Kallianos

Special Acknowledgments

This has been a collaborative project from the start. We gratefully acknowledge the thousands of thoughtful comments, corrections, and advice of the many medical students, international medical graduates, and faculty who have supported the authors in our continuing development of *First Aid for the USMLE Step 1*.

We provide special acknowledgment and thanks to the following individuals who made exemplary contributions to this edition through our voting, proofreading, and crowdsourcing platform: Huzaifa Ahmad, Ram Baboo, Kashif Badar, Nwamaka Bob-Ume, Paige Estave, Nathaniel Fitch, Panagiotis Kaparaliotis, Elaine Luther, Sarah Hamid Mian, Prashank Shree Neupane, Keyhan Piranviseh, Cindy Tsui, and Ankeet Vakharia.

For support and encouragement throughout the process, we are grateful to Thao Pham, Jinky Flang, and Jonathan Kirsch, Esq. Thanks to Louise Petersen for organizing and supporting the project. Thanks to our publisher, McGraw-Hill, for the valuable assistance of its staff, including Bob Boehringer, Christina Thomas, Jim Shanahan, Laura Libretti, and Jeffrey Herzich.

We are also very grateful to Dr. Fred Howell and Dr. Robert Cannon of Textensor Ltd for providing us extensive customization and support for their powerful Annotate.co collaborative editing platform (www.annotate.co), which allows us to efficiently manage thousands of contributions. Thanks to Dr. Richard Usatine and Dr. Kristine Krafts for their outstanding image contributions. Thanks also to Jean-Christophe Fournet (www.humpath.com), Dr. Ed Uthman, and Dr. Frank Gaillard (www.radiopaedia.org) for generously allowing us to access some of their striking photographs. Thank you to Dr. Brenda Zureick for her ophthalmology review. For faculty contributions, we thank Dr. Aditya Bardia, Dr. Christina Ciaccio, Dr. Stuart Flynn, Dr. Vicki Park, Dr. Jeannine Rahimian, Dr. Joseph Schindler, and Dr. Stephen Thung.

For exceptional editorial leadership, enormous thanks to Christine Diedrich, Emma Underdown, and Catherine Johnson. Thank you to our USMLE-Rx/ScholarRx team of editors, Linda Davoli, Jacqueline Mahon, Janene Matragrano, Erika Nein, Isabel Nogueira, Sally Rineker, Rebecca Stigall, Ashley Vaughn, and Hannah Warnshuis. Many thanks to Tara Price for page design and all-around InDesign expertise. Thank you to Ruthie Whittaker for assistance in reorganizing the Rapid Review section. Special thanks to our indexer Dr. Anne Fifer. We are also grateful to our medical illustrator, Hans Neuhart, for his creative work on the new and updated illustrations. Lastly, tremendous thanks to Rainbow Graphics, especially David Hommel and Donna Campbell, for remarkable ongoing editorial and production support under time pressure.

Louisville	Tao Le
Boracay	Vikas Bhushan
St. Louis	Matthew Sochat
New York City	Yash Chavda
Ann Arbor	Andrew Zureick
Pittsburgh	Mehboob Kalani
San Francisco	Kimberly Kallianos

General Acknowledgments

Each year we are fortunate to receive the input of thousands of medical students and graduates who provide new material, clarifications, and potential corrections through our website and our collaborative editing platform. This has been a tremendous help in clarifying difficult concepts, correcting errata from the previous edition, and minimizing new errata during the revision of the current edition. This reflects our long-standing vision of a true, student-to-student publication. We have done our best to thank each person individually below, but we recognize that errors and omissions are likely. Therefore, we will post an updated list of acknowledgments at our website, www.firstaidteam.com/bonus/. We will gladly make corrections if they are brought to our attention.

For submitting contributions and corrections, many thanks to Mohammad Abbasi, Ibrahim Abdelfattah, Mostafa Ahmed Abdellah, Omar Abdelrahim Alawadi, Sufyan Abdul Mujeeb, Omar Abu Slieh, Khalil Abu Zaina, Muhamed Abubacker, Ayman Abunimer, Terumbur Abwa, Jesus Mauricio Acero, Raghav Acharya, Rojan Adhikari, Anisha Adhikari, Shivani Adhyaru, Kristopher Aghemo, Cassandra Ahmed, Adiel Aizenberg, Dolani Ajanaku, Mythri AK, Ahmad Akhtar, Murad Al Masri, Mejbel Alazemi, Isam Albaba, Camilo José Albert Fernández, Khalil Ali, Muhammed Alikhan, Mohamed Ali, Murad Almasri, Luai Alsakkaf, Vivian V Altiery De Jesus, Fazilhan Altintas, Alvaro Alvarez, Farah Amer, Christopher Anderson, Gilberto Aquino, Jay Argue, Khashayar Arianpour, Fernando Daniel Arias, Lama Assi, Rizwan Attiq, Scarlett Austin, Carlos Andres Avila, Zaki Azam, Sara Azeem, Parag Badami, Nadia Badar, Louis Baeseman, Karsyn Bailey, Bryce Baird, Devin Baith, Matthew Balatbat, Vyshnavy Balendra, Ugur Berkay Balkanci, Josiah Ballantine, Muhammad Yasir Baloch, Melissa Banez, Hari Prasad Baral, Saira Bari, Elan Baskir, Jacqueline Bekhit, Leah Beland, Jackson Bell, Elizabeth Benge, Lauren Benning, Hussein Berjaoui, Maresa Dorothee Berns, Kulsajan Bhatia, Saravjit S. Bhatti, Navpreet Bhurji, M. Yaasen Bhutta, Jacques Bijon, Safal Bijukshe, Jeffrey Black, Christer Blindheim, Luigi Bonini, Peter Boucas, Mary Boulanger, Alexandre Boulos, Chantal Brand, Zachary Britstone, Aaron Brown, Conor Buckley, Natassia Buckridge, Omar Bukhari, Welland Burnside, Pavel Burskii, Avi Bursky-Tammam, David Buziashvili, Michael Byers, Adam Cadesky, Elizabeth Cai, Alexandra Calingo, Andrei Callejas, Francisco Caraballo, Jorge Carrasco, Esteban Casasola, Gabriel Castano, Yoly Angelina Castellanos, Marco A Castillo, Gabriel Castro Gueits, Rorigo Cavalcante, Natalie Cazeau, Harold Viviano Cedeño, Jesse Chait, Ingita Chand, Eric Chang, Fong-Wan Chau Zhou, Jaimini Chauhan, Mit Chauhan, Maureen Chavez, Mehmood Cheema, Christopher Chhoun, Youna Choi, Rebecca D. Chou, Erika Chow, Mahbub Chowdhury, Elizabeth Ann Chu, Jessica Chung, Katherine Chung, Benjamin Ciccarelli, Joseph Cioffi, John Coda, Zack Cohen, Lee Colaianni, Nahimarys Colón Hernández, Julijana Conic, Jeffrey Cooney, Erica Corredera, Cody Couperus, Eric Cox, Caitlin Crosier, Matthew Culbert, John Cummins, Abdul Dada, Christopher Dallo, Parnaz Daneshpajouhnejad, Jason Darr, Camille Davis, Solomon Dawson, James Dee, Matthew Derakhshesh, Rajat Dhand, Shreena Dhawan, Vijay Dhillon, Angel Joel Diaz Martinez, Luboslav Dimitrov, Lennox Din, Soraya Djadjo, Mustafa Rıdvan Dönmez, Hima Doppalapudi, Landry Dorsett, Morgan Drucker, Elena Duca, Wesley Durand, Aaron Dwan, Marc Egerman, Christopher El Mouhayyar, David Ellenbogen, Mahmoud Elmahdy, Ashley Ermann, Yashar Eshman, Mikael Fadoul, Joseph

Fahmy, Giselle Falconi, Matthew Farajzadeh, Behnam Faridian, Amelia Fatsi, Rachel Fayne, Anthony Febres, Jin Feng, Brittany Fera, Leila Ferreira, Anthony Findley, Eitan Fleischman, Thomas Flynn, Allison Forrest, Adisson Fortunel, Brandon Fram, Daniel Franco, Gabriel Franta, Jacob Fried, Yaakov Fried, Luis Alberto Ribeiro Froes Jr., Virginia Fuenmayor, Sudha Gade, Emily Gall, Max Galvan, Nick Gamboa, Dan Ganz, Fabian Garcia, Melanie Garcia, Okubit Gebreyonas, Nicholas Geiger, David Gelbart, Bill Gentry, Dylan Gerlach, Brielle Gerry, Nina Gertsvolf, Sara Ghoneim, Jake Gibbons, Gobind Gill, Victoria Gonzales, Alberto Gonzalez, Mounica Gooty, Barbara Gordon, Sophie Gottesman, Manjeet Goyal, Kylie Grady, Zacharia Grami, Mark Greenhill, Jora Singh Grewal, Harry Griffin, Maria Grig, Vincent Grzywacz, Jinglin Gu, Leidy Laura Guerrero Hernández, James Guirguis, Nikhil Gupta, Deepak Gupta, Zarar Hafeez, Ramez Maher Halaseh, Erik Haley, Mohanad Hamandi, Saffa Hamde, Mohammad Hamidi, Nicola Hampel, Alexandra Handy, Christine Hanish, Mary Hanna, Laura Harding, Maxwell Harley, Glenn R. Harris, Hasanain Hasan, Danial Hayek, Corrie Hays, Luke He, Jackson Hearn, Leif Helland, Ariana Hess, Joyce Ho, Walter Hodges, Tara Hogan, Brian Huang, Naureen Huda, Daniel Huff, Robert Huis in 't Veld, Frank Hurd, Zaid Hussain, Jordan Huxall, Elizabeth Hwang, Taylin Im, Mimoza Isufi, Frank Jackson, Banafsheh Jalalian, Abbas Jama, Nader Jamaleddine, David Janese, Jesse Jaremek, Ranjit Jasraj, Parth Javia, Kyu-Jin Jeon, Benjamin Hans Jeuk, Eric Jiang, Alfredo Joffre, Hollis Johanson, Ryan Johnson, Sarah Johnson, Gavin Jones, Gregory Jordan, Josefina Fernandez, Michael Joseph, Pavel Kacnov, Preethi Kamath, Irina Kanzafarova, Komal Kapoor, Egishe Karapetyan, Nikoloz Karazanashvili, Shalemar Ann Kasan, Matt Kasson, Orest Kayder, Chelsae Keeney, Kristen Kelly, Danielle Keyes, Fahad Khan, Tamer Khashab, Susie Kim, Ann Kim, Rachel Kim, Nikhar Kinger, Mark Kirane, Tamara Kliot, Walter Klyce, Sammy Knefati, Christopher Kocharians, Sam Kociola, Karthikram Komanduri, Nicholas Kondoleon, David Kowal, Robert Kowtoniuk, Leonardo Kozian, Oleksandr Kozlov, Alec Krosser, Judah Kupferman, Stephanie Kuschel, Stephanie Kwan, Nikola Kyuchukov, Ton La, Michael Landolfi, Wells LaRiviere, Matthew Lee, Sean Lee, Sun Yong Lee, Michael Lee, Daniel Leisman, Jacob Leroux, Solomon Levin, David Li, Yedda Li, Jonathan Lieberman, Viktor Limanskiy, Meng-Chen Vanessa Lin, David Liu, Serena Liu, Jason Livingstone, Mavis Lobo, José López, Zhuo Luan, Marcela Marie Luna, Nicolas Luzino, Miles Maassen, Emily MacDuffie, Robertson Mackenzie, Jonathan Macleod, Evan Madill, Sergio Magaña, Marielle Mahan, Hossen Mahmud, Nodari Maisuradze, Abdallah Malas, Genesis Maldonado, Madiha A. Malik, Margaret Maloney, Hassan Mandil, Taylor Maney, Navyata Mangu, Kori Mansfield, Lina Marenco, John Marinelli, Laurel Mast, Micah Mathai, Anita Mathew, Candler Mathews, Fasil Mathews, John Mayfield, Guillermo Maza, Lina Mazin, Benjamin McCormick, Luis Medina, Romy Megahed, Laura I Mendez Morente, Felipe Alonso Mercado, Haley Mertens, Raman Michael, Amanda Miller, Joseph Mininni, Andria Marcela Miranda Chada, Thomas Mitchell, Sarah Mizrachi, Ghady Moafa, Pezhman Mobasher, Mahmoud Mohamed, Syed Mohammad, Denelle Mohammed, Sarah Mohtadi, Agnes Mokrzycki, Guarina Molina, Austin Momii, Eric Mong, Edgar Moradel, Andreina Moreno, Zachary Mortensen, Rachel Moss, Zachary Mostel, Turna Mukherjee, Greg Muller, Nirav Mungalpara, John Myers, Louai Naddaf, Merna Naji, Rohit Nallani, Aram Namavar, Alex Nantsios, Anthony Naquin, Abeeha Naqvi, Haider Naqvi, Samir Narula, Suraj Narvekar, Iraj Nasrabadi, Steven Nevers, Norman Ng, Samuel Ng, Raye Ng, Brandon Nguyen, Brian Nguyen, Chi-Tam Nguyen, Doris Nguyen, Michael Nguyen, Vanessa Nguyen, Timothy Nguyen, Hosea Njoku, Jason Nosrati, Yoav Nudell, Agnes Nyeck, Onyeka Olisemeka, Foluwakemi Olufehinti, Oluyinka Olutoye II, Abdillahi Omar, Nuhah Omar, Michael O'Shea, Zonghao Pan, Abdullah Panchbhaya, Niranjan Pandey, Saurabh Pandit, Khang Wen Pang, Rajbir Singh Pannu, Brian Park, Anishinder Parkash, Om Parkash, Jordan Parker, Matt Partan, Aaron Parzuchowski, Arpan Patel, Dharti Patel, Harshkumar Patel, Neel Patel, Tejas Patel, Vanisha Patel, Yesha Patel, Vrutant Patel, Dwani Patel, Jayesh Patel, Savan Patel, Dipesh Patel, Shiv U. Patel, Jay Patel, Thomas Paterniti, Priya Pathak, Saikrishna Patibandla, Iqra Patoli, Fernando Pellerano, Luke Perry, Romela Petrosyan, Jimmy Tam Huy Pham, Suzanne Piccione, Saran Pillai, Vivek Podder, Dmitry Pokhvashchev, Marc Polanik, Chelsea Powell, Andrew Puckett, Abdulhameed Qashqary, Carlos Quinonez, Joshua Radparvar, Shahrose Rahman, Alia Raja, Vinaya Rajan, Shayan Rakhit, Ferza Raks, Devan Ramachandran, Bashar Ramadan, Gokul Ramani, Shandilya Ramdas, Jose Ramos, Rakin Rashid, Mikhail Rassokhin, Mohsin Raza, Yunus Raza,

Dheevena Reddy, Lenisse Miguelina Reyes Reyes, Peter Rezkalla, Beatriz Rivera, Dalianne Rivera, Chelsea Roberts, Moshe Roberts, Lydia Robles, Alexander Rodriguez, Daniel Rodriguez Benzo, Daniel Enrique Rodríguez Benzo, Evgeny Romanov, Lukas Ronner, Geoffrey Rosen, Max Rosenthal, Yuan Ross, Lindsay Rothfield, Cody Russell, Anas Saad, Rorita Sadhu, Anna Sadovnikova, Dev Sahni, Kamal Sahu, Hemamalini Sakthivel, Abid Saleem, Ololade Saliu, Julienne Sanchez, Mason Sanders, Roshun Sangani, Michael Santarelli, Theodore Schoenfeldt, Kyle Scott, Arshiya Sehgal, Anand Sewak, Congzhou Sha, Nazila Shafagati, Anna Shah, Nauman Shah, Shaili Shah, Ahmed Shah, Abdulla Shaheen, Milton Shapiro, Kanika Sharma, Elizabeth Shay, Derek Sheen, Daniel Sherwood, David Shieh, Scott Shuldiner, Sunober Siddiqi, Gabriel Silva, Matthew Simhon, Bhart Singal, Amadeldin Singer, Amitoj Singh, Chandandeep Singh, Shivreet Singh, Steven Siragusa, Ramzi Y. Skaik, Christina Small, Conor Smith, Destini Smith, Will Smith, Austen Smith, Benjamin Smood, Hannah Snyder, Anubhav Sood, Benjamin Rojas Soosiah, Wilfredo Soto-Fuentes, Matthew Spano, Phalguni Srivastava, Tina Stanco, Josiah Strawser, Thomas Strobel, Annie Suarez, Zoilo Karim Suarez Yeb, Akhil Sureen, Gorica Svalina, Kayley Swope, Laura Szczesniak, Aboud Tahanis, Jayul Tailor, Austin Tam, Ming Yao Jonavan Tan, Olive Tang, Asna Tasleem, Sara Tavarez, Claudia Tejera, Anand Tekriwal, Priyesh Thakurathi, Vaishakh Tharavath, Chris Thomas, Lanice Thomas, Karima Thompson, John Tiang-Leung, Alvin Trieu, Michelle Trieu, Birva Trivedi, Katie Truong, Akshit Tuli, Marcia E. Uddoh, Nneamaka Ukatu, Johnson Ukken, Claire Unruh, Adelynn Vadrar, Andrew Valliyil, Vivek Vallurupalli, Blanca Vargas, Vandana Vekariya, Erick Candido Velasquez Centellas, Michael Venincasa, Michael Villalba, Marcos Villarreal, Phuong Vo, Steven Vuu, William Waddell, Holden Wagstaff, Nicholas Walther, Tony Wang, Jason L. Wang, Jonathan Warczak, Jacob Warner, Eric Wei, Paul Wei, Ronald Weir, Garrett Welle, Matthew Wells, Allison Williams, Michael Winter, Adriana Wong, Donald Wright, Brian Wu, Lawrence Wu, Michael Wydeko, Catherine Xie, Tamar Yacoel, Dong-han Yao, Alexander Yevtukh, Jaemin Yim, Raquel Yokoda, Sadaf Younis, Christopher Yun, Nicholas Yurko, Mubarak Hassan Yusuf, Pavel Zagadailov, Alireza Zandifar, Batool Zehra, Xue Zhang, Eric Zhang, Angie Zhang, Jasmine Zhao, Mohammad Zmaili, Spyridon Zouridis, Andrew Zovath, and Kathleen Zuniga.

How to Contribute

This version of *First Aid for the USMLE Step 1* incorporates thousands of contributions and improvements suggested by student and faculty advisors. We invite you to participate in this process. Please send us your suggestions for:

- Study and test-taking strategies for the USMLE Step 1
- New facts, mnemonics, diagrams, and clinical images
- High-yield topics that may appear on future Step 1 exams
- Personal ratings and comments on review books, question banks, apps, videos, and courses

For each new entry incorporated into the next edition, you will receive up to a **$20 Amazon.com gift card** as well as personal acknowledgment in the next edition. Significant contributions will be compensated at the discretion of the authors. Also, let us know about material in this edition that you feel is low yield and should be deleted.

All submissions including potential errata should ideally be supported with hyperlinks to a dynamically updated Web resource such as UpToDate, AccessMedicine, and ClinicalKey.

We welcome potential errata on grammar and style if the change improves readability. Please note that *First Aid* style is somewhat unique; for example, we have fully adopted the *AMA Manual of Style* recommendations on eponyms ("We recommend that the possessive form be omitted in eponymous terms") and on abbreviations (no periods with eg, ie, etc).

The preferred way to submit new entries, clarifications, mnemonics, or potential corrections with a valid, authoritative reference is via our website: **www.firstaidteam.com**.

This website will be continuously updated with validated errata, new high-yield content, and a new online platform to contribute suggestions, mnemonics, diagrams, clinical images, and potential errata.

Alternatively, you can email us at: **firstaidteam@yahoo.com**.

Contributions submitted by **May 15, 2018**, receive priority consideration for the 2019 edition of *First Aid for the USMLE Step 1*. We thank you for taking the time to share your experience and apologize in advance that we cannot individually respond to all contributors as we receive thousands of contributions each year.

▶ NOTE TO CONTRIBUTORS

All contributions become property of the authors and are subject to editing and reviewing. Please verify all data and spellings carefully. Contributions should be supported by at least two high-quality references.

Check our website first to avoid duplicate submissions. In the event that similar or duplicate entries are received, only the first complete entry received with valid, authoritative references will be credited. Please follow the style, punctuation, and format of this edition as much as possible.

▶ JOIN THE FIRST AID TEAM

The *First Aid* author team is pleased to offer part-time and full-time paid internships in medical education and publishing to motivated medical students and physicians. Internships range from a few months (eg, a summer) up to a full year. Participants will have an opportunity to author, edit, and earn academic credit on a wide variety of projects, including the popular *First Aid* series.

For 2018, we are actively seeking passionate medical students and graduates with a specific interest in improving our medical illustrations, expanding our database of medical photographs, and developing the software that supports our crowdsourcing platform. We welcome people with prior experience and talent in these areas. Relevant skills include clinical imaging, digital photography, digital asset management, information design, medical illustration, graphic design, and software development.

Please email us at **firstaidteam@yahoo.com** with a CV and summary of your interest or sample work.

How to Use This Book

CONGRATULATIONS: You now possess the book that has guided nearly two million students to USMLE success for over 25 years. With appropriate care, the binding should last the useful life of the book. Keep in mind that putting excessive flattening pressure on any binding will accelerate its failure. If you purchased a book that you believe is defective, please **immediately** return it to the place of purchase. If you encounter ongoing issues, you can also contact Customer Service at our publisher, McGraw-Hill Education, at https://www.mheducation.com/contact.html.

START EARLY: Use this book as early as possible while learning the basic medical sciences. The first semester of your first year is not too early! Devise a study plan by reading Section I: Guide to Efficient Exam Preparation, and make an early decision on resources to use by checking Section IV: Top-Rated Review Resources. Note that *First Aid* is neither a textbook nor a comprehensive review book, and it is not a panacea for inadequate preparation.

CONSIDER *FIRST AID* YOUR ANNOTATION HUB: Annotate material from other resources, such as class notes or comprehensive textbooks, into your book. This will keep all the high-yield information you need in one place. Other tips on keeping yourself organized:

- For best results, use fine-tipped ballpoint pens (eg, BIC Pro+, Uni-Ball Jetstream Sports, Pilot Drawing Pen, Zebra F-301). If you like gel pens, try Pentel Slicci, and for markers that dry almost immediately, consider Staedtler Triplus Fineliner, Pilot Drawing Pen, and Sharpies.

- Consider using pens with different colors of ink to indicate different sources of information (eg, blue for USMLE-Rx Step 1 Qmax, green for UWorld Step 1 Qbank).

- Choose highlighters that are bright and dry quickly to minimize smudging and bleeding through the page (eg, Tombow Kei Coat, Sharpie Gel).

- Many students de-spine their book and get it 3-hole-punched. This will allow you to insert materials from other sources, including curricular materials.

INTEGRATE STUDY WITH CASES, FLASH CARDS, AND QUESTIONS: To broaden your learning strategy, consider integrating your *First Aid* study with case-based reviews (eg, *First Aid Cases for the USMLE Step 1*), flash cards (eg, First Aid Flash Facts), and practice questions (eg, the USMLE-Rx Step 1 Qmax). Read the chapter in the book, then test your comprehension by using cases, flash cards, and questions that cover the same topics. Maintain access to more comprehensive resources (eg, *First Aid for the Basic Sciences: General Principles* and *Organ Systems* and First Aid Express videos) for deeper review as needed.

PRIME YOUR MEMORY: Return to your annotated Sections II and III several days before taking the USMLE Step 1. The book can serve as a useful way of retaining key associations and keeping high-yield facts fresh in your memory just prior to the exam. The Rapid Review section includes high-yield topics to help guide your studying.

CONTRIBUTE TO FIRST AID: Reviewing the book immediately after your exam can help us improve the next edition. Decide what was truly high and low yield and send us your comments. Feel free to send us scanned images from your annotated *First Aid* book as additional support. Of course, always remember that **all examinees are under agreement with the NBME to not disclose the specific details of copyrighted test material.**

Selected USMLE Laboratory Values

* = Included in the Biochemical Profile (SMA-12)

Blood, Plasma, Serum	Reference Range	SI Reference Intervals
*Alanine aminotransferase (ALT, GPT at 30°C)	8–20 U/L	8–20 U/L
Amylase, serum	25–125 U/L	25–125 U/L
*Aspartate aminotransferase (AST, GOT at 30°C)	8–20 U/L	8–20 U/L
Bilirubin, serum (adult)		
Total // Direct	0.1–1.0 mg/dL // 0.0–0.3 mg/dL	2–17 µmol/L // 0–5 µmol/L
*Calcium, serum (Total)	8.4–10.2 mg/dL	2.1–2.8 mmol/L
*Cholesterol, serum (Total)	Rec: < 200 mg/dL	< 5.2 mmol/L
*Creatinine, serum (Total)	0.6–1.2 mg/dL	53–106 µmol/L
Electrolytes, serum		
Sodium (Na^+)	136–145 mEq/L	136–145 mmol/L
Chloride (Cl^-)	95–105 mEq/L	95–105 mmol/L
* Potassium (K^+)	3.5–5.0 mEq/L	3.5–5.0 mmol/L
Bicarbonate (HCO^{3-})	22–28 mEq/L	22–28 mmol/L
Magnesium (Mg^{2+})	1.5–2 mEq/L	0.75–1.0 mmol/L
Gases, arterial blood (room air)		
P_{O_2}	75–105 mm Hg	10.0–14.0 kPa
P_{CO_2}	33–45 mm Hg	4.4–5.9 kPa
pH	7.35–7.45	[H^+] 36–44 nmol/L
*Glucose, serum	Fasting: 70–110 mg/dL	3.8–6.1 mmol/L
	2-h postprandial: < 120 mg/dL	< 6.6 mmol/L
Growth hormone – arginine stimulation	Fasting: < 5 ng/mL	< 5 µg/L
	provocative stimuli: > 7 ng/mL	> 7 µg/L
Osmolality, serum	275–295 mOsm/kg	275–295 mOsm/kg
*Phosphatase (alkaline), serum (p-NPP at 30°C)	20–70 U/L	20–70 U/L
*Phosphorus (inorganic), serum	3.0–4.5 mg/dL	1.0–1.5 mmol/L
Prolactin, serum (hPRL)	< 20 ng/mL	< 20 µg/L
*Proteins, serum		
Total (recumbent)	6.0–7.8 g/dL	60–78 g/L
Albumin	3.5–5.5 g/dL	35–55 g/L
Globulins	2.3–3.5 g/dL	23–35 g/L
*Urea nitrogen, serum (BUN)	7–18 mg/dL	1.2–3.0 mmol/L
*Uric acid, serum	3.0–8.2 mg/dL	0.18–0.48 mmol/L

(continues)

Cerebrospinal Fluid	Reference Range	SI Reference Intervals
Glucose	40–70 mg/dL	2.2–3.9 mmol/L
Hematologic		
Erythrocyte count	Male: 4.3–5.9 million/mm^3 Female: 3.5–5.5 million/mm^3	$4.3–5.9 \times 10^{12}$/L $3.5–5.5 \times 10^{12}$/L
Erythrocyte sedimentation rate (Westergen)	Male: 0–15 mm/h Female: 0–20 mm/h	0–15 mm/h 0–20 mm/h
Hematocrit	Male: 41–53% Female: 36–46%	0.41–0.53 0.36–0.46
Hemoglobin, blood	Male: 13.5–17.5 g/dL Female: 12.0–16.0 g/dL	2.09–2.71 mmol/L 1.86–2.48 mmol/L
Hemoglobin, plasma	1–4 mg/dL	0.16–0.62 µmol/L
Leukocyte count and differential		
Leukocyte count	4,500–11,000/mm^3	$4.5–11.0 \times 10^9$/L
Segmented neutrophils	54–62%	0.54–0.62
Band forms	3–5%	0.03–0.05
Eosinophils	1–3%	0.01–0.03
Basophils	0–0.75%	0–0.0075
Lymphocytes	25–33%	0.25–0.33
Monocytes	3–7%	0.03–0.07
Mean corpuscular hemoglobin	25.4–34.6 pg/cell	0.39–0.54 fmol/cell
Mean corpuscular volume	80–100 µm^3	80–100 fL
Partial thromboplastin time (activated)	25–40 seconds	25–40 seconds
Platelet count	150,000–400,000/mm^3	$150–400 \times 10^9$/L
Prothrombin time	11–15 seconds	11–15 seconds
Reticulocyte count	0.5–1.5% of red cells	0.005–0.015
Sweat		
Chloride	0–35 mmol/L	0–35 mmol/L
Urine		
Creatine clearance	Male: 97–137 mL/min Female: 88–128 mL/min	
Osmolality	50–1,400 mOsmol/kg H_2O	
Proteins, total	< 150 mg/24 h	< 0.15 g/24 h

First Aid Checklist for the USMLE Step 1

This is an example of how you might use the information in Section I to prepare for the USMLE Step 1. Refer to corresponding topics in Section I for more details.

Years Prior
☐ Select top-rated review resources as study guides for first-year medical school courses.
☐ Ask for advice from those who have recently taken the USMLE Step 1.

Months Prior
☐ Review computer test format and registration information.
☐ Register six months in advance. Carefully verify name and address printed on scheduling permit. Call Prometric or go online for test date ASAP.
☐ Define goals for the USMLE Step 1 (eg, comfortably pass, beat the mean, ace the test).
☐ Set up a realistic timeline for study. Cover less crammable subjects first. Review subject-by-subject emphasis and clinical vignette format.
☐ Simulate the USMLE Step 1 to pinpoint strengths and weaknesses in knowledge and test-taking skills.
☐ Evaluate and choose study methods and materials (eg, review books, question banks).

Weeks Prior
☐ Simulate the USMLE Step 1 again. Assess how close you are to your goal.
☐ Pinpoint remaining weaknesses. Stay healthy (exercise, sleep).
☐ Verify information on admission ticket (eg, location, date).

One Week Prior
☐ Remember comfort measures (loose clothing, earplugs, etc).
☐ Work out test site logistics such as location, transportation, parking, and lunch.
☐ Call Prometric and confirm your exam appointment.

One Day Prior
☐ Relax.
☐ Lightly review short-term material if necessary. Skim high-yield facts.
☐ Get a good night's sleep.
☐ Make sure the name printed on your photo ID appears EXACTLY the same as the name printed on your scheduling permit.

Day of Exam
☐ Relax. Eat breakfast. Minimize bathroom breaks during the exam by avoiding excessive morning caffeine.
☐ Analyze and make adjustments in test-taking technique.

After the Exam
☐ Celebrate, regardless.
☐ Send feedback to us on our website at **www.firstaidteam.com**.

Guide to Efficient Exam Preparation

"I don't love studying. I hate studying. I like learning. Learning is beautiful."

—Natalie Portman

"Finally, from so little sleeping and so much reading, his brain dried up and he went completely out of his mind."

—Miguel de Cervantes Saavedra, *Don Quixote*

"Sometimes the questions are complicated and the answers are simple."

—Dr. Seuss

"He who knows all the answers has not been asked all the questions."

—Confucius

"It's what you learn after you know it all that counts."

—John Wooden

"A goal without a plan is just a wish."

—Antoine de Saint-Exupéry

"I was gratified to be able to answer promptly, and I did. I said I didn't know."

—Mark Twain

▶ INTRODUCTION

Relax.

This section is intended to make your exam preparation easier, not harder. Our goal is to reduce your level of anxiety and help you make the most of your efforts by helping you understand more about the United States Medical Licensing Examination, Step 1 (USMLE Step 1). As a medical student, you are no doubt familiar with taking standardized examinations and quickly absorbing large amounts of material. When you first confront the USMLE Step 1, however, you may find it all too easy to become sidetracked from your goal of studying with maximal effectiveness. Common mistakes that students make when studying for Step 1 include the following:

- Starting to study (including *First Aid*) too late
- Starting to study intensely too early and burning out
- Starting to prepare for boards before creating a knowledge foundation
- Using inefficient or inappropriate study methods
- Buying the wrong resources or buying too many resources
- Buying only one publisher's review series for all subjects
- Not using practice examinations to maximum benefit
- Not understanding how scoring is performed or what the score means
- Not using review books along with your classes
- Not analyzing and improving your test-taking strategies
- Getting bogged down by reviewing difficult topics excessively
- Studying material that is rarely tested on the USMLE Step 1
- Failing to master certain high-yield subjects owing to overconfidence
- Using *First Aid* as your sole study resource
- Trying to prepare for it all alone

In this section, we offer advice to help you avoid these pitfalls and be more productive in your studies.

> ▶ *The test at a glance:*
> - *8-hour exam*
> - *Up to a total of 280 multiple choice items*
> - *7 test blocks (60 min/block)*
> - *Up to 40 test items per block*
> - *45 minutes of break time, plus another 15 if you skip the tutorial*

▶ USMLE STEP 1—THE BASICS

The USMLE Step 1 is the first of three examinations that you must pass in order to become a licensed physician in the United States. The USMLE is a joint endeavor of the National Board of Medical Examiners (NBME) and the Federation of State Medical Boards (FSMB). The USMLE serves as the single examination system for US medical students and international medical graduates (IMGs) seeking medical licensure in the United States.

The Step 1 exam includes test items drawn from the following content areas[1]:

DISCIPLINE	ORGAN SYSTEM
Aging	Behavioral Health & Nervous Systems/Special Senses
Anatomy	
Behavioral Sciences	Biostatistics & Epidemiology/ Population Health/ Social Sciences
Biochemistry	
Biostatistics and Epidemiology	
Genetics	Blood & Lymphoreticular System
Immunology	Cardiovascular System
Microbiology	Endocrine System
Molecular and Cell Biology	Gastrointestinal System
Nutrition	General Principles of Foundational Science
Pathology	
Pharmacology	Immune System
Physiology	Multisystem Processes & Disorders
	Musculoskeletal, Skin, & Subcutaneous Tissue
	Renal/Urinary System
	Reproductive System
	Respiratory System

How Is the Computer-Based Test (CBT) Structured?

The CBT Step 1 exam consists of one "optional" tutorial/simulation block and seven "real" question blocks of up to 40 questions per block with no more than 280 questions in total, timed at 60 minutes per block. A short 11-question survey follows the last question block. The computer begins the survey with a prompt to proceed to the next block of questions.

Once an examinee finishes a particular question block on the CBT, he or she must click on a screen icon to continue to the next block. Examinees **cannot** go back and change their answers to questions from any previously completed block. However, changing answers is allowed **within** a block of questions as long as the block has not been ended and if time permits.

What Is the CBT Like?

Given the unique environment of the CBT, it's important that you become familiar ahead of time with what your test-day conditions will be like. In fact, you can easily add up to 15 minutes to your break time! This is because the 15-minute tutorial offered on exam day may be skipped if you are already familiar with the exam procedures and the testing interface. The 15 minutes is then added to your allotted break time of 45 minutes for a total of 1 hour of potential break time. You can download the tutorial from the USMLE website and do it before test day. This tutorial interface is very similar to the one you will use in the exam; learn it now and you can skip taking it during the exam, giving you up to 15 extra minutes of break time. You can also gain experience

> ▶ *If you know the format, you can skip the tutorial and add up to 15 minutes to your break time!*

with the CBT format by taking the 120 practice questions (3 blocks with 40 questions each) available online or by signing up for a practice session at a test center.

For security reasons, examinees are not allowed to bring any personal electronic equipment into the testing area. This includes both digital and analog watches, iPods, tablets, calculators, cell phones, and electronic paging devices. Examinees are also prohibited from carrying in their books, notes, pens/pencils, and scratch paper. Food and beverages are also prohibited in the testing area. The testing centers are monitored by audio and video surveillance equipment. However, most testing centers allot each examinee a small locker outside the testing area in which he or she can store snacks, beverages, and personal items.

Questions are typically presented in multiple choice format, with 4–5 possible answer options. There is a countdown timer on the lower left corner of the screen as well. There is also a button that allows the examinee to mark a question for review. If a given question happens to be longer than the screen (which occurs very rarely), a scroll bar will appear on the right, allowing the examinee to see the rest of the question. Regardless of whether the examinee clicks on an answer choice or leaves it blank, he or she must click the "Next" button to advance to the next question.

The USMLE features a small number of media clips in the form of audio and/or video. There may even be a question with a multimedia heart sound simulation. In these questions, a digital image of a torso appears on the screen, and the examinee directs a digital stethoscope to various auscultation points to listen for heart and breath sounds. The USMLE orientation materials include several practice questions in these formats. During the exam tutorial, examinees are given an opportunity to ensure that both the audio headphones and the volume are functioning properly. If you are already familiar with the tutorial and planning on skipping it, first skip ahead to the section where you can test your headphones. After you are sure the headphones are working properly, proceed to the exam.

The examinee can call up a window displaying normal laboratory values. In order to do so, he or she must click the "Lab" icon on the top part of the screen. Afterward, the examinee will have the option to choose between "Blood," "Cerebrospinal," "Hematologic," or "Sweat and Urine." The normal values screen may obscure the question if it is expanded. The examinee may have to scroll down to search for the needed lab values. You might want to memorize some common lab values so you spend less time on questions that require you to analyze these.

The CBT interface provides a running list of questions on the left part of the screen at all times. The software also permits examinees to highlight or cross out information by using their mouse. There is a "Notes" icon on the top part of the screen that allows students to write notes to themselves for review at a later time. Finally, the USMLE has recently added new functionality including text magnification and reverse color (white text on black background). Being

---

▶ Keyboard shortcuts:
  ▪ A, B, etc—letter choices
  ▪ Enter or spacebar—move to next question
  ▪ Esc—exit pop-up Lab and Exhibit windows
  ▪ Alt-T—countdown timers for current session and overall test

▶ Heart sounds are tested via media questions. Make sure you know how different heart diseases sound on auscultation.

▶ Be sure to test your headphones during the tutorial.

▶ Familiarize yourself with the commonly tested lab values (eg, Hgb, WBC, platelets, Na^+, K^+).

▶ Illustrations on the test include:
  ▪ Gross specimen photos
  ▪ Histology slides
  ▪ Medical imaging (eg, x-ray, CT, MRI)
  ▪ Electron micrographs
  ▪ Line drawings

familiar with these features can save time and may help you better view and organize the information you need to answer a question.

For those who feel they might benefit, the USMLE offers an opportunity to take a simulated test, or "CBT Practice Session" at a Prometric center. Students are eligible to register for this three-and-one-half-hour practice session after they have received their scheduling permit.

The same USMLE Step 1 sample test items (120 questions) available on the USMLE website, www.usmle.org, are used at these sessions. **No new items will be presented.** The practice session is available at a cost of $75 and is divided into a short tutorial and three 1-hour blocks of ~40 test items each. Students receive a printed percent-correct score after completing the session. **No explanations of questions are provided.**

You may register for a practice session online at www.usmle.org. A separate scheduling permit is issued for the practice session. Students should allow two weeks for receipt of this permit.

How Do I Register to Take the Exam?

Prometric test centers offer Step 1 on a year-round basis, except for the first two weeks in January and major holidays. The exam is given every day except Sunday at most centers. Some schools administer the exam on their own campuses. Check with the test center you want to use before making your exam plans.

US students can apply to take Step 1 at the NBME website. This application allows you to select one of 12 overlapping three-month blocks in which to be tested (eg, April–May–June, June–July–August). Choose your three-month eligibility period wisely. If you need to reschedule outside your initial three-month period, you can request a one-time extension of eligibility for the next contiguous three-month period, and pay a rescheduling fee. The application also includes a photo ID form that must be certified by an official at your medical school to verify your enrollment. After the NBME processes your application, it will send you a scheduling permit.

The scheduling permit you receive from the NBME will contain your USMLE identification number, the eligibility period in which you may take the exam, and two additional numbers. The first of these is known as your "scheduling number." You must have this number in order to make your exam appointment with Prometric. The second number is known as the "candidate identification number," or CIN. Examinees must enter their CINs at the Prometric workstation in order to access their exams. However, you will not be allowed to bring your permit into the exam and will be asked to copy your CIN onto your scratch paper. Prometric has no access to the codes. **Do not lose your permit!** You will not be allowed to take the exam unless you present this permit along with an unexpired, government-issued photo ID that includes your signature (such as a driver's license or passport). Make sure the name on your photo ID exactly matches the name that appears on your scheduling permit.

▶ *Ctrl-Alt-Delete are the keys of death during the exam. Don't touch them at the same time!*

▶ *You can take a shortened CBT practice test at a Prometric center.*

▶ *The Prometric Web site will display a calendar with open test dates.*

▶ The confirmation emails that Prometric and NBME send are not the same as the scheduling permit.

Once you receive your scheduling permit, you may access the Prometric website or call Prometric's toll-free number to arrange a time to take the exam. You may contact Prometric two weeks before the test date if you want to confirm identification requirements. Although requests for taking the exam may be completed more than six months before the test date, examinees will not receive their scheduling permits earlier than six months before the eligibility period. The eligibility period is the three-month period you have chosen to take the exam. Most medical students choose the April–June or June–August period. Because exams are scheduled on a "first-come, first-served" basis, it is recommended that you contact Prometric as soon as you receive your permit. After you've scheduled your exam, it's a good idea to confirm your exam appointment with Prometric at least one week before your test date. Prometric will provide appointment confirmation on a print-out and by email. Be sure to read the *2018 USMLE Bulletin of Information* for further details.

▶ Test scheduling is done on a "first-come, first-served" basis. It's important to call and schedule an exam date as soon as you receive your scheduling permit.

What If I Need to Reschedule the Exam?

You can change your test date and/or center by contacting Prometric at 1-800-MED-EXAM (1-800-633-3926) or www.prometric.com. Make sure to have your CIN when rescheduling. If you are rescheduling by phone, you must speak with a Prometric representative; leaving a voicemail message will not suffice. To avoid a rescheduling fee, you will need to request a change at least 31 calendar days before your appointment. Please note that your rescheduled test date must fall within your assigned three-month eligibility period.

When Should I Register for the Exam?

▶ Register six months in advance for seating and scheduling preference.

You should plan to register as far in advance as possible ahead of your desired test date (eg, six months), but, depending on your particular test center, new dates and times may open closer to the date. Scheduling early will guarantee that you will get either your test center of choice or one within a 50-mile radius of your first choice. For most US medical students, the desired testing window is in June, since most medical school curricula for the second year end in May or June. Thus, US medical students should plan to register before January in anticipation of a June test date. The timing of the exam is more flexible for IMGs, as it is related only to when they finish exam preparation. Talk with upperclassmen who have already taken the test so you have real-life experience from students who went through a similar curriculum, then formulate your own strategy.

Where Can I Take the Exam?

Your testing location is arranged with Prometric when you call for your test date (after you receive your scheduling permit). For a list of Prometric locations nearest you, visit www.prometric.com.

How Long Will I Have to Wait Before I Get My Scores?

The USMLE reports scores in three to four weeks, unless there are delays in score processing. Examinees will be notified via email when their scores are available. By following the online instructions, examinees will be able to view, download, and print their score report online for ~120 days after score notification, after which scores can only be obtained through requesting an official USMLE transcript. Additional information about score timetables and accessibility is available on the official USMLE website.

What About Time?

Time is of special interest on the CBT exam. Here's a breakdown of the exam schedule:

15 minutes	Tutorial (skip if familiar with test format and features)
7 hours	Seven 60-minute question blocks
45 minutes	Break time (includes time for lunch)

The computer will keep track of how much time has elapsed on the exam. However, the computer will show you only how much time you have remaining in a given block. Therefore, it is up to you to determine if you are pacing yourself properly (at a rate of approximately one question per 90 seconds).

▶ *Gain extra break time by skipping the tutorial or finishing a block early.*

The computer does not warn you if you are spending more than your allotted time for a break. You should therefore budget your time so that you can take a short break when you need one and have time to eat. You must be especially careful not to spend too much time in between blocks (you should keep track of how much time elapses from the time you finish a block of questions to the time you start the next block). After you finish one question block, you'll need to click to proceed to the next block of questions. If you do not click within 30 seconds, you will automatically be entered into a break period.

Break time for the day is 45 minutes, but you are not required to use all of it, nor are you required to use any of it. You can gain extra break time (but not extra time for the question blocks) by skipping the tutorial or by finishing a block ahead of the allotted time. Any time remaining on the clock when you finish a block gets added to your remaining break time. Once a new question block has been started, you may not take a break until you have reached the end of that block. If you do so, this will be recorded as an "unauthorized break" and will be reported on your final score report.

▶ *Be careful to watch the clock on your break time.*

Finally, be aware that it may take a few minutes of your break time to "check out" of the secure resting room and then "check in" again to resume testing, so plan accordingly. The "check-in" process may include fingerprints, pocket checks, and metal detector scanning. Some students recommend pocketless clothing on exam day to streamline the process.

If I Freak Out and Leave, What Happens to My Score?

Your scheduling permit shows a CIN that you will need to enter to start your exam. Entering the CIN is the same as breaking the seal on a test book, and you are considered to have started the exam when you do so. However, no score will be reported if you do not complete the exam. In fact, if you leave at any time from the start of the test to the last block, no score will be reported. The fact that you started but did not complete the exam, however, will appear on your USMLE score transcript. Even though a score is not posted for incomplete tests, examinees may still get an option to request that their scores be calculated and reported if they desire; unanswered questions will be scored as incorrect.

The exam ends when all question blocks have been completed or when their time has expired. As you leave the testing center, you will receive a printed test-completion notice to document your completion of the exam. To receive an official score, you must finish the entire exam.

What Types of Questions Are Asked?

> ▶ Nearly three fourths of Step 1 questions begin with a description of a patient.

All questions on the exam are **one-best-answer multiple choice items.** Most questions consist of a clinical scenario or a direct question followed by a list of five or more options. You are required to select the single best answer among the options given. There are no "except," "not," or matching questions on the exam. A number of options may be partially correct, in which case you must select the option that best answers the question or completes the statement. Additionally, keep in mind that experimental questions may appear on the exam, which do not affect your score.

How Is the Test Scored?

Each Step 1 examinee receives an electronic score report that includes the examinee's pass/fail status, a three-digit test score, and a graphic depiction of the examinee's performance by discipline and organ system or subject area. The actual organ system profiles reported may depend on the statistical characteristics of a given administration of the examination.

The USMLE score report is divided into two sections: performance by discipline and performance by organ system. Each of the questions (minus experimental questions) is tagged according to any or all relevant content areas. Your performance in each discipline and each organ system is represented by a line of X's, where the width of the line is related to the confidence interval for your performance, which is often a direct consequence of the total number of questions for each discipline/system. If any lines have an asterisk (*) at the far right, this means your performance was exemplary in that area—not necessarily representing a perfect score, but often close to it (see Figure 1).

The NBME provides a three-digit test score based on the total number of items answered correctly on the examination, which corresponds to a

FIGURE 1. Sample USMLE Step 1 Performance Profile.

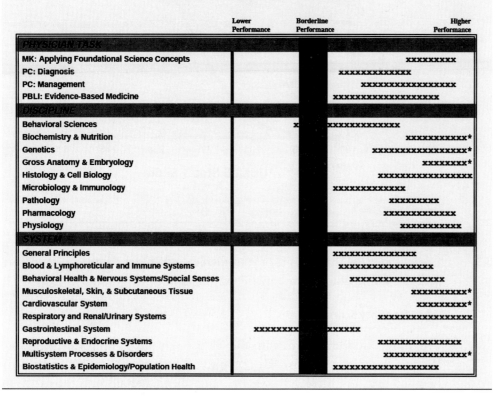

INFORMATION PROVIDED FOR EXAMINEE USE ONLY

The Performance Profile below is provided solely for the benefit of the examinee.
These profiles are developed as self-assessment tools for examinees only and will not be reported or verified to any third party.

USMLE STEP 1 PERFORMANCE PROFILE

	Lower Performance	Borderline Performance	Higher Performance
PHYSICIAN TASK			
MK: Applying Foundational Science Concepts			xxxxxxxxx
PC: Diagnosis		xxxxxxxxxxxxx	
PC: Management		xxxxxxxxxxxxxxxxx	
PBLI: Evidence-Based Medicine		xxxxxxxxxxxxxxxxxx	
DISCIPLINE			
Behavioral Sciences		x xxxxxxxxxxxxx	
Biochemistry & Nutrition			xxxxxxxxxxx*
Genetics			xxxxxxxxxxxxxxxxx*
Gross Anatomy & Embryology			xxxxxxxx*
Histology & Cell Biology			xxxxxxxxxxxxxxxxx
Microbiology & Immunology		xxxxxxxxxxxxx	
Pathology			xxxxxxxxx
Pharmacology			xxxxxxxxxxxx
Physiology			xxxxxxxxxxx
SYSTEM			
General Principles		xxxxxxxxxxxxxxx	
Blood & Lymphoreticular and Immune Systems		xxxxxxxxxxxxxxxxx	
Behavioral Health & Nervous Systems/Special Senses		xxxxxxxxxxxxxxxxx	
Musculoskeletal, Skin, & Subcutaneous Tissue			xxxxxxxxxx*
Cardiovascular System			xxxxxxxxxx*
Respiratory and Renal/Urinary Systems		xxxxxxxxxxxxxxxxx	
Gastrointestinal System	xxxxxxxx	xxxxxx	
Reproductive & Endocrine Systems		xxxxxxxxxxxxxx	
Multisystem Processes & Disorders		xxxxxxxxxxxxxxx*	
Biostatistics & Epidemiology/Population Health		xxxxxxxxxxxxxxxxxx	

particular percentile (see Figure 2). Your three-digit score will be qualified by the mean and standard deviation of US and Canadian medical school first-time examinees. The translation from the lines of X's and number of asterisks you receive on your report to the three-digit score is unclear, but higher three-digit scores are associated with more asterisks.

Since some questions may be experimental and are not counted, it is possible to get different scores for the same number of correct answers. In 2016, the mean score was 228 with a standard deviation of 21.

A score of **192** or higher is required to pass Step 1. The NBME does not report the minimum number of correct responses needed to pass, but estimates that it is roughly 60–70%. The NBME may adjust the minimum passing score in the future, so please check the USMLE website or www.firstaidteam.com for updates.

According to the USMLE, medical schools receive a listing of total scores and pass/fail results plus group summaries by discipline and organ system. Students can withhold their scores from their medical school if they wish. Official USMLE transcripts, which can be sent on request to residency programs, include only total scores, not performance profiles.

▶ The mean Step 1 score for US medical students continues to rise, from 200 in 1991 to 228 in 2016.

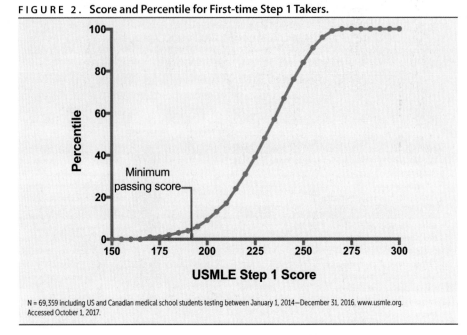

FIGURE 2. Score and Percentile for First-time Step 1 Takers.

N = 69,359 including US and Canadian medical school students testing between January 1, 2014–December 31, 2016. www.usmle.org. Accessed October 1, 2017.

Consult the USMLE website or your medical school for the most current and accurate information regarding the examination.

What Does My Score Mean?

The most important point with the Step 1 score is passing versus failing. Passing essentially means, "Hey, you're on your way to becoming a fully licensed doc." As Table 1 shows, the majority of students pass the exam, so remember, we told you to relax.

TABLE 1. Passing Rates for the 2015–2016 USMLE Step 1.[2]

	2015		2016	
	No. Tested	% Passing	No. Tested	% Passing
Allopathic 1st takers	20,213	96%	20,122	96%
Repeaters	898	68%	1,000	64%
Allopathic total	21,111	94%	21,122	94%
Osteopathic 1st takers	3,185	93%	3,398	94%
Repeaters	37	65%	56	75%
Osteopathic total	3,222	93%	3,454	93%
Total US/Canadian	24,333	94%	24,576	94%
IMG 1st takers	15,030	78%	15,031	78%
Repeaters	2,719	38%	2,575	39%
IMG total	17,749	72%	17,606	72%
Total Step 1 examinees	42,082	85%	42,182	88%

Beyond that, the main point of having a quantitative score is to give you a sense of how well you've done on the exam and to help schools and residencies rank their students and applicants, respectively.

Official NBME/USMLE Resources

The NBME offers a Comprehensive Basic Science Examination (CBSE) for practice that is a shorter version of the Step 1. The CBSE contains four blocks of 50 questions each and covers material that is typically learned during the basic science years. Scores range from 45 to 95 and correlate with a Step 1 equivalent (see Table 2). The standard error of measurement is approximately 3 points, meaning a score of 80 would estimate the student's proficiency is somewhere between 77 and 83. In other words, the actual Step 1 score could be predicted to be between 218 and 232. Of course, these values do not correlate exactly, and they do not reflect different test preparation methods. Many schools use this test to gauge whether a student is expected to pass Step 1. If this test is offered by your school, it is usually conducted at the end of regular didactic time before any dedicated Step 1 preparation. If you do not encounter the CBSE before your dedicated study time, you need not worry about taking it. Use the information to help set realistic goals and timetables for your success.

The NBME also offers six forms of Comprehensive Basic Science Self-Assessment (CBSSA). Students who prepared for the exam using this web-based tool reported that they found the format and content highly indicative of questions tested on the actual exam. In addition, the CBSSA is a fair predictor of USMLE performance (see Table 3). The test interface, however, does not match the actual USMLE test interface, so practicing with these forms alone is not advised.

The CBSSA exists in two formats: standard-paced and self-paced, both of which consist of four sections of 50 questions each (for a total of 200 multiple choice items). The standard-paced format allows the user up to 65 minutes to complete each section, reflecting time limits similar to the actual exam. By contrast, the self-paced format places a 4:20 time limit on answering all multiple choice questions. Every few years, a new form is released and an older one is retired, reflecting changes in exam content. Therefore, the newer exams tend to be more similar to the actual Step 1, and scores from these exams tend to provide a better estimation of exam day performance.

Keep in mind that this bank of questions is available only on the web. The NBME requires that users log on, register, and start the test within 30 days of registration. Once the assessment has begun, users are required to complete the sections within 20 days. Following completion of the questions, the CBSSA provides a performance profile indicating the user's relative strengths and weaknesses, much like the report profile for the USMLE Step 1 exam. The profile is scaled with an average score of 500 and a standard deviation of 100. In addition to the performance profile, examinees will be informed of the number of questions answered incorrectly. You will have the ability to review the text of the incorrect question with the correct answer. Explanations for

TABLE 2. CBSE to USMLE Score Prediction.

CBSE Score	Step 1 Equivalent
≥ 94	≥ 260
92	255
90	250
88	245
86	240
84	235
82	230
80	225
78	220
76	215
74	210
72	205
70	200
68	195
66	190
64	185
62	180
60	175
58	170
56	165
54	160
52	155
50	150
48	145
46	140
≤ 44	≤ 135

▶ *Practice questions may be easier than the actual exam.*

TABLE 3. CBSSA to USMLE Score Prediction.

CBSSA Score	Approximate USMLE Step 1 Score
150	155
200	165
250	175
300	186
350	196
400	207
450	217
500	228
550	238
600	248
650	259
700	269
750	280
800	290

the correct answer, however, will not be provided. The NBME charges $60 for assessments with expanded feedback. The fees are payable by credit card or money order. For more information regarding the CBSE and the CBSSA, visit the NBME's website at www.nbme.org.

The NBME scoring system is weighted for each assessment exam. While some exams seem more difficult than others, the score reported takes into account these inter-test differences when predicting Step 1 performance. Also, while many students report seeing Step 1 questions "word-for-word" out of the assessments, the NBME makes special note that no live USMLE questions are shown on any NBME assessment.

Lastly, the International Foundations of Medicine (IFOM) offers a Basic Science Examination (BSE) practice exam at participating Prometric test centers for $200. Students may also take the self-assessment test online for $35 through the NBME's website. The IFOM BSE is intended to determine an examinee's relative areas of strength and weakness in general areas of basic science—not to predict performance on the USMLE Step 1 exam—and the content covered by the two examinations is somewhat different. However, because there is substantial overlap in content coverage and many IFOM items were previously used on the USMLE Step 1, it is possible to roughly project IFOM performance onto the USMLE Step 1 score scale. More information is available at http://www.nbme.org/ifom/.

▶ DEFINING YOUR GOAL

It is useful to define your own personal performance goal when approaching the USMLE Step 1. Your style and intensity of preparation can then be matched to your goal. Furthermore, your goal may depend on your school's requirements, your specialty choice, your grades to date, and your personal assessment of the test's importance. Do your best to define your goals early so that you can prepare accordingly.

▶ *Some competitive residency programs place more weight on Step 1 scores when choosing candidates to interview.*

▶ *Fourth-year medical students have the best feel for how Step 1 scores factor into the residency application process.*

The value of the USMLE Step 1 score in selecting residency applicants remains controversial, and some have called for less emphasis to be placed on the score when selecting or screening applicants.[3] For the time being, however, it continues to be an important part of the residency application, and it is not uncommon for some specialties to implement filters that screen out applicants who score below a certain cutoff. This is more likely to be seen in competitive specialties (eg, orthopedic surgery, ophthalmology, dermatology, otolaryngology). Independent of your career goals, you can maximize your future options by doing your best to obtain the highest score possible (see Figure 3). At the same time, your Step 1 score is only one of a number of factors that are assessed when you apply for residency. In fact, many residency programs value other criteria such as letters of recommendation, third-year clerkship grades, honors, and research experience more than a high score on Step 1. Fourth-year medical students who have recently completed the residency application process can be a valuable resource in this regard.

FIGURE 3. Median USMLE Step 1 Score by Specialty for Matched US Seniors.[a,b]

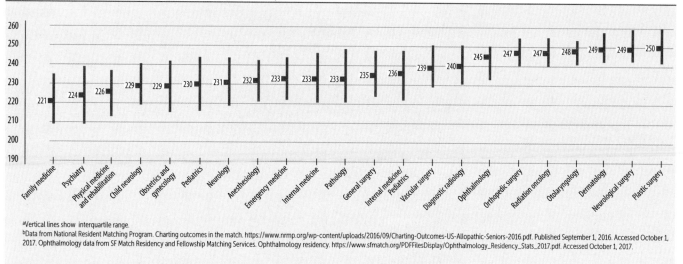

[a]Vertical lines show interquartile range.
[b]Data from National Resident Matching Program. Charting outcomes in the match. https://www.nrmp.org/wp-content/uploads/2016/09/Charting-Outcomes-US-Allopathic-Seniors-2016.pdf. Published September 1, 2016. Accessed October 1, 2017. Ophthalmology data from SF Match Residency and Fellowship Matching Services. Ophthalmology residency. https://www.sfmatch.org/PDFFilesDisplay/Ophthalmology_Residency_Stats_2017.pdf. Accessed October 1, 2017.

▶ LEARNING STRATEGIES

Many students feel overwhelmed during the preclinical years and struggle to find an effective learning strategy. Table 4 lists several learning strategies you can try and their estimated effectiveness for Step 1 preparation based on the literature (see References). These are merely suggestions, and it's important to take your learning preferences into account. Your comprehensive learning approach will contain a combination of strategies (eg, elaborative interrogation followed by practice testing, mnemonics review using spaced repetition, etc). Regardless of your choice, the foundation of knowledge you build during your basic science years is the most important resource for success on the USMLE Step 1.

> ▶ *The foundation of knowledge you build during your basic science years is the most important resource for success on the USMLE Step 1.*

HIGH EFFICACY

Practice Testing

Also called "retrieval practice," practice testing has both direct and indirect benefits to the learner.[4] Effortful retrieval of answers does not only identify weak spots—it directly strengthens long-term retention of material.[5] The more effortful the recall, the better the long-term retention. This advantage has been shown to result in higher test scores and GPAs.[6] In fact, research has shown a positive correlation between the number of boards-style practice questions completed and Step 1 scores among medical students.[7]

> ▶ *Research has shown a positive correlation between the number of boards-style practice questions completed and Step 1 scores among medical students.*

Practice testing should be done with "interleaving" (mixing of questions from different topics in a single session). Question banks often allow you to intermingle topics. Interleaved practice helps learners develop their ability to focus on the relevant concept when faced with many possibilities. Practicing topics in massed fashion (eg, all cardiology, then all dermatology) may seem intuitive, but there is strong evidence that interleaving correlates with longer-

TABLE 4. Effective Learning Strategies.

EFFICACY	STRATEGY	EXAMPLE RESOURCES
High efficacy	Practice testing	UWorld Qbank NBME Self-Assessments USMLE-Rx QMax Kaplan Qbank
	Distributed practice	USMLE-Rx Flash Facts Anki Firecracker Memorang Osmosis
Moderate efficacy	Mnemonics	*Pre-made:* SketchyMedical Picmonic *Self-made:* Mullen Memory
	Elaborative interrogation/ self-explanation	
	Concept mapping	Coggle FreeMind XMind MindNode
Low efficacy	Rereading	
	Highlighting/underlining	
	Summarization	

term retention and increased student achievement, especially on tasks that involve problem solving.[5]

In addition to using question banks, you can test yourself by arranging your notes in a question-answer format (eg, via flash cards). Testing these Q&As in random order allows you to reap the benefit of interleaved practice. Bear in mind that the utility of practice testing comes from the practice of information retrieval, so simply reading through Q&As will attenuate this benefit.

Distributed Practice

Also called "spaced repetition," distributed practice is the opposite of massed practice or "cramming." Learners review material at increasingly spaced out intervals (days to weeks to months). Massed learning may produce more short-term gains and satisfaction, but learners who use distributed practice have better mastery and retention over the long term.[5,9]

Flash cards are a simple way to incorporate both distributed practice and practice testing. Studies have linked spaced repetition learning with flash cards to improved long-term knowledge retention and higher exam scores.[6,8,10] Apps with automated spaced-repetition software (SRS) for flash cards exist for smartphones and tablets, so the cards are accessible anywhere. Proceed with caution: there is an art to making and reviewing cards. The ease of quickly downloading or creating digital cards can lead to flash card overload (it is unsustainable to make 50 flash cards per lecture!). Even at a modest pace, the thousands upon thousands of cards are too overwhelming for Step 1 preparation. Unless you have specific high-yield cards (and have checked the content with high-yield resources), stick to pre-made cards by reputable sources that curate the vast amount of knowledge for you.

> ▶ Studies have linked spaced repetition learning with flash cards to improved long-term knowledge retention and higher exam scores.

If you prefer pen and paper, consider using a planner or spreadsheet to organize your study material over time. Distributed practice allows for some forgetting of information, and the added effort of recall over time strengthens the learning.

MODERATE EFFICACY

Mnemonics

A "mnemonic" refers to any device that assists memory, such as acronyms, mental imagery (eg, keywords with or without memory palaces), etc. Keyword mnemonics have been shown to produce superior knowledge retention when compared with rote memorization in many scenarios. However, they are generally more effective when applied to memorization-heavy, keyword-friendly topics and may not be broadly suitable.[5] Keyword mnemonics may not produce long-term retention, so consider combining mnemonics with distributed, retrieval-based practice (eg, via flash cards with SRS).

Self-made mnemonics may have an advantage when material is simple and keyword friendly. If you can create your own mnemonic that accurately represents the material, this will be more memorable. When topics are complex and accurate mnemonics are challenging to create, pre-made mnemonics may be more effective, especially if you are inexperienced at creating mnemonics.[11]

Elaborative Interrogation/Self-Explanation

Elaborative interrogation ("why" questions) and self-explanation (general questioning) prompt learners to generate explanations for facts. When reading passages of discrete facts, consider using these techniques, which have been shown to be more effective than rereading (eg, improved recall and better problem-solving/diagnostic performance).[5,12,13]

> ▶ Elaborative interrogation and self-explanation prompt learners to generate explanations for facts, which improves recall and problem solving.

Concept Mapping

Concept mapping is a method for graphically organizing knowledge, with concepts enclosed in boxes and lines drawn between related concepts.

Creating or studying concept maps may be more effective than other activities (eg, writing or reading summaries/outlines). However, studies have reached mixed conclusions about its utility, and the small size of this effect raises doubts about its authenticity and pedagogic significance.[14]

LOW EFFICACY

Rereading

While the most commonly used method among surveyed students, rereading has not been shown to correlate with grade point average.[9] Due to its popularity, rereading is often a comparator in studies on learning. Other strategies that we have discussed (eg, practice testing) have been shown to be significantly more effective than rereading.

Highlighting/Underlining

Because this method is passive, it tends to be of minimal value for learning and recall. In fact, lower-performing students are more likely to use these techniques.[9] Students who highlight and underline do not learn how to actively recall learned information and thus find it difficult to apply knowledge to exam questions.

Summarization

While more useful for improving performance on generative measures (eg, free recall or essays), summarization is less useful for exams that depend on recognition (eg, multiple choice). Findings on the overall efficacy of this method have been mixed.[5]

▶ TIMELINE FOR STUDY

Before Starting

Your preparation for the USMLE Step 1 should begin when you enter medical school. Organize and commit to studying from the beginning so that when the time comes to prepare for the USMLE, you will be ready with a strong foundation.

Make a Schedule

After you have defined your goals, map out a study schedule that is consistent with your objectives, your vacation time, the difficulty of your ongoing coursework, and your family and social commitments (see Figure 4). Determine whether you want to spread out your study time or concentrate it into 14-hour study days in the final weeks. Then factor in your own history in

FIGURE 4. Typical Timeline for the USMLE Step 1.

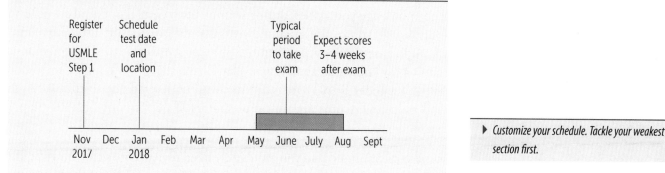

> ▶ Customize your schedule. Tackle your weakest section first.

preparing for standardized examinations (eg, SAT, MCAT). Talk to students at your school who have recently taken Step 1. Ask them for their study schedules, especially those who have study habits and goals similar to yours.

Typically, US medical schools allot between four and eight weeks for dedicated Step 1 preparation. The time you dedicate to exam preparation will depend on your target score as well as your success in preparing yourself during the first two years of medical school. Some students reserve about a week at the end of their study period for final review; others save just a few days. When you have scheduled your exam date, do your best to adhere to it. Studies show that a later testing date does not translate into a higher score, so avoid pushing back your test date without good reason.[15]

Make your schedule realistic, and set achievable goals. Many students make the mistake of studying at a level of detail that requires too much time for a comprehensive review—reading *Gray's Anatomy* in a couple of days is not a realistic goal! Have one catch-up day per week of studying. No matter how well you stick to your schedule, unexpected events happen. But don't let yourself procrastinate because you have catch-up days; stick to your schedule as closely as possible and revise it regularly on the basis of your actual progress. Be careful not to lose focus. Beware of feelings of inadequacy when comparing study schedules and progress with your peers. **Avoid others who stress you out.** Focus on a few top-rated resources that suit your learning style—not on some obscure books your friends may pass down to you. Accept the fact that you cannot learn it all.

> ▶ "Crammable" subjects should be covered later and less crammable subjects earlier.

You will need time for uninterrupted and focused study. Plan your personal affairs to minimize crisis situations near the date of the test. Allot an adequate number of breaks in your study schedule to avoid burnout. Maintain a healthy lifestyle with proper diet, exercise, and sleep.

> ▶ Avoid burnout. Maintain proper diet, exercise, and sleep habits.

Another important aspect of your preparation is your studying environment. **Study where you have always been comfortable studying.** Be sure to include everything you need close by (review books, notes, coffee, snacks, etc). If you're the kind of person who cannot study alone, form a study group with other students taking the exam. The main point here is to create a comfortable environment with minimal distractions.

Year(s) Prior

The knowledge you gained during your first two years of medical school and even during your undergraduate years should provide the groundwork on which to base your test preparation. Student scores on NBME subject tests (commonly known as "shelf exams") have been shown to be highly correlated with subsequent Step 1 scores.[16] Moreover, undergraduate science GPAs as well as MCAT scores are strong predictors of performance on the Step 1 exam.[17]

> ▶ Buy review books early (first year) and use while studying for courses.

We also recommend that you buy highly rated review books early in your first year of medical school and use them as you study throughout the two years. When Step 1 comes along, these books will be familiar and personalized to the way in which you learn. It is risky and intimidating to use unfamiliar review books in the final two or three weeks preceding the exam. Some students find it helpful to personalize and annotate *First Aid* throughout the curriculum.

Months Prior

Review test dates and the application procedure. Testing for the USMLE Step 1 is done on a year-round basis. If you have disabilities or special circumstances, contact the NBME as early as possible to discuss test accommodations (see the Section I Supplement at www.firstaidteam.com/bonus).

> ▶ Simulate the USMLE Step 1 under "real" conditions before beginning your studies.

Use this time to finalize your ideal schedule. Consider upcoming breaks and whether you want to relax or study. Work backward from your test date to make sure you finish at least one question bank. Also add time to redo missed or flagged questions (which may be half the bank). This is the time to build a structured plan with enough flexibility for the realities of life.

Begin doing blocks of questions from reputable question banks under "real" conditions. Don't use tutor mode until you're sure you can finish blocks in the allotted time. It is important to continue balancing success in your normal studies with the Step 1 test preparation process.

Weeks Prior (Dedicated Preparation)

> ▶ In the final two weeks, focus on review, practice questions, and endurance. Stay confident!

Your dedicated prep time may be one week or two months. You should have a working plan as you go into this period. Finish your schoolwork strong, take a day off, and then get to work. Start by simulating a full-length USMLE Step 1 if you haven't yet done so. Consider doing one NBME CBSSA and the free questions from the NBME website. Alternatively, you could choose 7 blocks of randomized questions from a commercial question bank. Make sure you get feedback on your strengths and weaknesses and adjust your studying accordingly. Many students study from review sources or comprehensive programs for part of the day, then do question blocks. Also, keep in mind that reviewing a question block can take upward of two hours. Feedback from CBSSA exams and question banks will help you focus on your weaknesses.

One Week Prior

Make sure you have your CIN (found on your scheduling permit) as well as other items necessary for the day of the examination, including a current driver's license or another form of photo ID with your signature (make sure the name on your **ID exactly** matches that on your scheduling permit). Confirm the Prometric testing center location and test time. Work out how you will get to the testing center and what parking and traffic problems you might encounter. Drive separately from other students taking the test on the same day, and exchange cell phone numbers in case of emergencies. If possible, visit the testing site to get a better idea of the testing conditions you will face. Determine what you will do for lunch. Make sure you have everything you need to ensure that you will be comfortable and alert at the test site. It may be beneficial to adjust your schedule to start waking up at the same time that you will on your test day. And of course, make sure to maintain a healthy lifestyle and get enough sleep.

> ▶ One week before the test:
> ■ Sleep according to the same schedule you'll use on test day
> ■ Review the CBT tutorial one last time
> ■ Call Prometric to confirm test date and time

One Day Prior

Try your best to relax and rest the night before the test. Double-check your admissions and test-taking materials as well as the comfort measures discussed earlier so that you will not have to deal with such details on the morning of the exam. At this point it will be more effective to review short-term memory material that you're already familiar with than to try to learn new material. The Rapid Review section at the end of this book is high yield for last-minute studying. Remember that regardless of how hard you have studied, you cannot know everything. There will be things on the exam that you have never even seen before, so do not panic. Do not underestimate your abilities.

Many students report difficulty sleeping the night prior to the exam. This is often exacerbated by going to bed much earlier than usual. Do whatever it takes to ensure a good night's sleep (eg, massage, exercise, warm milk, no back-lit screens at night). Do not change your daily routine prior to the exam. Exam day is not the day for a caffeine-withdrawal headache.

Morning of the Exam

On the morning of the Step 1 exam, wake up at your regular time and eat a normal breakfast. If you think it will help you, have a close friend or family member check to make sure you get out of bed. Make sure you have your scheduling permit admission ticket, test-taking materials, and comfort measures as discussed earlier. Wear loose, comfortable clothing. Plan for a variable temperature in the testing center. Arrive at the test site 30 minutes before the time designated on the admission ticket; however, do not come too early, as doing so may intensify your anxiety. When you arrive at the test site, the proctor should give you a USMLE information sheet that will explain critical factors such as the proper use of break time. Seating may be assigned, but ask to be reseated if necessary; you need to be seated in an area that

> ▶ No notes, books, calculators, pagers, cell phones, recording devices, or watches of any kind are allowed in the testing area, but they are allowed in lockers.

▶ *Arrive at the testing center 30 minutes before your scheduled exam time. If you arrive more than half an hour late, you will not be allowed to take the test.*

will allow you to remain comfortable and to concentrate. Get to know your testing station, especially if you have never been in a Prometric testing center before. Listen to your proctors regarding any changes in instructions or testing procedures that may apply to your test site.

Finally, remember that it is natural (and even beneficial) to be a little nervous. Focus on being mentally clear and alert. Avoid panic. When you are asked to begin the exam, take a deep breath, focus on the screen, and then begin. Keep an eye on the timer. Take advantage of breaks between blocks to stretch, maybe do some jumping jacks, and relax for a moment with deep breathing or stretching.

After the Test

After you have completed the exam, be sure to have fun and relax regardless of how you may feel. Taking the test is an achievement in itself. Remember, you are much more likely to have passed than not. Enjoy the free time you have before your clerkships. Expect to experience some "reentry" phenomena as you try to regain a real life. Once you have recovered sufficiently from the test (or from partying), we invite you to send us your feedback, corrections, and suggestions for entries, facts, mnemonics, strategies, resource ratings, and the like (see p. xvii, How to Contribute). Sharing your experience will benefit fellow medical students and IMGs.

▶ STUDY MATERIALS

Quality Considerations

Although an ever-increasing number of review books and software are now available on the market, the quality of such material is highly variable. Some common problems are as follows:

- Certain review books are too detailed to allow for review in a reasonable amount of time or cover subtopics that are not emphasized on the exam.
- Many sample question books were originally written years ago and have not been adequately updated to reflect recent trends.
- Some question banks test to a level of detail that you will not find on the exam.

▶ *If a given review book is not working for you, stop using it no matter how highly rated it may be or how much it costs.*

Review Books

In selecting review books, be sure to weigh different opinions against each other, read the reviews and ratings in Section IV of this guide, examine the books closely in the bookstore, and choose carefully. You are investing not only money but also your limited study time. Do not worry about finding the "perfect" book, as many subjects simply do not have one, and different students prefer different formats. Supplement your chosen books with personal notes from other sources, including what you learn from question banks.

There are two types of review books: those that are stand-alone titles and those that are part of a series. Books in a series generally have the same style, and you must decide if that style works for you. However, a given style is not optimal for every subject.

You should also find out which books are up to date. Some recent editions reflect major improvements, whereas others contain only cursory changes. Take into consideration how a book reflects the format of the USMLE Step 1.

▶ *Charts and diagrams may be the best approach for physiology and biochemistry, whereas tables and outlines may be preferable for microbiology.*

Apps

With the explosion of smartphones and tablets, apps are an increasingly popular way to review for the Step 1 exam. The majority of apps are compatible with both iOS and Android. Many popular Step 1 review resources (eg, UWorld, USMLE-Rx) have apps that are compatible with their software. Many popular web references (eg, UpToDate) also now offer app versions. All of these apps offer flexibility, allowing you to study while away from a computer (eg, while traveling).

Practice Tests

Taking practice tests provides valuable information about potential strengths and weaknesses in your fund of knowledge and test-taking skills. Some students use practice examinations simply as a means of breaking up the monotony of studying and adding variety to their study schedule, whereas other students rely almost solely on practice. You should also subscribe to one or more high-quality question banks. In addition, students report that many current practice-exam books have questions that are, on average, shorter and less clinically oriented than those on the current USMLE Step 1.

▶ *Most practice exams are shorter and less clinical than the real thing.*

Additionally, some students preparing for the Step 1 exam have started to incorporate case-based books intended primarily for clinical students on the wards or studying for the Step 2 CK exam. *First Aid Cases for the USMLE Step 1* aims to directly address this need.

After taking a practice test, spend time on each question and each answer choice whether you were right or wrong. There are important teaching points in each explanation. Knowing why a wrong answer choice is incorrect is just as important as knowing why the right answer is correct. Do not panic if your practice scores are low as many questions try to trick or distract you to highlight a certain point. Use the questions you missed or were unsure about to develop focused plans during your scheduled catch-up time.

▶ *Use practice tests to identify concepts and areas of weakness, not just facts that you missed.*

Textbooks and Course Syllabi

Limit your use of textbooks and course syllabi for Step 1 review. Many textbooks are too detailed for high-yield review and include material that is generally not tested on the USMLE Step 1 (eg, drug dosages, complex chemical structures). Syllabi, although familiar, are inconsistent across medical schools and frequently reflect the emphasis of individual faculty, which often does not correspond to that of the USMLE Step 1. Syllabi also tend to be less organized than top-rated books and generally contain fewer diagrams and study questions.

▶ TEST-TAKING STRATEGIES

Your test performance will be influenced by both your knowledge and your test-taking skills. You can strengthen your performance by considering each of these factors. Test-taking skills and strategies should be developed and perfected well in advance of the test date so that you can concentrate on the test itself. We suggest that you try the following strategies to see if they might work for you.

> ▶ Practice! Develop your test-taking skills and strategies well before the test date.

Pacing

You have seven hours to complete up to 280 questions. Note that each one-hour block contains up to 40 questions. This works out to approximately 90 seconds per question. We recommend following the "1 minute rule" to pace yourself. Spend no more than 1 minute on each question. If you are still unsure about the answer after this time, mark the question, make an educated guess, and move on. Following this rule, you should have approximately 20 minutes left after all questions are answered, which you can use to revisit all of your marked questions. Remember that some questions may be experimental and do not count for points (and reassure yourself that these experimental questions are the ones that are stumping you). In the past, pacing errors have been detrimental to the performance of even highly prepared examinees. The bottom line is to keep one eye on the clock at all times!

> ▶ Time management is an important skill for exam success.

Dealing with Each Question

There are several established techniques for efficiently approaching multiple choice questions; find what works for you. One technique begins with identifying each question as easy, workable, or impossible. Your goal should be to answer all easy questions, resolve all workable questions in a reasonable amount of time, and make quick and intelligent guesses on all impossible questions. Most students read the stem, think of the answer, and turn immediately to the choices. A second technique is to first skim the answer choices to get a context, then read the last sentence of the question (the lead-in), and then read through the passage quickly, extracting only information relevant to answering the question. This can be particularly helpful for questions with long clinical vignettes. Try a variety of techniques on practice exams and see what works best for you. If you get overwhelmed, remember that a 30-second time out to refocus may get you back on track.

Guessing

There is **no penalty** for wrong answers. Thus, **no test block should be left with unanswered questions.** A hunch is probably better than a random guess. If you have to guess, we suggest selecting an answer you recognize over one with which you are totally unfamiliar.

Changing Your Answer

The conventional wisdom is not to change answers that you have already marked unless there is a convincing and logical reason to do so—in other words, go with your "first hunch." Many question banks tell you how many questions you changed from right to wrong, wrong to wrong, and wrong to right. Use this feedback to judge how good a second-guesser you are. If you have extra time, reread the question stem and make sure you didn't misinterpret the question.

> ▶ Go with your first hunch, unless you are certain that you are a good second-guesser.

▶ CLINICAL VIGNETTE STRATEGIES

In recent years, the USMLE Step 1 has become increasingly clinically oriented. This change mirrors the trend in medical education toward introducing students to clinical problem solving during the basic science years. The increasing clinical emphasis on Step 1 may be challenging to those students who attend schools with a more traditional curriculum.

> ▶ Be prepared to read fast and think on your feet!

What Is a Clinical Vignette?

A clinical vignette is a short (usually paragraph-long) description of a patient, including demographics, presenting symptoms, signs, and other information concerning the patient. Sometimes this paragraph is followed by a brief listing of important physical findings and/or laboratory results. The task of assimilating all this information and answering the associated question in the span of one minute can be intimidating. So be prepared to read quickly and think on your feet. Remember that the question is often indirectly asking something you already know.

> ▶ Practice questions that include case histories or descriptive vignettes are critical for Step 1 preparation.

Strategy

Remember that Step 1 vignettes usually describe diseases or disorders in their most classic presentation. So look for cardinal signs (eg, malar rash for SLE or nuchal rigidity for meningitis) in the narrative history. Be aware that the question will contain classic signs and symptoms instead of buzzwords. Sometimes the data from labs and the physical exam will help you confirm or reject possible diagnoses, thereby helping you rule answer choices in or out. In some cases, they will be a dead giveaway for the diagnosis.

> ▶ Step 1 vignettes usually describe diseases or disorders in their most classic presentation.

Making a diagnosis from the history and data is often not the final answer. Not infrequently, the diagnosis is divulged at the end of the vignette, after you have just struggled through the narrative to come up with a diagnosis of your own. The question might then ask about a related aspect of the diagnosed disease. Consider skimming the answer choices and lead-in before diving into a long stem. However, be careful with skimming the answer choices; going too fast may warp your perception of what the vignette is asking.

▶ IF YOU THINK YOU FAILED

After the test, many examinees feel that they have failed, and most are at the very least unsure of their pass/fail status. There are several sensible steps you can take to plan for the future in the event that you do not achieve a passing score. First, save and organize all your study materials, including review books, practice tests, and notes. Familiarize yourself with the reapplication procedures for Step 1, including application deadlines and upcoming test dates.

▶ *If you pass Step 1 (score of 192 or above), you are not allowed to retake the exam.*

Make sure you know both your school's and the NBME's policies regarding retakes. The NBME allows a maximum of six attempts to pass each Step examination.[18] You may take Step 1 no more than three times within a 12-month period. Your fourth and subsequent attempts must be at least 12 months after your first attempt at that exam and at least six months after your most recent attempt at that exam.

The performance profiles on the back of the USMLE Step 1 score report provide valuable feedback concerning your relative strengths and weaknesses. Study these profiles closely. Set up a study timeline to strengthen gaps in your knowledge as well as to maintain and improve what you already know. Do not neglect high-yield subjects. It is normal to feel somewhat anxious about retaking the test, but if anxiety becomes a problem, seek appropriate counseling.

▶ TESTING AGENCIES

- **National Board of Medical Examiners (NBME) / USMLE Secretariat**
  Department of Licensing Examination Services
  3750 Market Street
  Philadelphia, PA 19104-3102
  (215) 590-9500 (operator) or
  (215) 590-9700 (automated information line)
  Fax: (215) 590-9457
  Email: webmail@nbme.org
  www.nbme.org

▪ **Educational Commission for Foreign Medical Graduates (ECFMG)**
3624 Market Street
Philadelphia, PA 19104-2685
(215) 386-5900
Fax: (215) 386-9196
Email: info@ecfmg.org
www.ecfmg.org

▶ REFERENCES

1. United States Medical Licensing Examination. Available from: http://www.usmle.org/bulletin/exam-content. Accessed September 25, 2017.
2. United States Medical Licensing Examination. 2016 Performance Data. Available from: http://www.usmle.org/performance-data/default.aspx#2015_step-1. Accessed September 25, 2017.
3. Prober CG, Kolars JC, First LR, et al. A plea to reassess the role of United States Medical Licensing Examination Step 1 scores in residency selection. *Acad Med.* 2016;91(1):12–15.
4. Roediger HL, Butler AC. The critical role of retrieval practice in long-term retention. *Trends Cogn Sci.* 2011;15(1):20–27.
5. Dunlosky J, Rawson KA, Marsh EJ, et al. Improving students' learning with effective learning techniques: promising directions from cognitive and educational psychology. *Psychol Sci Publ Int.* 2013;14(1):4–58.
6. Larsen DP, Butler AC, Lawson AL, et al. The importance of seeing the patient: test-enhanced learning with standardized patients and written tests improves clinical application of knowledge. *Adv Health Sci Educ.* 2013;18(3):409–425.
7. Panus PC, Stewart DW, Hagemeier NE, et al. A subgroup analysis of the impact of self-testing frequency on examination scores in a pathophysiology course. *Am J Pharm Educ.* 2014;78(9):165.
8. Deng F, Gluckstein JA, Larsen DP. Student-directed retrieval practice is a predictor of medical licensing examination performance. *Perspect Med Educ.* 2015;4(6):308–313.
9. McAndrew M, Morrow CS, Atiyeh L, et al. Dental student study strategies: are self-testing and scheduling related to academic performance? *J Dent Educ.* 2016;80(5):542–552.
10. Augustin M. How to learn effectively in medical school: test yourself, learn actively, and repeat in intervals. *Yale J Biol Med.* 2014;87(2):207–212.
11. Bellezza FS. Mnemonic devices: classification, characteristics, and criteria. *Rev Educ Res.* 1981;51(2):247–275.
12. Dyer J-O, Hudon A, Montpetit-Tourangeau K, et al. Example-based learning: comparing the effects of additionally providing three different integrative learning activities on physiotherapy intervention knowledge. *BMC Med Educ.* 2015;15:37.
13. Chamberland M, Mamede S, St-Onge C, et al. Self-explanation in learning clinical reasoning: the added value of examples and prompts. *Med Educ.* 2015;49(2):193–202.
14. Nesbit JC, Adesope OO. Learning with concept and knowledge maps: a meta-analysis. *Rev Educ Res.* 2006;76(3):413–448.

15. Pohl CA, Robeson MR, Hojat M, et al. Sooner or later? USMLE Step 1 performance and test administration date at the end of the second year. *Acad Med*. 2002;77(10):S17–S19.

16. Holtman MC, Swanson DB, Ripkey DR, et al. Using basic science subject tests to identify students at risk for failing Step 1. *Acad Med*. 2001;76(10):S48–S51.

17. Basco WT, Way DP, Gilbert GE, et al. Undergraduate institutional MCAT scores as predictors of USMLE Step 1 performance. *Acad Med*. 2002;77(10):S13–S16.

18. United States Medical Licensing Examination. 2018 USMLE Bulletin of Information. Available from: http://www.usmle.org/pdfs/bulletin/2018bulletin.pdf. Accessed September 25, 2017.

Special Situations

Please visit **www.firstaidteam.com/bonus/** to view this section.

▶ NOTES

SECTION II

High-Yield
General Principles

"There comes a time when for every addition of knowledge you forget something that you knew before. It is of the highest importance, therefore, not to have useless facts elbowing out the useful ones."
—Sir Arthur Conan Doyle, *A Study in Scarlet*

"Never regard study as a duty, but as the enviable opportunity to learn."
—Albert Einstein

"Live as if you were to die tomorrow. Learn as if you were to live forever."
—Gandhi

▶ HOW TO USE THE DATABASE

The 2018 edition of *First Aid for the USMLE Step 1* contains a revised and expanded database of basic science material that students, student authors, and faculty authors have identified as high yield for board review. The information is presented in a partially organ-based format. Hence, Section II is devoted to the foundational principles of biochemistry, microbiology, immunology, basic pathology, basic pharmacology, and public health sciences. Section III focuses on organ systems, with subsections covering the embryology, anatomy and histology, physiology, clinical pathology, and clinical pharmacology relevant to each. Each subsection is then divided into smaller topic areas containing related facts. Individual facts are generally presented in a three-column format, with the **Title** of the fact in the first column, the **Description** of the fact in the second column, and the **Mnemonic** or **Special Note** in the third column. Some facts do not have a mnemonic and are presented in a two-column format. Others are presented in list or tabular form in order to emphasize key associations.

The database structure used in Sections II and III is useful for reviewing material already learned. These sections are **not** ideal for learning complex or highly conceptual material for the first time.

The database of high-yield facts is not comprehensive. Use it to complement your core study material and not as your primary study source. The facts and notes have been condensed and edited to emphasize the essential material, and as a result, each entry is "incomplete" and arguably "over-simplified." Often, the more you research a topic, the more complex it becomes, with certain topics resisting simplification. Work with the material, add your own notes and mnemonics, and recognize that not all memory techniques work for all students.

We update the database of high-yield facts annually to keep current with new trends in boards emphasis, including clinical relevance. However, we must note that inevitably many other high-yield topics are not yet included in our database.

We actively encourage medical students and faculty to submit high-yield topics, well-written entries, diagrams, clinical images, and useful mnemonics so that we may enhance the database for future students. We also solicit recommendations of alternate tools for study that may be useful in preparing for the examination, such as charts, flash cards, apps, and online resources (see How to Contribute, p. xvii).

Image Acknowledgments

All images and diagrams marked with ℞ are © USMLE-Rx.com (MedIQ Learning, LLC) and reproduced here by special permission. All images marked with ℞ are © Dr. Richard P. Usatine, author of *The Color Atlas of Family Medicine*, *The Color Atlas of Internal Medicine*, and *The Color Atlas of Pediatrics*, and are reproduced here by special permission (www. usatinemedia.com). Images and diagrams marked with ✳ are adapted or reproduced with permission of other sources as listed on page 707. Images and diagrams with no acknowledgment are part of this book.

Disclaimer

The entries in this section reflect student opinions of what is high yield. Because of the diverse sources of material, no attempt has been made to trace or reference the origins of entries individually. We have regarded mnemonics as essentially in the public domain. Errata will gladly be corrected if brought to the attention of the authors, either through our online errata submission form at www.firstaidteam.com or directly by email to firstaidteam@yahoo.com.

▶ NOTES

Biochemistry

"Biochemistry is the study of carbon compounds that crawl."

—Mike Adams

"We think we have found the basic mechanism by which life comes from life."

—Francis H. C. Crick

"The biochemistry and biophysics are the notes required for life; they conspire, collectively, to generate the real unit of life, the organism."

—Ursula Goodenough

This high-yield material includes molecular biology, genetics, cell biology, and principles of metabolism (especially vitamins, cofactors, minerals, and single-enzyme-deficiency diseases). When studying metabolic pathways, emphasize important regulatory steps and enzyme deficiencies that result in disease, as well as reactions targeted by pharmacologic interventions. For example, understanding the defect in Lesch-Nyhan syndrome and its clinical consequences is higher yield than memorizing every intermediate in the purine salvage pathway. Do not spend time on hard-core organic chemistry, mechanisms, or physical chemistry. Detailed chemical structures are infrequently tested; however, many structures have been included here to help students learn reactions and the important enzymes involved. Familiarity with the biochemical techniques that have medical relevance—such as ELISA, immunoelectrophoresis, Southern blotting, and PCR—is useful. Review the related biochemistry when studying pharmacology or genetic diseases as a way to reinforce and integrate the material.

▸ BIOCHEMISTRY—MOLECULAR

Chromatin structure

DNA double-helix

H1 histone (linker)

DNA

Nucleosome (H2A, H2B, H3, H4) ×2

Euchromatin

Supercoiled structure

Heterochromatin

Metaphase chromosome

DNA exists in the condensed, chromatin form to fit into the nucleus. DNA loops twice around a histone octamer to form a nucleosome ("**beads on a string**"). H1 binds to the nucleosome and to "linker DNA," thereby stabilizing the chromatin fiber.

Phosphate groups give DNA a $\ominus$ charge. Lysine and arginine give histones a $\oplus$ charge.

In mitosis, DNA condenses to form chromosomes. DNA and histone synthesis occurs during S phase.

Mitochondria have their own DNA, which is circular and does not utilize histones.

Heterochromatin	Condensed, appears darker on EM (labeled H in **A**; Nu, nucleolus). Transcriptionally inactive, sterically inaccessible. ↑ methylation, ↓ acetylation.	HeteroChromatin = Highly Condensed. Barr bodies (inactive X chromosomes) may be visible on the periphery of nucleus.
Euchromatin	Less condensed, appears lighter on EM (labeled E in **A**). Transcriptionally active, sterically accessible.	*Eu* = true, "truly transcribed." Euchromatin is Expressed.
DNA methylation	Changes the expression of a DNA segment without changing the sequence. Involved with genomic imprinting, X-chromosome inactivation, repression of transposable elements, aging, and carcinogenesis.	DNA is methylated in imprinting. Methylation within gene promoter (CpG islands) typically represses gene transcription. CpG Methylation Makes DNA Mute.
Histone methylation	Usually causes reversible transcriptional suppression, but can also cause activation depending on location of methyl groups.	Histone Methylation Mostly Makes DNA Mute.
Histone acetylation	Relaxes DNA coiling, allowing for transcription.	Histone Acetylation makes DNA Active.

Nucleotides

NucleoSide = base + (deoxy)ribose (Sugar).

NucleoTide = base + (deoxy)ribose + phosphaTe; linked by 3′-5′ phosphodiester bond. 5′ end of incoming nucleotide bears the triphosphate (energy source for the bond). Triphosphate bond is target of 3′ hydroxyl attack.

PURines (A,G)—2 rings. PURe As Gold.

PYrimidines (C,U,T)—1 ring. CUT the PY (pie).

Thymine has a methyl.

Deamination of cytosine forms uracil. Deamination of adenine forms hypoxanthine. Deamination of guanine forms xanthine. Deamination of 5-methylcytosine forms thymine. G-C bond (3 H bonds) stronger than A-T bond (2 H bonds). ↑ G-C content → ↑ melting temperature of DNA. "C-G bonds are like Crazy Glue."

Uracil found in RNA; thymine in DNA. Methylation of uracil makes thymine.

Amino acids necessary for **pur**ine synthesis (Cats **purr** until they **GAG**):
Glycine
Aspartate
Glutamine

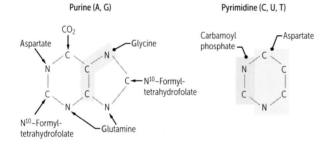

De novo pyrimidine and purine synthesis

Various immunosuppressive, antineoplastic, and antibiotic drugs function by interfering with nucleotide synthesis:

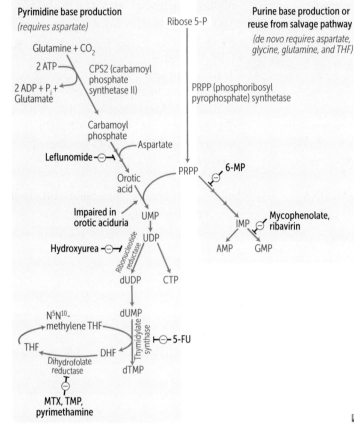

Pyrimidine synthesis:

- Leflunomide: inhibits dihydroorotate dehydrogenase
- Methotrexate (MTX), trimethoprim (TMP), and pyrimethamine: inhibit dihydrofolate reductase (↓ deoxythymidine monophosphate [dTMP]) in humans, bacteria, and protozoa, respectively
- 5-fluorouracil (5-FU) and its prodrug capecitabine: form 5-F-dUMP, which inhibits thymidylate synthase (↓ dTMP)

Purine synthesis:

- 6-mercaptopurine (6-MP) and its prodrug azathioprine: inhibit de novo purine synthesis
- Mycophenolate and ribavirin: inhibit inosine monophosphate dehydrogenase

Purine and pyrimidine synthesis:

- Hydroxyurea: inhibits ribonucleotide reductase

CPS1 = mItochondria (urea cycle)
CPS2 = cyTWOsol

Purine salvage deficiencies

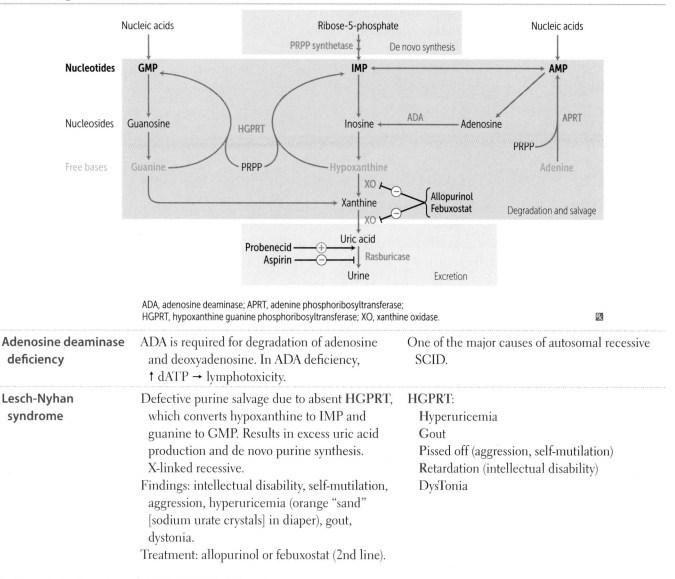

ADA, adenosine deaminase; APRT, adenine phosphoribosyltransferase; HGPRT, hypoxanthine guanine phosphoribosyltransferase; XO, xanthine oxidase.

Adenosine deaminase deficiency	ADA is required for degradation of adenosine and deoxyadenosine. In ADA deficiency, ↑ dATP → lymphotoxicity.	One of the major causes of autosomal recessive SCID.
Lesch-Nyhan syndrome	Defective purine salvage due to absent HGPRT, which converts hypoxanthine to IMP and guanine to GMP. Results in excess uric acid production and de novo purine synthesis. X-linked recessive. Findings: intellectual disability, self-mutilation, aggression, hyperuricemia (orange "sand" [sodium urate crystals] in diaper), gout, dystonia. Treatment: allopurinol or febuxostat (2nd line).	**HGPRT**: **H**yperuricemia **G**out **P**issed off (aggression, self-mutilation) **R**etardation (intellectual disability) Dys**T**onia

Genetic code features

Unambiguous	Each codon specifies only 1 amino acid.	
Degenerate/ redundant	Most amino acids are coded by multiple codons. **Wobble**—codons that differ in 3rd, "wobble" position may code for the same tRNA/amino acid. Specific base pairing is usually required only in the first 2 nucleotide positions of mRNA codon.	Exceptions: methionine (AUG) and tryptophan (UGG) encoded by only 1 codon.
Commaless, nonoverlapping	Read from a fixed starting point as a continuous sequence of bases.	Exceptions: some viruses.
Universal	Genetic code is conserved throughout evolution.	Exception in humans: mitochondria.

DNA replication	Eukaryotic DNA replication is more complex than the prokaryotic process but uses many enzymes analogous to those listed below. In both prokaryotes and eukaryotes, DNA replication is semiconservative, involves both continuous and discontinuous (Okazaki fragment) synthesis, and occurs in the 5′ → 3′ direction.	
Origin of replication A	Particular consensus sequence of base pairs in genome where DNA replication begins. May be single (prokaryotes) or multiple (eukaryotes).	AT-rich sequences (such as TATA box regions) are found in promoters and origins of replication.
Replication fork B	Y-shaped region along DNA template where leading and lagging strands are synthesized.	
Helicase C	Unwinds DNA template at replication fork.	Helicase Halves DNA.
Single-stranded binding proteins D	Prevent strands from reannealing.	
DNA topoisomerases E	Create a single- or double-stranded break in the helix to add or remove supercoils.	In eukaryotes: irinotecan/topotecan inhibit topoisomerase (TOP) I, etoposide/teniposide inhibit TOP II. In prokaryotes: fluoroquinolones inhibit TOP II (DNA gyrase) and TOP IV.
Primase F	Makes an RNA primer on which DNA polymerase III can initiate replication.	
DNA polymerase III G	Prokaryotes only. Elongates leading strand by adding deoxynucleotides to the 3′ end. Elongates lagging strand until it reaches primer of preceding fragment. 3′ → 5′ exonuclease activity "proofreads" each added nucleotide.	DNA polymerase III has 5′ → 3′ synthesis and proofreads with 3′ → 5′ exonuclease. Drugs blocking DNA replication often have a modified 3′ OH, thereby preventing addition of the next nucleotide ("chain termination").
DNA polymerase I H	Prokaryotic only. Degrades RNA primer; replaces it with DNA.	Same functions as DNA polymerase III, also excises RNA primer with 5′ → 3′ exonuclease.
DNA ligase I	Catalyzes the formation of a phosphodiester bond within a strand of double-stranded DNA.	Joins Okazaki fragments. Ligase Links DNA.
Telomerase	Eukaryotes only. A reverse transcriptase (RNA-dependent DNA polymerase) that adds DNA (**TTAGGG**) to 3′ ends of chromosomes to avoid loss of genetic material with every duplication.	Often dysregulated in cancer cells, allowing unlimited replication. Telomerase TAGs for Greatness and Glory.

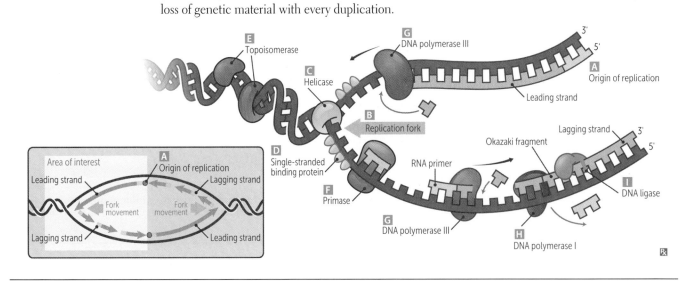

Mutations in DNA	Severity of damage: silent ≪ missense < nonsense < frameshift. For point (silent, missense, and nonsense) mutations: <ul><li>Transition—purine to purine (eg, A to G) or pyrimidine to pyrimidine (eg, C to T).</li><li>Transversion—purine to pyrimidine (eg, A to T) or pyrimidine to purine (eg, C to G).</li></ul>	
Silent	Nucleotide substitution but codes for same (synonymous) amino acid; often base change in 3rd position of codon (tRNA wobble).	
Missense	Nucleotide substitution resulting in changed amino acid (called conservative if new amino acid is similar in chemical structure).	Sickle cell disease (substitution of glutamic acid with valine).
Nonsense	Nucleotide substitution resulting in early **stop** codon (UAG, UAA, UGA). Usually results in nonfunctional protein.	Stop the **nonsense!**
Frameshift	Deletion or insertion of a number of nucleotides not divisible by 3, resulting in misreading of all nucleotides downstream. Protein may be shorter or longer, and its function may be disrupted or altered.	Duchenne muscular dystrophy, Tay-Sachs disease.
Splice site	Mutation at a splice site → retained intron in the mRNA → protein with impaired or altered function.	Rare cause of cancers, dementia, epilepsy, some types of β-thalassemia.

***Lac* operon**	Classic example of a genetic response to an environmental change. Glucose is the preferred metabolic substrate in *E coli*, but when glucose is absent and lactose is available, the *lac* operon is activated to switch to lactose metabolism. Mechanism of shift: <ul><li>Low glucose → ↑ adenylate cyclase activity → ↑ generation of cAMP from ATP → activation of catabolite activator protein (CAP) → ↑ transcription.</li><li>High lactose → unbinds repressor protein from repressor/operator site → ↑ transcription.</li></ul>

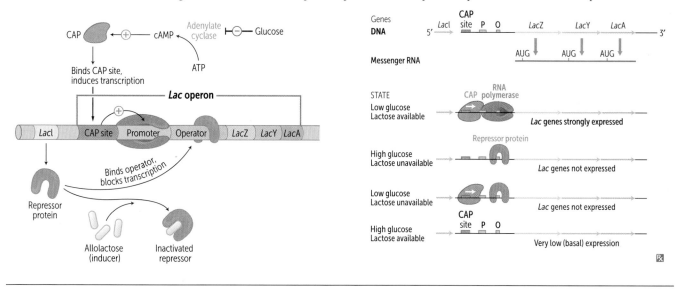

DNA repair

Single strand		
Nucleotide excision repair	Specific endonucleases release the oligonucleotides containing damaged bases; DNA polymerase and ligase fill and reseal the gap, respectively. Repairs bulky helix-distorting lesions. Occurs in G_1 phase of cell cycle.	Defective in xeroderma pigmentosum (inability to repair DNA pyrimidine dimers caused by UV exposure). Findings: dry skin, extreme light sensitivity, skin cancer.
Base excision repair	Base-specific Glycosylase removes altered base and creates AP site (apurinic/apyrimidinic). One or more nucleotides are removed by AP-Endonuclease, which cleaves the 5′ end. Lyase cleaves the 3′ end. DNA Polymerase-β fills the gap and DNA Ligase seals it. Occurs throughout cell cycle.	Important in repair of spontaneous/toxic deamination. "**GEL PL**ease"
Mismatch repair	Newly synthesized strand is recognized, mismatched nucleotides are removed, and the gap is filled and resealed. Occurs predominantly in S phase of cell cycle.	Defective in Lynch syndrome (hereditary nonpolyposis colorectal cancer [HNPCC]).
Double strand		
Nonhomologous end joining	Brings together 2 ends of DNA fragments to repair double-stranded breaks. No requirement for homology. Some DNA may be lost.	Defective in ataxia telangiectasia and Fanconi anemia.
Homologous recombination	Requires two homologous DNA duplexes. A strand from the damaged dsDNA is repaired using a complementary strand from the intact homologous dsDNA as a template. Restores duplexes accurately without loss of nucleotides.	Defective in breast/ovarian cancers with *BRCA1* mutation.

Start and stop codons

mRNA start codons	AUG (or rarely GUG).	**AUG** in**AUG**urates protein synthesis.
Eukaryotes	Codes for methionine, which may be removed before translation is completed.	
Prokaryotes	Codes for N-formylmethionine (fMet).	fMet stimulates neutrophil chemotaxis.
mRNA stop codons	UGA, UAA, UAG.	**UGA** = **U G**o **A**way. **UAA** = **U A**re **A**way. **UAG** = **U A**re **G**one.

Functional organization of a eukaryotic gene

Transcription start
(mRNA synthesized 5′ → 3′)

ATG = Start codon

CAAT box TATA box

Polyadenylation signal

DNA coding strand 5′ | CAAT | TATAAT | Exon 1 | GT | AG | Exon 2 | GT | AG | Exon 3 | AATAAA | 3′

Promoter   5′ UTR   Intron 1   Intron 2   3′ UTR

Regulation of gene expression

Promoter	Site where RNA polymerase II and multiple other transcription factors bind to DNA upstream from gene locus (AT-rich upstream sequence with TATA and CAAT boxes).	Promoter mutation commonly results in dramatic ↓ in level of gene transcription.
Enhancer	DNA locus where regulatory proteins ("activators") bind → increasing expression of a gene on the same chromosome.	Enhancers and silencers may be located close to, far from, or even within (in an intron) the gene whose expression it regulates.
Silencer	DNA locus where regulatory proteins ("repressors") bind → decreasing expression of a gene on the same chromosome.	

RNA polymerases

Eukaryotes	RNA polymerase I makes rRNA, the most common (rampant) type; present only in nucleolus. RNA polymerase II makes mRNA (largest RNA, massive). mRNA is read 5′ to 3′. RNA polymerase III makes 5S rRNA, tRNA (smallest RNA, tiny). No proofreading function, but can initiate chains. RNA polymerase II opens DNA at promoter site.	I, II, and III are numbered in the same order that their products are used in protein synthesis: rRNA, mRNA, then tRNA. α-amanitin, found in *Amanita phalloides* (death cap mushrooms), inhibits RNA polymerase II. Causes severe hepatotoxicity if ingested. Actinomycin D inhibits RNA polymerase in both prokaryotes and eukaryotes.
Prokaryotes	1 RNA polymerase (multisubunit complex) makes all 3 kinds of RNA.	Rifampin inhibits DNA-dependent RNA polymerase in prokaryotes.

RNA processing (eukaryotes)

Cap   Coding

5′
Gppp

3′
HO-AAAAA
Tail

Initial transcript is called heterogeneous nuclear RNA (hnRNA). hnRNA is then modified and becomes mRNA.
The following processes occur in the nucleus:
- Capping of 5′ end (addition of 7-methylguanosine cap)
- Polyadenylation of 3′ end (≈ 200 A's)
- Splicing out of introns

Capped, tailed, and spliced transcript is called mRNA.

mRNA is transported out of the nucleus into the cytosol, where it is translated.
mRNA quality control occurs at cytoplasmic processing bodies (P-bodies), which contain exonucleases, decapping enzymes, and microRNAs; mRNAs may be degraded or stored in P-bodies for future translation.
Poly-A polymerase does not require a template.
AAUAAA = polyadenylation signal.

Splicing of pre-mRNA

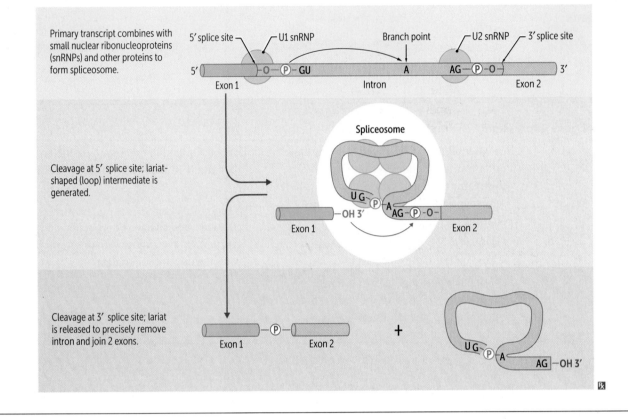

Primary transcript combines with small nuclear ribonucleoproteins (snRNPs) and other proteins to form spliceosome.

Cleavage at 5′ splice site; lariat-shaped (loop) intermediate is generated.

Cleavage at 3′ splice site; lariat is released to precisely remove intron and join 2 exons.

Introns vs exons

Exons contain the actual genetic information coding for protein.

Introns are intervening noncoding segments of DNA.

Different exons are frequently combined by alternative splicing to produce a larger number of unique proteins.

Alternative splicing can produce a variety of protein products from a single hnRNA sequence (eg, transmembrane vs secreted Ig, tropomyosin variants in muscle, dopamine receptors in the brain).

Introns are intervening sequences and stay in the nucleus, whereas exons exit and are expressed.

Variants in which splicing occurs abnormally are implicated in oncogenesis and many genetic disorders (eg, β-thalassemia, Gaucher disease, Tay-Sachs disease, Marfan syndrome).

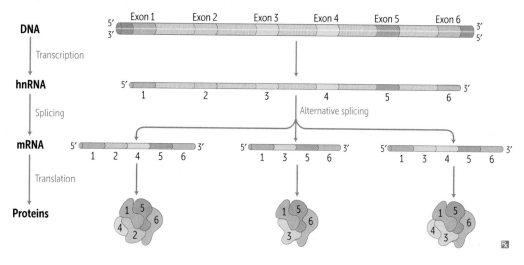

microRNAs

MicroRNAs (miRNAs) are small, conserved, noncoding RNA molecules that posttranscriptionally regulate gene expression by targeting the 3′ untranslated region of specific mRNAs for degradation or translational repression. Abnormal expression of miRNAs contributes to certain malignancies (eg, by silencing an mRNA from a tumor suppressor gene).

tRNA

Structure	75–90 nucleotides, 2° structure, cloverleaf form, anticodon end is opposite 3′ aminoacyl end. All tRNAs, both eukaryotic and prokaryotic, have CCA at 3′ end along with a high percentage of chemically modified bases. The amino acid is covalently bound to the 3′ end of the tRNA. **CCA Can Carry Amino acids.** T-arm: contains the TΨC (ribothymidine, pseudouridine, cytidine) sequence necessary for tRNA-ribosome binding. **T-arm Tethers** tRNA molecule to ribosome. D-arm: contains dihydrouridine residues necessary for tRNA recognition by the correct aminoacyl-tRNA synthetase. **D-arm Detects** the tRNA by aminoacyl-tRNA synthetase. Acceptor stem: the 5′-CCA-3′ is the amino acid acceptor site.
Charging	Aminoacyl-tRNA synthetase (1 per amino acid; "matchmaker"; uses ATP) scrutinizes amino acid before and after it binds to tRNA. If incorrect, bond is hydrolyzed. The amino acid-tRNA bond has energy for formation of peptide bond. A mischarged tRNA reads usual codon but inserts wrong amino acid. Aminoacyl-tRNA synthetase and binding of charged tRNA to the codon are responsible for accuracy of amino acid selection.

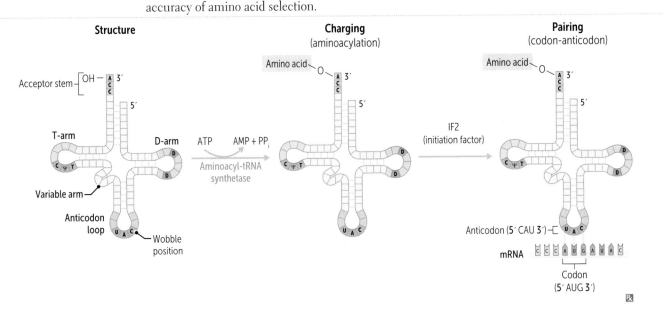

Protein synthesis

Initiation	Eukaryotic initiation factors (eIFs) identify either the 5′ cap or an internal ribosome entry site (IRES). IRES can be located at many places in an mRNA (most often 5′ UTR). The eIFs then help assemble the 40S ribosomal subunit with the initiator tRNA and are released when the mRNA and the ribosomal 60S subunit assemble with the complex. Requires GTP.	Eukaryotes: 40S + 60S → 80S (Even). PrOkaryotes: 30S + 50S → 70S (Odd). Synthesis occurs from N-terminus to C-terminus. ATP—tRNA Activation (charging). GTP—tRNA Gripping and Going places (translocation). Think of "going APE": A site = incoming Aminoacyl-tRNA. P site = accommodates growing Peptide. E site = holds Empty tRNA as it Exits.
Elongation	1. Aminoacyl-tRNA binds to A site (except for initiator methionine), requires an elongation factor and GTP 2. rRNA ("ribozyme") catalyzes peptide bond formation, transfers growing polypeptide to amino acid in A site 3. Ribosome advances 3 nucleotides toward 3′ end of mRNA, moving peptidyl tRNA to P site (translocation)	
Termination	Release factor recognizes stop codon and halts translation → completed polypeptide is released from ribosome. Requires GTP.	

Posttranslational modifications

Trimming	Removal of N- or C-terminal propeptides from zymogen to generate mature protein (eg, trypsinogen to trypsin).
Covalent alterations	Phosphorylation, glycosylation, hydroxylation, methylation, acetylation, and ubiquitination.

Chaperone protein	Intracellular protein involved in facilitating and/or maintaining protein folding. For example, in yeast, heat shock proteins (eg, HSP60) are expressed at high temperatures to prevent protein denaturing/misfolding.

▶ BIOCHEMISTRY—CELLULAR

Cell cycle phases	Checkpoints control transitions between phases of cell cycle. This process is regulated by cyclins, cyclin-dependent kinases (CDKs), and tumor suppressors. M phase (shortest phase of cell cycle) includes mitosis (prophase, prometaphase, metaphase, anaphase, telophase) and cytokinesis (cytoplasm splits in two). G_1 and G_0 are of variable duration.

REGULATION OF CELL CYCLE

Cyclin-dependent kinases	Constitutive and inactive.
Cyclins	Regulatory proteins that control cell cycle events; phase specific; activate CDKs.
Cyclin-CDK complexes	Phosphorylate other proteins to coordinate cell cycle progression; must be activated and inactivated at appropriate times for cell cycle to progress.
Tumor suppressors	p53 induces p21, which inhibits CDKs → hypophosphorylation (activation) of Rb → inhibition of G_1-S progression. Mutations in tumor suppressor genes can result in unrestrained cell division (eg, Li-Fraumeni syndrome). Growth factors (eg, insulin, PDGF, EPO, EGF) bind tyrosine kinase receptors to transition the cell from G_1 to S phase.

Rb, p53 modulate G_1 restriction point

CELL TYPES

Permanent	Remain in G_0, regenerate from stem cells.	Neurons, skeletal and cardiac muscle, RBCs.
Stable (quiescent)	Enter G_1 from G_0 when stimulated.	Hepatocytes, lymphocytes, PCT, periosteal cells.
Labile	Never go to G_0, divide rapidly with a short G_1. Most affected by chemotherapy.	Bone marrow, gut epithelium, skin, hair follicles, germ cells.

Rough endoplasmic reticulum	Site of synthesis of secretory (exported) proteins and of N-linked oligosaccharide addition to many proteins. Nissl bodies (RER in neurons)—synthesize peptide neurotransmitters for secretion. Free ribosomes—unattached to any membrane; site of synthesis of cytosolic and organellar proteins.	Mucus-secreting goblet cells of the small intestine and antibody-secreting plasma cells are rich in RER.
Smooth endoplasmic reticulum	Site of steroid synthesis and detoxification of drugs and poisons. Lacks surface ribosomes.	Liver hepatocytes and steroid hormone–producing cells of the adrenal cortex and gonads are rich in SER.

Cell trafficking

Golgi is the distribution center for proteins and lipids from the ER to the vesicles and plasma membrane. Modifies N-oligosaccharides on asparagine. Adds O-oligosaccharides on serine and threonine. Adds mannose-6-phosphate to proteins for trafficking to lysosomes.

Endosomes are sorting centers for material from outside the cell or from the Golgi, sending it to lysosomes for destruction or back to the membrane/Golgi for further use.

I-cell disease (inclusion cell disease/mucolipidosis type II)—inherited lysosomal storage disorder; defect in N-acetylglucosaminyl-1-phosphotransferase → failure of the Golgi to phosphorylate mannose residues (↓ mannose-6-phosphate) on glycoproteins → proteins are secreted extracellularly rather than delivered to lysosomes. Results in coarse facial features, gingival hyperplasia, clouded corneas, restricted joint movements, claw hand deformities, kyphoscoliosis, and high plasma levels of lysosomal enzymes. Often fatal in childhood.

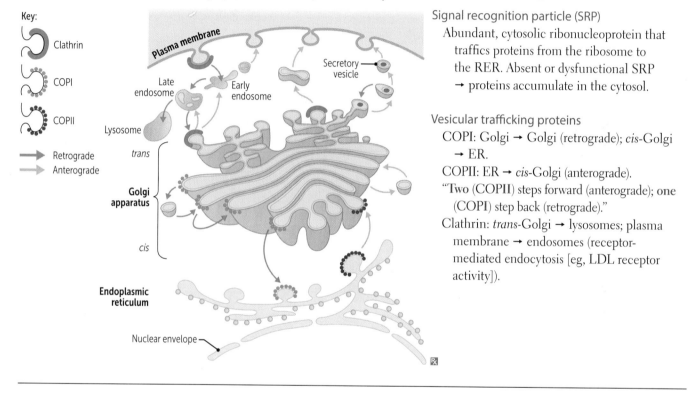

Signal recognition particle (SRP)

Abundant, cytosolic ribonucleoprotein that traffics proteins from the ribosome to the RER. Absent or dysfunctional SRP → proteins accumulate in the cytosol.

Vesicular trafficking proteins

COPI: Golgi → Golgi (retrograde); *cis*-Golgi → ER.

COPII: ER → *cis*-Golgi (anterograde).

"Two (COPII) steps forward (anterograde); one (COPI) step back (retrograde)."

Clathrin: *trans*-Golgi → lysosomes; plasma membrane → endosomes (receptor-mediated endocytosis [eg, LDL receptor activity]).

Peroxisome

Membrane-enclosed organelle involved in:

- β-oxidation of very-long-chain fatty acids (VLCFA)
- α-oxidation (strictly peroxisomal process)
- Catabolism of branched-chain fatty acids, amino acids, and ethanol
- Synthesis of cholesterol, bile acids, and plasmalogens (important membrane phospholipid, especially in white matter of brain)

Zellweger syndrome—autosomal recessive disorder of peroxisome biogenesis due to mutated *PEX* genes. Hypotonia, seizures, hepatomegaly, early death.

Refsum disease—autosomal recessive disorder of α-oxidation → phytanic acid not metabolized to pristanic acid. Scaly skin, ataxia, cataracts/night blindness, shortening of 4th toe, epiphyseal dysplasia. Treatment: diet, plasmapheresis.

Adrenoleukodystrophy—X-linked recessive disorder of β-oxidation → VLCFA buildup in **adrenal** glands, white (**leuko**) matter of brain, testes. Progressive disease that can lead to adrenal gland crisis, coma, and death.

Proteasome　　Barrel-shaped protein complex that degrades damaged or ubiquitin-tagged proteins. Defects in the ubiquitin-proteasome system have been implicated in some cases of Parkinson disease.

Cytoskeletal elements　　A network of protein fibers within the cytoplasm that supports cell structure, cell and organelle movement, and cell division.

TYPE OF FILAMENT	PREDOMINANT FUNCTION	EXAMPLES
Microfilaments	Muscle contraction, cytokinesis	Actin, microvilli.
Intermediate filaments	Maintain cell structure	Vimentin, desmin, cytokeratin, lamins, glial fibrillary acidic protein (GFAP), neurofilaments.
Microtubules	Movement, cell division	Cilia, flagella, mitotic spindle, axonal trafficking, centrioles.

Microtubule

Positive end (+)

Heterodimer

Protofilament

Negative end (−)

Cylindrical outer structure composed of a helical array of polymerized heterodimers of α- and β-tubulin. Each dimer has 2 GTP bound. Incorporated into flagella, cilia, mitotic spindles. Grows slowly, collapses quickly. Also involved in slow axoplasmic transport in neurons.

Molecular motor proteins—transport cellular cargo toward opposite ends of microtubule tracks.

- Dynein—retrograde to microtubule (+ → −).
- Kinesin—anterograde to microtubule (− → +).

Drugs that act on microtubules (Microtubules Get Constructed Very Poorly):

- Mebendazole (antihelminthic)
- Griseofulvin (antifungal)
- Colchicine (antigout)
- Vincristine/Vinblastine (anticancer)
- Paclitaxel (anticancer)

Negative end Near Nucleus
Positive end Points to Periphery

Cilia structure

9 doublet + 2 singlet arrangement of microtubules A.

Basal body (base of cilium below cell membrane) consists of 9 microtubule triplets B with no central microtubules.

Axonemal dynein—ATPase that links peripheral 9 doublets and causes bending of cilium by differential sliding of doublets.

Gap junctions enable coordinated ciliary movement.

Kartagener syndrome (1° ciliary dyskinesia)—immotile cilia due to a dynein arm defect. Autosomal recessive. Results in ↓ male and female fertility due to immotile sperm and dysfunctional fallopian tube cilia, respectively; ↑ risk of ectopic pregnancy. Can cause bronchiectasis, recurrent sinusitis, chronic ear infections, conductive hearing loss, and situs inversus (eg, dextrocardia on CXR C). (Kartagener's restaurant: take-out only, there's no dynein "dine-in").

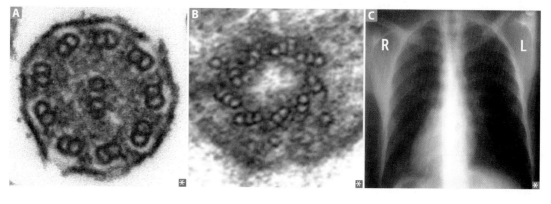

Sodium-potassium pump

Na^+-K^+ ATPase is located in the plasma membrane with ATP site on cytosolic side. For each ATP consumed, $3Na^+$ go out of the cell (pump phosphorylated) and $2K^+$ come into the cell (pump dephosphorylated).

Plasma membrane is an asymmetric lipid bilayer containing cholesterol, phospholipids, sphingolipids, glycolipids, and proteins.

Pumpkin = pump K^+ in.

Ouabain (a cardiac glycoside) inhibits by binding to K^+ site.

Cardiac glycosides (digoxin and digitoxin) directly inhibit the Na^+-K^+ ATPase, which leads to indirect inhibition of Na^+/Ca^{2+} exchange → ↑ $[Ca^{2+}]_i$ → ↑ cardiac contractility.

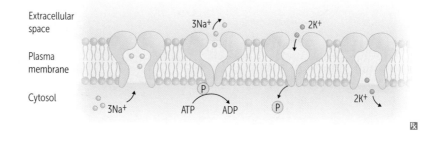

Collagen	Most abundant protein in the human body. Extensively modified by posttranslational modification. Organizes and strengthens extracellular matrix.	Be (So Totally) Cool, Read Books.
Type I	Most common (90%)—Bone (made by osteoblasts), Skin, Tendon, dentin, fascia, cornea, late wound repair.	Type I: bone. ↓ production in osteogenesis imperfecta type I.
Type II	Cartilage (including hyaline), vitreous body, nucleus pulposus.	Type II: cartWOlage.
Type III	Reticulin—skin, blood vessels, uterus, fetal tissue, granulation tissue.	Type III: deficient in the uncommon, vascular type of Ehlers-Danlos syndrome (ThreE D).
Type IV	Basement membrane, basal lamina, lens.	Type IV: under the floor (basement membrane). Defective in Alport syndrome; targeted by autoantibodies in Goodpasture syndrome.

Collagen synthesis and structure

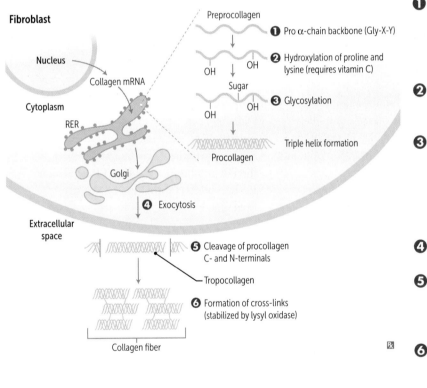

❶ Synthesis—translation of collagen α chains (preprocollagen)—usually Gly-X-Y (X and Y are proline or lysine). Glycine content best reflects collagen synthesis (collagen is ⅓ glycine).

❷ Hydroxylation—hydroxylation of specific proline and lysine residues. Requires vitamin C; deficiency → scurvy.

❸ Glycosylation—glycosylation of pro-α-chain hydroxylysine residues and formation of procollagen via hydrogen and disulfide bonds (triple helix of 3 collagen α chains). Problems forming triple helix → osteogenesis imperfecta.

❹ Exocytosis—exocytosis of procollagen into extracellular space.

❺ Proteolytic processing—cleavage of disulfide-rich terminal regions of procollagen → insoluble tropocollagen. Problems with cleavage → Ehlers-Danlos syndrome.

❻ Cross-linking—reinforcement of many staggered tropocollagen molecules by covalent lysine-hydroxylysine cross-linkage (by copper-containing lysyl oxidase) to make collagen fibrils. Problems with cross-linking → Ehlers-Danlos syndrome, Menkes disease.

Osteogenesis imperfecta

Genetic bone disorder (brittle bone disease) caused by a variety of gene defects (most commonly *COL1A1* and *COL1A2*).

Most common form is autosomal dominant with ↓ production of otherwise normal type I collagen. Manifestations can include:

- Multiple fractures with minimal trauma 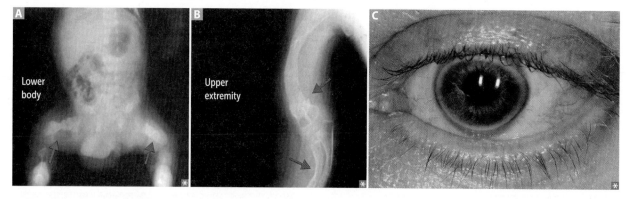 A B; may occur during the birth process
- Blue sclerae C due to the translucent connective tissue over choroidal veins
- Some forms have tooth abnormalities, including opalescent teeth that wear easily due to lack of dentin (dentinogenesis imperfecta)
- Hearing loss (abnormal ossicles)

May be confused with child abuse.

Treat with bisphosphonates to ↓ fracture risk.

Patients can't **BITE**:

Bones = multiple fractures

I (eye) = blue sclerae

Teeth = dental imperfections

Ear = hearing loss

Lower body

Upper extremity

Ehlers-Danlos syndrome

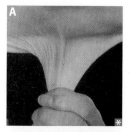
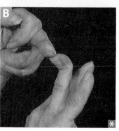

Faulty collagen synthesis causing hyperextensible skin A, hypermobile joints B, and tendency to bleed (easy bruising).

Multiple types. Inheritance and severity vary. Can be autosomal dominant or recessive. May be associated with joint dislocation, berry and aortic aneurysms, organ rupture.

Hypermobility type (joint instability): most common type.

Classical type (joint and skin symptoms): caused by a mutation in type V collagen (eg, *COL5A1*, *COL5A2*).

Vascular type (fragile tissues including vessels [eg, aorta], muscles, and organs that are prone to rupture): deficient type III procollagen.

Menkes disease   X-linked recessive connective tissue disease caused by impaired copper absorption and transport due to defective Menkes protein (ATP7A). Leads to ↓ activity of lysyl oxidase (copper is a necessary cofactor) → defective collagen. Results in brittle, "kinky" hair, growth retardation, and hypotonia.

Elastin   Stretchy protein within skin, lungs, large arteries, elastic ligaments, vocal cords, ligamenta flava (connect vertebrae → relaxed and stretched conformations).

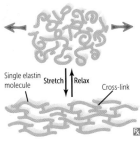

Single elastin molecule   Stretch ↕ Relax   Cross-link

Rich in nonhydroxylated proline, glycine, and lysine residues, vs the hydroxylated residues of collagen.

Tropoelastin with fibrillin scaffolding.

Cross-linking takes place extracellularly and gives elastin its elastic properties.

Broken down by elastase, which is normally inhibited by α_1-antitrypsin.

α_1-Antitrypsin deficiency results in unopposed elastase activity, which can cause emphysema.

Changes with aging: ↓ dermal collagen and elastin, ↓ synthesis of collagen fibrils; crosslinking remains normal.

Marfan syndrome—autosomal dominant connective tissue disorder affecting skeleton, heart, and eyes. *FBN1* gene mutation on chromosome 15 results in defective fibrillin, a glycoprotein that forms a sheath around elastin. Findings: tall with long extremities; pectus carinatum (more specific) or pectus excavatum; hypermobile joints; long, tapering fingers and toes (arachnodactyly); cystic medial necrosis of aorta; aortic incompetence and dissecting aortic aneurysms; floppy mitral valve. Subluxation of lenses, typically upward and temporally. (Look up at a ceiling fan.)

▶ BIOCHEMISTRY—LABORATORY TECHNIQUES

Polymerase chain reaction   Molecular biology lab procedure used to amplify a desired fragment of DNA. Useful as a diagnostic tool (eg, neonatal HIV, herpes encephalitis).

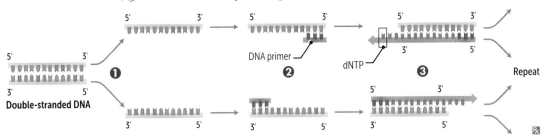

5'   3'   5'   3'   5'   3'
DNA primer   dNTP
❶   ❷   ❸   Repeat
5'   3'
Double-stranded DNA
3'   5'   3'   5'   3'   5'
3'   5'   3'   5'   3'   5'

❶ **Denaturation**—DNA is heated to ~95°C to separate the strands.

❷ **Annealing**—Sample is cooled to ~55°C. DNA primers, a heat-stable DNA polymerase (*Taq*), and deoxynucleotide triphosphates (dNTPs) are added. DNA primers anneal to the specific sequence to be amplified on each strand.

❸ **Elongation**—Temperature is increased to ~72°C. DNA polymerase attaches dNTPs to the strand to replicate the sequence after each primer.

Heating and cooling cycles continue until the DNA sample size is sufficient.

CRISPR/Cas9	A genome editing tool, derived from bacteria. Composed of an endonuclease (Cas9, which cleaves dsDNA) and a guide RNA (gRNA) sequence that binds to a complementary target DNA sequence. Cell DNA repair machinery (nonhomologous end joining) fills in the gap introduced by the system (knock-out) or a donor DNA can be added to the system to fill the gap (knock-in). The gRNA can be designed to target any DNA sequence.

Blotting procedures

Southern blot	1. **DNA** sample is enzymatically cleaved into smaller pieces, which are separated on a gel by electrophoresis, and then transferred to a filter. 2. Filter is exposed to radiolabeled DNA probe that recognizes and anneals to its complementary strand. 3. Resulting double-stranded, labeled piece of DNA is visualized when filter is exposed to film.	
Northern blot	Similar to Southern blot, except that an **RNA** sample is electrophoresed. Useful for studying mRNA levels, which are reflective of gene expression.	SNoW DRoP: Southern = DNA Northern = RNA Western = Protein
Western blot	Sample protein is separated via gel electrophoresis and transferred to a membrane. Labeled antibody is used to bind to relevant **protein**.	
Southwestern blot	Identifies **DNA-binding proteins** (eg, transcription factors) using labeled oligonucleotide probes.	

Flow cytometry

Laboratory technique to assess size, granularity, and protein expression (immunophenotype) of individual cells in a sample.

Commonly used in workup of hematologic abnormalities (eg, paroxysmal nocturnal hemoglobinuria, fetal RBCs in mother's blood) and immunodeficiencies (eg, CD4 cell count in HIV).

Cells are tagged with antibodies specific to surface or intracellular proteins. Antibodies are then tagged with a unique fluorescent dye. Sample is analyzed one cell at a time by focusing a laser on the cell and measuring light scatter and intensity of fluorescence.

Data are plotted either as histogram (one measure) or scatter plot (any two measures, as shown). In illustration:

- Cells in left lower quadrant ⊖ for both CD8 and CD3.
- Cells in right lower quadrant ⊕ for CD8 and ⊖ for CD3. Right lower quadrant is empty because all CD8-expressing cells also express CD3.
- Cells in left upper quadrant ⊕ for CD3 and ⊖ for CD8.
- Cells in right upper quadrant ⊕ for CD8 and CD3 (red + blue → purple).

Microarrays

Thousands of nucleic acid sequences are arranged in grids on glass or silicon. DNA or RNA probes are hybridized to the chip, and a scanner detects the relative amounts of complementary binding. Used to profile gene expression levels of thousands of genes simultaneously to study certain diseases and treatments. Able to detect single nucleotide polymorphisms (SNPs) and copy number variations (CNVs) for a variety of applications including genotyping, clinical genetic testing, forensic analysis, cancer mutations, and genetic linkage analysis.

Enzyme-linked immunosorbent assay

Immunologic test used to detect the presence of either a specific antigen (eg, HBsAg) or antibody (eg, anti-HBs) in a patient's blood sample. Detection involves the use of an antibody linked to an enzyme. Added substrate reacts with enzyme, producing a detectable signal. Can have high sensitivity and specificity, but is less specific than Western blot.

Direct ELISA tests for the antigen directly, while indirect ELISA tests for the antibody (thus indirectly testing for the antigen).

Karyotyping

A process in which metaphase chromosomes are stained, ordered, and numbered according to morphology, size, arm-length ratio, and banding pattern (arrows in A point to extensive abnormalities in a cancer cell).

Can be performed on a sample of blood, bone marrow, amniotic fluid, or placental tissue.

Used to diagnose chromosomal imbalances (eg, autosomal trisomies, sex chromosome disorders).

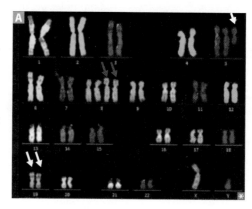

Fluorescence in situ hybridization

Fluorescent DNA or RNA probe binds to specific gene site of interest on chromosomes (arrows in A point to abnormalities in a cancer cell, whose karyotype is seen above; each fluorescent color represents a chromosome-specific probe).

Used for specific localization of genes and direct visualization of chromosomal anomalies at the molecular level.

- Microdeletion—no fluorescence on a chromosome compared to fluorescence at the same locus on the second copy of that chromosome
- Translocation—fluorescence signal that corresponds to one chromosome is found in a different chromosome (two white arrows in A show fragments of chromosome 17 that have translocated to chromosome 19)
- Duplication—a second copy of a chromosome, resulting in a trisomy or tetrasomy (two blue arrows show duplicated chromosomes 8, resulting in a tetrasomy)

Molecular cloning

Production of a recombinant DNA molecule in a bacterial host.

Steps:

1. Isolate eukaryotic mRNA (post-RNA processing) of interest.
2. Add reserve transcriptase (an RNA-dependent DNA polymerase) to produce complementary DNA (cDNA, lacks introns).
3. Insert cDNA fragments into bacterial plasmids containing antibiotic resistance genes.
4. Transform (insert) recombinant plasmid into bacteria.
5. Surviving bacteria on antibiotic medium produce cloned DNA (copies of cDNA).

Gene expression modifications	Transgenic strategies in mice involve: ▪ Random insertion of gene into mouse genome ▪ Targeted insertion or deletion of gene through homologous recombination with mouse gene	**Knock-out** = removing a gene, taking it out. **Knock-in** = inserting a gene. Random insertion—constitutive. Targeted insertion—conditional.
Cre-lox system	Can inducibly manipulate genes at specific developmental points (eg, to study a gene whose deletion causes embryonic death).	
RNA interference	dsRNA is synthesized that is complementary to the mRNA sequence of interest. When transfected into human cells, dsRNA separates and promotes degradation of target mRNA, "knocking down" gene expression.	

▶ BIOCHEMISTRY—GENETICS

Genetic terms

TERM	DEFINITION	EXAMPLE
Codominance	Both alleles contribute to the phenotype of the heterozygote.	Blood groups A, B, AB; α_1-antitrypsin deficiency; HLA groups.
Variable expressivity	Patients with the same genotype have varying phenotypes.	2 patients with neurofibromatosis type 1 (NF1) may have varying disease severity.
Incomplete penetrance	Not all individuals with a mutant genotype show the mutant phenotype. % penetrance × probability of inheriting genotype = risk of expressing phenotype.	*BRCA1* gene mutations do not always result in breast or ovarian cancer.
Pleiotropy	One gene contributes to multiple phenotypic effects.	Untreated phenylketonuria (PKU) manifests with light skin, intellectual disability, and musty body odor.
Anticipation	Increased severity or earlier onset of disease in succeeding generations.	Trinucleotide repeat diseases (eg, Huntington disease).
Loss of heterozygosity	If a patient inherits or develops a mutation in a tumor suppressor gene, the complementary allele must be deleted/mutated before cancer develops. This is not true of oncogenes.	Retinoblastoma and the "two-hit hypothesis," Lynch syndrome (HNPCC), Li-Fraumeni syndrome.
Dominant negative mutation	Exerts a dominant effect. A heterozygote produces a nonfunctional altered protein that also prevents the normal gene product from functioning.	Mutation of a transcription factor in its allosteric site. Nonfunctioning mutant can still bind DNA, preventing wild-type transcription factor from binding.
Linkage disequilibrium	Tendency for certain alleles at 2 linked loci to occur together more or less often than expected by chance. Measured in a population, not in a family, and often varies in different populations.	

Genetic terms *(continued)*

TERM	DEFINITION	EXAMPLE
Mosaicism	Presence of genetically distinct cell lines in the same individual. Somatic mosaicism—mutation arises from mitotic errors after fertilization and propagates through multiple tissues or organs. Gonadal mosaicism—mutation only in egg or sperm cells. If parents and relatives do not have the disease, suspect gonadal (or germline) mosaicism.	**McCune-Albright syndrome**—due to mutation affecting G-protein signaling. Presents with unilateral café-au-lait spots A with ragged edges, polyostotic fibrous dysplasia (bone is replaced by collagen and fibroblasts), and at least one endocrinopathy (eg, precocious puberty). Lethal if mutation occurs before fertilization (affecting all cells), but survivable in patients with mosaicism.
Locus heterogeneity	Mutations at different loci can produce a similar phenotype.	Albinism.
Allelic heterogeneity	Different mutations in the same locus produce the same phenotype.	β-thalassemia.
Heteroplasmy	Presence of both normal and mutated mtDNA, resulting in variable expression in mitochondrially inherited disease.	mtDNA passed from mother to all children.
Uniparental disomy	Offspring receives 2 copies of a chromosome from 1 parent and no copies from the other parent. HeterodIsomy (heterozygous) indicates a meiosis I error. IsodIsomy (homozygous) indicates a meiosis II error or postzygotic chromosomal duplication of one of a pair of chromosomes, and loss of the other of the original pair.	Uniparental is euploid (correct number of chromosomes). Most occurrences of uniparental disomy (UPD) → normal phenotype. Consider UPD in an individual manifesting a recessive disorder when only one parent is a carrier. Examples: Prader-Willi and Angelman syndromes.

Hardy-Weinberg population genetics

	pA	qa
pA	AA $p \times p = p^2$	Aa $p \times q$
qa	Aa $p \times q$	aa $q \times q = q^2$

If a population is in Hardy-Weinberg equilibrium and if p and q are the frequencies of separate alleles, then: $p^2 + 2pq + q^2 = 1$ and $p + q = 1$, which implies that:
p^2 = frequency of homozygosity for allele A
q^2 = frequency of homozygosity for allele a
$2pq$ = frequency of heterozygosity (carrier frequency, if an autosomal recessive disease).
The frequency of an X-linked recessive disease in males = q and in females = q^2.

Hardy-Weinberg law assumptions include:
- No mutation occurring at the locus
- Natural selection is not occurring
- Completely random mating
- No net migration

Disorders of imprinting	Imprinting—one gene copy is silenced by methylation, and only the other copy is expressed → parent-of-origin effects.	
Prader-Willi syndrome	Maternally derived genes are silenced (imprinted). Disease occurs when the Paternal allele is deleted or mutated. Results in hyperphagia, obesity, intellectual disability, hypogonadism, and hypotonia.	Associated with a mutation or deletion of chromosome 15 of paternal origin. 25% of cases due to maternal uniparental disomy.
AngelMan syndrome	Paternally derived *UBE3A* gene is silenced (imprinted). Disease occurs when the Maternal allele is deleted or mutated. Results in inappropriate laughter ("happy puppet"), seizures, ataxia, and severe intellectual disability.	Associated with mutation or deletion of the *UBE3A* gene on the maternal copy of chromosome 15. 5% of cases due to paternal uniparental disomy.

Modes of inheritance

Autosomal dominant	Often due to defects in structural genes. Many generations, both males and females are affected.	Often pleiotropic (multiple apparently unrelated effects) and variably expressive (different between individuals). Family history crucial to diagnosis. With one affected (heterozygous) parent, on average, ½ of children affected.
Autosomal recessive	Often due to enzyme deficiencies. Usually seen in only 1 generation.	Commonly more severe than dominant disorders; patients often present in childhood. ↑ risk in consanguineous families. With 2 carrier (heterozygous) parents, on average: ¼ of children will be affected (homozygous), ½ of children will be carriers, and ¼ of children will be neither affected nor carriers.
X-linked recessive	Sons of heterozygous mothers have a 50% chance of being affected. No male-to-male transmission. Skips generations.	Commonly more severe in males. Females usually must be homozygous to be affected.
X-linked dominant	Transmitted through both parents. Mothers transmit to 50% of daughters and sons; fathers transmit to all daughters but no sons.	**Hypophosphatemic rickets**—formerly known as vitamin D–resistant rickets. Inherited disorder resulting in ↑ phosphate wasting at proximal tubule. Results in rickets-like presentation. Other examples: fragile X syndrome, Alport syndrome.
Mitochondrial inheritance	Transmitted only through the mother. All offspring of affected females may show signs of disease.	Variable expression in a population or even within a family due to heteroplasmy. **Mitochondrial myopathies**—rare disorders; often present with myopathy, lactic acidosis, and CNS disease, eg, MELAS syndrome (mitochondrial encephalomyopathy, lactic acidosis, and stroke-like episodes). 2° to failure in oxidative phosphorylation. Muscle biopsy often shows "ragged red fibers" (due to accumulation of diseased mitochondria). **Leber hereditary optic neuropathy**—cell death in optic nerve neurons → subacute bilateral vision loss in teens/young adults, 90% males. Usually permanent.

☐ = unaffected male; ■ = affected male; ○ = unaffected female; ● = affected female.

Autosomal dominant diseases	Achondroplasia, autosomal dominant polycystic kidney disease, familial adenomatous polyposis, familial hypercholesterolemia, hereditary hemorrhagic telangiectasia (Osler-Weber-Rendu syndrome), hereditary spherocytosis, Huntington disease, Li-Fraumeni syndrome, Marfan syndrome, multiple endocrine neoplasias, myotonic muscular dystrophy, neurofibromatosis type 1 (von Recklinghausen disease), neurofibromatosis type 2, tuberous sclerosis, von Hippel-Lindau disease.
Autosomal recessive diseases	Albinism, autosomal recessive polycystic kidney disease (ARPKD), cystic fibrosis, Friedreich ataxia, glycogen storage diseases, hemochromatosis, Kartagener syndrome, mucopolysaccharidoses (except Hunter syndrome), phenylketonuria, sickle cell anemia, sphingolipidoses (except Fabry disease), thalassemias, Wilson disease.

Cystic fibrosis

GENETICS	Autosomal recessive; defect in *CFTR* gene on chromosome 7; commonly a deletion of Phe508. Most common lethal genetic disease in Caucasian population.
PATHOPHYSIOLOGY	*CFTR* encodes an ATP-gated Cl^- channel that secretes Cl^- in lungs and GI tract, and reabsorbs Cl^- in sweat glands. Most common mutation → misfolded protein → protein retained in RER and not transported to cell membrane, causing ↓ Cl^- (and H_2O) secretion; ↑ intracellular Cl^- results in compensatory ↑ Na^+ reabsorption via epithelial Na^+ channels → ↑ H_2O reabsorption → abnormally thick mucus secreted into lungs and GI tract. ↑ Na^+ reabsorption also causes more negative transepithelial potential difference.
DIAGNOSIS	↑ Cl^- concentration in pilocarpine-induced sweat test is diagnostic. Can present with contraction alkalosis and hypokalemia (ECF effects analogous to a patient taking a loop diuretic) because of ECF H_2O/Na^+ losses and concomitant renal K^+/H^+ wasting. ↑ immunoreactive trypsinogen (newborn screening).
COMPLICATIONS	Recurrent pulmonary infections (eg, *S aureus* [early infancy], *P aeruginosa* [adolescence]), chronic bronchitis and bronchiectasis → reticulonodular pattern on CXR, opacification of sinuses. Pancreatic insufficiency, malabsorption with steatorrhea, fat-soluble vitamin deficiencies (A, D, E, K), biliary cirrhosis, liver disease. Meconium ileus in newborns. Infertility in men (absence of vas deferens, spermatogenesis may be unaffected) and subfertility in women (amenorrhea, abnormally thick cervical mucus). Nasal polyps, clubbing of nails.
TREATMENT	Multifactorial: chest physiotherapy, albuterol, aerosolized dornase alfa (DNase), and hypertonic saline facilitate mucus clearance. Azithromycin used as anti-inflammatory agent. Ibuprofen slows disease progression. In patients with Phe508 deletion: combination of lumacaftor (corrects misfolded proteins and improves their transport to cell surface) and ivacaftor (opens Cl^- channels → improved chloride transport).

X-linked recessive disorders	Ornithine transcarbamylase deficiency, Fabry disease, Wiskott-Aldrich syndrome, Ocular albinism, G6PD deficiency, Hunter syndrome, Bruton agammaglobulinemia, Hemophilia A and B, Lesch-Nyhan syndrome, Duchenne (and Becker) muscular dystrophy. X-inactivation (lyonization)—female carriers variably affected depending on the pattern of inactivation of the X chromosome carrying the mutant vs normal gene.	**O**blivious **F**emale **W**ill **O**ften **G**ive **H**er **B**oys **H**er x-**L**inked **D**isorders Females with Turner syndrome (45,XO) are more likely to have an X-linked recessive disorder.

Muscular dystrophies

Duchenne	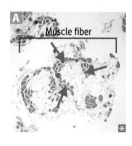 X-linked disorder typically due to **frameshift** or nonsense mutations → truncated or absent dystrophin protein → progressive myofiber damage. Weakness begins in pelvic girdle muscles and progresses superiorly. Pseudohypertrophy of calf muscles due to fibrofatty replacement of muscle A. Waddling gait. Onset before 5 years of age. Dilated cardiomyopathy is common cause of death. **Gower sign**—patient uses upper extremities to help stand up. Classically seen in Duchenne muscular dystrophy, but also seen in other muscular dystrophies and inflammatory myopathies (eg, polymyositis).	Duchenne = deleted dystrophin. Dystrophin gene (*DMD*) is the largest protein-coding human gene → ↑ chance of spontaneous mutation. Dystrophin helps anchor muscle fibers, primarily in skeletal and cardiac muscle. It connects the intracellular cytoskeleton (actin) to the transmembrane proteins α- and β-dystroglycan, which are connected to the extracellular matrix (ECM). Loss of dystrophin → myonecrosis. ↑ CK and aldolase; genetic testing confirms diagnosis. 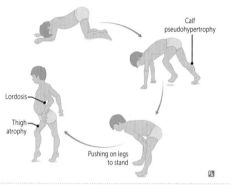
Becker	X-linked disorder typically due to **non-frameshift** deletions in dystrophin gene (partially functional instead of truncated). Less severe than Duchenne. Onset in adolescence or early adulthood.	Deletions can cause both Duchenne and Becker muscular dystrophies. ⅔ of cases have large deletions spanning one or more exons.
Myotonic type 1	Autosomal dominant. CTG trinucleotide repeat expansion in the *DMPK* gene → abnormal expression of myotonin protein kinase → myotonia, muscle wasting, cataracts, testicular atrophy, frontal balding, arrhythmia.	Cataracts, Toupee (early balding in men), Gonadal atrophy.

Rett syndrome	Sporadic disorder seen almost exclusively in girls (affected males die in utero or shortly after birth). Most cases are caused by de novo mutation of *MECP2* on X chromosome. Symptoms of **Rett** syndrome usually appear between ages 1–4 and are characterized by regression (**Rett**urn) in motor, verbal, and cognitive abilities; ataxia; seizures; growth failure; and stereotyped hand-wringing.

Fragile X syndrome	X-linked dominant inheritance. Trinucleotide repeat in *FMR1* gene → hypermethylation → ↓ expression. Most common cause of inherited intellectual disability and 2nd most common cause of genetically associated mental deficiency (after Down syndrome). Findings: post-pubertal macroorchidism (enlarged testes), long face with a large jaw, large everted ears, autism, mitral valve prolapse.	Trinucleotide repeat expansion [$(CGG)_n$] occurs during oogenesis.
Trinucleotide repeat expansion diseases	Huntington disease, myotonic dystrophy, fragile X syndrome, and Friedreich ataxia. May show genetic anticipation (disease severity ↑ and age of onset ↓ in successive generations).	**Try** (**tri**nucleotide) **hunting** for **my fragile** cage-free **eggs** (**X**).

DISEASE	TRINUCLEOTIDE REPEAT	MODE OF INHERITANCE	MNEMONIC
Huntington disease	$(CAG)_n$	AD	Caudate has ↓ ACh and GABA
Myotonic dystrophy	$(CTG)_n$	AD	Cataracts, Toupee (early balding in men), Gonadal atrophy
Fragile X syndrome	$(CGG)_n$	XD	Chin (protruding), Giant Gonads
Friedreich ataxia	$(GAA)_n$	AR	Ataxic GAAit

Autosomal trisomies

Down syndrome (trisomy 21)	Findings: intellectual disability, flat facies, prominent epicanthal folds, single palmar crease, gap between 1st 2 toes, duodenal atresia, Hirschsprung disease, congenital heart disease (eg, atrioventricular septal defect), Brushfield spots. Associated with early-onset Alzheimer disease (chromosome 21 codes for amyloid precursor protein) and ↑ risk of ALL and AML. 95% of cases due to meiotic nondisjunction (↑ with advanced maternal age; from 1:1500 in women < 20 to 1:25 in women > 45 years old). 4% of cases due to unbalanced Robertsonian translocation, most typically between chromosomes 14 and 21. Only 1% of cases are due to postfertilization mitotic error.	Incidence 1:700. Drinking age (21). Most common viable chromosomal disorder and most common cause of genetic intellectual disability. First-trimester ultrasound commonly shows ↑ nuchal translucency and hypoplastic nasal bone. The 5 A's of Down syndrome: ▪ Advanced maternal age ▪ Atresia (duodenal) ▪ Atrioventricular septal defect ▪ Alzheimer disease (early onset) ▪ AML/ALL
Edwards syndrome (trisomy 18)	Findings: **PRINCE** Edward—Prominent occiput, Rocker-bottom feet, Intellectual disability, Nondisjunction, Clenched fists (with overlapping fingers), low-set Ears, micrognathia (small jaw), congenital heart disease. Death usually occurs by age 1.	Incidence 1:8000. Election age (18). 2nd most common autosomal trisomy resulting in live birth (most common is Down syndrome).
Patau syndrome (trisomy 13)	Findings: severe intellectual disability, rocker-bottom feet, microphthalmia, microcephaly, cleft liP/Palate, holoProsencephaly, Polydactyly, cutis aPlasia, congenital heart disease, Polycystic kidney disease. Death usually occurs by age 1.	Incidence 1:15,000. Puberty (13).

Serum markers			
Trisomy	21	18	13
1st trimester			
β-hCG	↑	↓	↓
PAPP-A	↓	↓	↓
2nd trimester			
AFP	↓	↓	N
β-hCG	↑	↓	N
Estriol	↓	↓	N
Inhibin A	↑	N↓	N

N = normal.

Genetic disorders by chromosome

CHROMOSOME	SELECTED EXAMPLES
3	von Hippel-Lindau disease, renal cell carcinoma
4	ADPKD (*PKD2*), achondroplasia, Huntington disease
5	Cri-du-chat syndrome, familial adenomatous polyposis
6	Hemochromatosis (*HFE*)
7	Williams syndrome, cystic fibrosis
9	Friedreich ataxia, tuberous sclerosis (*TSC1*)
11	Wilms tumor, β-globin gene defects (eg, sickle cell disease, β-thalassemia), MEN1
13	Patau syndrome, Wilson disease, retinoblastoma (*RB1*), BRCA2
15	Prader-Willi syndrome, Angelman syndrome, Marfan syndrome
16	ADPKD (*PKD1*), α-globin gene defects (eg, α-thalassemia), tuberous sclerosis (*TSC2*)
17	Neurofibromatosis type 1, *BRCA1*, *p53*
18	Edwards syndrome
21	Down syndrome
22	Neurofibromatosis type 2, DiGeorge syndrome (22q11)
X	Fragile X syndrome, X-linked agammaglobulinemia, Klinefelter syndrome (XXY)

Robertsonian translocation

Chromosomal translocation that commonly involves chromosome pairs 13, 14, 15, 21, and 22. One of the most common types of translocation. Occurs when the long arms of 2 acrocentric chromosomes (chromosomes with centromeres near their ends) fuse at the centromere and the 2 short arms are lost.

Balanced translocations normally do not cause any abnormal phenotype. Unbalanced translocations can result in miscarriage, stillbirth, and chromosomal imbalance (eg, Down syndrome, Patau syndrome).

Cri-du-chat syndrome

Congenital deletion on short arm of chromosome 5 (46,XX or XY, 5p–).
Findings: microcephaly, moderate to severe intellectual disability, high-pitched **crying/ meowing**, epicanthal folds, cardiac abnormalities (VSD).

Cri du chat = **cry** of the **cat**.

Williams syndrome

Congenital microdeletion of long arm of chromosome 7 (deleted region includes elastin gene).
Findings: distinctive "**elfin**" facies, intellectual disability, hypercalcemia (↑ sensitivity to vitamin D), well-developed verbal skills, extreme friendliness with strangers, cardiovascular problems (eg, supravalvular aortic stenosis, renal artery stenosis). Think **Will** Ferrell in **Elf**.

| **22q11 deletion syndromes** | Microdeletion at chromosome 22q11 → variable presentations including Cleft palate, Abnormal facies, Thymic aplasia → T-cell deficiency, Cardiac defects, and Hypocalcemia 2° to parathyroid aplasia.
DiGeorge syndrome—thymic, parathyroid, and cardiac defects.
Velocardiofacial syndrome—palate, facial, and cardiac defects. | CATCH-22.
Due to aberrant development of 3rd and 4th branchial (pharyngeal) pouches. |

▸ BIOCHEMISTRY—NUTRITION

| **Vitamins: fat soluble** | A, D, E, K. Absorption dependent on gut and pancreas. Toxicity more common than for water-soluble vitamins because fat-soluble vitamins accumulate in fat. | Malabsorption syndromes with steatorrhea (eg, cystic fibrosis and celiac disease) or mineral oil intake can cause fat-soluble vitamin deficiencies. |
| **Vitamins: water soluble** | B_1 (thiamine: TPP)
B_2 (riboflavin: FAD, FMN)
B_3 (niacin: NAD^+)
B_5 (pantothenic acid: CoA)
B_6 (pyridoxine: PLP)
B_7 (biotin)
B_9 (folate)
B_{12} (cobalamin)
C (ascorbic acid) | All wash out easily from body except B_{12} and B_9 (folate). B_{12} stored in liver for ~ 3–4 years. B_9 stored in liver for ~ 3–4 months.
B-complex deficiencies often result in dermatitis, glossitis, and diarrhea.
Can be coenzymes (eg, ascorbic acid) or precursors to organic cofactors (eg, FAD, NAD^+). |

Vitamin A	Also called retinol.	
FUNCTION	Antioxidant; constituent of visual pigments (**retinal**); essential for normal differentiation of epithelial cells into specialized tissue (pancreatic cells, mucus-secreting cells); prevents squamous metaplasia. Used to treat measles and acute promyelocytic leukemia (APL).	**Retinol** is vitamin A, so think **retin-A** (used topically for wrinkles and Acne). Found in liver and leafy vegetables. Use oral isotretinoin to treat severe cystic acne. Use *all*-trans retinoic acid to treat acute promyelocytic leukemia.
DEFICIENCY	Night blindness (nyctalopia); dry, scaly skin (xerosis cutis); corneal degeneration (keratomalacia); Bitot spots (foamy appearance) on conjunctiva ; immunosuppression.	
EXCESS	Acute toxicity—nausea, vomiting, vertigo, and blurred vision. Chronic toxicity—alopecia, dry skin (eg, scaliness), hepatic toxicity and enlargement, arthralgias, and pseudotumor cerebri. Teratogenic (cleft palate, cardiac abnormalities), therefore a ⊖ pregnancy test and two forms of contraception are required before isotretinoin (vitamin A derivative) is prescribed.	Isotretinoin is teratogenic.

Vitamin B$_1$	Also called thiamine.	
FUNCTION	In thiamine pyrophosphate (TPP), a cofactor for several dehydrogenase enzyme reactions: ■ Pyruvate dehydrogenase (links glycolysis to TCA cycle) ■ α-ketoglutarate dehydrogenase (TCA cycle) ■ Transketolase (HMP shunt) ■ Branched-chain ketoacid dehydrogenase	Think ATP: α-ketoglutarate dehydrogenase, Transketolase, and Pyruvate dehydrogenase. Spell beriberi as Ber1Ber1 to remember vitamin B$_1$. Wernicke-Korsakoff syndrome—confusion, ophthalmoplegia, ataxia (classic triad) + confabulation, personality change, memory loss (permanent). Damage to medial dorsal nucleus of thalamus, mammillary bodies. Dry beriberi—polyneuropathy, symmetrical muscle wasting. Wet beriberi—high-output cardiac failure (dilated cardiomyopathy), edema.
DEFICIENCY	Impaired glucose breakdown → ATP depletion worsened by glucose infusion; highly aerobic tissues (eg, brain, heart) are affected first. In alcoholic or malnourished patients, give thiamine before dextrose to ↓ risk of precipitating Wernicke encephalopathy. Diagnosis made by ↑ in RBC transketolase activity following vitamin B$_1$ administration.	

Vitamin B$_2$	Also called riboflavin.	
FUNCTION	Component of flavins FAD and FMN, used as cofactors in redox reactions, eg, the succinate dehydrogenase reaction in the TCA cycle.	FAD and FMN are derived from riboFlavin (B$_2 \approx$ 2 ATP).
DEFICIENCY	Cheilosis (inflammation of lips, scaling and fissures at the corners of the mouth), Corneal vascularization.	The 2 C's of B$_2$.

Vitamin B$_3$	Also called niacin.	
FUNCTION	Constituent of NAD$^+$, NADP$^+$ (used in redox reactions). Derived from tryptophan. Synthesis requires vitamins B$_2$ and B$_6$. Used to treat dyslipidemia; lowers levels of VLDL and raises levels of HDL.	NAD derived from Niacin (B$_3 \approx$ 3 ATP).
DEFICIENCY	Glossitis. Severe deficiency leads to pellagra, which can also be caused by Hartnup disease, malignant carcinoid syndrome (↑ tryptophan metabolism), and isoniazid (↓ vitamin B$_6$). Symptoms of pellagra: Diarrhea, Dementia (also hallucinations), Dermatitis (C3/C4 dermatome circumferential "broad collar" rash [Casal necklace], hyperpigmentation of sun-exposed limbs).	The 3 D's of B$_3$. **Hartnup disease**—autosomal recessive. Deficiency of neutral amino acid (eg, tryptophan) transporters in proximal renal tubular cells and on enterocytes → neutral aminoaciduria and ↓ absorption from the gut → ↓ tryptophan for conversion to niacin → pellagra-like symptoms. Treat with high-protein diet and nicotinic acid. Deficiency of vitamin B$_3$ → **pell**agra.
EXCESS	Facial flushing (induced by prostaglandin, not histamine; can avoid by taking aspirin with niacin), hyperglycemia, hyperuricemia.	Excess of vitamin B$_3$ → **pod**agra.

Vitamin B$_5$	Also called pantothenic acid.	
FUNCTION	Essential component of coenzyme A (CoA, a cofactor for acyl transfers) and fatty acid synthase.	B$_5$ is "pento"thenic acid.
DEFICIENCY	Dermatitis, enteritis, alopecia, adrenal insufficiency.	

Vitamin B$_6$	Also called pyridoxine.
FUNCTION	Converted to pyridoxal phosphate (PLP), a cofactor used in transamination (eg, ALT and AST), decarboxylation reactions, glycogen phosphorylase. Synthesis of cystathionine, heme, niacin, histamine, and neurotransmitters including serotonin, epinephrine, norepinephrine (NE), dopamine, and GABA.
DEFICIENCY	Convulsions, hyperirritability, peripheral neuropathy (deficiency inducible by isoniazid and oral contraceptives), sideroblastic anemias (due to impaired hemoglobin synthesis and iron excess).

Vitamin B$_7$	Also called biotin.	
FUNCTION	Cofactor for carboxylation enzymes (which add a 1-carbon group): • Pyruvate carboxylase: pyruvate (3C) → oxaloacetate (4C) • Acetyl-CoA carboxylase: acetyl-CoA (2C) → malonyl-CoA (3C) • Propionyl-CoA carboxylase: propionyl-CoA (3C) → methylmalonyl-CoA (4C)	
DEFICIENCY	Relatively rare. Dermatitis, enteritis, alopecia. Caused by antibiotic use or excessive ingestion of raw egg whites.	"**Avidin** in egg whites **avidly** binds biotin."

Vitamin B$_9$	Also called folate.	
FUNCTION	Converted to tetrahydrofolic acid (THF), a coenzyme for 1-carbon transfer/methylation reactions. Important for the synthesis of nitrogenous bases in DNA and RNA.	Found in leafy green vegetables. Absorbed in jejunum. Folate from **foliage**. Small reserve pool stored primarily in the liver.
DEFICIENCY	Macrocytic, megaloblastic anemia; hypersegmented polymorphonuclear cells (PMNs); glossitis; no neurologic symptoms (as opposed to vitamin B$_{12}$ deficiency). Labs: ↑ homocysteine, normal methylmalonic acid levels. Seen in alcoholism and pregnancy.	Deficiency can be caused by several drugs (eg, phenytoin, sulfonamides, methotrexate). Supplemental maternal folic acid at least 1 month prior to conception and during early pregnancy to ↓ risk of neural tube defects. Give vitamin B$_9$ for the 9 months of pregnancy.

Vitamin B$_{12}$	Also called cobalamin.	
FUNCTION	Cofactor for methionine synthase (transfers CH$_3$ groups as methylcobalamin) and methylmalonyl-CoA mutase. Important for DNA synthesis.	Found in animal products. Synthesized only by microorganisms. Very large reserve pool (several years) stored primarily in the liver. Deficiency caused by malabsorption (eg, sprue, enteritis, *Diphyllobothrium latum*, achlorhydria, bacterial overgrowth, alcohol excess), lack of intrinsic factor (eg, pernicious anemia, gastric bypass surgery), absence of terminal ileum (surgical resection, eg, for Crohn disease), or insufficient intake (eg, veganism).
DEFICIENCY	Macrocytic, megaloblastic anemia; hypersegmented PMNs; paresthesias and subacute combined degeneration (degeneration of dorsal columns, lateral corticospinal tracts, and spinocerebellar tracts) due to abnormal myelin. Associated with ↑ serum homocysteine and methylmalonic acid levels, along with 2° folate deficiency. Prolonged deficiency → irreversible nerve damage.	Anti-intrinsic factor antibodies diagnostic for pernicious anemia. Folate supplementation can mask the hematologic symptoms of B$_{12}$ deficiency, but not the neurologic symptoms.

Vitamin C	Also called ascorbic acid.	
FUNCTION	Antioxidant; also facilitates iron absorption by reducing it to Fe^{2+} state. Necessary for hydroxylation of proline and lysine in collagen synthesis. Necessary for dopamine β-hydroxylase, which converts dopamine to NE.	Found in fruits and vegetables. Pronounce "**absorbic**" acid. Ancillary treatment for methemoglobinemia by reducing Fe^{3+} to Fe^{2+}.
DEFICIENCY	Scurvy—swollen gums, bruising, petechiae, hemarthrosis, anemia, poor wound healing, perifollicular and subperiosteal hemorrhages, "corkscrew" hair. Weakened immune response.	Vitamin C deficiency causes sCurvy due to a Collagen synthesis defect.
EXCESS	Nausea, vomiting, diarrhea, fatigue, calcium oxalate nephrolithiasis. Can ↑ iron toxicity in predisposed individuals by increasing dietary iron absorption (ie, can worsen hereditary hemochromatosis or transfusion-related iron overload).	

Vitamin D	D_3 (cholecalciferol) from exposure of skin (stratum basale) to sun, ingestion of fish, milk, plants. D_2 (ergocalciferol) from ingestion of plants, fungi, yeasts. Both converted to 25-OH D_3 (storage form) in liver and to the active form 1,25-$(OH)_2$ D_3 (calcitriol) in kidney.
FUNCTION	↑ intestinal absorption of Ca^{2+} and PO_4^{3}. ↑ bone mineralization at low levels. ↑ bone resorption at higher levels.
REGULATION	↑ PTH, ↓ Ca^{2+}, ↓ PO_4^{3-} → ↑ 1,25-$(OH)_2D_3$ production. 1,25-$(OH)_2D_3$ feedback inhibits its own production. ↑ PTH → ↑ Ca^{2+} reabsorption and ↓ PO_4^{3-} reabsorption in the kidney.
DEFICIENCY	Rickets in children (deformity, such as genu varum "bow legs" A), osteomalacia in adults (bone pain and muscle weakness), hypocalcemic tetany. Caused by malabsorption, ↓ sun exposure, poor diet, chronic kidney disease. Give oral vitamin D to breastfed infants. Deficiency is exacerbated by pigmented skin, premature birth.
EXCESS	Hypercalcemia, hypercalciuria, loss of appetite, stupor. Seen in granulomatous disease (↑ activation of vitamin D by epithelioid macrophages).

Vitamin E	Includes tocopherol, tocotrienol.	
FUNCTION	Antioxidant (protects RBCs and membranes from free radical damage).	High-dose supplementation may alter metabolism of vitamin K → enhanced anticoagulant effects of warfarin.
DEFICIENCY	Hemolytic anemia, acanthocytosis, muscle weakness, posterior column and spinocerebellar tract demyelination.	Neurologic presentation may appear similar to vitamin B_{12} deficiency, but without megaloblastic anemia, hypersegmented neutrophils, or ↑ serum methylmalonic acid levels.
EXCESS	Risk of enterocolitis in infants.	

Vitamin K	Includes phytomenadione, phylloquinone, phytonadione, menaquinone.	
FUNCTION	Activated by epoxide reductase to the reduced form, which is a cofactor for the γ-carboxylation of glutamic acid residues on various proteins required for blood clotting. Synthesized by intestinal flora.	**K** is for **K**oagulation. Necessary for the maturation of clotting factors II, VII, IX, X, and proteins C and S. Warfarin inhibits vitamin K–dependent synthesis of these factors and proteins.
DEFICIENCY	Neonatal hemorrhage with ↑ PT and ↑ aPTT but normal bleeding time (neonates have sterile intestines and are unable to synthesize vitamin K). Can also occur after prolonged use of broad-spectrum antibiotics.	Not in breast milk; neonates are given vitamin K injection at birth to prevent hemorrhagic disease of the newborn.

Zinc	
FUNCTION	Mineral essential for the activity of 100+ enzymes. Important in the formation of zinc fingers (transcription factor motif).
DEFICIENCY	Delayed wound healing, suppressed immunity, hypogonadism, ↓ adult hair (axillary, facial, pubic), dysgeusia, anosmia, acrodermatitis enteropathica **A**. May predispose to alcoholic cirrhosis.

Protein-energy malnutrition	
Kwashiorkor	Protein malnutrition resulting in skin lesions, edema due to ↓ plasma oncotic pressure, liver malfunction (fatty change due to ↓ apolipoprotein synthesis). Clinical picture is small child with swollen abdomen **A**. Kwashiorkor results from protein-deficient **MEALS**: **M**alnutrition **E**dema **A**nemia **L**iver (fatty) **S**kin lesions (eg, hyperkeratosis, dyspigmentation)
Marasmus	Malnutrition not causing edema. Diet is deficient in calories but no nutrients are entirely absent. Marasmus results in Muscle wasting **B**.

Ethanol metabolism

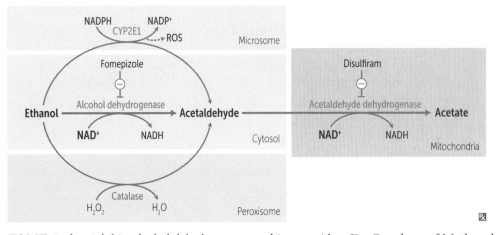

FOMEpizole—inhibits alcohol dehydrogenase and is an antidote For Overdoses of Methanol or Ethylene glycol.

Disulfiram—inhibits acetaldehyde dehydrogenase (acetaldehyde accumulates, contributing to hangover symptoms), discouraging drinking.

NAD^+ is the limiting reagent.

Alcohol dehydrogenase operates via zero-order kinetics.

Ethanol metabolism ↑ $NADH/NAD^+$ ratio in liver, causing:
- Pyruvate → lactate (lactic acidosis)
- Oxaloacetate → malate (prevents gluconeogenesis → fasting hypoglycemia)
- Dihydroxyacetone phosphate → glycerol-3-phosphate (combines with fatty acids to make triglycerides → hepatosteatosis)

Additionally, ↑ $NADH/NAD^+$ ratio disfavors TCA production of NADH → ↑ utilization of acetyl-CoA for ketogenesis (→ ketoacidosis) and lipogenesis (→ hepatosteatosis).

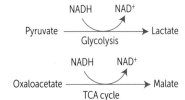

Metabolism sites

Mitochondria	Fatty acid oxidation (β-oxidation), acetyl-CoA production, TCA cycle, oxidative phosphorylation, ketogenesis.
Cytoplasm	Glycolysis, HMP shunt, and synthesis of steroids (SER), proteins (ribosomes, RER), fatty acids, cholesterol, and nucleotides.
Both	Heme synthesis, Urea cycle, Gluconeogenesis. HUGs take two (ie, both).

Enzyme terminology	An enzyme's name often describes its function. For example, glucokinase is an enzyme that catalyzes the phosphorylation of glucose using a molecule of ATP. The following are commonly used enzyme descriptors.
Kinase	Catalyzes transfer of a phosphate group from a high-energy molecule (usually ATP) to a substrate (eg, phosphofructokinase).
Phosphorylase	Adds inorganic phosphate onto substrate without using ATP (eg, glycogen phosphorylase).
Phosphatase	Removes phosphate group from substrate (eg, fructose-1,6-bisphosphatase).
Dehydrogenase	Catalyzes oxidation-reduction reactions (eg, pyruvate dehydrogenase).
Hydroxylase	Adds hydroxyl group (–OH) onto substrate (eg, tyrosine hydroxylase).
Carboxylase	Transfers CO_2 groups with the help of biotin (eg, pyruvate carboxylase).
Mutase	Relocates a functional group within a molecule (eg, vitamin B_{12}–dependent methylmalonyl-CoA mutase).
Synthase/synthetase	Joins two molecules together using a source of energy (eg, ATP, acetyl CoA, nucleotide sugar).

Rate-determining enzymes of metabolic processes

PROCESS	ENZYME	REGULATORS
Glycolysis	Phosphofructokinase-1 (PFK-1)	AMP ⊕, fructose-2,6-bisphosphate ⊕ ATP ⊖, citrate ⊖
Gluconeogenesis	Fructose-1,6-bisphosphatase	Citrate ⊕ AMP ⊖, fructose-2,6-bisphosphate ⊖
TCA cycle	Isocitrate dehydrogenase	ADP ⊕ ATP ⊖, NADH ⊖
Glycogenesis	Glycogen synthase	Glucose-6-phosphate ⊕, insulin ⊕, cortisol ⊕ Epinephrine ⊖, glucagon ⊖
Glycogenolysis	Glycogen phosphorylase	Epinephrine ⊕, glucagon ⊕, AMP ⊕ Glucose-6-phosphate ⊖, insulin ⊖, ATP ⊖
HMP shunt	Glucose-6-phosphate dehydrogenase (G6PD)	$NADP^+$ ⊕ NADPH ⊖
De novo pyrimidine synthesis	Carbamoyl phosphate synthetase II	ATP ⊕, PRPP ⊕ UTP ⊖
De novo purine synthesis	Glutamine-phosphoribosylpyrophosphate (PRPP) amidotransferase	AMP ⊖, inosine monophosphate (IMP) ⊖, GMP ⊖
Urea cycle	Carbamoyl phosphate synthetase I	N-acetylglutamate ⊕
Fatty acid synthesis	Acetyl-CoA carboxylase (ACC)	Insulin ⊕, citrate ⊕ Glucagon ⊖, palmitoyl-CoA ⊖
Fatty acid oxidation	Carnitine acyltransferase I	Malonyl-CoA ⊖
Ketogenesis	HMG-CoA synthase	
Cholesterol synthesis	HMG-CoA reductase	Insulin ⊕, thyroxine ⊕ Glucagon ⊖, cholesterol ⊖

Summary of pathways

1 Galactokinase *(mild galactosemia)*

2 Galactose-1-phosphate uridyltransferase *(severe galactosemia)*

3 Hexokinase/glucokinase

4 Glucose-6-phosphatase *(von Gierke disease)*

5 Glucose-6-phosphate dehydrogenase

6 Transketolase

7 Phosphofructokinase-1

8 Fructose-1,6-bisphosphatase

9 Fructokinase *(essential fructosuria)*

10 Aldolase B *(fructose intolerance)*

11 Aldolase B *(liver)*, A *(muscle)*

12 Triose phosphate isomerase

13 Pyruvate kinase

14 Pyruvate dehydrogenase

15 Pyruvate carboxylase

16 PEP carboxykinase

17 Citrate synthase

18 Isocitrate dehydrogenase

19 α-ketoglutarate dehydrogenase

20 Carbamoyl phosphate synthetase I

21 Ornithine transcarbamylase

22 Propionyl-CoA carboxylase

23 HMG-CoA reductase

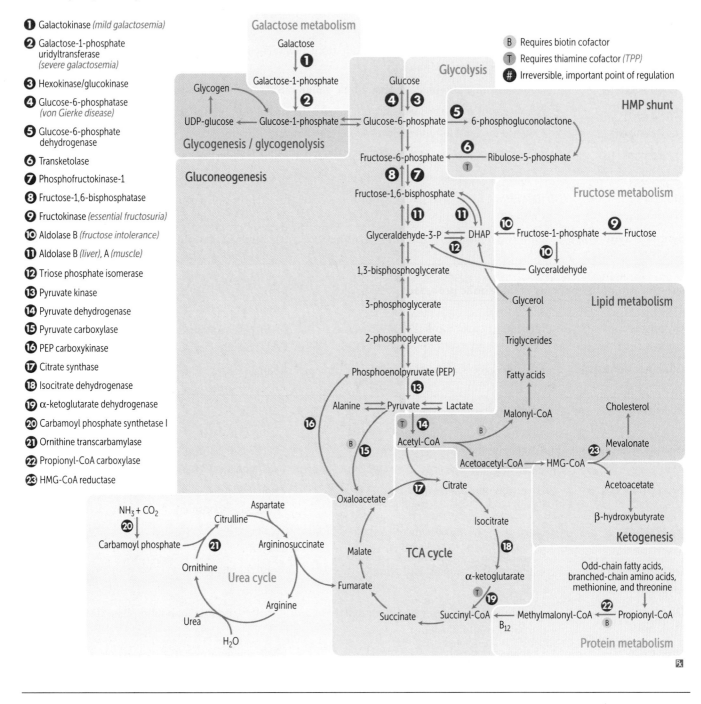

| ATP production | Aerobic metabolism of one glucose molecule produces 32 net ATP via malate-aspartate shuttle (heart and liver), 30 net ATP via glycerol-3-phosphate shuttle (muscle). Anaerobic glycolysis produces only 2 net ATP per glucose molecule. ATP hydrolysis can be coupled to energetically unfavorable reactions. | Arsenic causes glycolysis to produce zero net ATP. |

Activated carriers	CARRIER MOLECULE	CARRIED IN ACTIVATED FORM
	ATP	Phosphoryl groups
	NADH, NADPH, $FADH_2$	Electrons
	CoA, lipoamide	Acyl groups
	Biotin	CO_2
	Tetrahydrofolates	1-carbon units
	S-adenosylmethionine (SAM)	CH_3 groups
	TPP	Aldehydes

Universal electron acceptors	Nicotinamides (NAD^+, $NADP^+$ from vitamin B_3) and flavin nucleotides (FAD^+ from vitamin B_2). NAD^+ is generally used in **catabolic** processes to carry reducing equivalents away as NADH. NADPH is used in **anabolic** processes (eg, steroid and fatty acid synthesis) as a supply of reducing equivalents.	NADPH is a product of the HMP shunt. NADPH is used in: ▪ Anabolic processes ▪ Respiratory burst ▪ Cytochrome P-450 system ▪ Glutathione reductase

Hexokinase vs glucokinase

Phosphorylation of glucose to yield glucose-6-phosphate is catalyzed by glucokinase in the liver and hexokinase in other tissues. Hexokinase sequesters glucose in tissues, where it is used even when glucose concentrations are low. At high glucose concentrations, glucokinase helps to store glucose in liver.

	Hexokinase	Glucokinase
Location	Most tissues, except liver and pancreatic β cells	Liver, β cells of pancreas
K_m	Lower (↑ affinity)	Higher (↓ affinity)
V_{max}	Lower (↓ capacity)	Higher (↑ capacity)
Induced by insulin	No	Yes
Feedback-inhibited by glucose-6-phosphate	Yes	No

Glycolysis regulation, key enzymes	Net glycolysis (cytoplasm): Glucose + 2 P_i + 2 ADP + 2 NAD⁺ → 2 pyruvate + 2 ATP + 2 NADH + 2 H⁺ + 2 H_2O. Equation not balanced chemically, and exact balanced equation depends on ionization state of reactants and products.

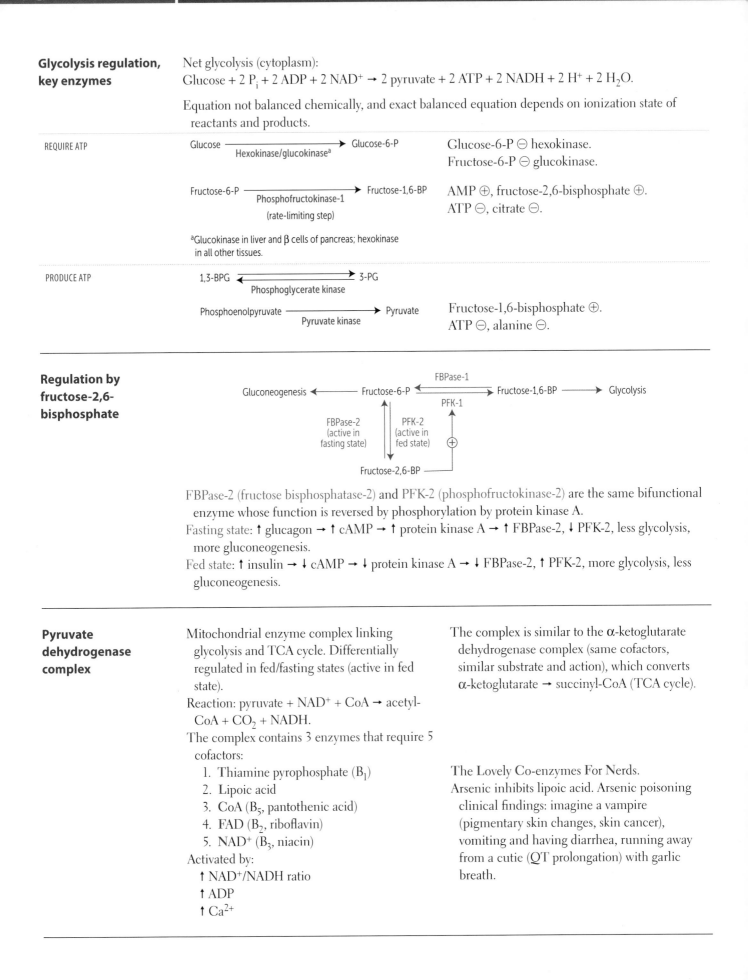

REQUIRE ATP

Glucose ——Hexokinase/glucokinase[a]——→ Glucose-6-P

Glucose-6-P ⊖ hexokinase.
Fructose-6-P ⊖ glucokinase.

Fructose-6-P ——Phosphofructokinase-1 (rate-limiting step)——→ Fructose-1,6-BP

AMP ⊕, fructose-2,6-bisphosphate ⊕.
ATP ⊖, citrate ⊖.

[a]Glucokinase in liver and β cells of pancreas; hexokinase in all other tissues.

PRODUCE ATP

1,3-BPG ←——Phosphoglycerate kinase——→ 3-PG

Phosphoenolpyruvate ——Pyruvate kinase——→ Pyruvate

Fructose-1,6-bisphosphate ⊕.
ATP ⊖, alanine ⊖.

Regulation by fructose-2,6-bisphosphate	Gluconeogenesis ← Fructose-6-P ⇄ (FBPase-1 / PFK-1) Fructose-1,6-BP → Glycolysis FBPase-2 (active in fasting state) / PFK-2 (active in fed state) ⊕ Fructose-2,6-BP FBPase-2 (fructose bisphosphatase-2) and PFK-2 (phosphofructokinase-2) are the same bifunctional enzyme whose function is reversed by phosphorylation by protein kinase A. Fasting state: ↑ glucagon → ↑ cAMP → ↑ protein kinase A → ↑ FBPase-2, ↓ PFK-2, less glycolysis, more gluconeogenesis. Fed state: ↑ insulin → ↓ cAMP → ↓ protein kinase A → ↓ FBPase-2, ↑ PFK-2, more glycolysis, less gluconeogenesis.

Pyruvate dehydrogenase complex	Mitochondrial enzyme complex linking glycolysis and TCA cycle. Differentially regulated in fed/fasting states (active in fed state).
	Reaction: pyruvate + NAD⁺ + CoA → acetyl-CoA + CO_2 + NADH.
	The complex contains 3 enzymes that require 5 cofactors:
	  1. Thiamine pyrophosphate (B_1)
	  2. Lipoic acid
	  3. CoA (B_5, pantothenic acid)
	  4. FAD (B_2, riboflavin)
	  5. NAD⁺ (B_3, niacin)
	Activated by:
	  ↑ NAD⁺/NADH ratio
	  ↑ ADP
	  ↑ Ca^{2+}
		The complex is similar to the α-ketoglutarate dehydrogenase complex (same cofactors, similar substrate and action), which converts α-ketoglutarate → succinyl-CoA (TCA cycle).
		
		The Lovely Co-enzymes For Nerds.
		Arsenic inhibits lipoic acid. Arsenic poisoning clinical findings: imagine a vampire (pigmentary skin changes, skin cancer), vomiting and having diarrhea, running away from a cutie (QT prolongation) with garlic breath.

Pyruvate dehydrogenase complex deficiency	Causes a buildup of pyruvate that gets shunted to lactate (via LDH) and alanine (via ALT). X-linked.
FINDINGS	Neurologic defects, lactic acidosis, ↑ serum alanine starting in infancy.
TREATMENT	↑ intake of ketogenic nutrients (eg, high fat content or ↑ lysine and leucine).

Pyruvate metabolism

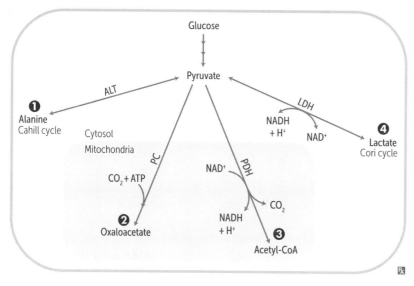

Functions of different pyruvate metabolic pathways (and their associated cofactors):

❶ Alanine aminotransferase (B_6): alanine carries amino groups to the liver from muscle

❷ Pyruvate carboxylase (biotin): oxaloacetate can replenish TCA cycle or be used in gluconeogenesis

❸ Pyruvate dehydrogenase (B_1, B_2, B_3, B_5, lipoic acid): transition from glycolysis to the TCA cycle

❹ Lactic acid dehydrogenase (B_3): end of anaerobic glycolysis (major pathway in RBCs, WBCs, kidney medulla, lens, testes, and cornea)

TCA cycle (Krebs cycle)

Pyruvate → acetyl-CoA produces 1 NADH, 1 CO_2.

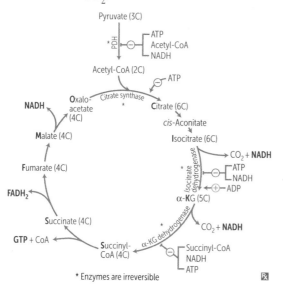

* Enzymes are irreversible

The TCA cycle produces 3 NADH, 1 $FADH_2$, 2 CO_2, 1 GTP per acetyl-CoA = 10 ATP/ acetyl-CoA (2× everything per glucose). TCA cycle reactions occur in the mitochondria.

α-ketoglutarate dehydrogenase complex requires the same cofactors as the pyruvate dehydrogenase complex (B_1, B_2, B_3, B_5, lipoic acid).

Citrate Is Krebs' Starting Substrate For Making Oxaloacetate.

Electron transport chain and oxidative phosphorylation

NADH electrons from glycolysis enter mitochondria via the malate-aspartate or glycerol-3-phosphate shuttle. $FADH_2$ electrons are transferred to complex II (at a lower energy level than NADH). The passage of electrons results in the formation of a proton gradient that, coupled to oxidative phosphorylation, drives the production of ATP.

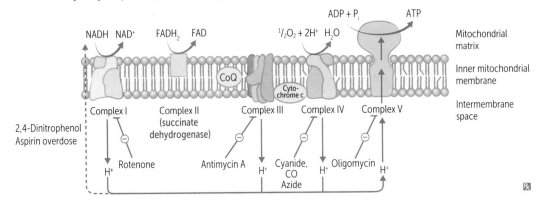

ATP PRODUCED VIA ATP SYNTHASE	
	1 NADH → 2.5 ATP; 1 $FADH_2$ → 1.5 ATP.

OXIDATIVE PHOSPHORYLATION POISONS		
Electron transport inhibitors	Directly inhibit electron transport, causing a ↓ proton gradient and block of ATP synthesis.	Rotenone: complex one inhibitor. "An-3-mycin" (antimycin) A: complex 3 inhibitor. Cyanide, carbon monoxide, azide (the -ides, 4 letters) inhibit complex IV.
ATP synthase inhibitors	Directly inhibit mitochondrial ATP synthase, causing an ↑ proton gradient. No ATP is produced because electron transport stops.	Oligomycin.
Uncoupling agents	↑ permeability of membrane, causing a ↓ proton gradient and ↑ O_2 consumption. ATP synthesis stops, but electron transport continues. Produces heat.	2,4-Dinitrophenol (used illicitly for weight loss), aspirin (fevers often occur after aspirin overdose), thermogenin in brown fat (has more mitochondria than white fat).

Gluconeogenesis, irreversible enzymes		Pathway Produces Fresh Glucose.
Pyruvate carboxylase	In mitochondria. Pyruvate → oxaloacetate.	Requires biotin, ATP. Activated by acetyl-CoA.
Phosphoenolpyruvate carboxykinase	In cytosol. Oxaloacetate → phosphoenolpyruvate.	Requires GTP.
Fructose-1,6-bisphosphatase	In cytosol. Fructose-1,6-bisphosphate → fructose-6-phosphate.	Citrate ⊕, AMP ⊖, fructose 2,6-bisphosphate ⊖.
Glucose-6-phosphatase	In ER. Glucose-6-phosphate → glucose.	

Occurs primarily in liver; serves to maintain euglycemia during fasting. Enzymes also found in kidney, intestinal epithelium. Deficiency of the key gluconeogenic enzymes causes hypoglycemia. (Muscle cannot participate in gluconeogenesis because it lacks glucose-6-phosphatase).

Odd-chain fatty acids yield 1 propionyl-CoA during metabolism, which can enter the TCA cycle (as succinyl-CoA), undergo gluconeogenesis, and serve as a glucose source. Even-chain fatty acids cannot produce new glucose, since they yield only acetyl-CoA equivalents.

HMP shunt (pentose phosphate pathway)	Provides a source of NADPH from abundantly available glucose-6-P (NADPH is required for reductive reactions, eg, glutathione reduction inside RBCs, fatty acid and cholesterol biosynthesis). Additionally, this pathway yields ribose for nucleotide synthesis. Two distinct phases (oxidative and nonoxidative), both of which occur in the cytoplasm. No ATP is used or produced. Sites: lactating mammary glands, liver, adrenal cortex (sites of fatty acid or steroid synthesis), RBCs.

REACTIONS	KEY ENZYMES	PRODUCTS
Oxidative (irreversible)		
Nonoxidative (reversible)		

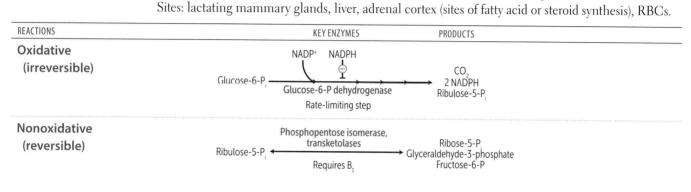

Glucose-6-phosphate dehydrogenase deficiency	NADPH is necessary to keep glutathione reduced, which in turn detoxifies free radicals and peroxides. ↓ NADPH in RBCs leads to hemolytic anemia due to poor RBC defense against oxidizing agents (eg, fava beans, sulfonamides, nitrofurantoin, primaquine/chloroquine, antituberculosis drugs). Infection (most common cause) can also precipitate hemolysis; inflammatory response produces free radicals that diffuse into RBCs, causing oxidative damage.	X-linked recessive disorder; most common human enzyme deficiency; more prevalent among African Americans. ↑ malarial resistance. Heinz bodies—denatured globin chains precipitate within RBCs due to oxidative stress. **Bite cells**—result from the phagocytic removal of **Heinz** bodies by splenic macrophages. Think, "**Bite** into some **Heinz** ketchup."

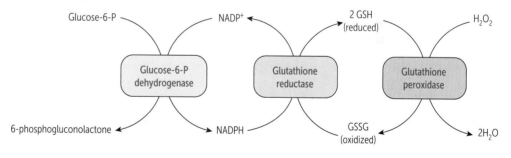

Disorders of fructose metabolism

Essential fructosuria	Involves a defect in **fructokinase**. Autosomal recessive. A benign, asymptomatic condition (fructokinase deficiency is kinder), since fructose is not trapped in cells. Hexokinase becomes 1° pathway for converting fructose to fructose-6-phosphate. Symptoms: fructose appears in blood and urine. Disorders of fructose metabolism cause milder symptoms than analogous disorders of galactose metabolism.
Hereditary fructose intolerance	Hereditary deficiency of **aldolase B**. Autosomal recessive. Fructose-1-phosphate accumulates, causing a ↓ in available phosphate, which results in inhibition of glycogenolysis and gluconeogenesis. Symptoms present following consumption of fruit, juice, or honey. Urine dipstick will be ⊖ (tests for glucose only); reducing sugar can be detected in the urine (nonspecific test for inborn errors of carbohydrate metabolism). Symptoms: hypoglycemia, jaundice, cirrhosis, vomiting. Treatment: ↓ intake of both fructose and sucrose (glucose + fructose).

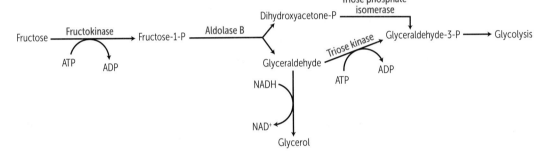

Fructose metabolism (liver)

Disorders of galactose metabolism

Galactokinase deficiency	Hereditary deficiency of **galactokinase**. Galactitol accumulates if galactose is present in diet. Relatively mild condition. Autosomal recessive. Symptoms: galactose appears in blood (galactosemia) and urine (galactosuria); infantile cataracts. May present as failure to track objects or to develop a social smile. Galactokinase deficiency is kinder (benign condition).
Classic galactosemia	Absence of **galactose-1-phosphate uridyltransferase**. Autosomal recessive. Damage is caused by accumulation of toxic substances (including galactitol, which accumulates in the lens of the eye). Symptoms develop when infant begins feeding (lactose present in breast milk and routine formula) and include failure to thrive, jaundice, hepatomegaly, infantile cataracts, intellectual disability. Can predispose to *E coli* sepsis in neonates. Treatment: exclude galactose and lactose (galactose + glucose) from diet.

Galactose metabolism

Galactokinase

Galactose → Galactose-1-P → Uridyltransferase → Glucose-1-P

ATP → ADP

UDP-Glu UDP-Gal

4-epimerase

Glycolysis/glycogenesis

Aldose reductase

Galactitol

Fructose is to Aldolase **B** as Galactose is to
UridylTransferase (**FAB GUT**).
The more serious defects lead to PO_4^{3-} depletion.

Sorbitol	An alternative method of trapping glucose in the cell is to convert it to its alcohol counterpart, sorbitol, via aldose reductase. Some tissues then convert sorbitol to fructose using sorbitol dehydrogenase; tissues with an insufficient amount/activity of this enzyme are at risk of intracellular sorbitol accumulation, causing osmotic damage (eg, cataracts, retinopathy, and peripheral neuropathy seen with chronic hyperglycemia in diabetes). High blood levels of galactose also result in conversion to the osmotically active galactitol via aldose reductase. Liver, Ovaries, and Seminal vesicles have both enzymes (they **LOSe** sorbitol).

$$\text{Glucose} \xrightarrow[\text{NADPH}]{\text{Aldose reductase}} \text{Sorbitol} \xrightarrow[\text{NAD}^+]{\text{Sorbitol dehydrogenase}} \text{Fructose}$$

Lens has primarily aldose reductase. Retina, Kidneys, and Schwann cells have only aldose reductase (**LuRKS**).

Lactase deficiency	Insufficient lactase enzyme → dietary lactose intolerance. Lactase functions on the intestinal brush border to digest lactose (in milk and milk products) into glucose and galactose. Primary: age-dependent decline after childhood (absence of lactase-persistent allele), common in people of Asian, African, or Native American descent. Secondary: loss of intestinal brush border due to gastroenteritis (eg, rotavirus), autoimmune disease, etc. Congenital lactase deficiency: rare, due to defective gene. Stool demonstrates ↓ pH and breath shows ↑ hydrogen content with lactose hydrogen breath test. Intestinal biopsy reveals normal mucosa in patients with hereditary lactose intolerance.
FINDINGS	Bloating, cramps, flatulence, osmotic diarrhea.
TREATMENT	Avoid dairy products or add lactase pills to diet; lactose-free milk.

Amino acids	Only L-amino acids are found in proteins.
Essential	**PVT TIM HaLL**: Phenylalanine, Valine, Tyrosine, Threonine, Isoleucine, Methionine, Histidine, Leucine, Lysine. Glucogenic: **M**ethionine, **his**tidine, **v**aline. **I met his v**alentine, she is so **sweet** (glucogenic). Glucogenic/ketogenic: Isoleucine, phenylalanine, threonine, tyrosine. Ketogenic: Leucine, Lysine. The on**L**y pure**L**y ketogenic amino acids.
Acidic	Aspartic **acid**, glutamic **acid**. Negatively charged at body pH.
Basic	Arginine, histidine, lysine. Arginine is most **basic**. Histidine has no charge at body pH. Arginine and histidine are required during periods of growth. Arginine and lysine are ↑ in histones which bind negatively charged DNA. **His lys** (lies) are basic.

Urea cycle

Amino acid catabolism results in the formation of common metabolites (eg, pyruvate, acetyl-CoA), which serve as metabolic fuels. Excess nitrogen generated by this process is converted to urea and excreted by the kidneys.

Ordinarily, Careless Crappers Are Also Frivolous About Urination.

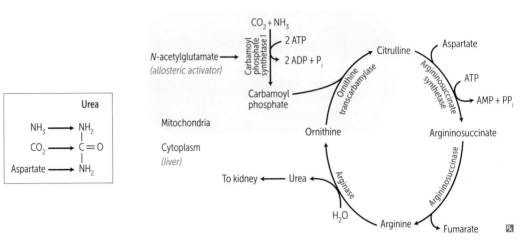

Urea

$$NH_3 \longrightarrow NH_2$$
$$CO_2 \longrightarrow C=O$$
$$Aspartate \longrightarrow NH_2$$

Transport of ammonia by alanine

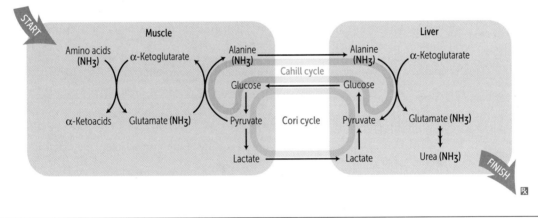

Hyperammonemia

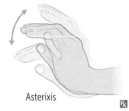

Asterixis

Can be acquired (eg, liver disease) or hereditary (eg, urea cycle enzyme deficiencies).
Excess NH_3 depletes glutamate (GABA) in the CNS and α-ketoglutarate → inhibition of TCA cycle.
Treatment: limit protein in diet.
May be given to ↓ ammonia levels:
- Lactulose to acidify the GI tract and trap NH_4^+ for excretion.
- Antibiotics (eg, rifaximin, neomycin) to ↓ colonic ammoniagenic bacteria.
- Benzoate, phenylacetate, or phenylbutyrate react with glycine or glutamine, forming products that are renally excreted.

Ammonia accumulation—flapping tremor (asterixis), slurring of speech, somnolence, vomiting, cerebral edema, blurring of vision.

Ornithine transcarbamylase deficiency	Most common urea cycle disorder. X-linked recessive (vs other urea cycle enzyme deficiencies, which are autosomal recessive). Interferes with the body's ability to eliminate ammonia. Often evident in the first few days of life, but may present later. Excess carbamoyl phosphate is converted to orotic acid (part of the pyrimidine synthesis pathway). Findings: ↑ orotic acid in blood and urine, ↓ BUN, symptoms of hyperammonemia. No megaloblastic anemia (vs orotic aciduria).

Amino acid derivatives

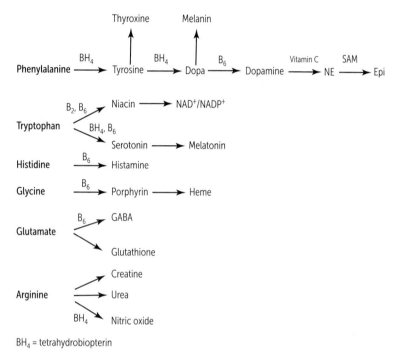

BH$_4$ = tetrahydrobiopterin

Catecholamine synthesis/tyrosine catabolism

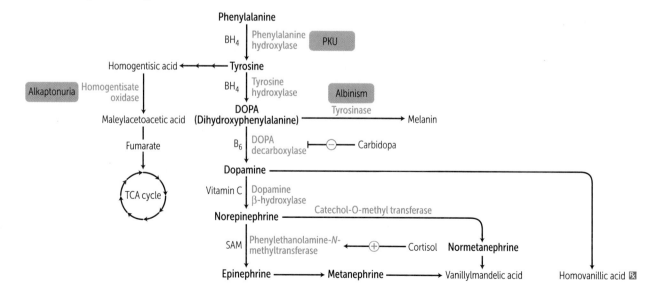

Phenylketonuria	Due to ↓ phenylalanine hydroxylase or ↓ tetrahydrobiopterin (BH_4) cofactor (malignant PKU). Tyrosine becomes essential. ↑ phenylalanine → excess phenyl ketones in urine. Findings: intellectual disability, growth retardation, seizures, fair complexion, eczema, musty body odor. Treatment: ↓ phenylalanine and ↑ tyrosine in diet, tetrahydrobiopterin supplementation. **Maternal PKU**—lack of proper dietary therapy during pregnancy. Findings in infant: microcephaly, intellectual disability, growth retardation, congenital heart defects.	Autosomal recessive. Incidence ≈ 1:10,000. Screening occurs 2–3 days after birth (normal at birth because of maternal enzyme during fetal life). Phenyl ketones—phenylacetate, phenyllactate, and phenylpyruvate. Disorder of **aromatic** amino acid metabolism → musty body **odor.** PKU patients must avoid the artificial sweetener aspartame, which contains phenylalanine.
Maple syrup urine disease	Blocked degradation of **branched** amino acids (Isoleucine, Leucine, Valine) due to ↓ branched-chain α-ketoacid dehydrogenase (B_1). Causes ↑ α-ketoacids in the blood, especially those of leucine. Causes severe CNS defects, intellectual disability, and death. Treatment: restriction of isoleucine, leucine, valine in diet, and thiamine supplementation.	Autosomal recessive. Presentation: vomiting, poor feeding, urine smells like maple syrup/burnt sugar. **I L**ove **V**ermont **maple syrup** from maple trees (with B_1**ranches**).
Alkaptonuria 	Congenital deficiency of homogentisate oxidase in the degradative pathway of tyrosine to fumarate → pigment-forming homogentisic acid accumulates in tissue **A**. Autosomal recessive. Usually benign. Findings: bluish-black connective tissue, ear cartilage, and sclerae (ochronosis); urine turns black on prolonged exposure to air. May have debilitating arthralgias (homogentisic acid toxic to cartilage).	
Homocystinuria	Types (all autosomal recessive): ■ Cystathionine synthase deficiency (treatment: ↓ methionine, ↑ cysteine, ↑ B_6, B_{12}, and folate in diet) ■ ↓ affinity of cystathionine synthase for pyridoxal phosphate (treatment: ↑↑ B_6 and ↑ cysteine in diet) ■ Methionine synthase (homocysteine methyltransferase) deficiency (treatment: ↑ methionine in diet)	All forms result in excess homocysteine. **HOMOCY**stinuria: ↑↑ **H**omocysteine in urine, **O**steoporosis, **M**arfanoid habitus, **O**cular changes (**d**ownward and **in**ward lens subluxation), **C**ardiovascular effects (thrombosis and atherosclerosis → stroke and MI), k**Y**phosis, intellectual disability. In homocystinuria, lens subluxes "down and in" (vs Marfan, "up and fans out").

Methionine ⟵ (Methionine synthase, B_{12}) ⟶ Homocysteine ⟶ (Cystathionine synthase, B_6, Serine) ⟶ Cystathionine ⟶ Cysteine

Cystinuria

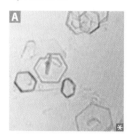

Hereditary defect of renal PCT and intestinal amino acid transporter that prevents reabsorption of Cystine, Ornithine, Lysine, and Arginine (**COLA**).

Excess cystine in the urine can lead to recurrent precipitation of hexagonal cystine stones 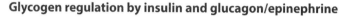. Treatment: urinary alkalinization (eg, potassium citrate, acetazolamide) and chelating agents (eg, penicillamine) ↑ solubility of cystine stones; good hydration.

Autosomal recessive. Common (1:7000). Urinary cyanide-nitroprusside test is diagnostic.

Cystine is made of 2 cysteines connected by a disulfide bond.

Glycogen regulation by insulin and glucagon/epinephrine

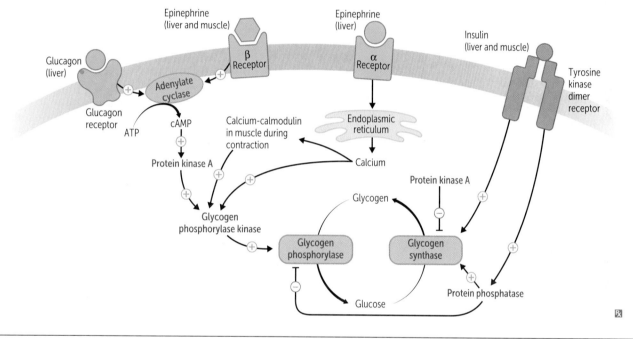

Glycogen	Branches have α-(1,6) bonds; linkages have α-(1,4) bonds.
Skeletal muscle	Glycogen undergoes glycogenolysis → glucose-1-phosphate → glucose-6-phosphate, which is rapidly metabolized during exercise.
Hepatocytes	Glycogen is stored and undergoes glycogenolysis to maintain blood sugar at appropriate levels. Glycogen phosphorylase ❹ liberates glucose-1-phosphate residues off branched glycogen until 4 glucose units remain on a branch. Then 4-α-D-glucanotransferase (debranching enzyme ❺) moves 3 of the 4 glucose units from the branch to the linkage. Then α-1,6-glucosidase (debranching enzyme ❻) cleaves off the last residue, liberating glucose.
	"Limit dextrin" refers to the one to four residues remaining on a branch after glycogen phosphorylase has already shortened it.

Note: A small amount of glycogen is degraded in lysosomes by ❼ α-1,4-glucosidase (acid maltase).

Glycogen storage diseases

At least 15 types have been identified, all resulting in abnormal glycogen metabolism and an accumulation of glycogen within cells. Periodic acid–Schiff stain identifies glycogen and is useful in identifying these diseases.

Very Poor Carbohydrate Metabolism. Types I, II, III, and V are autosomal recessive.

DISEASE	FINDINGS	DEFICIENT ENZYME	COMMENTS
Von Gierke disease (type I)	Severe fasting hypoglycemia, ↑↑ Glycogen in liver and kidneys, ↑ blood lactate, ↑ triglycerides, ↑ uric acid (Gout), and hepatomegaly, renomegaly. Liver does not regulate blood glucose.	Glucose-6-phosphatase	Treatment: frequent oral glucose/cornstarch; avoidance of fructose and galactose Impaired gluconeogenesis and glycogenolysis
Pompe disease (type II)	Cardiomegaly, hypertrophic cardiomyopathy, hypotonia, exercise intolerance, and systemic findings lead to early death.	Lysosomal acid α-1,4-glucosidase with α-1,6-glucosidase activity (acid maltase)	PomPe trashes the PumP (1,4) (heart, liver, and muscle)
Cori disease (type III)	Milder form of von Gierke (type I) with normal blood lactate levels. Accumulation of limit dextrin–like structures in cytosol.	Debranching enzyme (α-1,6-glucosidase)	Gluconeogenesis is intact
McArdle disease (type V)	↑ glycogen in muscle, but muscle cannot break it down → painful Muscle cramps, Myoglobinuria (red urine) with strenuous exercise, and arrhythmia from electrolyte abnormalities. Second-wind phenomenon noted during exercise due to ↑ muscular blood flow.	Skeletal muscle glycogen phosphorylase (Myophosphorylase) Hallmark is a flat venous lactate curve with normal rise in ammonia levels during exercise	Blood glucose levels typically unaffected McArdle = Muscle

Lysosomal storage diseases   Each is caused by a deficiency in one of the many lysosomal enzymes. Results in an accumulation of abnormal metabolic products.

DISEASE	FINDINGS	DEFICIENT ENZYME	ACCUMULATED SUBSTRATE	INHERITANCE
Sphingolipidoses				
Tay-Sachs disease	Progressive neurodegeneration, developmental delay, "cherry-red" spot on macula A, lysosomes with onion skin, no hepatosplenomegaly (vs Niemann-Pick).	❶ HeXosaminidase A ("TAy-SaX")	GM_2 ganglioside	AR
Fabry disease	Early: Triad of episodic peripheral neuropathy, angiokeratomas B, hypohidrosis. Late: progressive renal failure, cardiovascular disease.	❷ α-galactosidase A	Ceramide trihexoside	XR
Metachromatic leukodystrophy	Central and peripheral demyelination with ataxia, dementia.	❸ Arylsulfatase A	Cerebroside sulfate	AR
Krabbe disease	Peripheral neuropathy, destruction of oligodendrocytes, developmental delay, optic atrophy, globoid cells.	❹ Galactocerebrosidase	Galactocerebroside, psychosine	AR
Gaucher disease	Most common. Hepatosplenomegaly, pancytopenia, osteoporosis, avascular necrosis of femur, bone crises, Gaucher cells C (lipid-laden macrophages resembling crumpled tissue paper).	❺ Glucocerebrosidase (β-glucosidase); treat with recombinant glucocerebrosidase	Glucocerebroside	AR
Niemann-Pick disease	Progressive neurodegeneration, hepatosplenomegaly, foam cells (lipid-laden macrophages) D, "cherry-red" spot on macula A.	❻ Sphingomyelinase	Sphingomyelin	AR
Mucopolysaccharidoses				
Hurler syndrome	Developmental delay, gargoylism, airway obstruction, corneal clouding, hepatosplenomegaly.	α-L-iduronidase	Heparan sulfate, dermatan sulfate	AR
Hunter syndrome	Mild Hurler + aggressive behavior, no corneal clouding.	Iduronate-2-sulfatase	Heparan sulfate, dermatan sulfate	XR

GM₂   Ceramide trihexoside
❶↓   ❷↓
GM₃
Glucocerebroside
Sulfatides   ↓❺
❸↓   ❹→   Ceramide   ←❻   Sphingomyelin ℞
Galactocerebroside

No man picks (Niemann-Pick) his nose with his **sphinger** (**sphingomyelinase**).

Tay-SaX lacks he**X**osaminidase.

Hunters see clearly (no corneal clouding) and aggressively aim for the **X** (**X**-linked recessive).

↑ incidence of Tay-Sachs, Niemann-Pick, and some forms of Gaucher disease in Ashkenazi Jews.

Fatty acid metabolism

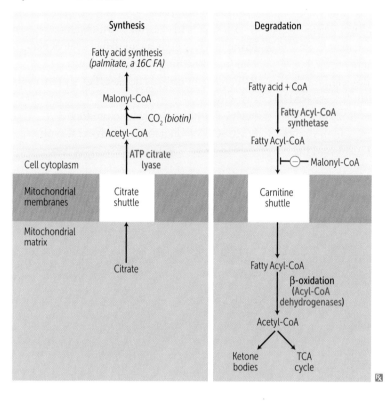

Fatty acid synthesis requires transport of citrate from mitochondria to cytosol. Predominantly occurs in liver, lactating mammary glands, and adipose tissue.

Long-chain fatty acid (LCFA) degradation requires carnitine-dependent transport into the mitochondrial matrix.

"SYtrate" = SYnthesis.
CARnitine = CARnage of fatty acids.

Systemic 1° carnitine deficiency—inherited defect in transport of LCFAs into the mitochondria → toxic accumulation. Causes weakness, hypotonia, and hypoketotic hypoglycemia.

Medium-chain acyl-CoA dehydrogenase deficiency—↓ ability to break down fatty acids into acetyl-CoA → accumulation of fatty acyl carnitines in the blood with hypoketotic hypoglycemia. Causes vomiting, lethargy, seizures, coma, liver dysfunction, hyperammonemia. Can lead to sudden death in infants or children. Treat by avoiding fasting.

Ketone bodies

In the liver, fatty acids and amino acids are metabolized to acetoacetate and β-hydroxybutyrate (to be used in muscle and brain).

In prolonged starvation and diabetic ketoacidosis, oxaloacetate is depleted for gluconeogenesis. In alcoholism, excess NADH shunts oxaloacetate to malate. Both processes cause a buildup of acetyl-CoA, which shunts glucose, amino acids, and FFAs toward the production of ketone bodies.

Ketone bodies: acetone, acetoacetate, β-hydroxybutyrate.

Breath smells like acetone (fruity odor).

Urine test for ketones can detect acetoacetate, but not β-hydroxybutyrate.

RBCs cannot utilize ketones; they strictly use glucose.

HMG-CoA lyase for ketone production.

HMG-CoA reductase for cholesterol synthesis.

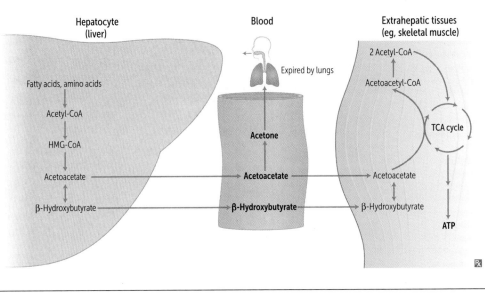

Metabolic fuel use

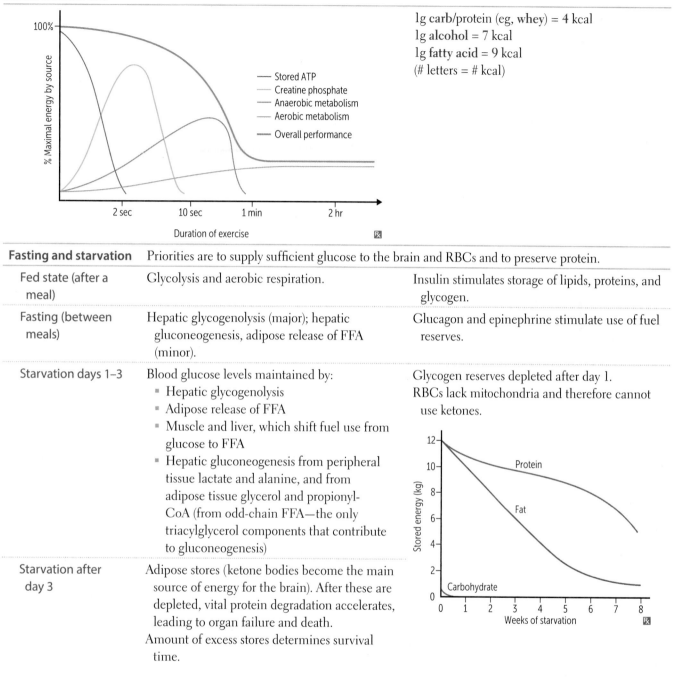

1g carb/protein (eg, whey) = 4 kcal
1g alcohol = 7 kcal
1g fatty acid = 9 kcal
(# letters = # kcal)

Fasting and starvation	Priorities are to supply sufficient glucose to the brain and RBCs and to preserve protein.	
Fed state (after a meal)	Glycolysis and aerobic respiration.	Insulin stimulates storage of lipids, proteins, and glycogen.
Fasting (between meals)	Hepatic glycogenolysis (major); hepatic gluconeogenesis, adipose release of FFA (minor).	Glucagon and epinephrine stimulate use of fuel reserves.
Starvation days 1–3	Blood glucose levels maintained by: ▪ Hepatic glycogenolysis ▪ Adipose release of FFA ▪ Muscle and liver, which shift fuel use from glucose to FFA ▪ Hepatic gluconeogenesis from peripheral tissue lactate and alanine, and from adipose tissue glycerol and propionyl-CoA (from odd-chain FFA—the only triacylglycerol components that contribute to gluconeogenesis)	Glycogen reserves depleted after day 1. RBCs lack mitochondria and therefore cannot use ketones.
Starvation after day 3	Adipose stores (ketone bodies become the main source of energy for the brain). After these are depleted, vital protein degradation accelerates, leading to organ failure and death. Amount of excess stores determines survival time.	

Lipid transport

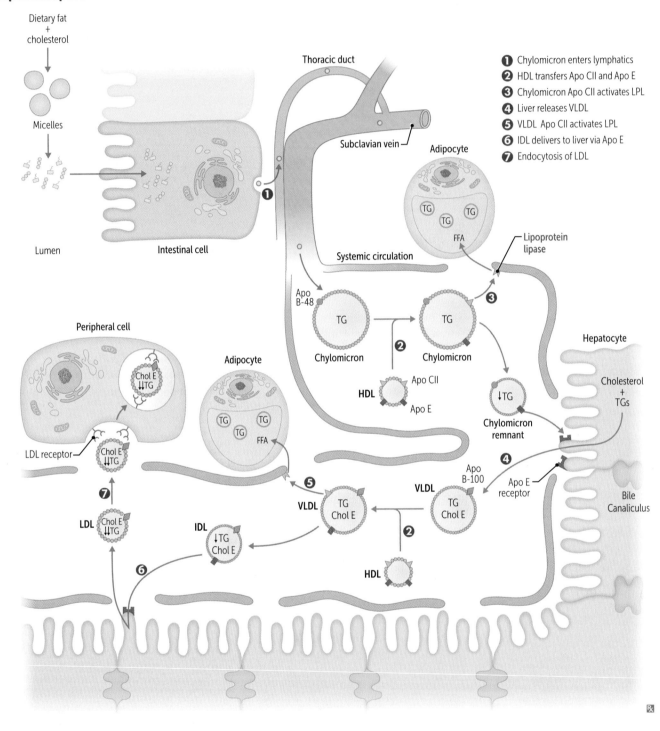

Dietary fat + cholesterol

Micelles

Lumen

Intestinal cell

Thoracic duct

Subclavian vein

Systemic circulation

Apo B-48

Chylomicron

Peripheral cell

LDL receptor

Chol E ↓↓TG

Adipocyte

TG   TG
   TG
      FFA

VLDL
TG
Chol E

IDL
↓TG
Chol E

LDL
Chol E
↓↓TG

HDL

Chylomicron

HDL
Apo CII
Apo E

Adipocyte

TG   TG
   TG
      FFA

Lipoprotein lipase

Hepatocyte

Cholesterol + TGs

Chylomicron remnant

↓TG

Apo B-100

Apo E receptor

Bile Canaliculus

VLDL
TG
Chol E

HDL

1. Chylomicron enters lymphatics
2. HDL transfers Apo CII and Apo E
3. Chylomicron Apo CII activates LPL
4. Liver releases VLDL
5. VLDL Apo CII activates LPL
6. IDL delivers to liver via Apo E
7. Endocytosis of LDL

Key enzymes in lipid transport	Cholesterol ester transfer protein mediates transfer of cholesterol esters to other lipoprotein particles.
Hepatic lipase	Degrades TGs remaining in IDL.
Hormone-sensitive lipase	Degrades TGs stored in adipocytes.
Lecithin-cholesterol acyltransferase	Catalyzes esterification of ⅔ of plasma cholesterol.
Lipoprotein lipase	Degrades TGs circulating chylomicrons and VLDLs. Found on vascular endothelial surface.
Pancreatic lipase	Degrades dietary TGs in small intestine.

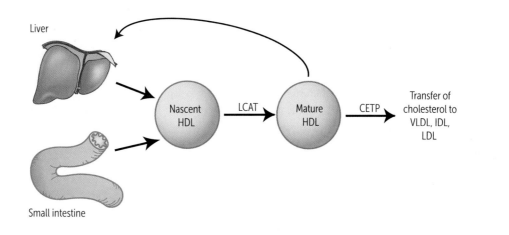

Major apolipoproteins

Apolipoprotein	Function	Chylomicron	Chylomicron remnant	VLDL	IDL	LDL	HDL
E	Mediates remnant uptake (Everything Except LDL)	✓	✓	✓	✓		✓
A-I	Activates LCAT						✓
C-II	Lipoprotein lipase Cofactor that Catalyzes Cleavage	✓		✓			✓
B-48	Mediates chylomicron secretion into lymphatics Only on particles originating from the intestines	✓	✓				
B-100	Binds LDL receptor Only on particles originating from the liver			✓	✓	✓	

Lipoprotein functions	Lipoproteins are composed of varying proportions of cholesterol, TGs, and phospholipids. LDL and HDL carry the most cholesterol.
	LDL transports cholesterol from liver to tissues. LDL is Lousy.
	HDL transports cholesterol from periphery to liver. HDL is Healthy.
Cholesterol	Needed to maintain cell membrane integrity and synthesize bile acid, steroids, and vitamin D.
Chylomicron	Delivers dietary TGs to peripheral tissues. Delivers cholesterol to liver in the form of chylomicron remnants, which are mostly depleted of their TGs. Secreted by intestinal epithelial cells.
VLDL	Delivers hepatic TGs to peripheral tissue. Secreted by liver.
IDL	Formed in the degradation of VLDL. Delivers TGs and cholesterol to liver.
LDL	Delivers hepatic cholesterol to peripheral tissues. Formed by hepatic lipase modification of IDL in the liver and peripheral tissue. Taken up by target cells via receptor-mediated endocytosis.
HDL	Mediates reverse cholesterol transport from periphery to liver. Acts as a repository for apolipoproteins C and E (which are needed for chylomicron and VLDL metabolism). Secreted from both liver and intestine. Alcohol ↑ synthesis.

Abetalipoproteinemia	Autosomal recessive. Chylomicrons, VLDL, LDL absent. Deficiency in ApoB-48, ApoB-100. Affected infants present with severe fat malabsorption, steatorrhea, failure to thrive. Later manifestations include retinitis pigmentosa, spinocerebellar degeneration due to vitamin E deficiency, progressive ataxia, acanthocytosis.
	Treatment: restriction of long-chain fatty acids, large doses of oral vitamin E.

Familial dyslipidemias

TYPE	INHERITANCE	PATHOGENESIS	↑ BLOOD LEVEL	CLINICAL
I—Hyper-chylomicronemia	AR	Lipoprotein lipase or apolipoprotein C-II deficiency	Chylomicrons, TG, cholesterol	Pancreatitis, hepatosplenomegaly, and eruptive/pruritic xanthomas (no ↑ risk for atherosclerosis). Creamy layer in supernatant.
II—Familial hyper-cholesterolemia	AD	Absent or defective LDL receptors, or defective ApoB-100	IIa: LDL, cholesterol IIb: LDL, cholesterol, VLDL	Heterozygotes (1:500) have cholesterol ≈ 300mg/dL; homozygotes (very rare) have cholesterol ≈ 700+ mg/dL. Accelerated atherosclerosis (may have MI before age 20), tendon (Achilles) xanthomas, and corneal arcus.
III—Dysbeta-lipoproteinemia	AR	Defective ApoE	Chylomicrons, VLDL	Premature atherosclerosis, tuberoeruptive xanthomas, palmar xanthomas.
IV—Hyper-triglyceridemia	AD	Hepatic overproduction of VLDL	VLDL, TG	Hypertriglyceridemia (> 1000 mg/dL) can cause acute pancreatitis. Related to insulin resistance.

Immunology

"I hate to disappoint you, but my rubber lips are immune to your charms."
—*Batman & Robin*

"An apple a day keeps the doctor away."

—English proverb

Understand how the many components of the immune system operate and interact in the normal immune response to infection at both the clinical and cellular levels. Know the immune mechanisms of responses to vaccines. Both congenital and acquired immunodeficiencies are very testable. Cell surface markers are high yield for understanding immune cell interactions and for laboratory diagnosis. Know the roles and functions of major cytokines and chemokines.

▶ IMMUNOLOGY—LYMPHOID STRUCTURES

Immune system organs	1° organs: ▪ Bone marrow—immune cell production, B cell maturation ▪ Thymus—T cell maturation 2° organs: ▪ Spleen, lymph nodes, tonsils, Peyer patches ▪ Allow immune cells to interact with antigen

Lymph node	A 2° lymphoid organ that has many afferents, 1 or more efferents. Encapsulated, with trabeculae. Functions are nonspecific filtration by macrophages, storage of B and T cells, and immune response activation.
Follicle	Site of B-cell localization and proliferation. In outer cortex. 1° follicles are dense and dormant. 2° follicles have pale central germinal centers and are active.
Medulla	Consists of medullary cords (closely packed lymphocytes and plasma cells) and medullary sinuses. Medullary sinuses communicate with efferent lymphatics and contain reticular cells and macrophages.
Paracortex	Houses T cells. Region of cortex between follicles and medulla. Contains high endothelial venules through which T and B cells enter from blood. Not well developed in patients with DiGeorge syndrome. Paracortex enlarges in an extreme cellular immune response (eg, viral infection).

Afferent lymphatic

Follicles (B cells)

Paracortex (T cells)

1° follicle

2° follicle

Germinal center

Mantle zone

Medullary cords (lymphocytes, plasma cells)

Postcapillary venule

Vein

Artery

Capillary supply

Efferent lymphatic

Trabecula

Medullary sinus (reticular cells, macrophages)

Capsule

Lymphatic drainage associations

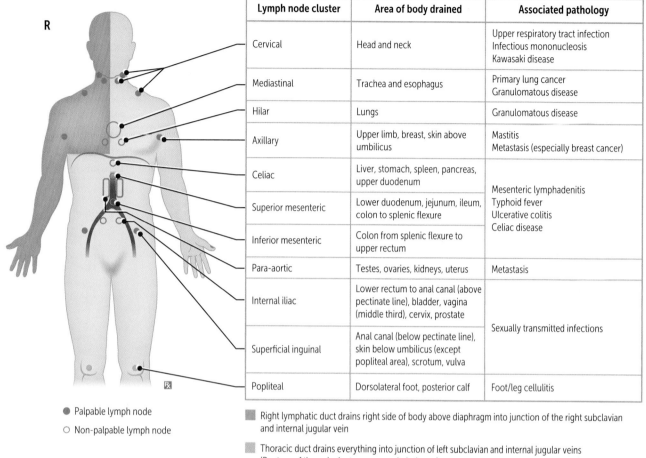

Lymph node cluster	Area of body drained	Associated pathology
Cervical	Head and neck	Upper respiratory tract infection Infectious mononucleosis Kawasaki disease
Mediastinal	Trachea and esophagus	Primary lung cancer Granulomatous disease
Hilar	Lungs	Granulomatous disease
Axillary	Upper limb, breast, skin above umbilicus	Mastitis Metastasis (especially breast cancer)
Celiac	Liver, stomach, spleen, pancreas, upper duodenum	Mesenteric lymphadenitis Typhoid fever Ulcerative colitis Celiac disease
Superior mesenteric	Lower duodenum, jejunum, ileum, colon to splenic flexure	
Inferior mesenteric	Colon from splenic flexure to upper rectum	
Para-aortic	Testes, ovaries, kidneys, uterus	Metastasis
Internal iliac	Lower rectum to anal canal (above pectinate line), bladder, vagina (middle third), cervix, prostate	Sexually transmitted infections
Superficial inguinal	Anal canal (below pectinate line), skin below umbilicus (except popliteal area), scrotum, vulva	
Popliteal	Dorsolateral foot, posterior calf	Foot/leg cellulitis

● Palpable lymph node

○ Non-palpable lymph node

▨ Right lymphatic duct drains right side of body above diaphragm into junction of the right subclavian and internal jugular vein

▨ Thoracic duct drains everything into junction of left subclavian and internal jugular veins (Rupture of thoracic duct can cause chylothorax)

Spleen

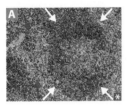

Located in LUQ of abdomen, anterior to left kidney, protected by 9th-11th ribs.

Sinusoids are long, vascular channels in red pulp (red arrows in) with fenestrated "barrel hoop" basement membrane.

- T cells are found in the periarteriolar lymphatic sheath (PALS) within the white pulp (white arrows in A).
- B cells are found in follicles within the white pulp.
- The marginal zone, in between the red pulp and white pulp, contains macrophages and specialized B cells, and is where antigen-presenting cells (APCs) capture blood-borne antigens for recognition by lymphocytes.

Splenic macrophages remove encapsulated bacteria.

Splenic dysfunction (eg, postsplenectomy state in sickle cell disease): ↓ IgM → ↓ complement activation → ↓ C3b opsonization → ↑ susceptibility to encapsulated organisms.

Postsplenectomy blood findings:
- Howell-Jolly bodies (nuclear remnants)
- Target cells
- Thrombocytosis (loss of sequestration and removal)
- Lymphocytosis (loss of sequestration)

Vaccinate patients undergoing splenectomy against encapsulated organisms (pneumococcal, Hib, meningococcal).

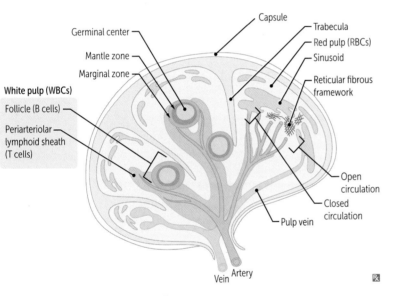

White pulp (WBCs)
Follicle (B cells)
Periarteriolar lymphoid sheath (T cells)

Germinal center
Mantle zone
Marginal zone

Capsule
Trabecula
Red pulp (RBCs)
Sinusoid
Reticular fibrous framework

Open circulation
Closed circulation
Pulp vein

Vein Artery

Thymus

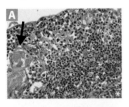

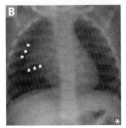

Located in the anterosuperior mediastinum. Site of T-cell differentiation and maturation. Encapsulated. **Thymus** is derived from the **Third** pharyngeal pouch. Lymphocytes of mesenchymal origin. Cortex is dense with immature T cells; medulla is pale with mature T cells and Hassall corpuscles A containing epithelial reticular cells.

Normal neonatal thymus "sail-shaped" on CXR B, involutes with age.

T cells = **T**hymus

B cells = **B**one marrow

Hypoplastic in DiGeorge syndrome and severe combined immunodeficiency (SCID).

Thymoma—neoplasm of thymus. Associated with myasthenia gravis and superior vena cava syndrome.

Innate vs adaptive immunity

	Innate immunity	Adaptive immunity
COMPONENTS	Neutrophils, macrophages, monocytes, dendritic cells, natural killer (NK) cells (lymphoid origin), complement, physical epithelial barriers, secreted enzymes.	T cells, B cells, circulating antibodies
MECHANISM	Germline encoded	Variation through V(D)J recombination during lymphocyte development
RESISTANCE	Resistance persists through generations; does not change within an organism's lifetime	Microbial resistance not heritable
RESPONSE TO PATHOGENS	Nonspecific Occurs rapidly (minutes to hours) No memory response	Highly specific, refined over time Develops over long periods; memory response is faster and more robust
SECRETED PROTEINS	Lysozyme, complement, C-reactive protein (CRP), defensins	Immunoglobulins
KEY FEATURES IN PATHOGEN RECOGNITION	Toll-like receptors (TLRs): pattern recognition receptors that recognize pathogen-associated molecular patterns (PAMPs) and lead to activation of NF-κB. Examples of PAMPs include LPS (gram ⊖ bacteria), flagellin (bacteria), nucleic acids (viruses).	Memory cells: activated B and T cells; subsequent exposure to a previously encountered antigen → stronger, quicker immune response

Major histocompatibility complex I and II

MHC encoded by HLA genes. Present antigen fragments to T cells and bind T-cell receptors (TCRs).

	MHC I	MHC II
LOCI	HLA-A, HLA-B, HLA-C MHC **I** loci have 1 letter	HLA-DP, HLA-DQ, HLA-DR MHC **II** loci have 2 letters
BINDING	TCR and CD8	TCR and CD4
STRUCTURE	1 long chain, 1 short chain	2 equal-length chains (2 α, 2 β)
EXPRESSION	All nucleated cells, APCs, platelets Not on RBCs	APCs
FUNCTION	Present endogenously synthesized antigens (eg, viral or cytosolic proteins) to CD8+ cytotoxic T cells	Present exogenously synthesized antigens (eg, bacterial proteins) to CD4+ helper T cells
ANTIGEN LOADING	Antigen peptides loaded onto MHC I in RER after delivery via TAP (transporter associated with antigen processing)	Antigen loaded following release of invariant chain in an acidified endosome
ASSOCIATED PROTEINS	β_2-microglobulin	Invariant chain
STRUCTURE		

HLA subtypes associated with diseases

HLA SUBTYPE	DISEASE	MNEMONIC
A3	Hemochromatosis	
B8	**Addison** disease, **my**asthenia gravis, **Graves** disease	Don't **Be** late(8), Dr. **Addison**, or else you'll send **my** patient to the **grave**.
B27	**P**soriatic arthritis, **A**nkylosing spondylitis, **I**BD-associated arthritis, **R**eactive arthritis	**PAIR**. Also known as seronegative arthropathies.
DQ2/DQ8	Celiac disease	I ate (8) too (2) much gluten at Dairy Queen.
DR2	**Multiple** sclerosis, **hay** fever, SLE, Good**pasture** syndrome	**Multiple hay pastures** have dirt.
DR3	Diabetes mellitus type 1, **SLE**, Graves disease, Hashimoto thyroiditis, Addison disease	2-3, S-L-E
DR4	**Rheum**atoid arthritis, diabetes mellitus type 1, Addison disease	There are 4 walls in a "**rheum**" (room).
DR5	Hashimoto thyroiditis	Hashimoto is an **odd** doctor (DR3, DR5).

Natural killer cells	Lymphocyte member of innate immune system.
	Use perforin and granzymes to induce apoptosis of virally infected cells and tumor cells.
	Activity enhanced by IL-2, IL-12, IFN-α, and IFN-β.
	Induced to kill when exposed to a nonspecific activation signal on target cell and/or to an absence of MHC I on target cell surface.
	Also kills via antibody-dependent cell-mediated cytotoxicity (CD16 binds Fc region of bound Ig, activating the NK cell).

Major functions of B and T cells

B cells	Humoral immunity.
	Recognize antigen—undergo somatic hypermutation to optimize antigen specificity.
	Produce antibody—differentiate into plasma cells to secrete specific immunoglobulins.
	Maintain immunologic memory—memory B cells persist and accelerate future response to antigen.
T cells	Cell-mediated immunity.
	CD4+ T cells help B cells make antibodies and produce cytokines to recruit phagocytes and activate other leukocytes.
	CD8+ T cells directly kill virus-infected cells.
	Delayed cell-mediated hypersensitivity (type IV).
	Acute and chronic cellular organ rejection.
	Rule of 8: MHC **II** × CD4 = 8; MHC **I** × CD8 = 8.

Differentiation of T cells

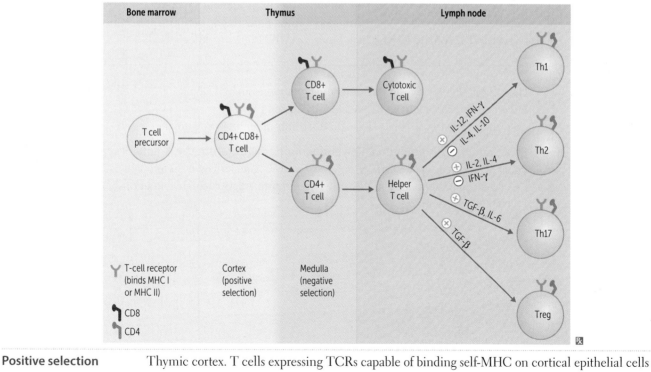

Positive selection	Thymic cortex. T cells expressing TCRs capable of binding self-MHC on cortical epithelial cells survive.
Negative selection	Thymic medulla. T cells expressing TCRs with high affinity for self antigens undergo apoptosis or become regulatory T cells. Tissue-restricted self-antigens are expressed in the thymus due to the action of autoimmune regulator (AIRE); deficiency leads to autoimmune polyendocrine syndrome-1.

T cell subsets

	Th1 cell	Th2 cell	Th17 cell	Treg
SECRETES	IFN-γ	**IL-4, IL-5**, IL-6, IL-10, **IL-13**	IL-17, IL-21, IL-22	TGF-ß, IL-10, IL-35
FUNCTION	Activates macrophages and cytotoxic T cells to kill phagocytosed microbes	Activate eosinophils and promote production of IgE for parasite defense	Immunity against extracellular microbes, through induction of neutrophilic inflammation	Prevent autoimmunity by maintaining tolerance to self-antigens
INDUCED BY	IFN-γ, IL-12	IL-2, IL-4	TGF-β, IL-1, IL-6	TGF-β, IL-2
INHIBITED BY	IL-4, IL-10 (from Th2 cell)	IFN-γ (from Th1 cell)	IFN-γ, IL-4	IL-6
IMMUNODEFICIENCY	Mendelian susceptibility to mycobacterial disease		Hyper-IgE syndrome	IPEX

Macrophage-lymphocyte interaction	Th1 cells secrete IFN-γ, which enhances the ability of monocytes and macrophages to kill microbes they ingest. This function is also enhanced by interaction of T cell CD40L with CD40 on macrophages.

Cytotoxic T cells	Kill virus-infected, neoplastic, and donor graft cells by inducing apoptosis. Release cytotoxic granules containing preformed proteins (eg, perforin, granzyme B). Cytotoxic T cells have CD8, which binds to MHC I on virus-infected cells.

Regulatory T cells	Help maintain specific immune tolerance by suppressing CD4 and CD8 T-cell effector functions. Identified by expression of CD3, CD4, CD25, and FOXP3. Activated regulatory T cells (Tregs) produce anti-inflammatory cytokines (eg, IL-10, TGF-β).
	IPEX (Immune dysregulation, Polyendocrinopathy, Enteropathy, X-linked) syndrome— genetic deficiency of FOXP3 → autoimmunity. Characterized by enteropathy, endocrinopathy, nail dystrophy, dermatitis, and/or other autoimmune dermatologic conditions. Associated with diabetes in male infants.

T- and B-cell activation   APCs: B cells, dendritic cells, Langerhans cells, macrophages.
Two signals are required for T-cell activation, B-cell activation, and class switching.

T-cell activation	❶ Dendritic cell (specialized APC) samples antigen, processes antigen, and migrates to the draining lymph node. ❷ T-cell activation (signal 1): antigen is presented on MHC II and recognized by TCR on Th (CD4+) cell. Endogenous or cross-presented antigen is presented on MHC I to Tc (CD8+) cell. ❸ Proliferation and survival (signal 2): costimulatory signal via interaction of B7 protein (CD80/86) on dendritic cell and CD28 on naïve T cell. ❹ Th cell activates and produces cytokines. Tc cell activates and is able to recognize and kill virus-infected cell.	
B-cell activation and class switching	❶ Th-cell activation as above. ❷ B-cell receptor–mediated endocytosis; foreign antigen is presented on MHC II and recognized by TCR on Th cell. ❸ CD40 receptor on B cell binds CD40 ligand (CD40L) on Th cell. ❹ Th cell secretes cytokines that determine Ig class switching of B cell. B cell activates and undergoes class switching, affinity maturation, and antibody production.	

▶ IMMUNOLOGY—IMMUNE RESPONSES

Antibody structure and function

Fab (containing the variable/hypervariable regions) consisting of light (L) and heavy (H) chains recognizes antigens. Fc region of IgM and IgG fixes complement. Heavy chain contributes to Fc and Fab regions. Light chain contributes only to Fab region.

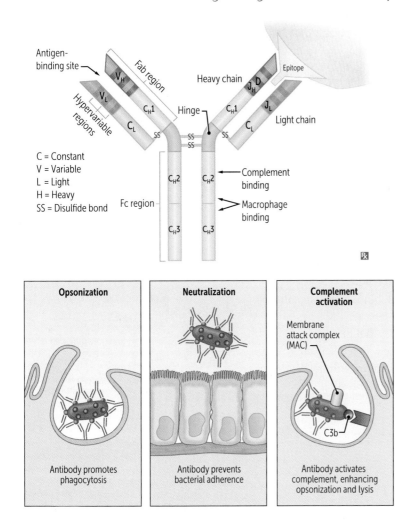

Fab:
- Fragment, antigen binding
- Determines idiotype: unique antigen-binding pocket; only 1 antigenic specificity expressed per B cell

Fc:
- Constant
- Carboxy terminal
- Complement binding
- Carbohydrate side chains
- Determines isotype (IgM, IgD, etc)

Generation of antibody diversity (antigen independent)
1. Random recombination of VJ (light-chain) or V(D)J (heavy-chain) genes
2. Random addition of nucleotides to DNA during recombination by terminal deoxynucleotidyl transferase (TdT)
3. Random combination of heavy chains with light chains

Generation of antibody specificity (antigen dependent)
4. Somatic hypermutation and affinity maturation (variable region)
5. Isotype switching (constant region)

Opsonization	Neutralization	Complement activation
Antibody promotes phagocytosis	Antibody prevents bacterial adherence	Antibody activates complement, enhancing opsonization and lysis

Immunoglobulin isotypes	All isotypes can exist as monomers. Mature, naive B cells prior to activation express IgM and IgD on their surfaces. They may differentiate in germinal centers of lymph nodes by isotype switching (gene rearrangement; induced by cytokines and CD40L) into plasma cells that secrete IgA, IgE, or IgG.
IgG	Main antibody in 2° response to an antigen. Most abundant isotype in serum. Fixes complement, opsonizes bacteria, neutralizes bacterial toxins and viruses. Only isotype that crosses the placenta (provides infants with passive immunity).
IgA	Prevents attachment of bacteria and viruses to mucous membranes; does not fix complement. Monomer (in circulation) or dimer (with J chain when secreted). Crosses epithelial cells by transcytosis. Produced in GI tract (eg, by Peyer patches) and protects against gut infections (eg, *Giardia*). Most produced antibody overall, but has lower serum concentrations. Released into secretions (tears, saliva, mucus) and breast milk. Picks up secretory component from epithelial cells, which protects the Fc portion from luminal proteases.
IgM	Produced in the 1° (**immediate**) response to an antigen. Fixes complement. Cannot cross the placenta. Antigen receptor on the surface of B cells. Monomer on B cell, pentamer with J chain when secreted. Pentamer enables avid binding to antigen while humoral response evolves.
IgD	Unclear function. Found on surface of many B cells and in serum.
IgE	Binds mast cells and basophils; cross-links when exposed to allergen, mediating immediate (type I) hypersensitivity through release of inflammatory mediators such as histamine. Contributes to immunity to parasites by activating eosinophils. Lowest concentration in serum.

Antigen type and memory

Thymus-independent antigens	Antigens lacking a peptide component (eg, lipopolysaccharides from gram ⊖ bacteria); cannot be presented by MHC to T cells. Weakly immunogenic; vaccines often require boosters and adjuvants (eg, pneumococcal polysaccharide vaccine).
Thymus-dependent antigens	Antigens containing a protein component (eg, diphtheria vaccine). Class switching and immunologic memory occur as a result of direct contact of B cells with Th cells.

Complement	System of hepatically synthesized plasma proteins that play a role in innate immunity and inflammation. Membrane attack complex (MAC) defends against gram ⊖ bacteria.	
ACTIVATION PATHWAYS	Classic—IgG or IgM mediated. Alternative—microbe surface molecules. Lectin—mannose or other sugars on microbe surface.	**GM** makes **classic** cars.
FUNCTIONS	C3b—opsonization. C3a, C4a, C5a—anaphylaxis. C5a—neutrophil chemotaxis. C5b-9—cytolysis by MAC.	C3b binds bacteria.
	Opsonins—C3b and IgG are the two 1° opsonins in bacterial defense; enhance phagocytosis. C3b also helps clear immune complexes.	
	Inhibitors—decay-accelerating factor (DAF, aka CD55) and C1 esterase inhibitor help prevent complement activation on self cells (eg, RBCs).	

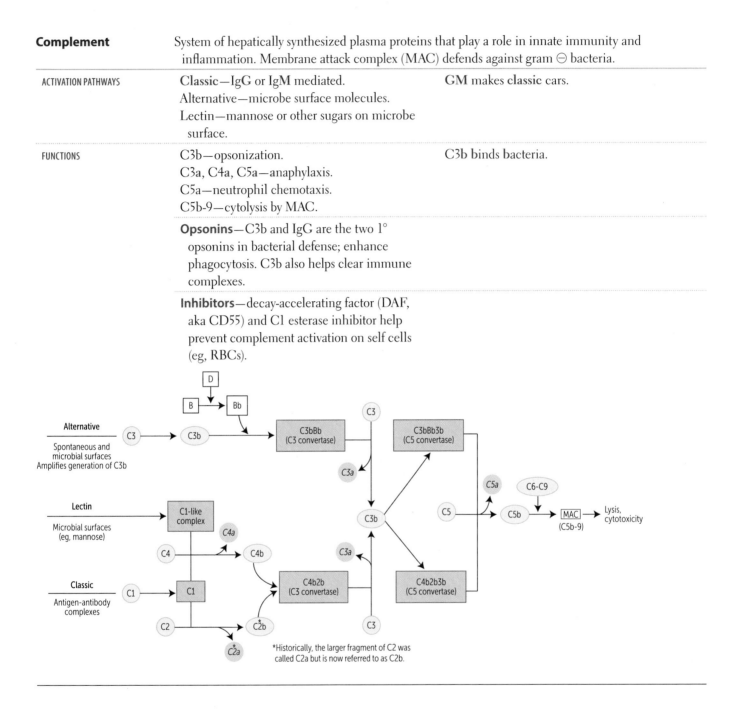

Complement disorders

Complement protein deficiencies	
Early complement deficiencies (C1-C4)	Increased risk of severe, recurrent pyogenic sinus and respiratory tract infections. Increased risk of SLE.
Terminal complement deficiencies (C5–C9)	Increased susceptibility to recurrent *Neisseria* bacteremia.

Complement regulatory protein deficiencies	
C1 esterase inhibitor deficiency	Causes hereditary angioedema due to unregulated activation of kallikrein → ↑ bradykinin. Characterized by ↓ C4 levels. ACE inhibitors are contraindicated.
Paroxysmal nocturnal hemoglobinuria	A defect in the *PIGA* gene preventing the formation of anchors for complement inhibitors, such as decay-accelerating factor (DAF/CD55) and membrane inhibitor of reactive lysis (MIRL/CD59). Causes complement-mediated lysis of RBCs.

Important cytokines

SECRETED BY MACROPHAGES		
Interleukin-1	Causes fever, acute inflammation. Activates endothelium to express adhesion molecules. Induces chemokine secretion to recruit WBCs. Also known as osteoclast-activating factor.	"Hot T-bone stEAK": IL-1: fever (**hot**). IL-2: stimulates **T** cells. IL-3: stimulates **bone** marrow. IL-4: stimulates IgE production. IL-5: stimulates IgA production. IL-6: stimulates a**K**ute-phase protein production.
Interleukin-6	Causes fever and stimulates production of acute-phase proteins.	
Interleukin-8	Major chemotactic factor for neutrophils.	"**Clean up on aisle 8**." Neutrophils are recruited by IL-8 to **clear** infections.
Interleukin-12	Induces differentiation of T cells into Th1 cells. Activates NK cells.	
Tumor necrosis factor-α	Activates endothelium. Causes WBC recruitment, vascular leak.	Causes cachexia in malignancy. Maintains granulomas in TB. IL-1, IL-6, TNF-α can mediate fever and sepsis.
SECRETED BY ALL T CELLS		
Interleukin-2	Stimulates growth of helper, cytotoxic, and regulatory T cells, and NK cells.	
Interleukin-3	Supports growth and differentiation of bone marrow stem cells. Functions like GM-CSF.	
FROM Th1 CELLS		
Interferon-γ	Secreted by NK cells and T cells in response to antigen or IL-12 from macrophages; stimulates macrophages to kill phagocytosed pathogens. Inhibits differentiation of Th2 cells.	Also activates NK cells to kill virus-infected cells. Increases MHC expression and antigen presentation by all cells.
FROM Th2 CELLS		
Interleukin-4	Induces differentiation of T cells into Th (helper) 2 cells. Promotes growth of B cells. Enhances class switching to IgE and IgG..	Ain't too proud 2 BEG 4 help.
Interleukin-5	Promotes growth and differentiation of B cells. Enhances class switching to IgA. Stimulates growth and differentiation of eosinophils.	
Interleukin-10	Attenuates inflammatory response. Decreases expression of MHC class II and Th1 cytokines. Inhibits activated macrophages and dendritic cells. Also secreted by regulatory T cells.	TGF-β and IL-10 both attenuate the immune response.

Respiratory burst (oxidative burst)	Involves the activation of the phagocyte NADPH oxidase complex (eg, in neutrophils, monocytes), which utilizes O_2 as a substrate. Plays an important role in the immune response → rapid release of reactive oxygen species (ROS). NADPH plays a role in both the creation and neutralization of ROS. Myeloperoxidase contains a blue-green heme-containing pigment that gives sputum its color.

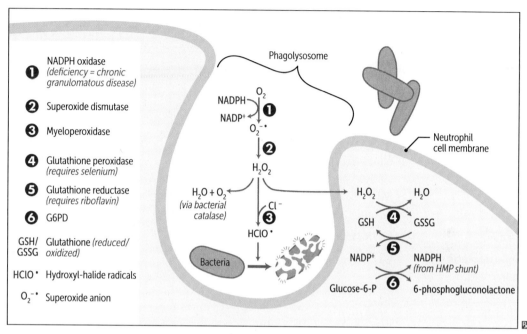

Phagocytes of patients with CGD can utilize H_2O_2 generated by invading organisms and convert it to ROS. Patients are at ↑ risk for infection by catalase ⊕ species (eg, *S aureus*, *Aspergillus*) capable of neutralizing their own H_2O_2, leaving phagocytes without ROS for fighting infections. Pyocyanin of *P aeruginosa* generates ROS to kill competing pathogens. Oxidative burst also leads to K^+ influx, which releases lysosomal enzymes from proteoglycans. Lactoferrin is a protein found in secretory fluids and neutrophils that inhibits microbial growth via iron chelation.

Interferon-α and -β	A part of innate host defense against both RNA and DNA viruses. Interferons are glycoproteins synthesized by virus-infected cells that act on local cells, "priming them" for viral defense by downregulating protein synthesis to resist potential viral replication and upregulating MHC expression to facilitate recognition of infected cells.	Interfere with viruses.

Cell surface proteins

T cells	TCR (binds antigen-MHC complex) CD3 (associated with TCR for signal transduction) CD28 (binds B7 on APC)	
Helper T cells	CD4, CD40L, CXCR4/CCR5 (co-receptor for HIV)	
Cytotoxic T cells	CD8	
Regulatory T cells	CD4, CD25	
B cells	Ig (binds antigen) CD19, CD20, CD21 (receptor for EBV), CD40 MHC II, B7	You can drink Beer at the Bar when you're 21: B cells, Epstein-Barr virus, CD21.
Macrophages	CD14 (receptor for PAMPs, eg, LPS), CD40 CCR5 MHC II, B7 (CD80/86) Fc and C3b receptors (enhanced phagocytosis)	
NK cells	CD16, CD56 (suggestive marker for NK)	
Hematopoietic stem cells	CD34	

Anergy	State during which a cell cannot become activated by exposure to its antigen. T and B cells become anergic when exposed to their antigen without costimulatory signal (signal 2). Another mechanism of self-tolerance.

Passive vs active immunity

	Passive	Active
MEANS OF ACQUISITION	Receiving preformed antibodies	Exposure to foreign antigens
ONSET	Rapid	Slow
DURATION	Short span of antibodies (half-life = 3 weeks)	Long-lasting protection (memory)
EXAMPLES	IgA in breast milk, maternal IgG crossing placenta, antitoxin, humanized monoclonal antibody	Natural infection, vaccines, toxoid
NOTES	After exposure to Tetanus toxin, Botulinum toxin, HBV, Varicella, Rabies virus, or diphtheria toxin, unvaccinated patients are given preformed antibodies (passive)—"To Be Healed Very Rapidly"	Combined passive and active immunizations can be given for hepatitis B or rabies exposure

Vaccination   Induces an active immune response (humoral and/or cellular) to specific pathogens.

VACCINE TYPE	DESCRIPTION	PROS/CONS	EXAMPLES
Live attenuated vaccine	Microorganism loses its pathogenicity but retains capacity for transient growth within inoculated host. Induces **cellular and humoral responses**. MMR and varicella vaccines can be given to HIV ⊕ patients without evidence of immunity if CD4 cell count ≥ 200 cells/mm^3.	Pros: induces strong, often lifelong immunity. Cons: may revert to virulent form. Often contraindicated in pregnancy and immunodeficiency.	Adenovirus (nonattenuated, given to military recruits), Polio (sabin), Varicella (chickenpox), Smallpox, BCG, Yellow fever, Influenza (intranasal), **MMR**, Rotavirus "Attention! Please Vaccinate **Small, Beautiful Young Infants with MMR Regularly!**"
Killed or inactivated vaccine	Pathogen is inactivated by heat or chemicals. Maintaining epitope structure on surface antigens is important for immune response. Mainly induces a **humoral response**.	Pros: safer than live vaccines. Cons: weaker immune response; booster shots usually required.	Rabies, Influenza (injection), Polio (Salk), hepatitis A **SalK = Killed** **RIP Always**
Subunit	Includes only the antigens that best stimulate the immune system.	Pros: lower chance of adverse reactions. Cons: expensive, weaker immune response.	HBV (antigen = HBsAg), HPV (types 6, 11, 16, and 18), acellular pertussis (aP), *Neisseria meningitidis* (various strains), *Streptococcus pneumoniae*, *Haemophilus influenzae* type b.
Toxoid	Denatured bacterial toxin with an intact receptor binding site. Stimulates the immune system to make antibodies without potential for causing disease.	Pros: protects against the bacterial toxins. Cons: antitoxin levels decrease with time, may require a booster.	*Clostridium tetani, Corynebacterium diphtheriae*

Hypersensitivity types	Four types (ABCD): Anaphylactic and Atopic (type I), AntiBody-mediated (type II), Immune Complex (type III), Delayed (cell-mediated, type IV). Types I, II, and III are all antibody-mediated.	
Type I hypersensitivity Allergen — Allergen-specific IgE Fc receptor for IgE Degranulation 〒	Anaphylactic and atopic—two phases: ▪ Immediate (minutes): antigen crosslinks preformed IgE on presensitized mast cells → immediate degranulation → release of histamine (a vasoactive amine) and tryptase (a marker of mast cell activation). ▪ Late (hours): chemokines (attract inflammatory cells, eg, eosinophils) and cytokines (eg, leukotrienes) from mast cells → inflammation and tissue damage.	First (type) and Fast (anaphylaxis). Test: skin test or blood test (ELISA) for allergen-specific IgE. Example: ▪ Anaphylaxis (eg, food, drug, or bee sting allergies)
Type II hypersensitivity NK cell Fc receptor for IgG Surface antigen Abnormal cell Antibody-dependent cellular cytotoxicity 〒	Antibodies bind to cell-surface antigens → cellular destruction, inflammation, and cellular dysfunction. Cellular destruction—cell is opsonized (coated) by antibodies, leading to either: ▪ Phagocytosis and/or activation of complement system. ▪ NK cell killing (antibody-dependent cellular cytotoxicity). Inflammation—binding of antibodies to cell surfaces → activation of complement system and Fc receptor-mediated inflammation. Cellular dysfunction—antibodies bind to cell surface receptors → abnormal blockade or activation of downstream process.	**Direct** Coombs test—detects antibodies attached **directly** to the RBC surface. Indirect Coombs test—detects presence of unbound antibodies in the serum Examples: ▪ Autoimmune-hemolytic anemia ▪ Immune thrombocytopenia ▪ Transfusion reactions ▪ Hemolytic disease of the newborn Examples: ▪ Goodpasture syndrome ▪ Rheumatic fever ▪ Hyperacute transplant rejection Examples: ▪ Myasthenia gravis ▪ Graves disease ▪ Pemphigus vulgaris

Hypersensitivity types (continued)

Type III hypersensitivity

Neutrophils

Enzymes from neutrophils damage endothelial cells

Immune complex—antigen-antibody (mostly IgG) complexes activate complement, which attracts neutrophils; neutrophils release lysosomal enzymes.

Can be associated with vasculitis and systemic manifestations.

Serum sickness—the prototype immune complex disease. Antibodies to foreign proteins are produced and 1–2 weeks later, antibody-antigen complexes form and deposit in tissues → complement activation → inflammation and tissue damage.

Arthus reaction—a local subacute immune complex-mediated hypersensitivity reaction. Intradermal injection of antigen into a presensitized (has circulating IgG) individual leads to immune complex formation in the skin. Characterized by edema, necrosis, and activation of complement.

In type III reaction, imagine an immune complex as 3 things stuck together: antigen-antibody-complement.

Examples:

- SLE
- Polyarteritis nodosa
- Poststreptococcal glomerulonephritis

Fever, urticaria, arthralgia, proteinuria, lymphadenopathy occur 1–2 weeks after antigen exposure. Serum sickness-like reactions are associated with some drugs (may act as haptens, eg, penicillin) and infections (eg, hepatitis B).

Type IV hypersensitivity

Antigen presenting cell

Antigen

Sensitized Th1 cell

Cytokines

Activated macrophage

Delayed-type hypersensitivity

Two mechanisms, each involving T cells:

1. Direct cell cytotoxicity: CD8+ cytotoxic T cells kill targeted cells.
2. Inflammatory reaction: effector CD4+ T cells recognize antigen and release inflammation-inducing cytokines (shown in illustration).

Response does not involve antibodies (vs types I, II, and III).

Examples: contact dermatitis (eg, poison ivy, nickel allergy) and graft-versus-host disease.

Tests (purpose): PPD (tuberculosis infection); patch test (cause of contact dermatitis); *Candida* extract (T cell immune function).

4T's: T cells, Transplant rejections, TB skin tests, Touching (contact dermatitis).

Fourth (type) and last (delayed).

Blood transfusion reactions

TYPE	PATHOGENESIS	CLINICAL PRESENTATION	TIMING
Allergic/anaphylactic reaction	Type I hypersensitivity reaction against plasma proteins in transfused blood. IgA-deficient individuals must receive blood products without IgA.	Urticaria, pruritus, fever, wheezing, hypotension, respiratory arrest, shock.	Within minutes to 2–3 hours
Febrile nonhemolytic transfusion reaction	Two known mechanisms: type II hypersensitivity reaction with host antibodies against donor HLA and WBCs; and induced by cytokines that are created and accumulate during the storage of blood products.	Fever, headaches, chills, flushing.	Within 1–6 hours
Acute hemolytic transfusion reaction	Type II hypersensitivity reaction. Intravascular hemolysis (ABO blood group incompatibility) or extravascular hemolysis (host antibody reaction against foreign antigen on donor RBCs).	Fever, hypotension, tachypnea, tachycardia, flank pain, hemoglobinuria (intravascular hemolysis), jaundice (extravascular).	Within 1 hour
Transfusion-related acute lung injury	Donor anti-leukocyte antibodies against recipient neutrophils and pulmonary endothelial cells.	Respiratory distress and noncardiogenic pulmonary edema.	Within 6 hours

Autoantibodies

AUTOANTIBODY	ASSOCIATED DISORDER
Anti-ACh receptor	Myasthenia gravis
Anti-presynaptic voltage-gated calcium channel	Lambert-Eaton myasthenic syndrome
Anti-β_2 glycoprotein	Antiphospholipid syndrome
Antinuclear (ANA)	Nonspecific screening antibody, often associated with SLE
Anticardiolipin, lupus anticoagulant	SLE, antiphospholipid syndrome
Anti-dsDNA, anti-Smith	SLE
Anti-histone	Drug-induced lupus
Anti-U1 RNP (ribonucleoprotein)	Mixed connective tissue disease
Rheumatoid factor (IgM antibody against IgG Fc region), anti-CCP (more specific)	Rheumatoid arthritis
Anti-Ro/SSA, anti-La/SSB	Sjögren syndrome
Anti-Scl-70 (anti-DNA topoisomerase I)	Scleroderma (diffuse)
Anticentromere	Limited scleroderma (CREST syndrome)
Antisynthetase (eg, anti-Jo-1), anti-SRP, anti-helicase (anti-Mi-2)	Polymyositis, dermatomyositis
Antimitochondrial 1° biliary cirrhosis	1° biliary cholangitis
Anti-smooth muscle	Autoimmune hepatitis type 1
MPO-ANCA/p-ANCA	Microscopic polyangiitis, eosinophilic granulomatosis with polyangiitis (Churg-Strauss syndrome), ulcerative colitis
PR3-ANCA/c-ANCA	Granulomatosis with polyangiitis (Wegener)
Anti-phospholipase A_2 receptor	1° membranous nephropathy
Anti-hemidesmosome	Bullous pemphigoid
Anti-desmoglein (anti-desmosome)	Pemphigus vulgaris
Antimicrosomal, antithyroglobulin, antithyroid peroxidase	Hashimoto thyroiditis
Anti-TSH receptor	Graves disease
IgA anti-endomysial, IgA anti-tissue transglutaminase, IgA and IgG deamidated gliadin peptide	Celiac disease
Anti-glutamic acid decarboxylase, islet cell cytoplasmic antibodies	Type 1 diabetes mellitus
Antiparietal cell, anti-intrinsic factor	Pernicious anemia
Anti-glomerular basement membrane	Goodpasture syndrome

Immunodeficiencies

DISEASE	DEFECT	PRESENTATION	FINDINGS
B-cell disorders			
X-linked (Bruton) agammaglobulinemia	Defect in *BTK*, a tyrosine kinase gene → no B-cell maturation. X-linked recessive (↑ in Boys).	Recurrent bacterial and enteroviral infections after 6 months (↓ maternal IgG).	Absent B cells in peripheral blood, ↓ Ig of all classes. Absent/scanty lymph nodes and tonsils. Live vaccines contraindicated.
Selective IgA deficiency	Unknown. Most common 1° immunodeficiency.	Majority Asymptomatic. Can see Airway and GI infections, Autoimmune disease, Atopy, Anaphylaxis to IgA-containing products.	↓ IgA with normal IgG, IgM levels. ↑ susceptibility to giardiasis.
Common variable immunodeficiency	Defect in B-cell differentiation. Cause is unknown in most cases.	Usually presents after age 2 and may be considerably delayed; ↑ risk of autoimmune disease, bronchiectasis, lymphoma, sinopulmonary infections.	↓ plasma cells, ↓ immunoglobulins.
T-cell disorders			
Thymic aplasia (DiGeorge syndrome)	22q11 deletion; failure to develop 3rd and 4th pharyngeal pouches → absent thymus and parathyroids.	Tetany (hypocalcemia), recurrent viral/fungal infections (T-cell deficiency), conotruncal abnormalities (eg, tetralogy of Fallot, truncus arteriosus).	↓ T cells, ↓ PTH, ↓ Ca^{2+}. Thymic shadow absent on CXR.
IL-12 receptor deficiency	↓ Th1 response. Autosomal recessive.	Disseminated mycobacterial and fungal infections; may present after administration of BCG vaccine.	↓ IFN-γ.
Autosomal dominant hyper-IgE syndrome (Job syndrome)	Deficiency of Th17 cells due to *STAT3* mutation → impaired recruitment of neutrophils to sites of infection.	FATED: coarse Facies, cold (noninflamed) staphylococcal Abscesses, retained primary Teeth, ↑ IgE, Dermatologic problems (eczema). Bone fractures from minor trauma.	↑ IgE. ↑ eosinophils.
Chronic mucocutaneous candidiasis	T-cell dysfunction. Can result from congenital genetic defects in IL-17 or IL-17 receptors.	Noninvasive *Candida albicans* infections of skin and mucous membranes.	Absent in vitro T-cell proliferation in response to *Candida* antigens. Absent cutaneous reaction to *Candida* antigens.

Immunodeficiencies (continued)

DISEASE	DEFECT	PRESENTATION	FINDINGS
B- and T-cell disorders			
Severe combined immunodeficiency	Several types including defective IL-2R gamma chain (most common, X-linked recessive), adenosine deaminase deficiency (autosomal recessive).	Failure to thrive, chronic diarrhea, thrush. Recurrent viral, bacterial, fungal, and protozoal infections. Treatment: avoid live vaccines, give antimicrobial prophylaxis and IVIG; bone marrow transplant curative (no concern for rejection).	↓ T-cell receptor excision circles (TRECs). Absence of thymic shadow (CXR), germinal centers (lymph node biopsy), and T cells (flow cytometry).
Ataxia-telangiectasia 	Defects in *ATM* gene → failure to detect DNA damage → failure to halt progression of cell cycle → mutations accumulate; autosomal recessive.	Triad: cerebellar defects (Ataxia), spider Angiomas (telangiectasia **A**), IgA deficiency.	↑ AFP. ↓ IgA, IgG, and IgE. Lymphopenia, cerebellar atrophy. ↑ risk of lymphoma and leukemia.
Hyper-IgM syndrome	Most commonly due to defective CD40L on Th cells → class switching defect; X-linked recessive.	Severe pyogenic infections early in life; opportunistic infection with *Pneumocystis*, *Cryptosporidium*, CMV.	Normal or ↑ IgM. ↓↓ IgG, IgA, IgE. Failure to make germinal centers.
Wiskott-Aldrich syndrome	Mutation in *WASp* gene; leukocytes and platelets unable to reorganize actin cytoskeleton → defective antigen presentation; X-linked recessive.	WATER: Wiskott-Aldrich: Thrombocytopenia, Eczema, Recurrent (pyogenic) infections. ↑ risk of autoimmune disease and malignancy.	↓ to normal IgG, IgM. ↑ IgE, IgA. Fewer and smaller platelets.
Phagocyte dysfunction			
Leukocyte adhesion deficiency (type 1)	Defect in LFA-1 integrin (CD18) protein on phagocytes; impaired migration and chemotaxis; autosomal recessive.	Recurrent skin and mucosal bacterial infections, absent pus, impaired wound healing, delayed (> 30 days) separation of umbilical cord.	↑ neutrophils in blood. Absence of neutrophils at infection sites.
Chédiak-Higashi syndrome 	Defect in lysosomal trafficking regulator gene (*LYST*). Microtubule dysfunction in phagosome-lysosome fusion; autosomal recessive.	PLAIN: Progressive neurodegeneration, Lymphohistiocytosis, Albinism (partial), recurrent pyogenic Infections by staphylococci and streptococci, peripheral Neuropathy.	Giant granules (**B**, arrows) in granulocytes and platelets. Pancytopenia. Mild coagulation defects.
Chronic granulomatous disease	Defect of NADPH oxidase → ↓ reactive oxygen species (eg, superoxide) and ↓ respiratory burst in neutrophils; X-linked form most common.	↑ susceptibility to catalase ⊕ organisms.	Abnormal dihydrorhodamine (flow cytometry) test (↓ green fluorescence). Nitroblue tetrazolium dye reduction test (obsolete) fails to turn blue.

Infections in immunodeficiency

PATHOGEN	↓ T CELLS	↓ B CELLS	↓ GRANULOCYTES	↓ COMPLEMENT
Bacteria	Sepsis	Encapsulated (Please **SHINE** my **SKiS**): *Pseudomonas aeruginosa*, *Streptococcus pneumoniae*, *Haemophilus Influenzae* type b, *Neisseria meningitidis*, *Escherichia coli*, *Salmonella*, *Klebsiella pneumoniae*, Group B *Streptococcus*	*Staphylococcus*, *Burkholderia cepacia*, *Pseudomonas aeruginosa*, *Serratia*, *Nocardia*	Encapsulated species with early complement deficiencies *Neisseria* with late complement (C5–C9) deficiencies
Viruses	CMV, EBV, JC virus, VZV, chronic infection with respiratory/GI viruses	Enteroviral encephalitis, poliovirus (live vaccine contraindicated)	N/A	N/A
Fungi/parasites	*Candida* (local), PCP, *Cryptococcus*	GI giardiasis (no IgA)	*Candida* (systemic), *Aspergillus*, *Mucor*	N/A

Note: B-cell deficiencies tend to produce recurrent bacterial infections, whereas T-cell deficiencies produce more fungal and viral infections.

Grafts

Autograft	From self.
Syngeneic graft (isograft)	From identical twin or clone.
Allograft	From nonidentical individual of same species.
Xenograft	From different species.

Transplant rejection

TYPE OF REJECTION	ONSET	PATHOGENESIS	FEATURES
Hyperacute	Within minutes	Pre-existing recipient antibodies react to donor antigen (type II hypersensitivity reaction), activate complement.	Widespread thrombosis of graft vessels → ischemia/necrosis. Graft must be removed.
Acute	Weeks to months	Cellular: CD8+ T cells and/ or CD4+ T cells activated against donor MHCs (type IV hypersensitivity reaction). Humoral: similar to hyperacute, except antibodies develop after transplant.	Vasculitis of graft vessels with dense interstitial lymphocytic infiltrate. Prevent/reverse with immunosuppressants.
Chronic	Months to years	CD4+ T cells respond to recipient APCs presenting donor peptides, including allogeneic MHC. Both cellular and humoral components (type II and IV hypersensitivity reactions).	Recipient T cells react and secrete cytokines → proliferation of vascular smooth muscle, parenchymal atrophy, interstitial fibrosis. Dominated by arteriosclerosis. Organ-specific examples: ▪ Bronchiolitis obliterans (lung) ▪ Accelerated atherosclerosis (heart) ▪ Chronic graft nephropathy (kidney) ▪ Vanishing bile duct syndrome (liver)
Graft-versus-host disease	Varies	Grafted immunocompetent T cells proliferate in the immunocompromised host and reject host cells with "foreign" proteins → severe organ dysfunction. Type IV hypersensitivity reaction.	Maculopapular rash, jaundice, diarrhea, hepatosplenomegaly. Usually in bone marrow and liver transplants (rich in lymphocytes). Potentially beneficial in bone marrow transplant for leukemia (graft-versus-tumor effect).

▶ IMMUNOLOGY—IMMUNOSUPPRESSANTS

Immunosuppressants　Agents that block lymphocyte activation and proliferation. Reduce acute transplant rejection by suppressing cellular immunity (used as prophylaxis). Frequently combined to achieve greater efficacy with ↓ toxicity. Chronic suppression ↑ risk of infection and malignancy.

DRUG	MECHANISM	OTHER USE	TOXICITY	NOTES
Cyclosporine	Calcineurin inhibitor; binds cyclophilin. Blocks T-cell activation by **preventing IL-2 transcription.**	Psoriasis, rheumatoid arthritis.	**Nephrotoxicity,** hypertension, hyperlipidemia, neurotoxicity, gingival hyperplasia, hirsutism.	Both calcineurin inhibitors are highly nephrotoxic.
Tacrolimus (FK506)	Calcineurin inhibitor; binds FK506 binding protein (FKBP). Blocks T-cell activation by **preventing IL-2 transcription.**		Similar to cyclosporine, ↑ risk of diabetes and neurotoxicity; no gingival hyperplasia or hirsutism.	
Sirolimus (Rapamycin)	mTOR inhibitor; binds FKBP. Blocks T-cell activation and B-cell differentiation by **preventing response to IL-2.**	Kidney transplant rejection prophylaxis specifically.	"PanSirtopenia" (pancytopenia), insulin resistance, hyperlipidemia; **not nephrotoxic.**	Kidney "sir-vives." Synergistic with cyclosporine. Also used in drug-eluting stents.
Basiliximab	Monoclonal antibody; blocks IL-2R.		Edema, hypertension, tremor.	
Azathioprine	Antimetabolite precursor of 6-mercaptopurine. Inhibits lymphocyte proliferation by blocking nucleotide synthesis.	Rheumatoid arthritis, Crohn disease, glomerulonephritis, other autoimmune conditions.	Pancytopenia.	6-MP degraded by xanthine oxidase; toxicity ↑ by allopurinol. Pronounce "azathio-purine."
Mycophenolate Mofetil	Reversibly inhibits IMP dehydrogenase, preventing purine synthesis of B and T cells.	Lupus nephritis.	GI upset, pancytopenia, hypertension, hyperglycemia. Less nephrotoxic and neurotoxic.	Associated with invasive CMV infection.
Glucocorticoids	Inhibit NF-κB. Suppress both B- and T-cell function by ↓ transcription of many cytokines. Induce T cell apoptosis.	Many autoimmune and inflammatory disorders, adrenal insufficiency, asthma, CLL, non-Hodgkin lymphoma.	Cushing syndrome, osteoporosis, hyperglycemia, diabetes, amenorrhea, adrenocortical atrophy, peptic ulcers, psychosis, cataracts, avascular necrosis (femoral head).	Demargination of WBCs causes artificial leukocytosis. Adrenal insufficiency may develop if drug is stopped abruptly after chronic use.

Immunosuppression targets

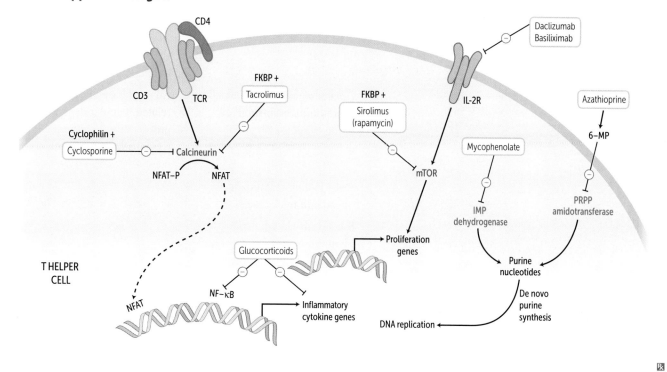

Recombinant cytokines and clinical uses

CYTOKINE	AGENT	CLINICAL USES
Bone marrow stimulation		
Erythropoietin	Epoetin alfa (EPO analog)	Anemias (especially in renal failure)
Colony stimulating factors	Filgrastim (G-CSF), Sargramostim (GM-CSF)	Leukopenia; recovery of granulocyte and monocyte counts
Thrombopoietin	Romiplostim (TPO analog), eltrombopag (TPO receptor agonist)	Autoimmune thrombocytopenia
Immunotherapy		
Interleukin-2	Aldesleukin	Renal cell carcinoma, metastatic melanoma
Interferon	IFN-α	Chronic hepatitis C (not preferred) and B, renal cell carcinoma
	IFN-β	Multiple sclerosis
	IFN-γ	Chronic granulomatous disease

Therapeutic antibodies

AGENT	TARGET	CLINICAL USE	NOTES
Cancer therapy			
Alemtuzumab	CD52	CLL, MS	"Alymtuzumab"—chronic lymphocytic leukemia
Bevacizumab	VEGF	Colorectal cancer, renal cell carcinoma, non-small cell lung cancer	Also used for neovascular age-related macular degeneration, proliferative diabetic retinopathy, and macular edema
Cetuximab	EGFR	Stage IV colorectal cancer, head and neck cancer	
Rituximab	CD20	B-cell non-Hodgkin lymphoma, CLL, rheumatoid arthritis, ITP, multiple sclerosis	
Trastuzumab	HER2	Breast cancer, gastric cancer	HER2—"tras2zumab"
Autoimmune disease therapy			
Adalimumab, certolizumab, golimumab, infliximab	Soluble TNF-α	IBD, rheumatoid arthritis, ankylosing spondylitis, psoriasis	Etanercept is a decoy TNF-α receptor and not a monoclonal antibody
Daclizumab	CD25 (part of IL-2 receptor)	Relapsing multiple sclerosis	
Eculizumab	Complement protein C5	Paroxysmal nocturnal hemoglobinuria	
Natalizumab	α4-integrin	Multiple sclerosis, Crohn disease	α4-integrin: WBC adhesion Risk of PML in patients with JC virus
Ustekinumab	IL-12/IL-23	Psoriasis, psoriatic arthritis	
Other applications			
Abciximab	Platelet glycoproteins IIb/IIIa	Antiplatelet agent for prevention of ischemic complications in patients undergoing percutaneous coronary intervention	IIb times IIIa equals "absiximab"
Denosumab	RANKL	Osteoporosis; inhibits osteoclast maturation (mimics osteoprotegerin)	Denosumab affects osteoclasts
Digoxin immune Fab	Digoxin	Antidote for digoxin toxicity	
Omalizumab	IgE	Refractory allergic asthma; prevents IgE binding to FcεRI	
Palivizumab	RSV F protein	RSV prophylaxis for high-risk infants	PaliVIzumab—VIrus

Microbiology

"Support bacteria. They're the only culture some people have."
—Steven Wright

"What lies behind us and what lies ahead of us are tiny matters compared to what lies within us."
—Henry S. Haskins

"Infectious disease is merely a disagreeable instance of a widely prevalent tendency of all living creatures to save themselves the bother of building, by their own efforts, the things they require."
—Hans Zinsser

Microbiology questions on the Step 1 exam often require two (or more) steps: Given a certain clinical presentation, you will first need to identify the most likely causative organism, and you will then need to provide an answer regarding some feature of that organism. For example, a description of a child with fever and a petechial rash will be followed by a question that reads, "From what site does the responsible organism usually enter the blood?"

This section therefore presents organisms in two major ways: in individual microbial "profiles" and in the context of the systems they infect and the clinical presentations they produce. You should become familiar with both formats. When reviewing the systems approach, remind yourself of the features of each microbe by returning to the individual profiles. Also be sure to memorize the laboratory characteristics that allow you to identify microbes.

▶ MICROBIOLOGY—BASIC BACTERIOLOGY

Bacterial structures

STRUCTURE	CHEMICAL COMPOSITION	FUNCTION
Appendages		
Flagellum	Proteins.	Motility.
Pilus/fimbria	Glycoprotein.	Mediate adherence of bacteria to cell surface; sex pilus forms during conjugation.
Specialized structures		
Spore	Keratin-like coat; dipicolinic acid; peptidoglycan, DNA.	Gram ⊕ only. Survival: resist dehydration, heat, chemicals.
Cell envelope		
Capsule	Organized, discrete polysaccharide layer (except poly-D-glutamate on *B anthracis*).	Protects against phagocytosis.
Glycocalyx	Loose network of polysaccharides.	Mediates adherence to surfaces, especially foreign surfaces (eg, indwelling catheters).
Outer membrane	Outer leaflet: contains endotoxin (LPS/LOS). Embedded proteins: porins and other outer membrane proteins (OMPs) Inner leaflet: phospholipids.	Gram ⊖ only. Endotoxin: lipid A induces TNF and IL-1; antigenic O polysaccharide component. Most OMPs are antigenic. Porins: transport across outer membrane.
Periplasm	Space between cytoplasmic membrane and outer membrane in gram ⊖ bacteria. (Peptidoglycan in middle.)	Accumulates components exiting gram ⊖ cells, including hydrolytic enzymes (eg, β-lactamases).
Cell wall	Peptidoglycan is a sugar backbone with peptide side chains cross-linked by transpeptidase.	Net-like structure gives rigid support, protects against osmotic pressure damage.
Cytoplasmic membrane	Phospholipid bilayer sac with embedded proteins (eg, penicillin-binding proteins [PBPs]) and other enzymes. Lipoteichoic acids (gram ⊕ only) extend from membrane to exterior.	Site of oxidative and transport enzymes; PBPs involved in cell wall synthesis. Lipoteichoic acids induce TNF-α and IL-1.

Cell envelope

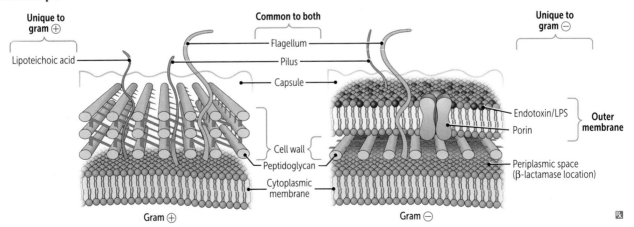

Bacterial taxonomy

MORPHOLOGY	Gram ⊕ examples	Gram ⊖ examples
Spherical (coccus)	*Staphylococcus* (clusters) *Streptococcus* (chains or pairs) *Enterococcus* (pairs or short chains)	*Moraxella catarrhalis* *Neisseria*
Rod (bacillus)	*Bacillus* *Clostridium* *Corynebacterium* *Gardnerella* (gram variable) *Lactobacillus* *Listeria* *Mycobacterium* (acid fast) *Cutibacterium* (formerly *Propionibacterium*)	Enterics: ▪ *Bacteroides* ▪ *Campylobacter* ▪ *E coli* ▪ *Enterobacter* ▪ *Fusobacterium* ▪ *Helicobacter* ▪ *Klebsiella* ▪ *Proteus* ▪ *Pseudomonas* ▪ *Salmonella* ▪ *Serratia* ▪ *Shigella* ▪ *Vibrio* ▪ *Yersinia* Respiratory: ▪ *Acinetobacter baumannii* ▪ *Bordetella* ▪ *Burkholderia cepacia* ▪ *Haemophilus* (pleomorphic) ▪ *Legionella* (silver stain) Zoonotic: ▪ *Bartonella* ▪ *Brucella* ▪ *Francisella* ▪ *Pasteurella*
Branching filamentous	*Actinomyces* *Nocardia* (weakly acid fast)	
Pleomorphic (no cell wall)		*Anaplasma, Ehrlichia* *Chlamydiae* (Giemsa) *Rickettsiae* (Giemsa) *Mycoplasma* (contains sterols, which do not Gram stain), *Ureaplasma*
Spiral		Spirochetes: ▪ *Borrelia* (Giemsa) ▪ *Leptospira* ▪ *Treponema*

Stains

Gram stain	First-line lab test in bacterial identification. Bacteria with thick peptidoglycan layer retain crystal violet dye (gram ⊕); bacteria with thin peptidoglycan layer turn red or pink (gram ⊖) with counterstain. These bugs do not Gram stain well (These Little Microbes May Unfortunately Lack Real Color But Are Everywhere).	
	Treponema, *Leptospira*	Too thin to be visualized.
	Mycobacteria	Cell wall has high lipid content.
	Mycoplasma, Ureaplasma	No cell wall.
	Legionella, Rickettsia, Chlamydia, Bartonella, Anaplasma, Ehrlichia	Primarily intracellular; also, *Chlamydia* lack classic peptidoglycan because of ↓ muramic acid.
Giemsa stain	*Rickettsia, Chlamydia*, Trypanosomes **A**, *Plasmodium, Borrelia*	Ricky got *Chlamydia* as he Tried to Please the Bored "Geisha."
Periodic acid–Schiff stain	Stains glycogen, mucopolysaccharides; used to diagnose Whipple disease (*Tropheryma whipplei* **B**)	PaSs the sugar.
Ziehl-Neelsen stain (carbol fuchsin)	Acid-fast bacteria (eg, *Mycobacteria* **C**, *Nocardia*; stains mycolic acid in cell wall); protozoa (eg, *Cryptosporidium* oocysts)	Auramine-rhodamine stain is more often used for screening (inexpensive, more sensitive).
India ink stain	*Cryptococcus neoformans* **D**; mucicarmine can also be used to stain thick polysaccharide capsule red	
Silver stain	Fungi (eg, *Coccidioides* **E**, *Pneumocystis jirovecii*), *Legionella, Helicobacter pylori*	
Fluorescent antibody stain	Used to identify many bacteria and viruses.	Example is FTA-ABS for syphilis.

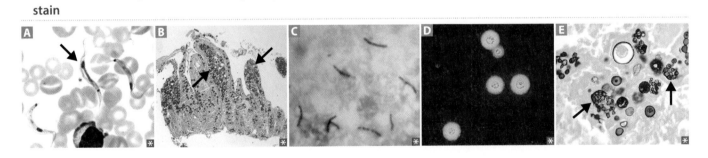

Properties of growth media

Properties of growth media	The same type of media can possess both (or neither) of these properties.
Selective media	Favors the growth of particular organism while preventing growth of other organisms, eg, Thayer-Martin agar contains antibiotics that allow the selective growth of *Neisseria* by inhibiting the growth of other sensitive organisms.
Indicator (differential) media	Yields a color change in response to the metabolism of certain organisms, eg, MacConkey agar contains a pH indicator; a lactose fermenter like *E coli* will convert lactose to acidic metabolites → color change.

Special culture requirements

BUG	MEDIA USED FOR ISOLATION	MEDIA CONTENTS/OTHER
H influenzae	Chocolate agar	Factors V (NAD$^+$) and X (hematin)
N gonorrhoeae, N meningitidis	Thayer-Martin agar	Selectively favors growth of *Neisseria* by inhibiting growth of gram ⊕ organisms with **V**ancomycin, gram ⊖ organisms except *Neisseria* with **T**rimethoprim and **C**olistin, and fungi with **N**ystatin **V**ery **T**ypically **C**ultures **N**eisseria
B pertussis	Bordet-Gengou agar (**Bordet** for *Bordetella*) Regan-Lowe medium	Potato extract Charcoal, blood, and antibiotic
C diphtheriae	Tellurite agar, Löffler medium	
M tuberculosis	Löwenstein-Jensen agar	
M pneumoniae	Eaton agar	Requires cholesterol
Lactose-fermenting enterics	MacConkey agar	Fermentation produces acid, causing colonies to turn pink
E coli	Eosin–methylene blue (EMB) agar	Colonies with green metallic sheen
Legionella	Charcoal yeast extract agar buffered with cysteine and iron	
Fungi	Sabouraud agar	"Sab's a **fun guy!**"

Aerobes	Use an O_2-dependent system to generate ATP. Examples include *Nocardia*, *Pseudomonas aeruginosa*, and **M**yco**B**acterium *tuberculosis*. Reactivation of *M tuberculosis* (eg, after immunocompromise or TNF-α inhibitor use) has a predilection for the apices of the lung.	**N**agging **P**ests **M**ust **B**reathe.
Anaerobes	Examples include *Clostridium*, *Bacteroides*, *Fusobacterium*, and *Actinomyces israelii*. They lack catalase and/or superoxide dismutase and are thus susceptible to oxidative damage. Generally foul smelling (short-chain fatty acids), are difficult to culture, and produce gas in tissue (CO_2 and H_2).	**A**naerobes **C**an't **B**reathe **F**resh **A**ir. Anaerobes are normal flora in GI tract, typically pathogenic elsewhere. AminO_2glycosides are ineffective against anaerobes because these antibiotics require O_2 to enter into bacterial cell.
Facultative anaerobes	May use O_2 as a terminal electron acceptor to generate ATP, but can also use fermentation and other O_2-independent pathways.	Streptococci, staphylococci, and enteric gram ⊖ bacteria.

Intracellular bugs

Obligate intracellular	*Rickettsia*, *CHlamydia*, *COxiella*. Rely on host ATP.	Stay inside (cells) when it is Really CHilly and COld.
Facultative intracellular	*Salmonella*, *Neisseria*, *Brucella*, *Mycobacterium*, *Listeria*, *Francisella*, *Legionella*, *Yersinia pestis*.	Some Nasty Bugs May Live FacultativeLY.

Encapsulated bacteria 	Examples are *Pseudomonas aeruginosa*, *Streptococcus pneumoniae* **A**, *Haemophilus influenzae* type b, *Neisseria meningitidis*, *Escherichia coli*, *Salmonella*, *Klebsiella pneumoniae*, and group B Strep. Their capsules serve as an antiphagocytic virulence factor. Capsular polysaccharide + protein conjugate serves as an antigen in vaccines.	Please SHiNE my SKiS. Are opsonized, and then cleared by spleen. Asplenics (No Spleen Here) have ↓ opsonizing ability and thus ↑ risk for severe infections; need vaccines to protect against: ▪ *N meningitidis* ▪ *S pneumoniae* ▪ *H influenzae*
Encapsulated bacteria vaccines	Some vaccines containing polysaccharide capsule antigens are conjugated to a carrier protein, enhancing immunogenicity by promoting T-cell activation and subsequent class switching. A polysaccharide antigen alone cannot be presented to T cells.	Pneumococcal vaccines: PCV13 (pneumococcal conjugate vaccine), PPSV23 (pneumococcal polysaccharide vaccine with no conjugated protein) *H influenzae* type b (conjugate vaccine) Meningococcal vaccine (conjugate vaccine)
Urease-positive organisms	*Proteus*, *Cryptococcus*, *H pylori*, *Ureaplasma*, *Nocardia*, *Klebsiella*, *S epidermidis*, *S saprophyticus*. Urease hydrolyzes urea to release ammonia and $CO_2 \rightarrow$ ↑ pH. Predisposes to struvite (ammonium magnesium phosphate) stones, particularly *Proteus*.	Pee CHUNKSS.
Catalase-positive organisms 	Catalase degrades H_2O_2 into H_2O and bubbles of O_2 **A** before it can be converted to microbicidal products by the enzyme myeloperoxidase. People with chronic granulomatous disease (NADPH oxidase deficiency) have recurrent infections with certain catalase ⊕ organisms. Examples: *Nocardia*, *Pseudomonas*, *Listeria*, *Aspergillus*, *Candida*, *E coli*, Staphylococci, *Serratia*, *B cepacia*, *H pylori*.	Cats Need **PLACESS** to Belch their Hairballs.

Pigment-producing bacteria	*Actinomyces israelii*—yellow "sulfur" granules, which are composed of filaments of bacteria.	Israel has yellow sand.
	S aureus—yellow pigment.	*Aureus* (Latin) = gold.
	P aeruginosa—blue-green pigment (pyocyanin and pyoverdin).	Aerugula is green.
	Serratia marcescens—red pigment.	Think **red Sriracha** hot sauce.

In vivo biofilm-producing bacteria	*S epidermidis*	Catheter and prosthetic device infections
	Viridans streptococci (*S mutans, S sanguinis*)	Dental plaques, infective endocarditis
	P aeruginosa	Respiratory tree colonization in patients with cystic fibrosis, ventilator-associated pneumonia Contact lens–associated keratitis
	Nontypeable (unencapsulated) *H influenzae*	Otitis media

Bacterial virulence factors	These promote evasion of host immune response.
Protein A	Binds Fc region of IgG. Prevents opsonization and phagocytosis. Expressed by *S aureus*.
IgA protease	Enzyme that cleaves IgA, allowing bacteria to adhere to and colonize mucous membranes. Secreted by *S pneumoniae, H influenzae* type b, and *Neisseria* (**SHiN**).
M protein	Helps prevent phagocytosis. Expressed by group A streptococci. Shares similar epitopes to human cellular proteins (molecular mimicry); possibly underlies the autoimmune response seen in acute rheumatic fever.

Type III secretion system	Also known as "injectisome." Needle-like protein appendage facilitating direct delivery of toxins from certain gram ⊖ bacteria (eg, *Pseudomonas, Salmonella, Shigella, E coli*) to eukaryotic host cell.

Bacterial genetics

Transformation

Competent bacteria can bind and import short pieces of environmental naked bacterial chromosomal DNA (from bacterial cell lysis). The transfer and expression of newly transferred genes is called transformation. A feature of many bacteria, especially *S pneumoniae*, *H influenzae* type b, and *Neisseria* (**SHiN**).

Adding deoxyribonuclease degrades naked DNA, preventing transformation.

Naked DNA   Recipient cell   Transformed cell

Conjugation

$F^+ \times F^-$

F^+ plasmid contains genes required for sex pilus and conjugation. Bacteria without this plasmid are termed F^-. Sex pilus on F^+ bacterium contacts F^- bacterium. A single strand of plasmid DNA is transferred across the conjugal bridge ("mating bridge"). No transfer of chromosomal DNA.

F^+ cell F^- cell F^+ cell F^- cell F^+ cell F^+ cell

$Hfr \times F^-$

F^+ plasmid can become incorporated into bacterial chromosomal DNA, termed high-frequency recombination (Hfr) cell. Transfer of leading part of plasmid and a few flanking chromosomal genes. High-frequency recombination may integrate some of those bacterial genes. Recipient cell remains F^- but now may have new bacterial genes.

F^+ cell F^- cell   Hfr cell F^- cell   Hfr cell F^- cell   Hfr cell   Recombinant F^- cell

Transduction

Generalized

A packaging "error." Lytic phage infects bacterium, leading to cleavage of bacterial DNA. Parts of bacterial chromosomal DNA may become packaged in phage capsid. Phage infects another bacterium, transferring these genes.

Release of new phage   Infects other   Phage's genes
from lysed cell   bacteria   transferred

Specialized

An "excision" event. Lysogenic phage infects bacterium; viral DNA incorporates into bacterial chromosome. When phage DNA is excised, flanking bacterial genes may be excised with it. DNA is packaged into phage capsid and can infect another bacterium.

Genes for the following 5 bacterial toxins are encoded in a lysogenic phage (**ABCD'S**): Group A strep erythrogenic toxin, Botulinum toxin, Cholera toxin, Diphtheria toxin, Shiga toxin.

Release of new phage   Infects other   Genes different from
from lysed cell   bacteria   donor and recipient

Bacterial genetics *(continued)*

Transposition	Segment of DNA (eg, transposon) that can "jump" (copy/excise and reinsert) from one location to another, can transfer genes from plasmid to chromosome and vice versa. This is a critical process in creating plasmids with multiple antibiotic resistance which can be transferred across species lines (eg, Tn*1546* carrying *vanA* gene from vancomycin-resistant *Enterococcus* to *S aureus*).	

Spore-forming bacteria	Some bacteria can form spores **A** when nutrients are limited. Spores lack metabolic activity. Spores are highly resistant to heat and chemicals. Core contains dipicolinic acid. Must autoclave to kill spores (as is done to surgical equipment) by steaming at 121°C for 15 minutes.	*Bacillus anthracis* *Bacillus cereus* *Clostridium botulinum* *Clostridium difficile* *Clostridium perfringens* *Clostridium tetani*	Anthrax Food poisoning Botulism Pseudomembranous colitis Gas gangrene Tetanus

Main features of exotoxins and endotoxins

	Exotoxins	Endotoxin
SOURCE	Certain species of gram ⊕ and gram ⊖ bacteria	Outer cell membrane of most gram ⊖ bacteria
SECRETED FROM CELL	Yes	No
CHEMISTRY	Polypeptide	Lipid A component of LPS (structural part of bacteria; released when lysed)
LOCATION OF GENES	Plasmid or bacteriophage	Bacterial chromosome
ADVERSE EFFECTS	High (fatal dose on the order of 1 µg)	Low (fatal dose on the order of hundreds of micrograms)
CLINICAL EFFECTS	Various effects (see following pages)	Fever, shock (hypotension), DIC
MODE OF ACTION	Various modes (see following pages)	Induces TNF, IL-1, and IL-6
ANTIGENICITY	Induces high-titer antibodies called antitoxins	Poorly antigenic
VACCINES	Toxoids used as vaccines	No toxoids formed and no vaccine available
HEAT STABILITY	Destroyed rapidly at 60°C (except staphylococcal enterotoxin and *E coli* heat-stable toxin)	Stable at 100°C for 1 hr
TYPICAL DISEASES	Tetanus, botulism, diphtheria	Meningococcemia; sepsis by gram ⊖ rods

Bugs with exotoxins

BACTERIA	TOXIN	MECHANISM	MANIFESTATION
Inhibit protein synthesis			
Corynebacterium diphtheriae	Diphtheria toxin[a]	Inactivate elongation factor (EF-2)	Pharyngitis with pseudomembranes in throat and severe lymphadenopathy (bull neck)
Pseudomonas aeruginosa	Exotoxin A[a]		Host cell death
Shigella spp.	Shiga toxin (ST)[a]	Inactivate 60S ribosome by removing adenine from rRNA	GI mucosal damage → dysentery; ST also enhances cytokine release, causing hemolytic-uremic syndrome (HUS)
Enterohemorrhagic *E coli*	Shiga-like toxin (SLT)[a]		SLT enhances cytokine release, causing HUS (prototypically in EHEC serotype O157:H7). Unlike *Shigella*, EHEC does not invade host cells
Increase fluid secretion			
Enterotoxigenic *E coli*	Heat-labile toxin (LT)[a]	Overactivates adenylate cyclase (↑ cAMP) → ↑ Cl⁻ secretion in gut and H_2O efflux	Watery diarrhea: "**labile** in the **Air** (**A**denylate cyclase), **stable** on the **Ground** (**G**uanylate cyclase)"
	Heat-stable toxin (ST)	Overactivates guanylate cyclase (↑ cGMP) → ↓ resorption of NaCl and H_2O in gut	
Bacillus anthracis	Edema toxin[a]	Mimics adenylate cyclase (↑ cAMP)	Likely responsible for characteristic edematous borders of black eschar in cutaneous anthrax
Vibrio cholerae	Cholera toxin[a]	Overactivates adenylate cyclase (↑ cAMP) by permanently activating G_s → ↑ Cl⁻ secretion in gut and H_2O efflux	Voluminous "rice-water" diarrhea
Inhibit phagocytic ability			
Bordetella pertussis	Pertussis toxin[a]	Overactivates adenylate cyclase (↑ cAMP) by disabling G_i, impairing phagocytosis to permit survival of microbe	Whooping cough—child coughs on expiration and "whoops" on inspiration (toxin may not actually be a cause of cough; can cause "100-day cough" in adults)
Inhibit release of neurotransmitter			
Clostridium tetani	Tetanospasmin[a]	Both are proteases that cleave SNARE (soluble NSF attachment protein receptor), a set of proteins required for neurotransmitter release via vesicular fusion	Toxin prevents release of **inhibitory** (GABA and glycine) neurotransmitters from Renshaw cells in spinal cord → spastic paralysis, risus sardonicus, trismus (lockjaw)
Clostridium botulinum	Botulinum toxin[a]		Toxin prevents release of **stimulatory** (ACh) signals at neuromuscular junction → flaccid paralysis (floppy baby)

[a]An AB toxin (aka, two-component toxin [or three for anthrax]) with **B** enabling binding and triggering uptake (endocytosis) of the active **A** component. The A components are usually ADP ribosyltransferases; others have enzymatic activities as listed in chart.

Bugs with exotoxins *(continued)*

BACTERIA	TOXIN	MECHANISM	MANIFESTATION
Lyse cell membranes			
Clostridium perfringens	Alpha toxin	Phospholipase (lecithinase) that degrades tissue and cell membranes	Degradation of phospholipids → myonecrosis ("gas gangrene") and hemolysis ("double zone" of hemolysis on blood agar)
Streptococcus pyogenes	Streptolysin O	Protein that degrades cell membrane	Lyses RBCs; contributes to β-hemolysis; host antibodies against toxin (ASO) used to diagnose rheumatic fever (do not confuse with immune complexes of poststreptococcal glomerulonephritis)
Superantigens causing shock			
Staphylococcus aureus	Toxic shock syndrome toxin (TSST-1)	Cross-links β region of TCR to MHC class II on APCs outside of the antigen binding site → overwhelming release of IL-1, IL-2, IFN-γ, and TNF-α → shock	Toxic shock syndrome: fever, rash, shock; other toxins cause scalded skin syndrome (exfoliative toxin) and food poisoning (heat-stable enterotoxin)
Streptococcus pyogenes	Erythrogenic exotoxin A		Toxic shock–like syndrome: fever, rash, shock; scarlet fever

Endotoxin	LPS found in outer membrane of gram ⊖ bacteria (both cocci and rods). Composed of O antigen + core polysaccharide + lipid A (the toxic component).	**ENDOTOXINS:**
	Released upon cell lysis or by living cells by blebs detaching from outer surface membrane (vs exotoxin, which is actively secreted).	**E**dema
		Nitric oxide
	Three main effects: macrophage activation (TLR4/CD14), complement activation, and tissue factor activation.	**D**IC/**D**eath
		Outer membrane
		TNF-α
		O-antigen + core polysaccharide + lipid A
		e**X**tremely heat stable
		IL-1 and IL-6
		Neutrophil chemotaxis
		Shock

▶ MICROBIOLOGY—CLINICAL BACTERIOLOGY

Gram-positive lab algorithm

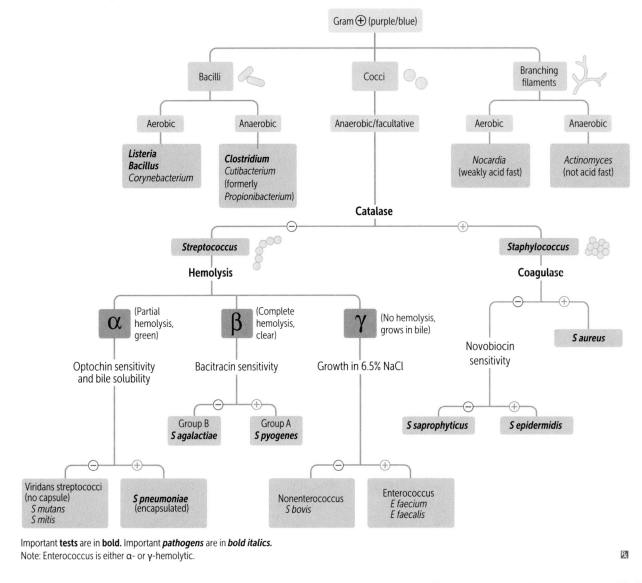

Important **tests** are in **bold**. Important ***pathogens*** are in ***bold italics.***
Note: Enterococcus is either α- or γ-hemolytic.

Gram-positive cocci antibiotic tests

Staphylococci	**NO**vobiocin—*Saprophyticus* is **R**esistant; *Epidermidis* is **S**ensitive.	On the office's "**staph**" retreat, there was **NO StRES**s.
Streptococci	**O**ptochin—*Viridans* is **R**esistant; *Pneumoniae* is **S**ensitive.	**OVRPS** (overpass).
	Bacitracin—group **B** strep are **R**esistant; group **A** strep are **S**ensitive.	**B-BRAS**.

α-hemolytic bacteria

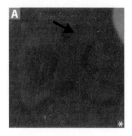

Gram ⊕ cocci. Partial reduction of hemoglobin causes greenish or brownish color without clearing around growth on blood agar ▲. Include the following organisms:
- *Streptococcus pneumoniae* (catalase ⊖ and optochin sensitive)
- Viridans streptococci (catalase ⊖ and optochin resistant)

β-hemolytic bacteria

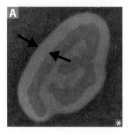

Gram ⊕ cocci. Complete lysis of RBCs → clear area surrounding colony on blood agar ▲. Include the following organisms:
- *Staphylococcus aureus* (catalase and coagulase ⊕)
- *Streptococcus pyogenes*—group A strep (catalase ⊖ and bacitracin sensitive)
- *Streptococcus agalactiae*—group B strep (catalase ⊖ and bacitracin resistant)

Staphylococcus aureus

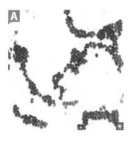

Gram ⊕, β-hemolytic, catalase ⊕, coagulase ⊕ cocci in clusters ▲. Protein A (virulence factor) binds Fc-IgG, inhibiting complement activation and phagocytosis. Commonly colonizes the nares, ears, axilla, and groin. Causes:
- Inflammatory disease—skin infections, organ abscesses, pneumonia (often after influenza virus infection), endocarditis, septic arthritis, and osteomyelitis.
- Toxin-mediated disease—toxic shock syndrome (TSST-1), scalded skin syndrome (exfoliative toxin), rapid-onset food poisoning (enterotoxins).
- MRSA (methicillin-resistant *S aureus*)— important cause of serious nosocomial and community-acquired infections; resistant to methicillin and nafcillin because of altered penicillin-binding protein.

TSST-1 is a superantigen that binds to MHC II and T-cell receptor, resulting in polyclonal T-cell activation.

Staphylococcal toxic shock syndrome (TSS)— fever, vomiting, rash, desquamation, shock, end-organ failure. TSS results in ↑ AST, ↑ ALT, ↑ bilirubin. Associated with prolonged use of vaginal tampons or nasal packing.

Compare with *Streptococcus pyogenes* TSS (a toxic shock–like syndrome associated with painful skin infection).

S aureus food poisoning due to ingestion of preformed toxin → short incubation period (2–6 hr) followed by nonbloody diarrhea and emesis. Enterotoxin is heat stable → not destroyed by cooking.

Bad staph (*aureus*) make coagulase and toxins. Forms fibrin clot around self → abscess.

Staphylococcus epidermidis

Gram ⊕, catalase ⊕, coagulase ⊖, urease ⊕ cocci in clusters. Novobiocin sensitive. Does not ferment mannitol (vs *S aureus*).

Normal flora of skin; contaminates blood cultures.

Infects prosthetic devices (eg, hip implant, heart valve) and IV catheters by producing adherent biofilms.

Staphylococcus saprophyticus

Gram ⊕, catalase ⊕, coagulase ⊖, urease ⊕ cocci in clusters. Novobiocin resistant.
Normal flora of female genital tract and perineum.
Second most common cause of uncomplicated UTI in young women (most common is *E coli*).

Streptococcus pneumoniae

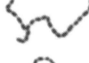

Gram ⊕, lancet-shaped diplococci .
Encapsulated. IgA protease. Optochin sensitive. Most common cause of:
- Meningitis
- Otitis media (in children)
- Pneumonia
- Sinusitis

Pneumococcus is associated with "rusty" sputum, sepsis in patients with sickle cell disease, and asplenic patients.
No virulence without capsule.
MOPS commonly spread pneumonia.

Viridans group streptococci

Gram ⊕, α-hemolytic cocci. Resistant to optochin, differentiating them from *S pneumoniae* which is α-hemolytic but optochin sensitive. Normal flora of the oropharynx.
Streptococcus mutans and *S mitis* cause dental caries.
S sanguinis makes dextrans that bind to fibrin-platelet aggregates on damaged **heart** valves, causing subacute bacterial endocarditis.

Viridans group strep live in the mouth, because they are not afraid of-the-chin (op-to-chin resistant).
Sanguinis = blood. Think, "there is lots of blood in the heart" (endocarditis).

Streptococcus pyogenes (group A streptococci)

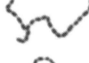

Gram ⊕ cocci in chains . Group A strep cause:
- Pyogenic—pharyngitis, cellulitis, impetigo ("honey-crusted" lesions), erysipelas
- Toxigenic—scarlet fever, toxic shock–like syndrome, necrotizing fasciitis
- Immunologic—rheumatic fever, glomerulonephritis

Bacitracin sensitive, β-hemolytic, pyrrolidonyl arylamidase (PYR) ⊕. Hyaluronic acid capsule and M protein inhibit phagocytosis. Antibodies to M protein enhance host defenses against *S pyogenes* but can give rise to rheumatic fever.
ASO titer or anti-DNase B antibodies indicate recent *S pyogenes* infection.

Pharyngitis can result in rheumatic "phever" and glomerulonephritis.
Strains causing impetigo can induce glomerulonephritis.
Scarlet fever—blanching, sandpaper-like body rash, strawberry tongue, and circumoral pallor in the setting of group A streptococcal pharyngitis (erythrogenic toxin ⊕).

***Streptococcus agalactiae* (group B streptococci)**	Gram ⊕ cocci, bacitracin resistant, β-hemolytic, colonizes vagina; causes pneumonia, meningitis, and sepsis, mainly in babies. Produces CAMP factor, which enlarges the area of hemolysis formed by *S aureus*. (Note: CAMP stands for the authors of the test, not cyclic AMP.) Hippurate test ⊕. PYR ⊖. Screen pregnant women at 35–37 weeks of gestation with rectal and vaginal swabs. Patients with ⊕ culture receive intrapartum penicillin prophylaxis.	Group B for Babies!
Streptococcus bovis	Gram ⊕ cocci, colonizes the gut. *S gallolyticus* (*S bovis* biotype 1) can cause bacteremia and subacute endocarditis and is associated with colon cancer.	Bovis in the blood = cancer in the colon.
Enterococci	Gram ⊕ cocci. Enterococci (*E faecalis* and *E faecium*) are normal colonic flora that are penicillin G resistant and cause UTI, biliary tract infections, and subacute endocarditis (following GI/GU procedures). Catalase ⊖, PYR ⊕, variable hemolysis. VRE (vancomycin-resistant enterococci) are an important cause of nosocomial infection.	Enterococci are more resilient than streptococci, can grow in 6.5% NaCl and bile (lab test). *Entero* = intestine, *faecalis* = feces, *strepto* = twisted (chains), *coccus* = berry.

Bacillus anthracis	Gram ⊕, spore-forming rod that produces anthrax toxin. The only bacterium with a polypeptide capsule (contains D-glutamate). Colonies show a halo of projections, sometimes referred to as "medusa head" appearance.
Cutaneous anthrax	Painless papule surrounded by vesicles → ulcer with black eschar (Ⓐ) (painless, necrotic) → uncommonly progresses to bacteremia and death.
Pulmonary anthrax	Inhalation of spores → flu-like symptoms that rapidly progress to fever, pulmonary hemorrhage, mediastinitis, and shock. Also known as woolsorter's disease. CXR may show widened mediastinum.

Bacillus cereus	Gram ⊕ rod. Causes food poisoning. Spores survive cooking rice (also known as reheated rice syndrome). Keeping rice warm results in germination of spores and enterotoxin formation. Emetic type usually seen with rice and pasta. Nausea and vomiting within 1–5 hr. Caused by cereulide, a preformed toxin. Diarrheal type causes watery, nonbloody diarrhea and GI pain within 8–18 hr.	
Clostridia (with exotoxins)	Gram ⊕, spore-forming, obligate anaerobic rods.	
C tetani	Produces tetanospasmin, an exotoxin causing tetanus. Tetanus toxin (and botulinum toxin) are proteases that cleave SNARE proteins for neurotransmitters. Blocks release of inhibitory neurotransmitters, GABA and glycine, from Renshaw cells in spinal cord. Causes spastic paralysis, trismus (lockjaw), risus sardonicus (raised eyebrows and open grin), opisthotonos (spasms of spinal extensors). Prevent with tetanus vaccine. Treat with antitoxin +/− vaccine booster, antibiotics, diazepam (for muscle spasms), and wound debridement.	Tetanus is tetanic paralysis.
C botulinum	Produces a heat-labile toxin that inhibits ACh release at the neuromuscular junction, causing botulism. In adults, disease is caused by ingestion of preformed toxin. In babies, ingestion of spores (eg, in honey) leads to disease (floppy baby syndrome). Treat with human botulinum immunoglobulin.	Symptoms of botulism (the 4 D's): Diplopia, Dysarthria, Dysphagia, Dyspnea. *Botulinum* is from bad bottles of food, juice, and honey (causes a descending flaccid paralysis). Local botox injections used to treat focal dystonia, achalasia, and muscle spasms. Also used for cosmetic reduction of facial wrinkles.
C perfringens	Produces α toxin (lecithinase, a phospholipase) that can cause myonecrosis (gas gangrene A; presents as soft tissue crepitus) and hemolysis. Spores can survive in undercooked food; when ingested, bacteria release heat-labile enterotoxin → food poisoning.	*Perfringens* perforates a gangrenous leg.
C difficile	Produces 2 toxins. Toxin A, an enterotoxin, binds to brush border of gut and alters fluid secretion. Toxin B, a cytotoxin, disrupts cytoskeleton via actin depolymerization. Both toxins lead to diarrhea → pseudomembranous colitis B. Often 2° to antibiotic use, especially clindamycin or ampicillin; associated with PPIs. Diagnosed by PCR or antigen detection of one or both toxins in stool.	*Difficile* causes diarrhea. Treatment: metronidazole or oral vancomycin. For recurrent cases, consider repeating prior regimen, fidaxomicin, or fecal microbiota transplant.

Corynebacterium diphtheriae

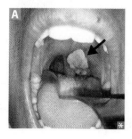

Gram ⊕ rod; transmitted via respiratory droplets. Causes diphtheria via exotoxin encoded by β-prophage. Potent exotoxin inhibits protein synthesis via ADP-ribosylation of EF-2.

Symptoms include pseudomembranous pharyngitis (grayish-white membrane **A**) with lymphadenopathy, myocarditis, and arrhythmias.

Lab diagnosis based on gram ⊕ rods with metachromatic (blue and red) granules and ⊕ Elek test for toxin.

Toxoid vaccine prevents diphtheria.

Coryne = club shaped.
Black colonies on cystine-tellurite agar.
ABCDEFG:
  ADP-ribosylation
  β-prophage
  Corynebacterium
  Diphtheriae
  Elongation Factor 2
  Granules

Listeria monocytogenes

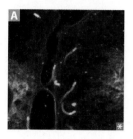

Gram ⊕, facultative intracellular rod; acquired by ingestion of unpasteurized dairy products and cold deli meats, via transplacental transmission, or by vaginal transmission during birth. Grows well at refrigeration temperatures (4°–10°C; "cold enrichment").

Forms "rocket tails" (red in **A**) via actin polymerization that allow intracellular movement and cell-to-cell spread across cell membranes, thereby avoiding antibody. Characteristic tumbling motility in broth.

Can cause amnionitis, septicemia, and spontaneous abortion in pregnant women; granulomatosis infantiseptica; neonatal meningitis; meningitis in immunocompromised patients; mild, self-limited gastroenteritis in healthy individuals.

Treatment: ampicillin.

Nocardia vs Actinomyces

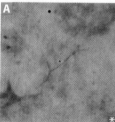

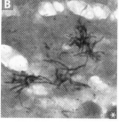

Both are gram ⊕ and form long, branching filaments resembling fungi.

Nocardia	Actinomyces
Aerobe	Anaerobe
Acid fast (weak) **A**	Not acid fast **B**
Found in soil	Normal oral, reproductive, and GI flora
Causes pulmonary infections in immunocompromised (can mimic TB but with ⊖ PPD); cutaneous infections after trauma in immunocompetent; can spread to CNS	Causes oral/facial abscesses that drain through sinus tracts; often associated with dental caries/extraction and other maxillofacial trauma; forms yellow "sulfur granules"; can also cause PID with IUDs
Treat with sulfonamides (TMP-SMX)	Treat with penicillin

Treatment is a **SNAP**: Sulfonamides—*Nocardia*; *Actinomyces*—Penicillin

Mycobacteria

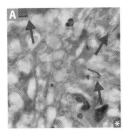

Mycobacterium tuberculosis (TB, often resistant to multiple drugs).

M avium–intracellulare (causes disseminated, non-TB disease in AIDS; often resistant to multiple drugs). Prophylaxis with azithromycin when CD4+ count < 50 cells/mm^3.

M scrofulaceum (cervical lymphadenitis in children).

M marinum (hand infection in aquarium handlers).

All mycobacteria are acid-fast organisms (pink rods; arrows in).

TB symptoms include fever, night sweats, weight loss, cough (nonproductive or productive), hemoptysis.

Cord factor creates a "serpentine cord" appearance in virulent *M tuberculosis* strains; activates macrophages (promoting granuloma formation) and induces release of TNF-α. Sulfatides (surface glycolipids) inhibit phagolysosomal fusion.

Tuberculosis

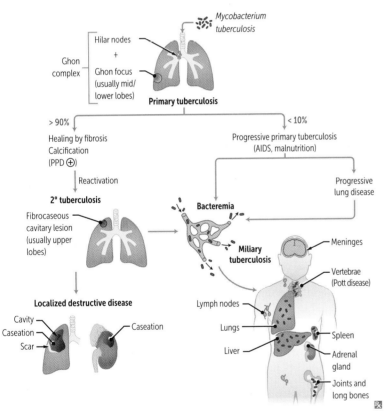

PPD ⊕ if current infection or past exposure.

PPD ⊖ if no infection and in sarcoidosis or HIV infection (especially with low CD4+ cell count).

Interferon-γ release assay (IGRA) has fewer false positives from BCG vaccination.

Caseating granulomas with central necrosis and Langhans giant cell (single example in 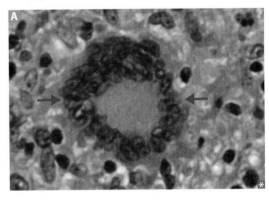) are characteristic of 2° tuberculosis.

Leprosy (Hansen disease)

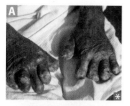

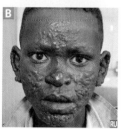

Caused by *Mycobacterium leprae*, an acid-fast bacillus that likes cool temperatures (infects skin and superficial nerves—"glove and stocking" loss of sensation 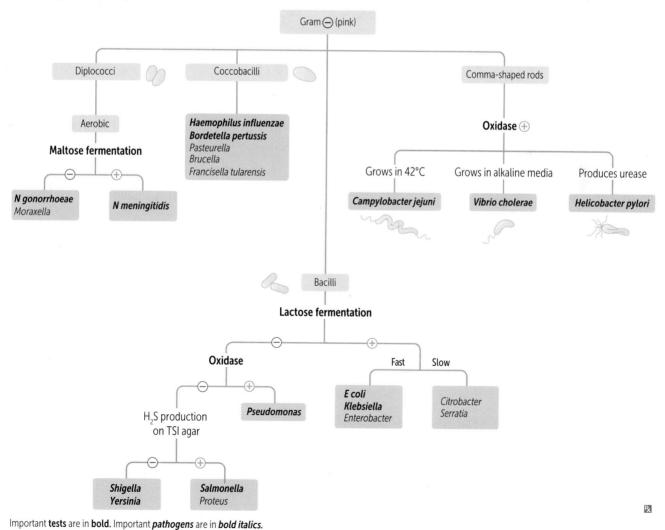A) and cannot be grown in vitro. Diagnosed via skin biopsy or tissue PCR. Reservoir in United States: armadillos.

Hansen disease has 2 forms (many cases fall temporarily between two extremes):

- Lepromatous—presents diffusely over the skin, with leonine (lion-like) facies B, and is communicable (high bacterial load); characterized by low cell-mediated immunity with a humoral Th2 response. Lepromatous form can be lethal.
- Tuberculoid—limited to a few hypoesthetic, hairless skin plaques; characterized by high cell-mediated immunity with a largely Th1-type immune response and low bacterial load.

Treatment: dapsone and rifampin for tuberculoid form; clofazimine is added for lepromatous form.

Gram-negative lab algorithm

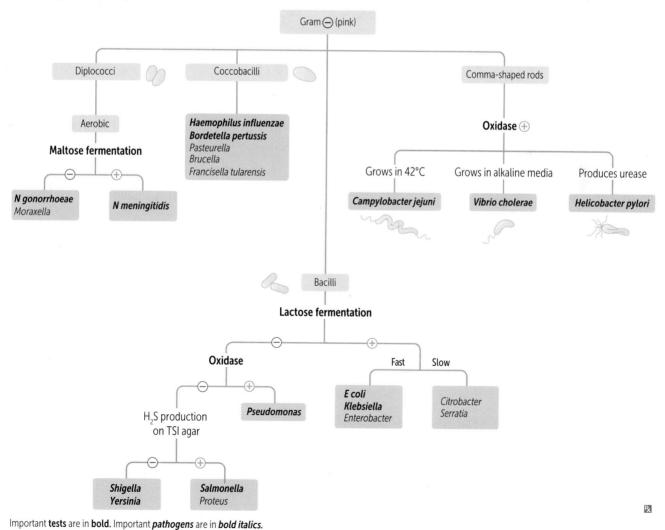

Important **tests** are in **bold**. Important ***pathogens*** are in ***bold italics***.

Neisseria

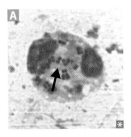

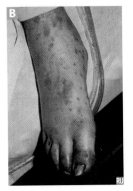

Gram ⊖ diplococci. Metabolize glucose and produce IgA proteases. Contain lipooligosaccharides (LOS) with strong endotoxin activity. *N gonorrhoeae* is often intracellular (within neutrophils) **A**.

MeninGococci ferment Maltose and Glucose. Gonococci ferment Glucose.

Gonococci	Meningococci
No polysaccharide capsule	Polysaccharide capsule
Maltose not fermented	Maltose fermentation
No vaccine due to antigenic variation of pilus proteins	Vaccine (type B vaccine not widely available)
Sexually or perinatally transmitted	Transmitted via respiratory and oral secretions
Causes gonorrhea, septic arthritis, neonatal conjunctivitis (2–5 days after birth), pelvic inflammatory disease (PID), and Fitz-Hugh–Curtis syndrome	Causes meningococcemia with petechial hemorrhages and gangrene of toes **B**, meningitis, Waterhouse-Friderichsen syndrome (adrenal insufficiency, fever, DIC, shock)
Condoms ↓ sexual transmission, erythromycin eye ointment prevents neonatal blindness	Rifampin, ciprofloxacin, or ceftriaxone prophylaxis in close contacts
Treatment: ceftriaxone (+ azithromycin or doxycycline, for possible chlamydial coinfection)	Treatment: ceftriaxone or penicillin G

Haemophilus influenzae

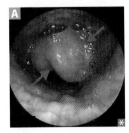

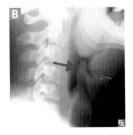

Small gram ⊖ (coccobacillary) rod. Aerosol transmission. Nontypeable (unencapsulated) strains are the most common cause of mucosal infections (otitis media, conjunctivitis, bronchitis) as well as invasive infections since the vaccine for capsular type b was introduced. Produces IgA protease.

Culture on chocolate agar, which contains factors V (NAD⁺) and X (hematin) for growth; can also be grown with *S aureus*, which provides factor V via RBC hemolysis.

HaEMOPhilus causes Epiglottitis (endoscopic appearance in **A**, can be "cherry red" in children; "thumb sign" on lateral neck x-ray **B**), Meningitis, Otitis media, and Pneumonia.

Treatment: amoxicillin +/– clavulanate for mucosal infections; ceftriaxone for meningitis; rifampin prophylaxis for close contacts.

Vaccine contains type b capsular polysaccharide (polyribosylribitol phosphate) conjugated to diphtheria toxoid or other protein. Given between 2 and 18 months of age.

Does not cause the flu (influenza virus does).

Bordetella pertussis	Gram ⊖, aerobic coccobacillus. Virulence factors include pertussis toxin (disables G_i), adenylate cyclase toxin (↑ cAMP), and tracheal cytotoxin. Three clinical stages:

- Catarrhal—low-grade fevers, Coryza.
- Paroxysmal—paroxysms of intense cough followed by inspiratory "whooP" ("whooping cough"), posttussive vomiting.
- Convalescent—gradual recovery of chronic cough.

Prevented by Tdap, DTaP vaccines. May be mistaken as viral infection due to lymphocytic infiltrate resulting from immune response.

Legionella pneumophila

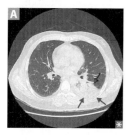

Gram ⊖ rod. Gram stains poorly—use **silver** stain. Grow on **charcoal** yeast extract medium with **iron** and **cysteine**. Detected by presence of antigen in urine. Labs may show hyponatremia.

Aerosol transmission from environmental water source habitat (eg, air conditioning systems, hot water tanks). No person-to-person transmission.

Treatment: macrolide or quinolone.

Legionnaires' disease—severe pneumonia (often unilateral and lobar), fever, GI and CNS symptoms. Common in smokers and in chronic lung disease.

Pontiac fever—mild flu-like syndrome.

Think of a French **legionnaire** (soldier) with his **silver** helmet, sitting around a campfire (**charcoal**) with his **iron** dagger—he is no **sissy** (cysteine).

Pseudomonas aeruginosa

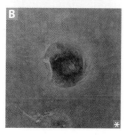

Aeruginosa—aerobic; motile, gram ⊖ rod. Non-lactose fermenting. Oxidase ⊕. Frequently found in water. Has a grape-like odor.

PSEUDOMONAS is associated with: **P**neumonia, **S**epsis, **E**cthyma gangrenosum, **U**TIs, **D**iabetes, **O**steomyelitis, **M**ucoid polysaccharide capsule, **O**titis externa (swimmer's ear), **N**osocomial infections (eg, catheters, equipment), **A**ddicts (drug abusers), **S**kin infections (eg, hot tub folliculitis, wound infection in burn victims).

Mucoid polysaccharide capsule may contribute to chronic pneumonia in cystic fibrosis patients due to biofilm formation.

Produces **PEEP**: **P**hospholipase C (degrades cell membranes); **E**ndotoxin (fever, shock); **E**xotoxin A (inactivates EF-2); **P**igments: pyoverdine and pyocyanin (blue-green pigment ; also generates reactive oxygen species).

Corneal ulcers/keratitis in contact lens wearers/ minor eye trauma.

Ecthyma gangrenosum—rapidly progressive, necrotic cutaneous lesion **B** caused by *Pseudomonas* bacteremia. Typically seen in immunocompromised patients.

Treatments include "CAMPFIRE" drugs:

- **C**arbapenems
- **A**minoglycosides
- **M**onobactams
- **P**olymyxins (eg, polymyxin B, colistin)
- **F**luoroquinolones (eg, ciprofloxacin, levofloxacin)
- Th**IR**d- and fourth-generation cephalosporins (eg, ceftazidime, cefepime)
- **E**xtended-spectrum penicillins (eg, piperacillin, ticarcillin)

Salmonella vs Shigella   Both *Salmonella* and *Shigella* are gram ⊖ rods, non-lactose fermenters, oxidase ⊖, and can invade the GI tract via M cells of Peyer patches.

	Salmonella typhi	*Salmonella* spp. (except *S typhi*)	*Shigella*
RESERVOIRS	Humans only	Humans and animals	Humans only
SPREAD	Can disseminate hematogenously	Can disseminate hematogenously	Cell to cell; no hematogenous spread
H_2S PRODUCTION	Yes	Yes	No
FLAGELLA	Yes (**salmon swim**)	Yes (**salmon swim**)	No
VIRULENCE FACTORS	Endotoxin; Vi capsule	Endotoxin	Endotoxin; Shiga toxin (enterotoxin)
INFECTIOUS DOSE (ID_{50})	High—large inoculum required; acid-labile (inactivated by gastric acids)	High	Low—very small inoculum required; acid stable (resistant to gastric acids)
EFFECT OF ANTIBIOTICS ON FECAL EXCRETION	Prolongs duration	Prolongs duration	Shortens duration
IMMUNE RESPONSE	Primarily monocytes	PMNs in disseminated disease	Primarily PMN infiltration
GI MANIFESTATIONS	Constipation, followed by diarrhea	Diarrhea (possibly bloody)	Bloody diarrhea (bacillary dysentery)
VACCINE	Oral vaccine contains live attenuated *S typhi* IM vaccine contains Vi capsular polysaccharide	No vaccine	No vaccine
UNIQUE PROPERTIES	▪ Causes typhoid fever (rose spots on abdomen, constipation, abdominal pain, fever); treat with ceftriaxone or fluoroquinolone ▪ Carrier state with gallbladder colonization	▪ Poultry, eggs, pets, and turtles are common sources ▪ Antibiotics not indicated ▪ Gastroenteritis is usually caused by non-typhoidal *Salmonella*	▪ **Four F's: Fingers, Flies, Food, Feces** ▪ In order of decreasing severity (less toxin produced): *S dysenteriae*, *S flexneri*, *S boydii*, *S sonnei* ▪ Invasion of M cells is key to pathogenicity: organisms that produce little toxin can cause disease

Yersinia enterocolitica   Gram ⊖ rod. Usually transmitted from pet feces (eg, puppies), contaminated milk, or pork. Causes acute diarrhea or pseudoappendicitis (right lower abdominal pain due to mesenteric adenitis and/or terminal ileitis).

Lactose-fermenting enteric bacteria   Fermentation of lactose → pink colonies on MacConkey agar. Examples include *Citrobacter*, *Klebsiella*, *E coli*, *Enterobacter*, and *Serratia* (weak fermenter). *E coli* produces β-galactosidase, which breaks down lactose into glucose and galactose.

Lactose is key.
Test with MacCon**KEE'S** agar.
EMB agar—lactose fermenters grow as purple/black colonies. *E coli* grows colonies with a green sheen.

Escherichia coli

Gram ⊖ rod. *E coli* virulence factors: fimbriae—cystitis and pyelonephritis (P-pili); K capsule—pneumonia, neonatal meningitis; LPS endotoxin—septic shock.

STRAIN	TOXIN AND MECHANISM	PRESENTATION
Enteroinvasive *E coli*	Microbe invades intestinal mucosa and causes necrosis and inflammation.	EIEC is Invasive; dysentery. Clinical manifestations similar to *Shigella*.
Enterotoxigenic *E coli*	Produces heat-labile and heat-stable enteroToxins. No inflammation or invasion.	ETEC; Traveler's diarrhea (watery).
Enteropathogenic *E coli*	No toxin produced. Adheres to apical surface, flattens villi, prevents absorption.	Diarrhea, usually in children (think EPEC and Pediatrics).
Enterohemorrhagic *E coli*	O157:H7 is most common serotype in US. Often transmitted via undercooked meat, raw leafy vegetables. Shiga-like toxin causes hemolytic-uremic syndrome: triad of anemia, thrombocytopenia, and acute renal failure due to microthrombi forming on damaged endothelium → mechanical hemolysis (with schistocytes on peripheral blood smear), platelet consumption, and ↓ renal blood flow.	Dysentery (toxin alone causes necrosis and inflammation). Does not ferment sorbitol (vs other *E coli*). Hemorrhagic, Hamburgers, Hemolytic-uremic syndrome.

Klebsiella

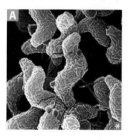

Gram ⊖ rod; intestinal flora that causes lobar pneumonia in alcoholics and diabetics when aspirated. Very mucoid colonies 🅰 caused by abundant polysaccharide capsules. Dark red "currant jelly" sputum (blood/mucus).

Also cause of nosocomial UTIs. Associated with evolution of multidrug resistance (MDR).

5 A's of *KlebsiellA*:
Aspiration pneumonia
Abscess in lungs and liver
Alcoholics
DiAbetics
"CurrAnt jelly" sputum

Campylobacter jejuni

Gram ⊖, comma or S shaped (with polar flagella) 🅰, oxidase ⊕, grows at 42°C ("*Campylobacter* likes the **hot campfire**").

Major cause of bloody diarrhea, especially in children. Fecal-oral transmission through person-to-person contact or via ingestion of undercooked contaminated poultry or meat, unpasteurized milk. Contact with infected animals (dogs, cats, pigs) is also a risk factor.

Common antecedent to Guillain-Barré syndrome and reactive arthritis.

Vibrio cholerae

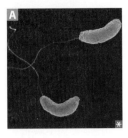

Gram ⊖, flagellated, comma shaped , oxidase ⊕, grows in alkaline media. Endemic to developing countries. Produces profuse rice-water diarrhea via enterotoxin that permanently activates G_s, ↑ cAMP. Sensitive to stomach acid (acid labile); requires large inoculum (high ID_{50}) unless host has ↓ gastric acidity. Transmitted via ingestion of contaminated water or uncooked food (eg, raw shellfish). Treat promptly with oral rehydration solution.

Helicobacter pylori

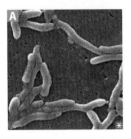

Curved, flagellated (motile), gram ⊖ rod that is **triple** ⊕: catalase ⊕, oxidase ⊕, and urease ⊕ (can use urea breath test or fecal antigen test for diagnosis). Urease produces ammonia, creating an alkaline environment, which helps *H pylori* survive in acidic mucosa. Colonizes mainly antrum of stomach; causes gastritis and peptic ulcers (especially duodenal). Risk factor for peptic ulcer disease, gastric adenocarcinoma, and MALT lymphoma.

Most common initial treatment is **triple** therapy: Amoxicillin (metronidazole if penicillin allergy) + Clarithromycin + Proton pump inhibitor; Antibiotics Cure *Pylori*.

Spirochetes

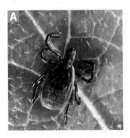

Spiral-shaped bacteria 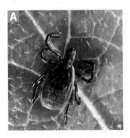 with axial filaments. Includes *Borrelia* (big size), *Leptospira*, and *Treponema*. Only *Borrelia* can be visualized using aniline dyes (Wright or Giemsa stain) in light microscopy due to size. *Treponema* is visualized by dark-field microscopy or direct fluorescent antibody (DFA) microscopy.

BLT.
Borrelia is Big.

Lyme disease

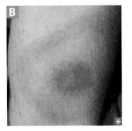

Caused by *Borrelia burgdorferi*, which is transmitted by the *Ixodes* deer tick (also vector for *Anaplasma* spp. and protozoa *Babesia*). Natural reservoir is the mouse (and important to tick life cycle).

Common in northeastern United States.

Stage 1—early localized: erythema migrans (typical "bulls-eye" configuration **B** is pathognomonic but not always present), flu-like symptoms.

Stage 2—early disseminated: secondary lesions, carditis, AV block, facial nerve (Bell) palsy, migratory myalgias/transient arthritis.

Stage 3—late disseminated: encephalopathy, chronic arthritis.

A Key Lyme pie to the FACE:
  Facial nerve palsy (typically bilateral)
  Arthritis
  Cardiac block
  Erythema migrans
Treatment: doxycycline (1st line); amoxicillin and cefuroxime in pregnant women and children.

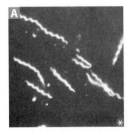

Leptospira interrogans	Spirochete with hook-shaped ends found in water contaminated with animal urine.
	Leptospirosis—flu-like symptoms, myalgias (classically of calves), jaundice, photophobia with conjunctival suffusion (erythema without exudate). Prevalent among surfers and in tropics (eg, Hawaii).
	Weil disease (icterohemorrhagic leptospirosis)—severe form with jaundice and azotemia from liver and kidney dysfunction, fever, hemorrhage, and anemia.

Syphilis	Caused by spirochete *Treponema pallidum*.
Primary syphilis	Localized disease presenting with **painless** chancre **A**. If available, use dark-field microscopy to visualize treponemes in fluid from chancre **B**. VDRL ⊕ in ~ 80%.
Secondary syphilis	Disseminated disease with constitutional symptoms, maculopapular rash **C** (including palms **D** and soles), condylomata lata **E** (smooth, painless, wart-like white lesions on genitals), lymphadenopathy, patchy hair loss; also confirmable with dark-field microscopy. Serologic testing: VDRL/RPR (nonspecific), confirm diagnosis with specific test (eg, FTA-ABS). Secondary syphilis = Systemic. Latent syphilis (⊕ serology without symptoms) may follow.
Tertiary syphilis	Gummas **F** (chronic granulomas), aortitis (vasa vasorum destruction), neurosyphilis (tabes dorsalis, "general paresis"), Argyll Robertson pupil (constricts with accommodation but is not reactive to light; also called "prostitute's pupil" since it accommodates but does not react). Signs: broad-based ataxia, ⊕ Romberg, Charcot joint, stroke without hypertension. For neurosyphilis: test spinal fluid with VDRL, FTA-ABS, and PCR.
Congenital syphilis	Presents with facial abnormalities such as rhagades (linear scars at angle of mouth, black arrow in **G**), snuffles (nasal discharge, red arrow in **G**), saddle nose, notched (Hutchinson) teeth **H**, mulberry molars, and short maxilla; saber shins; CN VIII deafness. To prevent, treat mother early in pregnancy, as placental transmission typically occurs after first trimester.

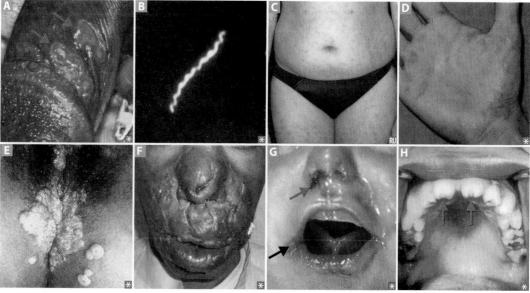

VDRL false positives

VDRL detects nonspecific antibody that reacts with beef cardiolipin. Quantitative, inexpensive, and widely available test for syphilis (sensitive but not specific).

False-Positive results on **VDRL** with:
 Pregnancy
 Viral infection (eg, EBV, hepatitis)
 Drugs
 Rheumatic fever
 Lupus and leprosy

Jarisch-Herxheimer reaction

Flu-like syndrome (fever, chills, headache, myalgia) after antibiotics are started; due to killed bacteria (usually spirochetes) releasing toxins.

Gardnerella vaginalis

A pleomorphic, gram-variable rod involved in bacterial vaginosis. Presents as a gray vaginal discharge with a **fishy** smell; nonpainful (vs vaginitis). Associated with sexual activity, but not sexually transmitted. Bacterial vaginosis is also characterized by overgrowth of certain anaerobic bacteria in vagina. **Clue** cells (vaginal epithelial cells covered with *Gardnerella*) have stippled appearance along outer margin (arrow in A).
Treatment: metronidazole or clindamycin.

I don't have a **clue** why I smell **fish** in the vagina **garden**!
Amine whiff test—mixing discharge with 10% KOH enhances fishy odor.

Chlamydiae

Chlamydiae cannot make their own ATP. They are obligate intracellular organisms that cause mucosal infections. 2 forms:
 - Elementary body (small, dense) is "Enfectious" and Enters cell via Endocytosis; transforms into reticulate body.
 - Reticulate body Replicates in cell by fission; Reorganizes into elementary bodies.

Chlamydia trachomatis causes reactive arthritis (Reiter syndrome), neonatal and follicular adult conjunctivitis A, nongonococcal urethritis, and PID.
Chlamydophila pneumoniae and *Chlamydophila psittaci* cause atypical pneumonia; transmitted by aerosol.
Treatment: azithromycin (favored because one-time treatment) or doxycycline (+ ceftriaxone for possible concomitant gonorrhea).

Chlamys = cloak (intracellular).
C psittaci—has an avian reservoir (parrots), causes atypical pneumonia.
Lab diagnosis: PCR, nucleic acid amplification test. Cytoplasmic inclusions (reticulate bodies) seen on Giemsa or fluorescent antibody–stained smear.
The chlamydial cell wall lacks classic peptidoglycan (due to reduced muramic acid), rendering β-lactam antibiotics ineffective.

Chlamydia trachomatis serotypes

Types A, B, and C	Chronic infection, cause blindness due to follicular conjunctivitis in Africa.	ABC = Africa, Blindness, Chronic infection.
Types D–K	Urethritis/PID, ectopic pregnancy, neonatal pneumonia (staccato cough) with eosinophilia, neonatal conjunctivitis (1–2 weeks after birth).	D–K = everything else. Neonatal disease can be acquired during passage through infected birth canal.
Types L1, L2, and L3	Lymphogranuloma venereum—small, painless ulcers on genitals → swollen, painful inguinal lymph nodes that ulcerate (buboes). Treat with doxycycline.	

Zoonotic bacteria

Zoonosis: infectious disease transmitted between animals and humans.

SPECIES	DISEASE	TRANSMISSION AND SOURCE
Anaplasma spp.	Anaplasmosis	*Ixodes* ticks (live on deer and mice)
Bartonella spp.	Cat scratch disease, bacillary angiomatosis	Cat scratch
Borrelia burgdorferi	Lyme disease	*Ixodes* ticks (live on deer and mice)
Borrelia recurrentis	**Relapsing** fever	Louse (recurrent due to variable surface antigens)
Brucella spp.	Brucellosis/**undulant** fever	Unpasteurized dairy
Campylobacter	Bloody diarrhea	Feces from infected pets/animals; contaminated meats/foods/hands
Chlamydophila psittaci	Psittacosis	Parrots, other birds
Coxiella burnetii	Q fever	Aerosols of cattle/sheep amniotic fluid
Ehrlichia chaffeensis	Ehrlichiosis	*Amblyomma* (Lone Star tick)
Francisella tularensis	Tularemia	Ticks, rabbits, deer flies
Leptospira spp.	Leptospirosis	Animal urine in water; recreational water use
Mycobacterium leprae	Leprosy	Humans with lepromatous leprosy; armadillo (rare)
Pasteurella multocida	Cellulitis, osteomyelitis	Animal bite, cats, dogs
Rickettsia prowazekii	Epidemic typhus	Human to human via human body louse
Rickettsia rickettsii	Rocky Mountain spotted fever	*Dermacentor* (dog tick)
Rickettsia typhi	Endemic typhus	Fleas
Salmonella spp. (except *S typhi*)	Diarrhea (which may be bloody), vomiting, fever, abdominal cramps	Reptiles and poultry
Yersinia pestis	Plague	Fleas (rats and prairie dogs are reservoirs)

Rickettsial diseases and vector-borne illnesses

Treatment: doxycycline (caution during pregnancy; alternative is chloramphenicol).

RASH COMMON

Rocky Mountain spotted fever	*Rickettsia rickettsii*, vector is tick. Despite its name, disease occurs primarily in the South Atlantic states, especially North Carolina. Rash typically starts at wrists 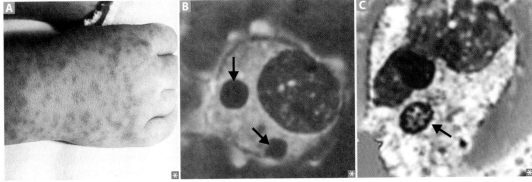 A and ankles and then spreads to trunk, palms, and soles.	Classic triad—headache, fever, rash (vasculitis). **Palms** and **soles** rash is seen in Coxsackievirus A infection (hand, foot, and mouth disease), Rocky Mountain spotted fever, and 2° Syphilis (you drive **CARS** using your **palms** and **soles**).
Typhus	Endemic (fleas)—*R typhi*. Epidemic (human body louse)—*R prowazekii*. Rash starts centrally and spreads out, sparing palms and soles.	*Rickettsii* on the w**R**ists, **T**yphus on the **T**runk.

RASH RARE

Ehrlichiosis	*Ehrlichia*, vector is tick. Monocytes with morulae B (mulberry-like inclusions) in cytoplasm.	**MEGA** berry— Monocytes = **E**hrlichiosis Granulocytes = **A**naplasmosis
Anaplasmosis	*Anaplasma*, vector is tick. Granulocytes with morulae C in cytoplasm.	
Q fever	*Coxiella burnetii*, no arthropod vector. Spores inhaled as aerosols from cattle/sheep amniotic fluid. Presents as pneumonia. Common cause of culture ⊖ endocarditis.	**Q** fever is **Q**ueer because it has no rash or vector and its causative organism can survive outside in its endospore form. Not in the *Rickettsia* genus, but closely related.

Mycoplasma pneumoniae 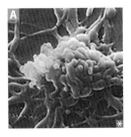	Classic cause of atypical "walking" pneumonia (insidious onset, headache, nonproductive cough, patchy or diffuse interstitial infiltrate). X-ray looks worse than patient. High titer of **cold** agglutinins (IgM), which can agglutinate RBCs. Grown on Eaton agar. Treatment: macrolides, doxycycline, or fluoroquinolone (penicillin ineffective since *Mycoplasma* have no cell wall).	No cell wall. Not seen on Gram stain. Pleomorphic A. Bacterial membrane contains sterols for stability. Mycoplasmal pneumonia is more common in patients < 30 years old. Frequent outbreaks in military recruits and prisons. *Mycoplasma* gets **cold** without a **coat** (cell wall).

▶ MICROBIOLOGY—MYCOLOGY

Systemic mycoses

All of the following can cause pneumonia and can disseminate.

All are caused by dimorphic fungi: **cold** (20°C) = **mold**; **heat** (37°C) = **yeast**. Only exception is *Coccidioides*, which is a spherule (not yeast) in tissue.

Systemic mycoses can form granulomas (like TB); cannot be transmitted person-to-person (unlike TB).

Treatment: fluconazole or itraconazole for **local** infection; amphotericin B for **systemic** infection.

DISEASE	ENDEMIC LOCATION	PATHOLOGIC FEATURES	UNIQUE SIGNS/SYMPTOMS	NOTES
Histoplasmosis	Mississippi and Ohio River Valleys	Macrophage filled with *Histoplasma* (smaller than RBC) **A**	Palatal/tongue ulcers, splenomegaly	Histo hides (within macrophages) Bird (eg, starlings) or bat droppings Diagnosis via urine/serum antigen
Blastomycosis	Eastern and Central US	**Broad**-based budding of *Blastomyces* (same size as RBC) **B**	Inflammatory lung disease, can disseminate to skin/bone Verrucous skin lesions can simulate SCC Forms granulomatous nodules	Blasto buds broadly
Coccidioidomycosis	Southwestern US, California	Spherule (much larger than RBC) filled with endospores of *Coccidioides* **C**	Disseminates to skin/bone Erythema nodosum (desert bumps) or multiforme Arthralgias (desert rheumatism) Can cause meningitis	
Para-coccidioidomycosis	Latin America	Budding yeast of *Paracoccidioides* with "captain's wheel" formation (much larger than RBC) **D**	Similar to blastomycosis, males > females	Paracoccidio parasails with the **captain's wheel** all the way to **Latin America**

Cutaneous mycoses

Tinea (dermatophytes)	Clinical name for dermatophyte (cutaneous fungal) infections. Dermatophytes include *Microsporum*, *Trichophyton*, and *Epidermophyton*. Branching septate hyphae visible on KOH preparation with blue fungal stain **A**. Associated with pruritus.
Tinea capitis	Occurs on head, scalp. Associated with lymphadenopathy, alopecia, scaling **B**.
Tinea corporis	Occurs on torso. Characterized by erythematous scaling rings ("ringworm") and central clearing **C**. Can be acquired from contact with an infected cat or dog.
Tinea cruris	Occurs in inguinal area **D**. Often does not show the central clearing seen in tinea corporis.
Tinea pedis	Three varieties: ▪ Interdigital **E**; most common ▪ Moccasin distribution **F** ▪ Vesicular type
Tinea unguium	Onychomycosis; occurs on nails.
Tinea (pityriasis) versicolor	Caused by *Malassezia* spp. (*Pityrosporum* spp.), a yeast-like fungus (not a dermatophyte despite being called tinea). Degradation of lipids produces acids that damage melanocytes and cause hypopigmented **G**, hyperpigmented, and/or pink patches. Less pruritic than dermatophytes. Can occur any time of year, but more common in summer (hot, humid weather). "Spaghetti and meatballs" appearance on microscopy **H**. Treatment: selenium sulfide, topical and/or oral antifungal medications.

Opportunistic fungal infections

Candida albicans	*alba* = white. Dimorphic; forms pseudohyphae and budding yeasts at 20°C 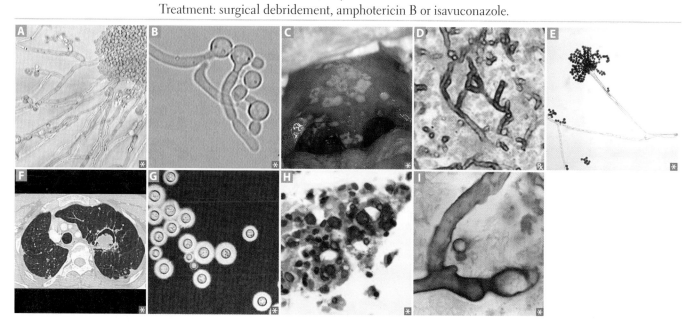A, germ tubes at 37°C B. Systemic or superficial fungal infection. Causes oral C and esophageal thrush in immunocompromised (neonates, steroids, diabetes, AIDS), vulvovaginitis (diabetes, use of antibiotics), diaper rash, endocarditis (IV drug users), disseminated candidiasis (especially in neutropenic patients), chronic mucocutaneous candidiasis. Treatment: oral fluconazole/topical azole for vaginal; nystatin, fluconazole, or echinocandins for oral/esophageal; fluconazole, echinocandins, or amphotericin B for systemic.
Aspergillus fumigatus	Monomorphic septate hyphae that branch at 45° Acute Angle D E. Causes invasive aspergillosis in immunocompromised patients, neutrophil dysfunction (eg, chronic granulomatous disease). Can cause aspergillomas in pre-existing lung cavities, especially after TB infection. Some species of *Aspergillus* produce Aflatoxins (associated with hepatocellular carcinoma). Allergic bronchopulmonary aspergillosis (ABPA) F—hypersensitivity response associated with asthma and cystic fibrosis; may cause bronchiectasis and eosinophilia.
Cryptococcus neoformans	5–10 μm with narrow budding. Heavily encapsulated yeast. Not dimorphic. Found in soil, pigeon droppings. Acquired through inhalation with hematogenous dissemination to meninges. Culture on Sabouraud agar. Highlighted with India ink (clear halo G) and mucicarmine (red inner capsule H). Latex agglutination test detects polysaccharide capsular antigen and is more specific. Causes cryptococcosis, cryptococcal meningitis, cryptococcal encephalitis ("soap bubble" lesions in brain), primarily in immunocompromised. Treatment: amphotericin B + flucytosine followed by fluconazole for cryptococcal meningitis.
Mucor and *Rhizopus* spp.	Irregular, broad, nonseptate hyphae branching at wide angles I. Causes mucormycosis, mostly in ketoacidotic diabetic and/or neutropenic patients (eg, leukemia). Inhalation of spores → fungi proliferate in blood vessel walls, penetrate cribriform plate, and enter brain. Rhinocerebral, frontal lobe abscess; cavernous sinus thrombosis. Headache, facial pain, black necrotic eschar on face; may have cranial nerve involvement. Treatment: surgical debridement, amphotericin B or isavuconazole.

Pneumocystis jirovecii

Causes *Pneumocystis* pneumonia (PCP), a diffuse interstitial pneumonia 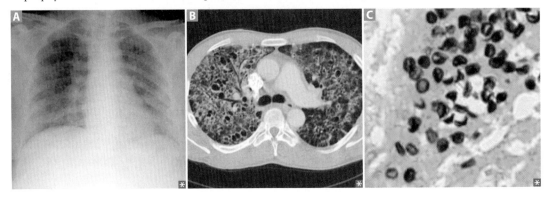. Yeast-like fungus (originally classified as protozoan). Most infections are asymptomatic. Immunosuppression (eg, AIDS) predisposes to disease. Diffuse, bilateral ground-glass opacities on CXR/CT, with pneumatoceles **B**. Diagnosed by lung biopsy or lavage. Disc-shaped yeast seen on methenamine silver stain of lung tissue **C**.

Treatment/prophylaxis: TMP-SMX, pentamidine, dapsone (prophylaxis only), atovaquone. Start prophylaxis when CD4+ count drops to < 200 cells/mm^3 in HIV patients.

Sporothrix schenckii

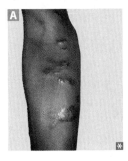

Sporotrichosis. Dimorphic, **cigar**-shaped budding yeast that grows in branching hyphae with rosettes of conidia; lives on vegetation. When spores are traumatically introduced into the skin, typically by a thorn ("**rose gardener**'s disease"), causes local pustule or ulcer with nodules along draining lymphatics (ascending lymphangitis **A**). Disseminated disease possible in immunocompromised host.

Treatment: itraconazole or **pot**assium iodide.

Think of a **rose gardener** who smokes a **cigar** and **pot**.

▶ MICROBIOLOGY—PARASITOLOGY

Protozoa—gastrointestinal infections

ORGANISM	DISEASE	TRANSMISSION	DIAGNOSIS	TREATMENT
Giardia lamblia	**Giardiasis**—bloating, flatulence, foul-smelling, fatty diarrhea (often seen in campers/hikers)—think fat-rich **Ghirardelli** chocolates for **fatty** stools of *Giardia*	Cysts in water	Multinucleated trophozoites **A** or cysts **B** in stool, antigen detection	Metronidazole
Entamoeba histolytica	**Amebiasis**—bloody diarrhea (dysentery), liver abscess ("anchovy paste" exudate), RUQ pain; histology of colon biopsy shows flask-shaped ulcers	Cysts in water	Serology, antigen testing, and/or trophozoites (with engulfed RBCs **C** in the cytoplasm) or cysts with up to 4 nuclei in stool **D**; **E**ntamoeba **E**ats **E**rythrocytes	Metronidazole; paromomycin or iodoquinol for asymptomatic cyst passers
Cryptosporidium	Severe diarrhea in AIDS Mild disease (watery diarrhea) in immunocompetent hosts	Oocysts in water	Oocysts on acid-fast stain **E**, antigen detection	Prevention (by filtering city water supplies); nitazoxanide in immunocompetent hosts

Protozoa—CNS infections

ORGANISM	DISEASE	TRANSMISSION	DIAGNOSIS	TREATMENT
Toxoplasma gondii	Immunocompetent: mononucleosis-like symptoms, ⊖ heterophile antibody test. Reactivation in AIDS → brain abscesses usually seen as multiple ring-enhancing lesions on MRI **A**. Congenital toxoplasmosis: classic triad of chorioretinitis, hydrocephalus, and intracranial calcifications.	Cysts in meat (most common); oocysts in cat feces; crosses placenta (pregnant women should avoid cats)	Serology, biopsy (tachyzoite) **B**	Sulfadiazine + pyrimethamine
Naegleria fowleri	Rapidly fatal meningoencephalitis	Swimming in warm **freshwater** (think **Nalgene** bottle filled with **fresh water** containing *Naegleria*); enters via cribriform plate	Amoebas in CSF **C**	Amphotericin B has been effective for a few survivors
Trypanosoma brucei	**African sleeping sickness**— enlarged lymph nodes, recurring fever (due to antigenic variation), somnolence, coma	Tsetse fly, a painful bite	Trypomastigote in blood smear **D**	Suramin for blood-borne disease or **melarsoprol** for CNS penetration ("**I sure am mellow when I'm sleeping**"; remember **melatonin** helps with **sleep**)

Protozoa—hematologic infections

ORGANISM	DISEASE	TRANSMISSION	DIAGNOSIS	TREATMENT
Plasmodium *P vivax/ovale* *P falciparum* *P malariae* 	**Malaria**—fever, headache, anemia, splenomegaly *P vivax/ovale*—48-hr cycle (tertian; includes fever on first day and third day, thus fevers are actually 48 hr apart); dormant form (hypnozoite) in liver *P falciparum*—severe; irregular fever patterns; parasitized RBCs occlude capillaries in brain (cerebral malaria), kidneys, lungs *P malariae*—72-hr cycle (quartan)	*Anopheles* mosquito	Blood smear: trophozoite ring form within RBC **A**, schizont containing merozoites; red granules (Schüffner stippling) **B** throughout RBC cytoplasm seen with *P vivax/ovale*	Chloroquine (for sensitive species), which blocks *Plasmodium* heme polymerase; if resistant, use mefloquine or atovaquone/ proguanil If life-threatening, use intravenous quinidine or artesunate (test for G6PD deficiency) For *P vivax/ovale*, add primaquine for hypnozoite (test for G6PD deficiency)
Babesia 	**Babesiosis**—fever and hemolytic anemia; predominantly in northeastern United States; asplenia ↑ risk of severe disease	*Ixodes* tick (same as *Borrelia burgdorferi* of Lyme disease; may often coinfect humans)	Blood smear: ring form **C1**, "Maltese cross" **C2**; PCR	Atovaquone + azithromycin

Protozoa—others

ORGANISM	DISEASE	TRANSMISSION	DIAGNOSIS	TREATMENT
Visceral infections				
Trypanosoma cruzi	**Chagas disease**—dilated cardiomyopathy with apical atrophy, megacolon, megaesophagus; predominantly in South America Unilateral periorbital swelling (Romaña sign) characteristic of acute stage	Triatomine ("**kissing**") bug, a type of reduviid bug, deposits feces in a painless bite (much like a **kiss**)	Trypomastigote in blood smear 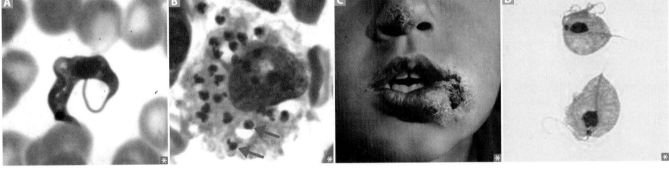A	Benznidazole or nifurtimox; *cruz*ing in my **Benz**, with a **fur** coat on
Leishmania donovani	**Visceral leishmaniasis (kala-azar)**—spiking fevers, hepatosplenomegaly, pancytopenia **Cutaneous leishmaniasis**—skin ulcers C	Sandfly	Macrophages containing amastigotes B	Amphotericin B, sodium stibogluconate
Sexually transmitted infections				
Trichomonas vaginalis	**Vaginitis**—foul-smelling, greenish discharge; itching and burning; do not confuse with *Gardnerella vaginalis*, a gram-variable bacterium associated with bacterial vaginosis	Sexual (cannot exist outside human because it cannot form cysts)	Trophozoites (motile) D on wet mount; "strawberry cervix"	Metronidazole for patient and partner (prophylaxis)

Nematode routes of infection	Ingested—*Enterobius, Ascaris, Toxocara, Trichinella, Trichuris* Cutaneous—*Strongyloides, Ancylostoma, Necator* Bites—*Loa loa, Onchocerca volvulus, Wuchereria bancrofti*	You'll get sick if you **EATTT** these! These get into your feet from the **SAN**d. Lay **LOW** to avoid getting bitten.

Nematodes (roundworms)

ORGANISM	DISEASE	TRANSMISSION	TREATMENT
Intestinal			
Enterobius vermicularis (pinworm)	Causes anal pruritus (diagnosed by seeing egg 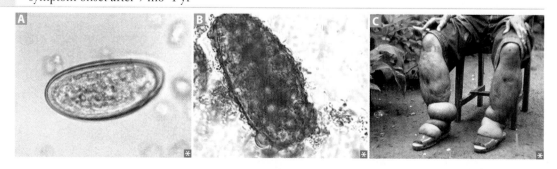 A via the tape test)	Fecal-oral	Pyrantel pamoate or **bend**azoles (because worms are **bend**y)
Ascaris lumbricoides (giant roundworm)	May cause obstruction at ileocecal valve, biliary obstruction, intestinal perforation, migrates from nose/mouth	Fecal-oral; knobby-coated, oval eggs seen in feces under microscope B	Bendazoles
Strongyloides stercoralis (threadworm)	Autoinfection: rarely, some larvae may penetrate the intestinal wall to enter the bloodstream without leaving the body	Larvae in soil penetrate skin; rhabditiform larvae seen in feces under microscope	Ivermectin or bendazoles
Ancylostoma duodenale, Necator americanus (hookworms)	Cause anemia by sucking blood from intestinal wall Cutaneous larva migrans—pruritic, serpiginous rash from walking barefoot on contaminated beach	Larvae penetrate skin	Bendazoles or pyrantel pamoate
Trichinella spiralis	Larvae enter bloodstream, encyst in striated muscle → muscle inflammation Trichinosis—fever, vomiting, nausea, periorbital edema, myalgia	Undercooked meat (especially pork); fecal-oral (less likely)	Bendazoles
Trichuris trichiura (whipworm)	Often asymptomatic; loose stools, anemia, rectal prolapse in children (heavy infection)	Fecal-oral	Bendazoles
Tissue			
Toxocara canis	Visceral larva migrans—nematodes migrate to blood through intestinal wall → inflammation and damage. Often affects heart (myocarditis), liver, eyes (visual impairment, blindness), and CNS (seizures, coma)	Fecal-oral	Bendazoles
Onchocerca volvulus	Skin changes, loss of elastic fibers, and river blindness (**black** flies, **black** skin nodules, "**black** sight"); allergic reaction to microfilaria possible	Female blackfly	Ivermectin (**iver**mectin for **river** blindness)
Loa loa	Swelling in skin, worm in conjunctiva	Deer fly, horse fly, mango fly	Diethylcarbamazine
Wuchereria bancrofti	Lymphatic filariasis (elephantiasis)—worms invade lymph nodes → inflammation → lymphedema C; symptom onset after 9 mo–1 yr	Female mosquito	Diethylcarbamazine

Cestodes (tapeworms)

ORGANISM	DISEASE	TRANSMISSION	TREATMENT
Taenia solium **A**	Intestinal tapeworm	Ingestion of larvae encysted in undercooked pork	Praziquantel
	Cysticercosis, neurocysticercosis (cystic CNS lesions, seizures) **B**	Ingestion of eggs in food contaminated with human feces	Praziquantel; albendazole for neurocysticercosis
Diphyllobothrium latum	Vitamin B_{12} deficiency (tapeworm competes for B_{12} in intestine) → megaloblastic anemia	Ingestion of larvae in raw freshwater fish	Praziquantel
Echinococcus granulosus **C**	Hydatid cysts **D** ("eggshell calcification") in liver **E**; cyst rupture can cause anaphylaxis	Ingestion of eggs in food contaminated with dog feces Sheep are an intermediate host	Albendazole

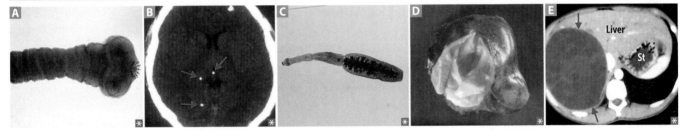

Trematodes (flukes)

ORGANISM	DISEASE	TRANSMISSION	TREATMENT
Schistosoma **A** **B**	Liver and spleen enlargement (*S mansoni*, egg with lateral spine **A**), fibrosis, inflammation, portal hypertension Chronic infection with *S haematobium* (egg with terminal spine **B**) can lead to squamous cell carcinoma of the bladder (painless hematuria) and pulmonary hypertension	Snails are intermediate host; cercariae penetrate skin of humans in contact with contaminated fresh water (eg, swimming or bathing)	Praziquantel
Clonorchis sinensis	Biliary tract inflammation → pigmented gallstones Associated with cholangiocarcinoma	Undercooked fish	Praziquantel

Ectoparasites

Sarcoptes scabiei 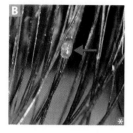	Mite burrow into stratum corneum and cause **scabies**—pruritus (worse at night) and serpiginous burrows (lines) in webspace of hands and feet **A**.	Common in children, crowded populations (jails, nursing homes); transmission through skin-to-skin contact (most common) or via fomites. Treatment: permethrin cream, washing/drying all clothing/bedding, treat close contacts.
Pediculus humanus/ Phthirus pubis	Blood-sucking lice that cause intense pruritus with associated excoriations, commonly on scalp and neck (head lice) or waistband and axilla (body lice).	Can transmit *Rickettsia prowazekii* (epidemic typhus), *Borrelia recurrentis* (relapsing fever), *Bartonella quintana* (trench fever). Treatment includes pyrethroids, malathion, or ivermectin lotion, and nit **B** combing. Children with head lice can be treated at home without interrupting school attendance.

Parasite hints

ASSOCIATIONS	ORGANISM
Biliary tract disease, cholangiocarcinoma	*Clonorchis sinensis*
Brain cysts, seizures	*Taenia solium* (neurocysticercosis)
Hematuria, squamous cell bladder cancer	*Schistosoma haematobium*
Liver (hydatid) cysts	*Echinococcus granulosus*
Microcytic anemia	*Ancylostoma, Necator*
Myalgias, periorbital edema	*Trichinella spiralis*
Perianal pruritus	*Enterobius*
Portal hypertension	*Schistosoma mansoni, Schistosoma japonicum*
Vitamin B_{12} deficiency	*Diphyllobothrium latum*

▸ MICROBIOLOGY—VIROLOGY

Viral structure—general features

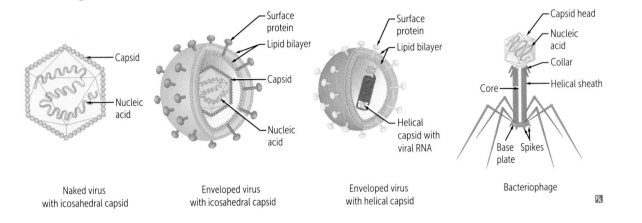

Naked virus
with icosahedral capsid

Enveloped virus
with icosahedral capsid

Enveloped virus
with helical capsid

Bacteriophage

Viral genetics

Recombination	Exchange of genes between 2 chromosomes by crossing over within regions of significant base sequence homology.
Reassortment	When viruses with segmented genomes (eg, influenza virus) exchange genetic material. For example, the 2009 novel H1N1 influenza A pandemic emerged via complex viral reassortment of genes from human, swine, and avian viruses. Has potential to cause antigenic shift.
Complementation	When 1 of 2 viruses that infect the cell has a mutation that results in a nonfunctional protein, the nonmutated virus "complements" the mutated one by making a functional protein that serves both viruses. For example, hepatitis D virus requires the presence of replicating hepatitis B virus to supply HBsAg, the envelope protein for HDV.
Phenotypic mixing	Occurs with simultaneous infection of a cell with 2 viruses. Genome of virus A can be partially or completely coated (forming pseudovirion) with the surface proteins of virus B. Type B protein coat determines the tropism (infectivity) of the hybrid virus. However, the progeny from this infection have a type A coat that is encoded by its type A genetic material.

DNA viral genomes	All DNA viruses have dsDNA genomes except Parvoviridae (ssDNA). All are linear except papilloma-, polyoma-, and hepadnaviruses (circular).	All are dsDNA (like our cells), except "part-of-a-virus" (**parvovirus**) is ssDNA. *Parvus* = small.
RNA viral genomes	All RNA viruses have ssRNA genomes except Reoviridae (dsRNA). ⊕ stranded RNA viruses: I went to a **retro** (**retrovirus**) **toga** (**togavirus**) party, where I drank flavored (**flavivirus**) **Corona** (**coronavirus**) and ate **hippie** (**hepevirus**) California (**calicivirus**) **pickles** (**picornavirus**).	All are ssRNA, except "repeato-virus" (**reovirus**) is dsRNA.

Naked viral genome infectivity

Purified nucleic acids of most dsDNA (except poxviruses and HBV) and ⊕ strand ssRNA (≈ mRNA) viruses are infectious. Naked nucleic acids of ⊖ strand ssRNA and dsRNA viruses are not infectious. They require polymerases contained in the complete virion.

Viral envelopes

Generally, enveloped viruses acquire their envelopes from plasma membrane when they exit from cell. Exceptions include herpesviruses, which acquire envelopes from nuclear membrane.

Naked (nonenveloped) viruses include Papillomavirus, Adenovirus, Parvovirus, Polyomavirus, Calicivirus, Picornavirus, Reovirus, and Hepevirus.

DNA = **PAPP**; RNA = **CPR** and **hepevirus**. Give **PAPP** smears and **CPR** to a **naked hippie** (hepevirus).

DNA virus characteristics

Some general rules—all DNA viruses:

GENERAL RULE	COMMENTS
Are **HHAPPPP**y viruses	Hepadna, Herpes, Adeno, Pox, Parvo, Papilloma, Polyoma.
Are double stranded	Except parvo (single stranded).
Have linear genomes	Except papilloma and polyoma (circular, supercoiled) and hepadna (circular, incomplete).
Are icosahedral	Except pox (complex).
Replicate in the nucleus	Except pox (carries own DNA-dependent RNA polymerase).

DNA viruses

All replicate in the nucleus (except poxvirus). "**Pox** is out of the **box** (nucleus)."

VIRAL FAMILY	ENVELOPE	DNA STRUCTURE	MEDICAL IMPORTANCE
Herpesviruses	Yes	DS and linear	See Herpesviruses entry
Poxvirus	Yes	DS and linear (largest DNA virus)	Smallpox eradicated world wide by use of the live-attenuated vaccine Cowpox ("milkmaid blisters") **Molluscum contagiosum**—flesh-colored papule with central umbilication
Hepadnavirus	Yes	Partially DS and circular	HBV: ▪ Acute or chronic hepatitis ▪ Not a retrovirus but has reverse transcriptase
Adenovirus 	No	DS and linear	Febrile pharyngitis **A**—sore throat Acute hemorrhagic cystitis Pneumonia Conjunctivitis—"pink eye" Gastroenteritis Myocarditis
Papillomavirus	No	DS and circular	HPV–warts (serotypes 1, 2, 6, 11), CIN, cervical cancer (most commonly 16, 18)
Polyomavirus	No	DS and circular	JC virus—progressive multifocal leukoencephalopathy (PML) in HIV BK virus—transplant patients, commonly targets kidney **JC**: **J**unky **C**erebrum; **BK**: **B**ad **K**idney
Parvovirus	No	SS and linear (smallest DNA virus)	B19 virus—aplastic crises in sickle cell disease, "slapped cheek" rash in children (erythema infectiosum, or fifth disease) RBC destruction in fetus leads to hydrops fetalis and death, in adults leads to pure RBC aplasia and rheumatoid arthritis–like symptoms

Herpesviruses

Enveloped, DS, and linear viruses

VIRUS	ROUTE OF TRANSMISSION	CLINICAL SIGNIFICANCE	NOTES
Herpes simplex virus-1	Respiratory secretions, saliva	Gingivostomatitis, keratoconjunctivitis **A**, herpes labialis **B**, herpetic whitlow on finger, temporal lobe encephalitis, esophagitis, erythema multiforme.	Most commonly latent in trigeminal ganglia. Most common cause of sporadic encephalitis, can present as altered mental status, seizures, and/or aphasia.
Herpes simplex virus-2	Sexual contact, perinatal	Herpes genitalis **C**, neonatal herpes.	Most commonly latent in sacral ganglia. Viral meningitis more common with HSV-2 than with HSV-1.
Varicella-Zoster virus (HHV-3)	Respiratory secretions	Varicella-zoster (chickenpox **D**, shingles **E**), encephalitis, pneumonia. Most common complication of shingles is post-herpetic neuralgia.	Latent in dorsal root or trigeminal ganglia; CN V_1 branch involvement can cause herpes zoster ophthalmicus.

Herpesviruses *(continued)*

VIRUS	ROUTE OF TRANSMISSION	CLINICAL SIGNIFICANCE	NOTES
Epstein-Barr virus (HHV-4)	Respiratory secretions, saliva; aka "kissing disease," (common in teens, young adults)	**Mononucleosis**—fever, hepatosplenomegaly 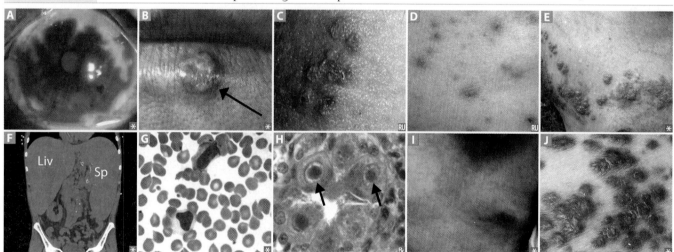, pharyngitis, and lymphadenopathy (especially posterior cervical nodes). Avoid contact sports until resolution due to risk of splenic rupture. Associated with lymphomas (eg, endemic Burkitt lymphoma), nasopharyngeal carcinoma (especially Asian adults), lymphoproliferative disease in transplant patients.	Infects B cells through CD21. Atypical lymphocytes on peripheral blood smear G—not infected B cells but reactive cytotoxic T cells. ⊕ Monospot test—heterophile antibodies detected by agglutination of sheep or horse RBCs. Use of amoxicillin in mononucleosis can cause characteristic maculopapular rash.
Cytomegalo-virus (HHV-5)	Congenital transfusion, sexual contact, saliva, urine, transplant	Mononucleosis (⊖ Monospot) in immunocompetent patients; infection in immunocompromised, especially pneumonia in transplant patients; esophagitis; AIDS **retinitis** ("**sight**omegalovirus"): hemorrhage, cotton-wool exudates, vision loss. Congenital CMV	Infected cells have characteristic "owl eye" intranuclear inclusions H. Latent in mononuclear cells.
Human herpes-viruses 6 and 7	Saliva	Roseola infantum (exanthem subitum): high fevers for several days that can cause seizures, followed by diffuse macular rash I.	**Roseola**: fever first, **Rosy** (rash) **later**. HHV-7—less common cause of roseola.
Human herpesvirus 8	Sexual contact	Kaposi sarcoma (neoplasm of endothelial cells). Seen in HIV/AIDS and transplant patients. Dark/violaceous plaques or nodules J representing vascular proliferations.	Can also affect GI tract and lungs.

HSV identification

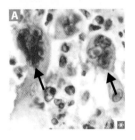

Viral culture for skin/genitalia.

CSF PCR for herpes encephalitis.

Tzanck test—a smear of an opened skin vesicle to detect multinucleated giant cells A commonly seen in HSV-1, HSV-2, and VZV infection. PCR of skin lesions is test of choice.

Tzanck heavens I do not have herpes.

Intranuclear eosinophilic Cowdry A inclusions also seen with HSV-1, HSV-2, VZV.

Receptors used by viruses

VIRUS	RECEPTORS
CMV	Integrins (heparan sulfate)
EBV	CD21
HIV	CD4, CXCR4, CCR5
Parvovirus B19	P antigen on RBCs
Rabies	Nicotinic AChR
Rhinovirus	ICAM-1

RNA viruses

All replicate in the cytoplasm (except **retrovirus** and **influenza virus**). "**Retro flu** is outta **cyt** (sight)."

VIRAL FAMILY	ENVELOPE	RNA STRUCTURE	CAPSID SYMMETRY	MEDICAL IMPORTANCE
Reoviruses	No	DS linear 10–12 segments	Icosahedral (double)	Coltivirus[a]—Colorado tick fever Rotavirus—cause of fatal diarrhea in children
Picornaviruses	No	SS ⊕ linear	Icosahedral	Poliovirus—polio-Salk/Sabin vaccines—IPV/OPV Echovirus—aseptic meningitis Rhinovirus—"common cold" Coxsackievirus—aseptic meningitis; herpangina (mouth blisters, fever); hand, foot, and mouth disease; myocarditis; pericarditis HAV—acute viral hepatitis **PERCH**
Hepevirus	No	SS ⊕ linear	Icosahedral	HEV
Caliciviruses	No	SS ⊕ linear	Icosahedral	Norovirus—viral gastroenteritis
Flaviviruses	Yes	SS ⊕ linear	Icosahedral	HCV Yellow fever[a] Dengue[a] St. Louis encephalitis[a] West Nile virus[a]—meningoencephalitis Zika virus[a]
Togaviruses	Yes	SS ⊕ linear	Icosahedral	Rubella Western and Eastern equine encephalitis[a] Chikungunya virus[a]
Retroviruses	Yes	SS ⊕ linear 2 copies	Icosahedral (HTLV), complex and conical (HIV)	Have reverse transcriptase HTLV—T-cell leukemia HIV—AIDS
Coronaviruses	Yes	SS ⊕ linear	Helical	"Common cold," SARS, MERS
Orthomyxoviruses	Yes	SS ⊖ linear 8 segments	Helical	Influenza virus

Paramyxoviruses	Yes	SS ⊖ linear Nonsegmented	Helical	PaRaMyxovirus:
				    Parainfluenza—croup
				    RSV—bronchiolitis in babies
				    Measles, Mumps

Rhabdoviruses	Yes	SS ⊖ linear	Helical	Rabies
Filoviruses	Yes	SS ⊖ linear	Helical	Ebola/Marburg hemorrhagic fever—often fatal.
Arenaviruses	Yes	SS ⊕ and ⊖ circular 2 segments	Helical	LCMV—lymphocytic choriomeningitis virus Lassa fever encephalitis—spread by rodents
Bunyaviruses	Yes	SS ⊖ circular 3 segments	Helical	California encephalitis[a] Sandfly/Rift Valley fevers[a] Crimean-Congo hemorrhagic fever[a] Hantavirus—hemorrhagic fever, pneumonia
Delta virus	Yes	SS ⊖ circular	Uncertain	HDV is a "defective" virus that requires the presence of HBV to replicate

SS, single-stranded; DS, double-stranded; ⊕, positive sense; ⊖, negative sense; [a]= **arbovirus, arthropod** borne (mosquitoes, ticks).

Negative-stranded viruses	Must transcribe ⊖ strand to ⊕. Virion brings its own RNA-dependent RNA polymerase. They include Arenaviruses, Bunyaviruses, Paramyxoviruses, Orthomyxoviruses, Filoviruses, and Rhabdoviruses.	Always Bring Polymerase Or Fail Replication.
Segmented viruses	All are RNA viruses. They include Bunyaviruses, Orthomyxoviruses (influenza viruses), Arenaviruses, and Reoviruses.	BOAR.
Picornavirus	Includes Poliovirus, Echovirus, Rhinovirus, Coxsackievirus, and HAV. RNA is translated into 1 large polypeptide that is cleaved by proteases into functional viral proteins. Can cause aseptic (viral) meningitis (except rhinovirus and HAV). All are enteroviruses except rhinovirus and HAV.	PicoRNAvirus = small RNA virus. PERCH on a "peak" (pico).
Rhinovirus	A picornavirus. Nonenveloped RNA virus. Cause of common cold; > 100 serologic types. Acid labile—destroyed by stomach acid; therefore, does not infect the GI tract (unlike the other picornaviruses).	Rhino has a runny nose.
Yellow fever virus	A flavivirus (also an arbovirus) transmitted by *Aedes* mosquitoes. Virus has a monkey or human reservoir. Symptoms: high fever, black vomitus, and jaundice. May see Councilman bodies (eosinophilic apoptotic globules) on liver biopsy.	*Flavi* = yellow, jaundice.
Rotavirus	Segmented dsRNA virus (a reovirus) . Most important global cause of infantile gastroenteritis. Major cause of acute diarrhea in the United States during winter, especially in day care centers, kindergartens. Villous destruction with atrophy leads to ↓ absorption of Na⁺ and loss of K⁺.	ROTAvirus = Right Out The Anus. CDC recommends routine vaccination of all infants except those with a history of intussusception or SCID.

Influenza viruses	Orthomyxoviruses. Enveloped, ⊖ ssRNA viruses with 8-segment genome. Contain hemagglutinin (binds sialic acid and promotes viral entry) and neuraminidase (promotes progeny virion release) antigens. Patients at risk for fatal bacterial superinfection, most commonly *S aureus, S pneumoniae*, and *H influenzae*.	Reformulated vaccine ("the flu shot") contains viral strains most likely to appear during the flu season, due to the virus' rapid genetic change. Killed viral vaccine is most frequently used. Live attenuated vaccine contains temperature-sensitive mutant that replicates in the nose but not in the lung; administered intranasally.
Genetic/antigenic shift 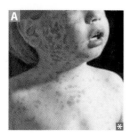 Reassortment	Causes pandemics. Reassortment of viral genome segments, such as when segments of human flu A virus reassort with swine flu A virus.	Sudden shift is more deadly than gradual drift.
Genetic/antigenic drift Random mutations	Causes epidemics. Minor (antigenic drift) changes based on random mutation in hemagglutinin or neuraminidase genes.	

Rubella virus	A togavirus. Causes rubella, once known as German (3-day) measles. Fever, postauricular and other lymphadenopathy, arthralgias, and fine, maculopapular rash that starts on face and spreads centrifugally to involve trunk and extremities A. Causes mild disease in children but serious congenital disease (a ToRCHeS infection). Congenital rubella findings include "blueberry muffin" appearance due to dermal extramedullary hematopoiesis.

Paramyxoviruses

Paramyxoviruses cause disease in children. They include those that cause parainfluenza (croup), mumps, measles, RSV, and human metapneumovirus, which causes respiratory tract infection (bronchiolitis, pneumonia) in infants. All contain surface F (fusion) protein, which causes respiratory epithelial cells to fuse and form multinucleated cells. Palivizumab (monoclonal antibody against F protein) prevents pneumonia caused by RSV infection in premature infants. Palivizumab for Paramyxovirus (RSV) Prophylaxis in Preemies.

Croup (acute laryngo-tracheobronchitis)

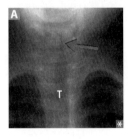

Caused by parainfluenza viruses, which are paramyxoviruses. Virus membrane contains hemagglutinin (binds sialic acid and promotes viral entry) and neuraminidase (promotes progeny virion release) antigens. Results in a "seal-like" barking cough and inspiratory stridor. Narrowing of upper trachea and subglottis leads to characteristic steeple sign on x-ray A. Severe croup can result in pulsus paradoxus 2° to upper airway obstruction.

Measles (rubeola) virus

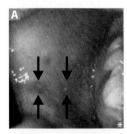

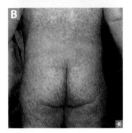

A paramyxovirus that causes measles. Usual presentation involves prodromal fever with cough, coryza, and conjunctivitis, then eventually Koplik spots (bright red spots with blue-white center on buccal mucosa A), followed 1–2 days later by a maculopapular rash B that starts at the head/neck and spreads downward.
Lymphadenitis with Warthin-Finkeldey giant cells (fused lymphocytes) in a background of paracortical hyperplasia. Possible sequelae:
- SSPE (subacute sclerosing panencephalitis, occurring years later)
- Encephalitis (1:2000)
- Giant cell pneumonia (rare except in immunosuppressed)

3 C's of measles:
  Cough
  Coryza
  Conjunctivitis
Vitamin A supplementation can reduce morbidity and mortality from measles, particularly in malnourished children.

Mumps virus

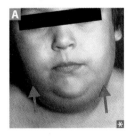

A paramyxovirus that causes mumps, uncommon due to effectiveness of MMR vaccine.
Symptoms: Parotitis A, Orchitis (inflammation of testes), aseptic Meningitis, and Pancreatitis. Can cause sterility (especially after puberty).

Mumps makes your parotid glands and testes as big as POM-Poms.

Rabies virus

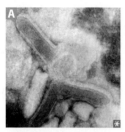

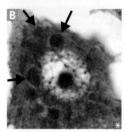

Bullet-shaped virus . Negri bodies (cytoplasmic inclusions **B**) commonly found in Purkinje cells of cerebellum and in hippocampal neurons. Rabies has long incubation period (weeks to months) before symptom onset. Postexposure prophylaxis is wound cleaning plus immunization with killed vaccine and rabies immunoglobulin. Example of passive-active immunity.

Travels to the CNS by migrating in a retrograde fashion (via dynein motors) up nerve axons after binding to ACh receptors.

Progression of disease: fever, malaise → agitation, photophobia, hydrophobia, hypersalivation → paralysis, coma → death.

Infection more commonly from bat, raccoon, and skunk bites than from dog bites in the United States; aerosol transmission (eg, bat caves) also possible.

Ebola virus

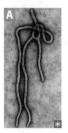

A filovirus **A** that targets endothelial cells, phagocytes, hepatocytes. Following an incubation period of up to 21 days, presents with abrupt onset of flu-like symptoms, diarrhea/vomiting, high fever, myalgia. Can progress to DIC, diffuse hemorrhage, shock. Diagnosed with RT-PCR within 48 hr of symptom onset. High mortality rate.

Transmission requires direct contact with bodily fluids, fomites (including dead bodies), infected bats or primates (apes/monkeys); high incidence of nosocomial infection.

Supportive care, no definitive treatment. Strict isolation of infected individuals and barrier practices for health care workers are key to preventing transmission.

Zika virus

A flavivirus most commonly transmitted by *Aedes* mosquito bites. Causes conjunctivitis, low-grade pyrexia, and itchy rash in 20% of cases. Can lead to congenital microcephaly or miscarriage if transmitted in utero. Diagnose with RT-PCR or serology.

Sexual and vertical transmission possible. Outbreaks more common in tropical and subtropical climates. Supportive care, no definitive treatment.

Hepatitis viruses

Signs and symptoms of all hepatitis viruses: episodes of fever, jaundice, ↑ ALT and AST. Naked viruses (HAV and HEV) lack an envelope and are not destroyed by the gut: the **vowels** hit your **bowels**.

HBV DNA polymerase has DNA- and RNA-dependent activities. Upon entry into nucleus, the polymerase completes the partial dsDNA. Host RNA polymerase transcribes mRNA from viral DNA to make viral proteins. The DNA polymerase then reverse transcribes viral RNA to DNA, which is the genome of the progeny virus.

HCV lacks 3′-5′ exonuclease activity → no proofreading ability → variation in antigenic structures of HCV envelope proteins. Host antibody production lags behind production of new mutant strains of HCV.

Virus	HAV	HBV	HCV	HDV	HEV
FAMILY	RNA picornavirus	DNA hepadnavirus	RNA flavivirus	RNA deltavirus	RNA hepevirus
TRANSMISSION	Fecal-oral (shellfish, travelers, day care)	Parenteral (Blood), sexual (Baby-making), perinatal (Birthing)	Primarily blood (IVDU, post-transfusion)	Parenteral, sexual, perinatal	Fecal-oral, especially waterborne
INCUBATION	Short (weeks)	Long (months)	Long	Superinfection (HDV after HBV) = short Coinfection (HDV with HBV) = long	Short
CLINICAL COURSE	Asymptomatic (usually), Acute	Initially like serum sickness (fever, arthralgias, rash); may progress to carcinoma	May progress to Cirrhosis or Carcinoma	Similar to HBV	Fulminant hepatitis in Expectant (pregnant) women
PROGNOSIS	Good	Adults → mostly full resolution; neonates → worse prognosis	Majority develop stable, Chronic hepatitis C	Superinfection → worse prognosis	High mortality in pregnant women
HCC RISK	No	Yes	Yes	Yes	No
LIVER BIOPSY	Hepatocyte swelling, monocyte infiltration, Councilman bodies	Granular eosinophilic "ground glass" appearance; cytotoxic T cells mediate damage	Lymphoid aggregates with focal areas of macrovesicular steatosis	Similar to HBV	Patchy necrosis
NOTES	No carrier state ("Alone")	Carrier state common	Carrier state very common	Defective virus, Depends on HBV HBsAg coat for entry into hepatocytes	Enteric, Epidemic, no carrier state

Extrahepatic manifestations of hepatitis B and C

	Hepatitis B	Hepatitis C
HEMATOLOGIC	Aplastic anemia	Essential mixed cryoglobulinemia, ↑ risk B-cell NHL, ITP, autoimmune hemolytic anemia
RENAL	Membranous GN > membranoproliferative GN	Membranoproliferative GN > membranous GN
VASCULAR	Polyarteritis nodosa	Leukocytoclastic vasculitis
DERMATOLOGIC		Sporadic porphyria cutanea tarda, lichen planus
ENDOCRINE		↑ risk of diabetes mellitus, autoimmune hypothyroidism

Hepatitis serologic markers

Anti-HAV (IgM)	IgM antibody to HAV; best test to detect acute hepatitis A.
Anti-HAV (IgG)	IgG antibody indicates prior HAV infection and/or prior vaccination; protects against reinfection.
HBsAg	Antigen found on surface of HBV; indicates hepatitis B infection.
Anti-HBs	Antibody to HBsAg; indicates immunity to hepatitis B due to vaccination or recovery from infection.
HBcAg	Antigen associated with core of HBV.
Anti-HBc	Antibody to HBcAg; IgM = acute/recent infection; IgG = prior exposure or chronic infection. IgM anti-HBc may be the sole ⊕ marker of infection during window period.
HBeAg	Secreted by infected hepatocyte into circulation. Not part of mature HBV virion. Indicates active viral replication and therefore high transmissibility and poorer prognosis.
Anti-HBe	Antibody to HBeAg; indicates low transmissibility.

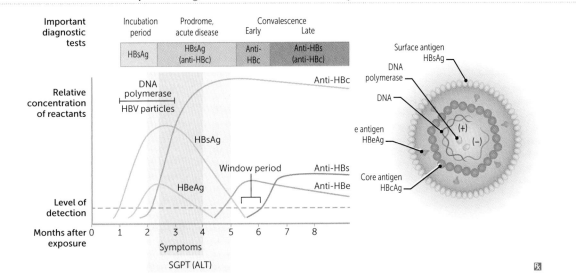

	HBsAg	Anti-HBs	HBeAg	Anti-HBe	Anti-HBc
Acute HBV	✓		✓		IgM
Window				✓	IgM
Chronic HBV (high infectivity)	✓		✓		IgG
Chronic HBV (low infectivity)	✓			✓	IgG
Recovery		✓		✓	IgG
Immunized		✓			

HIV

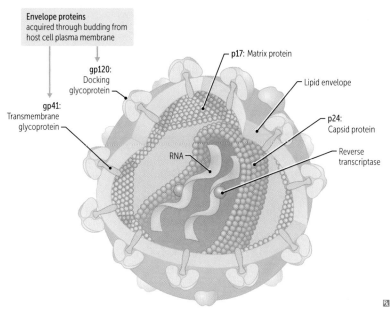

Envelope proteins acquired through budding from host cell plasma membrane

gp120: Docking glycoprotein

gp41: Transmembrane glycoprotein

p17: Matrix protein

Lipid envelope

p24: Capsid protein

Reverse transcriptase

RNA

Diploid genome (2 molecules of RNA).
The 3 structural genes (protein coded for):
- *env* (gp120 and gp41):
  - Formed from cleavage of gp160 to form envelope glycoproteins.
  - gp120—attachment to host CD4+ T cell.
  - gp41—fusion and entry.
- *gag* (p24 and p17)—capsid and matrix proteins, respectively.
- *pol*—reverse transcriptase, aspartate protease, integrase.

Reverse transcriptase synthesizes dsDNA from genomic RNA; dsDNA integrates into host genome.

Virus binds CD4 as well as a coreceptor, either CCR5 on macrophages (early infection) or CXCR4 on T cells (late infection).

Homozygous CCR5 mutation = immunity.
Heterozygous CCR5 mutation = slower course.

HIV diagnosis	Presumptive diagnosis made with HIV-1/2 Ag/Ab immunoassays. These immunoassays detect viral p24 Ag capsid protein and IgG Abs to HIV-1/2. Very high sensitivity/specificity. ⊕ tests are confirmed with HIV-1/2 Ab-differentiation immunoassays which determine whether patient has HIV-1 or HIV-2.

Presumptive diagnosis made with HIV-1/2 Ag/Ab immunoassays. These immunoassays detect viral p24 Ag capsid protein and IgG Abs to HIV-1/2. Very high sensitivity/specificity.

⊕ tests are confirmed with HIV-1/2 Ab-differentiation immunoassays which determine whether patient has HIV-1 or HIV-2.

If inconclusive differentiation assay, an HIV-1 nucleic acid amplification test (NAAT) is performed; if the NAAT is ⊖, patient had false positive initial Ag/Ab immunoassay.

Viral load tests determine the amount of viral RNA in the plasma. High viral load associated with poor prognosis. Also use viral load to monitor effect of drug therapy. Use HIV genotyping to determine appropriate therapy.

AIDS diagnosis ≤ 200 CD4+ cells/mm^3 (normal: 500–1500 cells/mm^3). HIV ⊕ with AIDS-defining condition (eg, *Pneumocystis* pneumonia) or CD4+ percentage < 14%.

Western blot tests are no longer recommended by the CDC for confirmatory testing.

HIV-1/2 Ag/Ab testing is not recommended in babies with suspected HIV due to maternally transferred antibody. Use HIV viral load instead.

Time course of untreated HIV infection

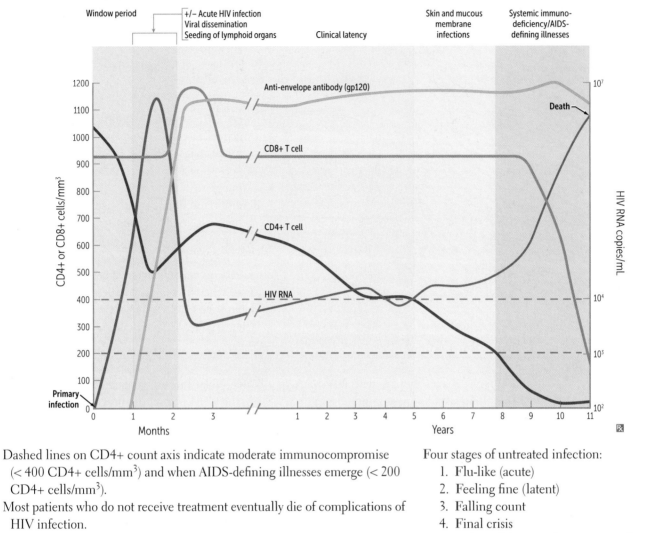

Dashed lines on CD4+ count axis indicate moderate immunocompromise (< 400 CD4+ cells/mm³) and when AIDS-defining illnesses emerge (< 200 CD4+ cells/mm³).

Most patients who do not receive treatment eventually die of complications of HIV infection.

Four stages of untreated infection:
1. Flu-like (acute)
2. Feeling fine (latent)
3. Falling count
4. Final crisis

During clinical latency phase, virus replicates in lymph nodes

Common diseases of HIV-positive adults

As CD4+ cell count ↓, risks of reactivation of past infections (eg, TB, HSV, shingles), dissemination of bacterial infections and fungal infections (eg, coccidioidomycosis), and non-Hodgkin lymphomas ↑.

PATHOGEN	PRESENTATION	FINDINGS
CD4+ cell count < 500/mm³		
Candida albicans	Oral thrush	Scrapable white plaque, pseudohyphae on microscopy
EBV	Oral hairy leukoplakia	Unscrapable white plaque on lateral tongue
HHV-8	Kaposi sarcoma	Biopsy with lymphocytic inflammation
HPV	Squamous cell carcinoma, commonly of anus (men who have sex with men) or cervix (women)	
CD4+ cell count < 200/mm³		
Histoplasma capsulatum	Fever, weight loss, fatigue, cough, dyspnea, nausea, vomiting, diarrhea	Oval yeast cells within macrophages
HIV	Dementia	
JC virus (reactivation)	Progressive multifocal leukoencephalopathy	Nonenhancing areas of demyelination on MRI
Pneumocystis jirovecii	*Pneumocystis* pneumonia	"Ground-glass" opacities on CXR
CD4+ cell count < 100/mm³		
Aspergillus fumigatus	Hemoptysis, pleuritic pain	Cavitation or infiltrates on chest imaging
Bartonella henselae	Bacillary angiomatosis	Biopsy with neutrophilic inflammation
Candida albicans	Esophagitis	White plaques on endoscopy; yeast and pseudohyphae on biopsy
CMV	Retinitis, esophagitis, colitis, pneumonitis, encephalitis	Linear ulcers on endoscopy, cotton-wool spots on fundoscopy. Biopsy reveals cells with intranuclear (owl eye) inclusion bodies
Cryptococcus neoformans	Meningitis	Encapsulated yeast on India ink stain or capsular antigen ⊕
Cryptosporidium spp.	Chronic, watery diarrhea	Acid-fast oocysts in stool
EBV	B-cell lymphoma (eg, non-Hodgkin lymphoma, CNS lymphoma)	CNS lymphoma—ring enhancing, may be solitary (vs *Toxoplasma*)
Mycobacterium avium–intracellulare, Mycobacterium avium complex	Nonspecific systemic symptoms (fever, night sweats, weight loss) or focal lymphadenitis	
Toxoplasma gondii	Brain abscesses	Multiple ring-enhancing lesions on MRI

Prions

Prion diseases are caused by the conversion of a normal (predominantly α-helical) protein termed prion protein (PrP^c) to a β-pleated form (PrP^{sc}), which is transmissible via CNS-related tissue (iatrogenic CJD) or food contaminated by BSE-infected animal products (variant CJD). PrP^{sc} resists protease degradation and facilitates the conversion of still more PrP^c to PrP^{sc}. Resistant to standard sterilizing procedures, including standard autoclaving. Accumulation of PrP^{sc} results in spongiform encephalopathy and dementia, ataxia, and death.

Creutzfeldt-Jakob disease—rapidly progressive dementia, typically sporadic (some familial forms).

Bovine spongiform encephalopathy—also known as "mad cow disease."

Kuru—acquired prion disease noted in tribal populations practicing human cannibalism.

▸ MICROBIOLOGY—SYSTEMS

Normal flora: dominant

Neonates delivered by C-section have no flora but are rapidly colonized after birth.

LOCATION	MICROORGANISM
Skin	S epidermidis
Nose	S epidermidis; colonized by S aureus
Oropharynx	Viridans group streptococci
Dental plaque	S mutans
Colon	B fragilis > E coli
Vagina	Lactobacillus; colonized by E coli and group B strep

Bugs causing food-borne illness

S aureus and B cereus food poisoning starts quickly and ends quickly.

MICROORGANISM	SOURCE OF INFECTION
B cereus	Reheated rice. "Food poisoning from reheated rice? **Be serious!**" (**B cereus**)
C botulinum	Improperly canned foods (toxins), raw honey (spores)
C perfringens	Reheated meat
E coli O157:H7	Undercooked meat
L monocytogenes	Deli meats, soft cheeses
Salmonella	Poultry, meat, and eggs
S aureus	Meats, mayonnaise, custard; preformed toxin
V parahaemolyticus and V vulnificus[a]	Contaminated seafood

[a] V vulnificus can also cause wound infections from contact with contaminated water or shellfish.

Bugs causing diarrhea

Bloody diarrhea	
Campylobacter	Comma- or S-shaped organisms; growth at 42°C
E histolytica	Protozoan; amebic dysentery; liver abscess
Enterohemorrhagic *E coli*	O157:H7; can cause HUS; makes Shiga-like toxin
Enteroinvasive *E coli*	Invades colonic mucosa
Salmonella (non-typhoidal)	Lactose $\ominus$; flagellar motility; has animal reservoir, especially poultry and eggs
Shigella	Lactose $\ominus$; very low ID_{50}; produces Shiga toxin (human reservoir only); bacillary dysentery
Y enterocolitica	Day care outbreaks; pseudoappendicitis

Watery diarrhea	
C difficile	Pseudomembranous colitis; associated with antibiotics and PPIs; occasionally bloody diarrhea
C perfringens	Also causes gas gangrene
Enterotoxigenic *E coli*	Travelers' diarrhea; produces heat-labile (LT) and heat-stable (ST) toxins
Protozoa	*Giardia, Cryptosporidium*
V cholerae	Comma-shaped organisms; rice-water diarrhea; often from infected seafood
Viruses	Rotavirus, norovirus, enteric adenovirus

Common causes of pneumonia

NEONATES (< 4 WK)	CHILDREN (4 WK–18 YR)	ADULTS (18–40 YR)	ADULTS (40–65 YR)	ELDERLY
Group B streptococci *E coli*	Viruses (**RSV**) *Mycoplasma* *C trachomatis* (infants–3 yr) *C pneumoniae* (school-aged children) *S pneumoniae* Runts May Cough Chunky Sputum	*Mycoplasma* *C pneumoniae* *S pneumoniae* Viruses (eg, influenza)	*S pneumoniae* *H influenzae* Anaerobes Viruses *Mycoplasma*	*S pneumoniae* Influenza virus Anaerobes *H influenzae* Gram $\ominus$ rods

Special groups	
Alcoholic	*Klebsiella*, anaerobes usually due to aspiration (eg, *Peptostreptococcus, Fusobacterium, Prevotella, Bacteroides*)
IV drug users	*S pneumoniae, S aureus*
Aspiration	Anaerobes
Atypical	*Mycoplasma, Chlamydophila, Legionella*, viruses (RSV, CMV, influenza, adenovirus)
Cystic fibrosis	*Pseudomonas, S aureus, S pneumoniae, Burkholderia cepacia*
Immunocompromised	*S aureus*, enteric gram $\ominus$ rods, fungi, viruses, *P jirovecii* (with HIV)
Nosocomial (hospital acquired)	*S aureus, Pseudomonas*, other enteric gram $\ominus$ rods
Postviral	*S pneumoniae, S aureus, H influenzae*

Common causes of meningitis

NEWBORN (0–6 MO)	CHILDREN (6 MO–6 YR)	6–60 YR	60 YR +
Group B streptococci	*S pneumoniae*	*S pneumoniae*	*S pneumoniae*
E coli	*N meningitidis*	*N meningitidis* (#1 in teens)	Gram ⊖ rods
Listeria	*H influenzae* type b	Enteroviruses	*Listeria*
	Enteroviruses	HSV	

Give ceftriaxone and vancomycin empirically (add ampicillin if *Listeria* is suspected).

Viral causes of meningitis: enteroviruses (especially coxsackievirus), HSV-2 (HSV-1 = encephalitis), HIV, West Nile virus (also causes encephalitis), VZV.

In HIV: *Cryptococcus* spp.

Note: Incidence of *H influenzae* meningitis has ↓ greatly due to conjugate *H influenzae* vaccinations. Today, cases are usually seen in unimmunized children.

Cerebrospinal fluid findings in meningitis

	OPENING PRESSURE	CELL TYPE	PROTEIN	GLUCOSE
Bacterial	↑	↑ PMNs	↑	↓
Fungal/TB	↑	↑ lymphocytes	↑	↓
Viral	Normal/↑	↑ lymphocytes	Normal/↑	Normal

Infections causing brain abscess	Most commonly viridans streptococci and *Staphylococcus aureus*. If dental infection or extraction precedes abscess, oral anaerobes commonly involved. Multiple abscesses are usually from bacteremia; single lesions from contiguous sites: otitis media and mastoiditis → temporal lobe and cerebellum; sinusitis or dental infection → frontal lobe. *Toxoplasma* reactivation in AIDS.

Osteomyelitis

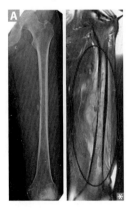

RISK FACTOR	ASSOCIATED INFECTION
Assume if no other information is available	*S aureus* (most common overall)
Sexually active	*Neisseria gonorrhoeae* (rare), septic arthritis more common
Sickle cell disease	*Salmonella* and *S aureus*
Prosthetic joint replacement	*S aureus* and *S epidermidis*
Vertebral involvement	*S aureus, Mycobacterium tuberculosis* (Pott disease)
Cat and dog bites	*Pasteurella multocida*
IV drug abuse	*S aureus*; also *Pseudomonas, Candida*

Elevated C-reactive protein (CRP) and erythrocyte sedimentation rate common but nonspecific. Radiographs are insensitive early but can be useful in chronic osteomyelitis (A, left). MRI is best for detecting acute infection and detailing anatomic involvement (A, right).

Urinary tract infections	Cystitis presents with dysuria, frequency, urgency, suprapubic pain, and WBCs (but not WBC casts) in urine. Primarily caused by ascension of microbes from urethra to bladder. Ascension to kidney results in pyelonephritis, which presents with fever, chills, flank pain, costovertebral angle tenderness, hematuria, and WBC casts.
	Ten times more common in women (shorter urethras colonized by fecal flora). Other predisposing factors: obstruction, kidney surgery, catheterization, GU malformation, diabetes, pregnancy. Males—infants with congenital defects, vesicoureteral reflux. Elderly—enlarged prostate.

SPECIES	FEATURES	COMMENTS
Escherichia coli	Leading cause of UTI. Colonies show strong pink lactose-fermentation on MacConkey agar.	Diagnostic markers:
Staphylococcus saprophyticus	2nd leading cause of UTI in sexually active women.	⊕ Leukocyte esterase = evidence of WBC activity. ⊕ Nitrite test = reduction of urinary nitrates by bacterial species (eg, *E coli*).
Klebsiella pneumoniae	3rd leading cause of UTI. Large mucoid capsule and viscous colonies.	⊕ Urease test = urease-producing bugs (eg, *S saprophyticus*, *Proteus*, *Klebsiella*).
Serratia marcescens	Some strains produce a red pigment; often nosocomial and drug resistant.	
Enterococcus	Often nosocomial and drug resistant.	
Proteus mirabilis	Motility causes "swarming" on agar; associated with struvite stones.	
Pseudomonas aeruginosa	Blue-green pigment and fruity odor; usually nosocomial and drug resistant.	

Common vaginal infections

	Bacterial vaginosis	***Trichomonas* vaginitis**	***Candida* vulvovaginitis**
SIGNS AND SYMPTOMS	No inflammation Thin, white discharge **A** with fishy odor	Inflammation ("strawberry cervix") Frothy, yellow-green, foul-smelling discharge	Inflammation Thick, white, "cottage cheese" discharge **C**
LAB FINDINGS	Clue cells pH > 4.5	Motile trichomonads **B** pH > 4.5	Pseudohyphae pH normal (4.0–4.5)
TREATMENT	Metronidazole or clindamycin	Metronidazole Treat sexual partner(s)	Azoles

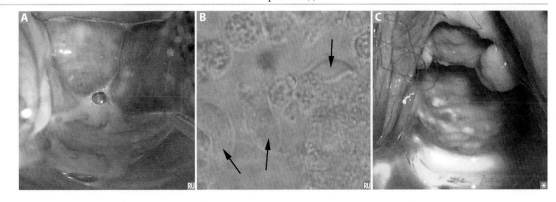

ToRCHeS infections　Microbes that may pass from mother to fetus. Transmission is transplacental in most cases, or via delivery (especially HSV-2). Nonspecific signs common to many ToRCHeS infections include hepatosplenomegaly, jaundice, thrombocytopenia, and growth retardation.

Other important infectious agents include *Streptococcus agalactiae* (group B streptococci), *E coli*, and *Listeria monocytogenes*—all causes of meningitis in neonates. Parvovirus B19 causes hydrops fetalis.

AGENT	MODES OF MATERNAL TRANSMISSION	MATERNAL MANIFESTATIONS	NEONATAL MANIFESTATIONS
Toxoplasma gondii	Cat feces or ingestion of undercooked meat	Usually asymptomatic; lymphadenopathy (rarely)	Classic triad: chorioretinitis, hydrocephalus, and intracranial calcifications, +/− "blueberry muffin" rash A.
Rubella	Respiratory droplets	Rash, lymphadenopathy, polyarthritis, polyarthralgia	Classic triad: abnormalities of **eye** (cataract) and **ear** (deafness) and congenital **heart** disease (PDA); ± "blueberry muffin" rash. "**I** (eye) ♥ **ruby** (**rubella**) **earrings**."
Cytomegalovirus	Sexual contact, organ transplants	Usually asymptomatic; mononucleosis-like illness	Hearing loss, seizures, petechial rash, "blueberry muffin" rash, chorioretinitis, periventricular calcifications B
HIV	Sexual contact, needlestick	Variable presentation depending on CD4+ cell count	Recurrent infections, chronic diarrhea
Herpes simplex virus-2	Skin or mucous membrane contact	Usually asymptomatic; herpetic (vesicular) lesions	Meningoencephalitis, herpetic (vesicular) lesions
Syphilis	Sexual contact	Chancre (1°) and disseminated rash (2°) are the two stages likely to result in fetal infection	Often results in stillbirth, hydrops fetalis; if child survives, presents with facial abnormalities (eg, notched teeth, saddle nose, short maxilla), saber shins, CN VIII deafness

Red rashes of childhood

AGENT	ASSOCIATED SYNDROME/DISEASE	CLINICAL PRESENTATION
Coxsackievirus type A	Hand-foot-mouth disease	Oval-shaped vesicles on palms and soles 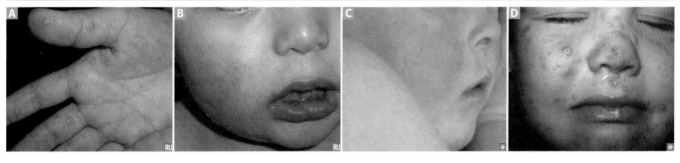; vesicles and ulcers in oral mucosa
Human herpesvirus 6	Roseola (exanthem subitum)	Asymptomatic rose-colored macules appear on body after several days of high fever; can present with febrile seizures; usually affects infants
Measles virus	Measles (rubeola)	Confluent rash beginning at head and moving down; preceded by cough, coryza, conjunctivitis, and blue-white (Koplik) spots on buccal mucosa
Parvovirus B19	Erythema infectiosum (fifth disease)	"Slapped cheek" rash on face B (can cause hydrops fetalis in pregnant women)
Rubella virus	Rubella	Pink macules and papules begin at head and move down, remain discrete → fine desquamating truncal rash; postauricular lymphadenopathy
Streptococcus pyogenes	Scarlet fever	Flushed cheeks and circumoral pallor C on the face; erythematous, sandpaper-like rash from neck to trunk and extremities; fever and sore throat
Varicella-Zoster virus	Chickenpox	Vesicular rash begins on trunk; spreads to face D and extremities with lesions of different stages

Sexually transmitted infections

DISEASE	CLINICAL FEATURES	ORGANISM
AIDS	Opportunistic infections, Kaposi sarcoma, lymphoma	HIV
Chancroid	Painful genital ulcer with exudate, inguinal adenopathy	*Haemophilus ducreyi* (it's so painful, you "do cry")
Chlamydia	Urethritis, cervicitis, epididymitis, conjunctivitis, reactive arthritis, PID	*Chlamydia trachomatis* (D–K)
Condylomata acuminata	Genital warts, koilocytes	HPV-6 and -11
Genital herpes	Painful penile, vulvar, or cervical vesicles and ulcers; can cause systemic symptoms such as fever, headache, myalgia	HSV-2, less commonly HSV-1
Gonorrhea	Urethritis, cervicitis, PID, prostatitis, epididymitis, arthritis, creamy purulent discharge	*Neisseria gonorrhoeae*
Granuloma inguinale (Donovanosis)	Painless, beefy red ulcer that bleeds readily on contact A Uncommon in US	*Klebsiella (Calymmatobacterium) granulomatis*; cytoplasmic Donovan bodies (bipolar staining) seen on microscopy
Hepatitis B	Jaundice	HBV
Lymphogranuloma venereum	Infection of lymphatics; painless genital ulcers, painful lymphadenopathy (ie, buboes)	*C trachomatis* (L1–L3)
Primary syphilis	Painless chancre	*Treponema pallidum*
Secondary syphilis	Fever, lymphadenopathy, skin rashes, condylomata lata	
Tertiary syphilis	Gummas, tabes dorsalis, general paresis, aortitis, Argyll Robertson pupil	
Trichomoniasis	Vaginitis, strawberry cervix, motile in wet prep	*Trichomonas vaginalis*

Pelvic inflammatory disease

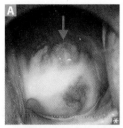
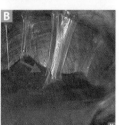

Top bugs—*Chlamydia trachomatis* (subacute, often undiagnosed), *Neisseria gonorrhoeae* (acute).

C trachomatis—most common bacterial STI in the United States.

Signs include cervical motion tenderness, adnexal tenderness, purulent cervical discharge A.

PID may include salpingitis, endometritis, hydrosalpinx, and tubo-ovarian abscess.

Salpingitis is a risk factor for ectopic pregnancy, infertility, chronic pelvic pain, and adhesions. Can lead to perihepatitis (**Fitz-Hugh–Curtis syndrome**)—infection and inflammation of liver capsule and "violin string" adhesions of peritoneum to liver B.

Nosocomial infections

E coli (UTI) and *S aureus* (wound infection) are the two most common causes.

RISK FACTOR	PATHOGEN	UNIQUE SIGNS/SYMPTOMS
Antibiotic use	*Clostridium difficile*	Watery diarrhea, leukocytosis
Aspiration (2° to altered mental status, old age)	Polymicrobial, gram ⊖ bacteria, often anaerobes	Right lower lobe infiltrate or right upper/ middle lobe (patient recumbent); purulent malodorous sputum
Decubitus ulcers, surgical wounds, drains	*S aureus* (including MRSA), gram ⊖ anaerobes (*Bacteroides, Prevotella, Fusobacterium*)	Erythema, tenderness, induration, drainage from surgical wound sites
Intravascular catheters	*S aureus* (including MRSA), *S epidermidis* (long term), *Enterobacter*	Erythema, induration, tenderness, drainage from access sites
Mechanical ventilation, endotracheal intubation	Late onset: *P aeruginosa, Klebsiella, Acinetobacter, S aureus*	New infiltrate on CXR, ↑ sputum production; sweet odor (*Pseudomonas*)
Renal dialysis unit, needlestick	HBV, HCV	
Urinary catheterization	*Proteus* spp, *E coli, Klebsiella* (infections in your PEcKer)	Dysuria, leukocytosis, flank pain or costovertebral angle tenderness
Water aerosols	*Legionella*	Signs of pneumonia, GI symptoms (diarrhea, nausea, vomiting), neurologic abnormalities

Bugs affecting unvaccinated children

CLINICAL PRESENTATION	FINDINGS/LABS	PATHOGEN
Dermatologic		
Rash	Beginning at head and moving down with postauricular lymphadenopathy	Rubella virus
	Beginning at head and moving down; rash preceded by cough, coryza, conjunctivitis, and blue-white (Koplik) spots on buccal mucosa	Measles virus
Neurologic		
Meningitis	Microbe colonizes nasopharynx	*H influenzae* type b
	Can also lead to myalgia and paralysis	Poliovirus
Respiratory		
Epiglottitis	Fever with dysphagia, drooling, and difficulty breathing due to edematous "cherry red" epiglottis; "thumbprint sign" on x-ray	*H influenzae* type b (also capable of causing epiglottitis in fully immunized children)
Pharyngitis	Grayish oropharyngeal exudate ("pseudomembranes" may obstruct airway); painful throat	*Corynebacterium diphtheriae* (elaborates toxin that causes necrosis in pharynx, cardiac, and CNS tissue)

Bug hints	CHARACTERISTIC	ORGANISM
	Asplenic patient (due to surgical splenectomy or autosplenectomy, eg, chronic sickle cell disease)	Encapsulated microbes, especially **SHiN** (*S pneumoniae* >> *H influenzae* type b > *N meningitidis*)
	Branching rods in oral infection, sulfur granules	*Actinomyces israelii*
	Chronic granulomatous disease	Catalase ⊕ microbes, especially *S aureus*
	"Currant jelly" sputum	*Klebsiella*
	Dog or cat bite	*Pasteurella multocida*
	Facial nerve palsy (typically bilateral)	*Borrelia burgdorferi* (Lyme disease)
	Fungal infection in diabetic or immunocompromised patient	*Mucor* or *Rhizopus* spp.
	Health care provider	HBV, HCV (from needlestick)
	Neutropenic patients	*Candida albicans* (systemic), *Aspergillus*
	Organ transplant recipient	CMV
	PAS ⊕	*Tropheryma whipplei* (Whipple disease)
	Pediatric infection	*Haemophilus influenzae* (including epiglottitis)
	Pneumonia in cystic fibrosis, burn infection	*Pseudomonas aeruginosa*
	Pus, empyema, abscess	*S aureus*
	Rash on hands and feet	Coxsackie A virus, *Treponema pallidum*, *Rickettsia rickettsii*
	Sepsis/meningitis in newborn	Group B strep
	Surgical wound	*S aureus*
	Traumatic open wound	*Clostridium perfringens*

▶ MICROBIOLOGY—ANTIMICROBIALS

Antimicrobial therapy

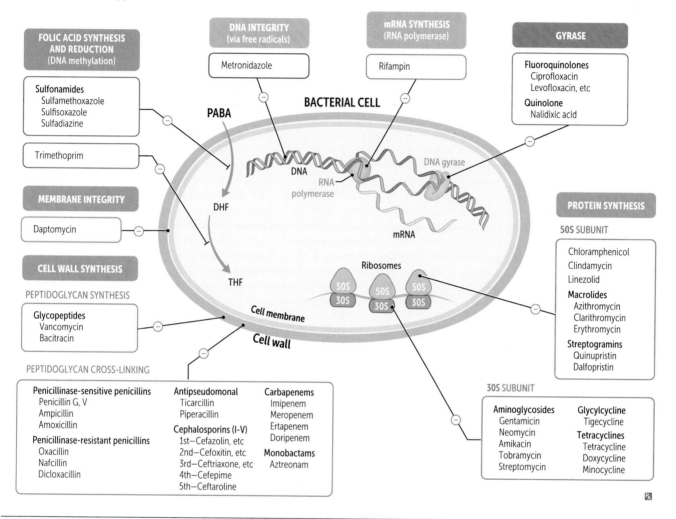

Penicillin G, V	Penicillin G (IV and IM form), penicillin V (oral). Prototype β-lactam antibiotics.
MECHANISM	D-Ala-D-Ala structural analog. Bind penicillin-binding proteins (transpeptidases). Block transpeptidase cross-linking of peptidoglycan in cell wall. Activate autolytic enzymes.
CLINICAL USE	Mostly used for gram ⊕ organisms (*S pneumoniae*, *S pyogenes*, *Actinomyces*). Also used for gram ⊖ cocci (mainly *N meningitidis*) and spirochetes (namely *T pallidum*). Bactericidal for gram ⊕ cocci, gram ⊕ rods, gram ⊖ cocci, and spirochetes. β-lactamase sensitive.
ADVERSE EFFECTS	Hypersensitivity reactions, direct Coombs ⊕ hemolytic anemia, drug-induced interstitial nephritis.
RESISTANCE	β-lactamase cleaves the β-lactam ring. Mutations in penicillin-binding proteins.

Penicillinase-sensitive penicillins	Amoxicillin, ampicillin; aminopenicillins.	
MECHANISM	Same as penicillin. Wider spectrum; penicillinase sensitive. Also combine with clavulanic acid to protect against destruction by β-lactamase.	AMinoPenicillins are AMPed-up penicillin. AmOxicillin has greater Oral bioavailability than ampicillin.
CLINICAL USE	Extended-spectrum penicillin—*H influenzae*, *H pylori*, *E coli*, *Listeria monocytogenes*, *Proteus mirabilis*, *Salmonella*, *Shigella*, enterococci.	Coverage: ampicillin/amoxicillin HHELPSS kill enterococci.
ADVERSE EFFECTS	Hypersensitivity reactions, rash, pseudomembranous colitis.	
MECHANISM OF RESISTANCE	Penicillinase (a type of β-lactamase) cleaves β-lactam ring.	

Penicillinase-resistant penicillins	Dicloxacillin, nafcillin, oxacillin.	
MECHANISM	Same as penicillin. Narrow spectrum; penicillinase resistant because bulky R group blocks access of β-lactamase to β-lactam ring.	
CLINICAL USE	*S aureus* (except MRSA).	"Use naf (nafcillin) for staph."
ADVERSE EFFECTS	Hypersensitivity reactions, interstitial nephritis.	
MECHANISM OF RESISTANCE	MRSA has altered penicillin-binding protein target site.	

Antipseudomonal penicillins	Piperacillin, ticarcillin.	
MECHANISM	Same as penicillin. Extended spectrum. Penicillinase sensitive; use with β-lactamase inhibitors.	
CLINICAL USE	*Pseudomonas* spp. and gram ⊖ rods.	
ADVERSE EFFECTS	Hypersensitivity reactions.	

β-lactamase inhibitors	Include Clavulanic acid, Avibactam, Sulbactam, Tazobactam. Often added to penicillin antibiotics to protect the antibiotic from destruction by β-lactamase (penicillinase).	CAST.

Cephalosporins

MECHANISM	β-lactam drugs that inhibit cell wall synthesis but are less susceptible to penicillinases. Bactericidal.	Organisms typically not covered by 1st–4th generation cephalosporins are **LAME**: *Listeria*, Atypicals (*Chlamydia*, *Mycoplasma*), **MRSA**, and Enterococci.
CLINICAL USE	1st generation (cefazolin, cephalexin)—gram ⊕ cocci, *Proteus mirabilis*, *E coli*, *Klebsiella pneumoniae*. Cefazolin used prior to surgery to prevent *S aureus* wound infections.	1st generation—**PEcK**.
	2nd generation (cefaclor, cefoxitin, cefuroxime, cefotetan)—gram ⊕ cocci, *H influenzae*, *Enterobacter aerogenes*, *Neisseria* spp., *Serratia marcescens*, *Proteus mirabilis*, *E coli*, *Klebsiella pneumoniae*.	2nd graders wear fake fox fur to tea parties. 2nd generation—**HENS PEcK**.
	3rd generation (ceftriaxone, cefotaxime, cefpodoxime, ceftazidime)—serious gram ⊖ infections resistant to other β-lactams.	Can cross blood-brain barrier. Ceftriaxone—meningitis, gonorrhea, disseminated Lyme disease. Ceftazidime—*Pseudomonas*.
	4th generation (cefepime)—gram ⊖ organisms, with ↑ activity against *Pseudomonas* and gram ⊕ organisms.	
	5th generation (ceftaroline)—broad gram ⊕ and gram ⊖ organism coverage; unlike 1st–4th generation cephalosporins, ceftaroline covers *Listeria*, MRSA, and *Enterococcus faecalis*—does not cover *Pseudomonas*.	
ADVERSE EFFECTS	Hypersensitivity reactions, autoimmune hemolytic anemia, disulfiram-like reaction, vitamin K deficiency. Low rate of cross-reactivity even in penicillin-allergic patients. ↑ nephrotoxicity of aminoglycosides.	
MECHANISM OF RESISTANCE	Inactivated by cephalosporinases (a type of β-lactamase). Structural change in penicillin-binding proteins (transpeptidases).	

Carbapenems

Doripenem, Imipenem, Meropenem, Ertapenem (**DIME** antibiotics are given when there is a 10/10 [life-threatening] infection).

MECHANISM	Imipenem is a broad-spectrum, β-lactamase–resistant carbapenem. Always administered with cilastatin (inhibitor of renal dehydropeptidase I) to ↓ inactivation of drug in renal tubules.	With imipenem, "the kill is **lastin'** with cilastatin." Newer carbapenems include ertapenem (limited *Pseudomonas* coverage) and doripenem.
CLINICAL USE	Gram ⊕ cocci, gram ⊖ rods, and anaerobes. Wide spectrum and significant side effects limit use to life-threatening infections or after other drugs have failed. Meropenem has a ↓ risk of seizures and is stable to dehydropeptidase I.	
ADVERSE EFFECTS	GI distress, rash, and CNS toxicity (seizures) at high plasma levels.	

Monobactams

Aztreonam

MECHANISM	Less susceptible to β-lactamases. Prevents peptidoglycan cross-linking by binding to penicillin-binding protein 3. Synergistic with aminoglycosides. No cross-allergenicity with penicillins.
CLINICAL USE	Gram ⊖ rods only—no activity against gram ⊕ rods or anaerobes. For penicillin-allergic patients and those with renal insufficiency who cannot tolerate aminoglycosides.
ADVERSE EFFECTS	Usually nontoxic; occasional GI upset.

Vancomycin

MECHANISM	Inhibits cell wall peptidoglycan formation by binding D-Ala-D-Ala portion of cell wall precursors. Bactericidal against most bacteria (bacteriostatic against *C difficile*). Not susceptible to β-lactamases.
CLINICAL USE	Gram ⊕ bugs only—serious, multidrug-resistant organisms, including MRSA, *S epidermidis*, sensitive *Enterococcus* species, and *Clostridium difficile* (oral dose for pseudomembranous colitis).
ADVERSE EFFECTS	Well tolerated in general—but **NOT** trouble free. Nephrotoxicity, Ototoxicity, Thrombophlebitis, diffuse flushing—red man syndrome **A** (largely preventable by pretreatment with antihistamines and slow infusion rate), drug reaction with eosinophilia and systemic symptoms (DRESS syndrome).
MECHANISM OF RESISTANCE	Occurs in bacteria (eg, *Enterococcus*) via amino acid modification of D-Ala-D-Ala to **D-Ala-D-Lac**. "If you **Lack** a **D-Ala** (dollar), you can't ride the **van** (vancomycin)."

Protein synthesis inhibitors

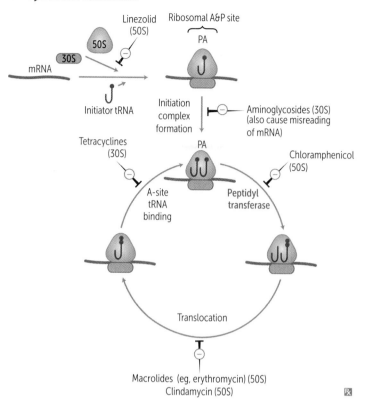

Specifically target smaller bacterial ribosome (70S, made of 30S and 50S subunits), leaving human ribosome (80S) unaffected.
All are bacteriostatic, except aminoglycosides (bactericidal) and linezolid (variable).

30S inhibitors
Aminoglycosides
Tetracyclines

50S inhibitors
Chloramphenicol, Clindamycin
Erythromycin (macrolides)
Linezolid

"Buy **AT 30, CCEL** (sell) at **50**."

Aminoglycosides	Gentamicin, Neomycin, Amikacin, Tobramycin, Streptomycin.	"**Mean**" (aminoglycoside) **GNATS** ca**NNOT** kill anaerobes.
MECHANISM	Bactericidal; irreversible inhibition of initiation complex through binding of the 30S subunit. Can cause misreading of mRNA. Also block translocation. Require O_2 for uptake; therefore ineffective against anaerobes.	
CLINICAL USE	Severe gram ⊖ rod infections. Synergistic with β-lactam antibiotics. Neomycin for bowel surgery.	
ADVERSE EFFECTS	Nephrotoxicity, Neuromuscular blockade, Ototoxicity (especially when used with loop diuretics). Teratogen.	
MECHANISM OF RESISTANCE	Bacterial transferase enzymes inactivate the drug by acetylation, phosphorylation, or adenylation.	

Tetracyclines	Tetracycline, doxycycline, minocycline.
MECHANISM	Bacteriostatic; bind to 30S and prevent attachment of aminoacyl-tRNA. Limited CNS penetration. Doxycycline is fecally eliminated and can be used in patients with renal failure. Do not take tetracyclines with milk (Ca^{2+}), antacids (Ca^{2+} or Mg^{2+}), or iron-containing preparations because divalent cations inhibit drugs' absorption in the gut.
CLINICAL USE	*Borrelia burgdorferi, M pneumoniae.* Drugs' ability to accumulate intracellularly makes them very effective against *Rickettsia* and *Chlamydia.* Also used to treat acne. Doxycycline effective against MRSA.
ADVERSE EFFECTS	GI distress, discoloration of teeth and inhibition of bone growth in children, photosensitivity. Contraindicated in pregnancy.
MECHANISM OF RESISTANCE	↓ uptake or ↑ efflux out of bacterial cells by plasmid-encoded transport pumps.

Glycylcyclines	Tigecycline.
MECHANISM	Tetracycline derivative. Binds to 30S, inhibiting protein synthesis. Generally bacteriostatic.
CLINICAL USE	Broad-spectrum anaerobic, gram ⊖, and gram ⊕ coverage. Multidrug-resistant organisms (MRSA, VRE) or infections requiring deep tissue penetration.
ADVERSE EFFECTS	GI symptoms: nausea, vomiting.

Chloramphenicol	
MECHANISM	Blocks peptidyltransferase at 50S ribosomal subunit. Bacteriostatic.
CLINICAL USE	Meningitis (*Haemophilus influenzae, Neisseria meningitidis, Streptococcus pneumoniae*) and rickettsial diseases (eg, Rocky Mountain spotted fever [*Rickettsia rickettsii*]). Limited use due to toxicity but often still used in developing countries because of low cost.
ADVERSE EFFECTS	Anemia (dose dependent), aplastic anemia (dose independent), gray baby syndrome (in premature infants because they lack liver UDP-glucuronosyltransferase).
MECHANISM OF RESISTANCE	Plasmid-encoded acetyltransferase inactivates the drug.

Clindamycin		
MECHANISM	Blocks peptide transfer (translocation) at 50S ribosomal subunit. Bacteriostatic.	
CLINICAL USE	Anaerobic infections (eg, *Bacteroides* spp., *Clostridium perfringens*) in aspiration pneumonia, lung abscesses, and oral infections. Also effective against invasive group A streptococcal infection.	Treats anaerobic infections **above** the diaphragm vs metronidazole (anaerobic infections **below** diaphragm).
ADVERSE EFFECTS	Pseudomembranous colitis (*C difficile* overgrowth), fever, diarrhea.	

Oxazolidinones	Linezolid.
MECHANISM	Inhibit protein synthesis by binding to 50S subunit and preventing formation of the initiation complex.
CLINICAL USE	Gram ⊕ species including MRSA and VRE.
ADVERSE EFFECTS	Bone marrow suppression (especially thrombocytopenia), peripheral neuropathy, serotonin syndrome.
MECHANISM OF RESISTANCE	Point mutation of ribosomal RNA.

Macrolides	Azithromycin, clarithromycin, erythromycin.
MECHANISM	Inhibit protein synthesis by blocking translocation ("macro**slides**"); bind to the 23S rRNA of the 50S ribosomal subunit. Bacteriostatic.
CLINICAL USE	Atypical pneumonias (*Mycoplasma, Chlamydia, Legionella*), STIs (*Chlamydia*), gram ⊕ cocci (streptococcal infections in patients allergic to penicillin), and *B pertussis*.
ADVERSE EFFECTS	**MACRO**: Gastrointestinal **M**otility issues, **A**rrhythmia caused by prolonged QT interval, acute **C**holestatic hepatitis, **R**ash, e**O**sinophilia. Increases serum concentration of theophylline, oral anticoagulants. Clarithromycin and erythromycin inhibit cytochrome P-450.
MECHANISM OF RESISTANCE	Methylation of 23S rRNA-binding site prevents binding of drug.

Polymyxins	Colistin (polymyxin E), polymyxin B.
MECHANISM	Cation polypeptides that bind to phospholipids on cell membrane of gram ⊖ bacteria. Disrupt cell membrane integrity → leakage of cellular components → cell death.
CLINICAL USE	Salvage therapy for multidrug-resistant gram ⊖ bacteria (eg, *P aeruginosa, E coli, K pneumoniae*). Polymyxin B is a component of a triple antibiotic ointment used for superficial skin infections.
ADVERSE EFFECTS	Nephrotoxicity, neurotoxicity (eg, slurred speech, weakness, paresthesias), respiratory failure.

Sulfonamides	Sulfamethoxazole (SMX), sulfisoxazole, sulfadiazine.
MECHANISM	Inhibit dihydropteroate synthase, thus inhibiting folate synthesis. Bacteriostatic (bactericidal when combined with trimethoprim).
CLINICAL USE	Gram ⊕, gram ⊖, *Nocardia*. TMP-SMX for simple UTI.
ADVERSE EFFECTS	Hypersensitivity reactions, hemolysis if G6PD deficient, nephrotoxicity (tubulointerstitial nephritis), photosensitivity, Stevens-Johnson syndrome, kernicterus in infants, displace other drugs from albumin (eg, warfarin).
MECHANISM OF RESISTANCE	Altered enzyme (bacterial dihydropteroate synthase), ↓ uptake, or ↑ PABA synthesis.

PABA + Pteridine

Dihydropteroate synthase ⊢ ─⊖── **Sulfonamides, dapsone**

Dihydropteroic acid

↓

Dihydrofolic acid

Dihydrofolate reductase ⊢ ─⊖── **Trimethoprim, pyrimethamine**

Tetrahydrofolic acid

Purines   Thymidine   Methionine

DNA, RNA   DNA   Protein   ℞

Dapsone	
MECHANISM	Similar to sulfonamides, but structurally distinct agent.
CLINICAL USE	Leprosy (lepromatous and tuberculoid), *Pneumocystis jirovecii* prophylaxis.
ADVERSE EFFECTS	Hemolysis if G6PD deficient, methemoglobinemia.

Trimethoprim	
MECHANISM	Inhibits bacterial dihydrofolate reductase. Bacteriostatic.
CLINICAL USE	Used in combination with sulfonamides (trimethoprim-sulfamethoxazole [TMP-SMX]), causing sequential block of folate synthesis. Combination used for UTIs, *Shigella*, *Salmonella*, *Pneumocystis jirovecii* pneumonia treatment and prophylaxis, toxoplasmosis prophylaxis.
ADVERSE EFFECTS	Megaloblastic anemia, leukopenia, granulocytopenia, which may be avoided with coadministration of folinic acid. **TMP** Treats **M**arrow **P**oorly.

Fluoroquinolones	Ciprofloxacin, enoxacin, norfloxacin, ofloxacin; respiratory fluoroquinolones—gemifloxacin, levofloxacin, moxifloxacin.	
MECHANISM	Inhibit prokaryotic enzymes topoisomerase II (DNA gyrase) and topoisomerase IV. Bactericidal. Must not be taken with antacids.	
CLINICAL USE	Gram ⊖ rods of urinary and GI tracts (including *Pseudomonas*), some gram ⊕ organisms, otitis externa.	
ADVERSE EFFECTS	GI upset, superinfections, skin rashes, headache, dizziness. Less commonly, can cause leg cramps and myalgias. Contraindicated in pregnant women, nursing mothers, and children < 18 years old due to possible damage to cartilage. Some may prolong QT interval. May cause tendonitis or tendon rupture in people > 60 years old and in patients taking prednisone. Ciprofloxacin inhibits cytochrome P-450.	**Fluoroquinolones** hurt attachments to your **bones**.
MECHANISM OF RESISTANCE	Chromosome-encoded mutation in DNA gyrase, plasmid-mediated resistance, efflux pumps.	

Daptomycin		
MECHANISM	Lipopeptide that disrupts cell membranes of gram ⊕ cocci by creating transmembrane channels.	
CLINICAL USE	*S aureus* skin infections (especially MRSA), bacteremia, endocarditis, VRE.	Not used for pneumonia (avidly binds to and is inactivated by surfactant).
ADVERSE EFFECTS	Myopathy, rhabdomyolysis.	

Metronidazole		
MECHANISM	Forms toxic free radical metabolites in the bacterial cell that damage DNA. Bactericidal, antiprotozoal.	
CLINICAL USE	Treats *Giardia, Entamoeba, Trichomonas, Gardnerella vaginalis,* Anaerobes (*Bacteroides, C difficile*). Can be used in place of amoxicillin in *H pylori* "triple therapy" in case of penicillin allergy.	**GET GAP** on the **Metro** with **metronidazole**! Treats anaerobic infection **below** the diaphragm vs clindamycin (anaerobic infections **above** diaphragm).
ADVERSE EFFECTS	Disulfiram-like reaction (severe flushing, tachycardia, hypotension) with alcohol; headache, metallic taste.	

Antimycobacterial drugs

BACTERIUM	PROPHYLAXIS	TREATMENT
M tuberculosis	Isoniazid	Rifampin, Isoniazid, Pyrazinamide, Ethambutol (**RIPE** for treatment)
M avium–intracellulare	Azithromycin, rifabutin	More drug resistant than *M tuberculosis*. Azithromycin or clarithromycin + ethambutol. Can add rifabutin or ciprofloxacin.
M leprae	N/A	Long-term treatment with dapsone and rifampin for tuberculoid form. Add clofazimine for lepromatous form.

MYCOBACTERIAL CELL

Rifamycins

Rifampin, rifabutin.

MECHANISM	Inhibit DNA-dependent RNA polymerase.
CLINICAL USE	*Mycobacterium tuberculosis*; delay resistance to dapsone when used for leprosy. Used for meningococcal prophylaxis and chemoprophylaxis in contacts of children with *H influenzae* type b.
ADVERSE EFFECTS	Minor hepatotoxicity and drug interactions (↑ cytochrome P-450); orange body fluids (nonhazardous side effect). Rifabutin favored over rifampin in patients with HIV infection due to less cytochrome P-450 stimulation.
MECHANISM OF RESISTANCE	Mutations reduce drug binding to RNA polymerase. Monotherapy rapidly leads to resistance.

Rifampin's 4 R's:
   RNA polymerase inhibitor
   Ramps up microsomal cytochrome P-450
   Red/orange body fluids
   Rapid resistance if used alone
Rifampin **ramps** up cytochrome P-450, but rifabutin does not.

Isoniazid

MECHANISM	↓ synthesis of mycolic acids. Bacterial catalase-peroxidase (encoded by KatG) needed to convert INH to active metabolite.	
CLINICAL USE	*Mycobacterium tuberculosis.* The only agent used as solo prophylaxis against TB. Also used as monotherapy for latent TB.	Different INH half-lives in fast vs slow acetylators.
ADVERSE EFFECTS	Hepatotoxicity, P-450 inhibition, drug-induced SLE, anion gap metabolic acidosis, vitamin B_6 deficiency (peripheral neuropathy, sideroblastic anemia). Administer with pyridoxine (B_6).	**INH** **I**njures **N**eurons and **H**epatocytes.
MECHANISM OF RESISTANCE	Mutations leading to underexpression of KatG.	

Pyrazinamide

MECHANISM	Mechanism uncertain. Pyrazinamide is a prodrug that is converted to the active compound pyrazinoic acid. Works best at acidic pH (eg, in host phagolysosomes).
CLINICAL USE	*Mycobacterium tuberculosis.*
ADVERSE EFFECTS	Hyperuricemia, hepatotoxicity.

Ethambutol

MECHANISM	↓ carbohydrate polymerization of mycobacterium cell wall by blocking arabinosyltransferase.
CLINICAL USE	*Mycobacterium tuberculosis.*
ADVERSE EFFECTS	Optic neuropathy (red-green color blindness). Pronounce "eyethambutol."

Streptomycin

MECHANISM	Interferes with 30S component of ribosome.
CLINICAL USE	*Mycobacterium tuberculosis* (2nd line).
ADVERSE EFFECTS	Tinnitus, vertigo, ataxia, nephrotoxicity.

Antimicrobial prophylaxis

CLINICAL SCENARIO	MEDICATION
High risk for endocarditis and undergoing surgical or dental procedures	Amoxicillin
Exposure to gonorrhea	Ceftriaxone
History of recurrent UTIs	TMP-SMX
Exposure to meningococcal infection	Ceftriaxone, ciprofloxacin, or rifampin
Pregnant woman carrying group B strep	Intrapartum penicillin G or ampicillin
Prevention of gonococcal conjunctivitis in newborn	Erythromycin ointment on eyes
Prevention of postsurgical infection due to S aureus	Cefazolin
Prophylaxis of strep pharyngitis in child with prior rheumatic fever	Benzathine penicillin G or oral penicillin V
Exposure to syphilis	Benzathine penicillin G

Prophylaxis in HIV patients

CELL COUNT	PROPHYLAXIS	INFECTION
CD4 < 200 cells/mm^3	TMP-SMX	*Pneumocystis* pneumonia
CD4 < 100 cells/mm^3	TMP-SMX	*Pneumocystis* pneumonia and toxoplasmosis
CD4 < 50 cells/mm^3	Azithromycin or clarithromycin	*Mycobacterium avium* complex

Treatment of highly resistant bacteria

MRSA: vancomycin, daptomycin, linezolid, tigecycline, ceftaroline, doxycycline.
VRE: linezolid and streptogramins (quinupristin, dalfopristin).
Multidrug-resistant *P aeruginosa*, multidrug-resistant *Acinetobacter baumannii*: polymyxins B and E (colistin).

Antifungal therapy

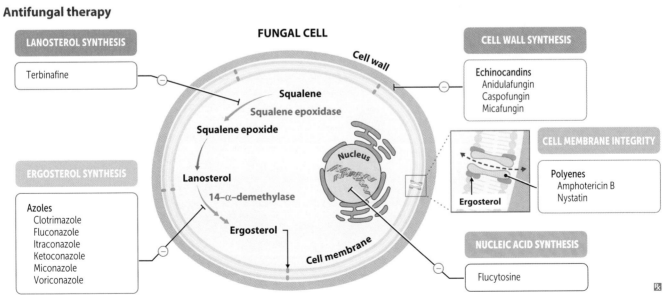

Amphotericin B

MECHANISM	Binds ergosterol (unique to fungi); forms membrane pores that allow leakage of electrolytes.	Amphotericin "tears" holes in the fungal membrane by forming pores.
CLINICAL USE	Serious, systemic mycoses. *Cryptococcus* (amphotericin B with/without flucytosine for cryptococcal meningitis), *Blastomyces*, *Coccidioides*, *Histoplasma*, *Candida*, *Mucor*. Intrathecally for fungal meningitis. Supplement K^+ and Mg^{2+} because of altered renal tubule permeability.	
ADVERSE EFFECTS	Fever/chills ("shake and bake"), hypotension, nephrotoxicity, arrhythmias, anemia, IV phlebitis ("**amphoterrible**"). Hydration ↓ nephrotoxicity. Liposomal amphotericin ↓ toxicity.	

Nystatin

MECHANISM	Same as amphotericin B. Topical use only as too toxic for systemic use.
CLINICAL USE	"Swish and swallow" for oral candidiasis (thrush); topical for diaper rash or vaginal candidiasis.

Flucytosine

MECHANISM	Inhibits DNA and RNA biosynthesis by conversion to 5-fluorouracil by cytosine deaminase.
CLINICAL USE	Systemic fungal infections (especially meningitis caused by *Cryptococcus*) in combination with amphotericin B.
ADVERSE EFFECTS	Bone marrow suppression.

Azoles

	Clotrimazole, fluconazole, isavuconazole, itraconazole, ketoconazole, miconazole, voriconazole.
MECHANISM	Inhibit fungal sterol (ergosterol) synthesis by inhibiting the cytochrome P-450 enzyme that converts lanosterol to ergosterol.
CLINICAL USE	Local and less serious systemic mycoses. Fluconazole for chronic suppression of cryptococcal meningitis in AIDS patients and candidal infections of all types. Itraconazole for *Blastomyces*, *Coccidioides*, *Histoplasma*. Clotrimazole and miconazole for topical fungal infections. Voriconazole for *Aspergillus* and some *Candida*. Isavuconazole for serious *Aspergillus* and *Mucor* infections.
ADVERSE EFFECTS	Testosterone synthesis inhibition (gynecomastia, especially with ketoconazole), liver dysfunction (inhibits cytochrome P-450).

Terbinafine

MECHANISM	Inhibits the fungal enzyme squalene epoxidase.
CLINICAL USE	Dermatophytoses (especially onychomycosis—fungal infection of finger or toe nails).
ADVERSE EFFECTS	GI upset, headaches, hepatotoxicity, taste disturbance.

Echinocandins	Anidulafungin, caspofungin, micafungin.
MECHANISM	Inhibit cell wall synthesis by inhibiting synthesis of β-glucan.
CLINICAL USE	Invasive aspergillosis, *Candida*.
ADVERSE EFFECTS	GI upset, flushing (by histamine release).

Griseofulvin	
MECHANISM	Interferes with microtubule function; disrupts mitosis. Deposits in keratin-containing tissues (eg, nails).
CLINICAL USE	Oral treatment of superficial infections; inhibits growth of dermatophytes (tinea, ringworm).
ADVERSE EFFECTS	Teratogenic, carcinogenic, confusion, headaches, disulfiram-like reaction, ↑ cytochrome P-450 and warfarin metabolism.

Antiprotozoal therapy	Pyrimethamine (toxoplasmosis), suramin and melarsoprol (*Trypanosoma brucei*), nifurtimox (*T cruzi*), sodium stibogluconate (leishmaniasis).

Anti-mite/louse therapy	Permethrin (inhibits Na⁺ channel deactivation → neuronal membrane depolarization), malathion (acetylcholinesterase inhibitor), lindane (blocks GABA channels → neurotoxicity). Used to treat scabies (*Sarcoptes scabiei*) and lice (*Pediculus* and *Pthirus*).	Treat **PML** (Pesty Mites and Lice) with **PML** (Permethrin, Malathion, Lindane), because they **NAG** you (Na, AChE, GABA blockade).

Chloroquine	
MECHANISM	Blocks detoxification of heme into hemozoin. Heme accumulates and is toxic to plasmodia.
CLINICAL USE	Treatment of plasmodial species other than *P falciparum* (frequency of resistance in *P falciparum* is too high). Resistance due to membrane pump that ↓ intracellular concentration of drug. Treat *P falciparum* with artemether/lumefantrine or atovaquone/proguanil. For life-threatening malaria, use quinidine in US (quinine elsewhere) or artesunate.
ADVERSE EFFECTS	Retinopathy; pruritus (especially in dark-skinned individuals).

Antihelminthic therapy	Pyrantel pamoate, Ivermectin, Mebendazole (microtubule inhibitor), Praziquantel, Diethylcarbamazine. Helminths get **PIMP'D**.

Antiviral therapy

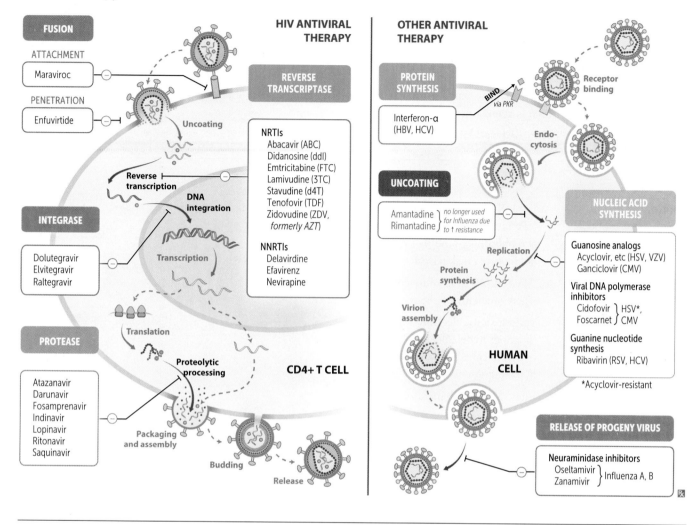

Oseltamivir, zanamivir

MECHANISM	Inhibit influenza neuraminidase → ↓ release of progeny virus.
CLINICAL USE	Treatment and prevention of both influenza A and B. Beginning therapy within 48 hours of symptom onset may shorten duration of illness.

Acyclovir, famciclovir, valacyclovir

MECHANISM	Guanosine analogs. Monophosphorylated by HSV/VZV thymidine kinase and not phosphorylated in uninfected cells → few adverse effects. Triphosphate formed by cellular enzymes. Preferentially inhibit viral DNA polymerase by chain termination.
CLINICAL USE	HSV and VZV. Weak activity against EBV. No activity against CMV. Used for HSV-induced mucocutaneous and genital lesions as well as for encephalitis. Prophylaxis in immunocompromised patients. No effect on latent forms of HSV and VZV. Valacyclovir, a prodrug of acyclovir, has better oral bioavailability. For herpes zoster, use famciclovir.
ADVERSE EFFECTS	Obstructive crystalline nephropathy and acute renal failure if not adequately hydrated.
MECHANISM OF RESISTANCE	Mutated viral thymidine kinase.

Ganciclovir

MECHANISM	5′-monophosphate formed by a CMV viral kinase. Guanosine analog. Triphosphate formed by cellular kinases. Preferentially inhibits viral DNA polymerase.
CLINICAL USE	CMV, especially in immunocompromised patients. Valganciclovir, a prodrug of ganciclovir, has better oral bioavailability.
ADVERSE EFFECTS	Bone marrow suppression (leukopenia, neutropenia, thrombocytopenia), renal toxicity. More toxic to host enzymes than acyclovir.
MECHANISM OF RESISTANCE	Mutated viral kinase.

Foscarnet

MECHANISM	Viral DNA/RNA polymerase inhibitor and HIV reverse transcriptase inhibitor. Binds to pyrophosphate-binding site of enzyme. Does not require any kinase activation.	Foscarnet = pyrofosphate analog.
CLINICAL USE	CMV retinitis in immunocompromised patients when ganciclovir fails; acyclovir-resistant HSV.	
ADVERSE EFFECTS	Nephrotoxicity, electrolyte abnormalities (hypo- or hypercalcemia, hypo- or hyperphosphatemia, hypokalemia, hypomagnesemia) can lead to seizures.	
MECHANISM OF RESISTANCE	Mutated DNA polymerase.	

Cidofovir

MECHANISM	Preferentially inhibits viral DNA polymerase. Does not require phosphorylation by viral kinase.
CLINICAL USE	CMV retinitis in immunocompromised patients; acyclovir-resistant HSV. Long half-life.
ADVERSE EFFECTS	Nephrotoxicity (coadminister with probenecid and IV saline to ↓ toxicity).

HIV therapy

Highly active antiretroviral therapy (HAART): often initiated at the time of HIV diagnosis. Strongest indication for patients presenting with AIDS-defining illness, low CD4+ cell counts (< 500 cells/mm^3), or high viral load. Regimen consists of 3 drugs to prevent resistance: 2 NRTIs and preferably an integrase inhibitor.

DRUG	MECHANISM	TOXICITY
NRTIs		
Abacavir (ABC) Didanosine (ddI) Emtricitabine (FTC) Lamivudine (3TC) Stavudine (d4T) Tenofovir (TDF) Zidovudine (ZDV, formerly AZT)	Competitively inhibit nucleotide binding to reverse transcriptase and terminate the DNA chain (lack a 3′ OH group). Tenofovir is a nucleoTide; the others are nucleosides. All need to be phosphorylated to be active. ZDV can be used for general prophylaxis and during pregnancy to ↓ risk of fetal transmission. Have you dined (vudine) with my **nuclear (nucleosides)** family?	Bone marrow suppression (can be reversed with granulocyte colony-stimulating factor [G-CSF] and erythropoietin), peripheral neuropathy, lactic acidosis (nucleosides), anemia (ZDV), pancreatitis (didanosine). Abacavir contraindicated if patient has HLA-B*5701 mutation due to ↑ risk of hypersensitivity.
NNRTIs		
Delavirdine Efavirenz Nevirapine	Bind to reverse transcriptase at site different from NRTIs. Do not require phosphorylation to be active or compete with nucleotides.	Rash and hepatotoxicity are common to all NNRTIs. Vivid dreams and CNS symptoms are common with efavirenz. Delavirdine and efavirenz are contraindicated in pregnancy.
Protease inhibitors		
Atazanavir Darunavir Fosamprenavir Indinavir Lopinavir Ritonavir Saquinavir	Assembly of virions depends on HIV-1 protease (*pol* gene), which cleaves the polypeptide products of HIV mRNA into their functional parts. Thus, protease inhibitors prevent maturation of new viruses. Ritonavir can "boost" other drug concentrations by inhibiting cytochrome P-450. **Navir** (never) **tease a protease**.	Hyperglycemia, GI intolerance (nausea, diarrhea), lipodystrophy (Cushing-like syndrome). Nephropathy, hematuria, thrombocytopenia (indinavir). Rifampin (potent CYP/UGT inducer) reduces protease inhibitor concentrations; use rifabutin instead.
Integrase inhibitors		
Dolutegravir Elvitegravir Raltegravir	Inhibits HIV genome integration into host cell chromosome by reversibly inhibiting HIV integrase.	↑ creatine kinase.
Fusion inhibitors		
Enfuvirtide	Binds gp41, inhibiting viral entry.	Skin reaction at injection sites. Enfuvirtide inhibits fusion.
Maraviroc	Binds CCR-5 on surface of T cells/monocytes, inhibiting interaction with gp120.	Maraviroc inhibits docking.

Interferons

MECHANISM	Glycoproteins normally synthesized by virus-infected cells, exhibiting a wide range of antiviral and antitumoral properties.
CLINICAL USE	Chronic HBV and HVC, Kaposi sarcoma, hairy cell leukemia, condyloma acuminatum, renal cell carcinoma, malignant melanoma, multiple sclerosis, chronic granulomatous disease.
ADVERSE EFFECTS	Flu-like symptoms, depression, neutropenia, myopathy.

Hepatitis C therapy

Chronic HCV infection is treated with different combinations of the following drugs; none is approved as monotherapy. Ribavirin also used to treat RSV (palivizumab preferred in children).

DRUG	MECHANISM	ADVERSE EFFECTS
Ledipasvir	Viral phosphoprotein (NS5A) inhibitor; NS5A plays important role in replication.	
Ribavirin	Inhibits synthesis of guanine nucleotides by competitively inhibiting inosine monophosphate dehydrogenase.	Hemolytic anemia, severe teratogen.
Simeprevir	HCV protease (NS3/4A); prevents viral replication.	Photosensitivity reactions, rash.
Sofosbuvir	Inhibits HCV RNA-dependent RNA polymerase (NS5B) acting as a chain terminator.	Fatigue, headache, nausea.

Disinfection and sterilization

Goals include the reduction of pathogenic organism counts to safe levels (disinfection) and the inactivation of all microbes including spores (sterilization).

Autoclave	Pressurized steam at > 120°C. Sporicidal. May not reliably inactivate prions.
Alcohols	Denature proteins and disrupt cell membranes. Not sporicidal.
Chlorhexidine	Denatures proteins and disrupts cell membranes. Not sporicidal.
Chlorine	Oxidizes and denatures proteins. Sporicidal.
Hydrogen peroxide	Free radical oxidation. Sporicidal.
Iodine and iodophors	Halogenation of DNA, RNA, and proteins. May be sporicidal.
Quaternary amines	Impair permeability of cell membranes. Not sporicidal.

Antimicrobials to avoid in pregnancy

ANTIMICROBIAL	ADVERSE EFFECT
Sulfonamides	Kernicterus
Aminoglycosides	Ototoxicity
Fluoroquinolones	Cartilage damage
Clarithromycin	Embryotoxic
Tetracyclines	Discolored teeth, inhibition of bone growth
Ribavirin	Teratogenic
Griseofulvin	Teratogenic
Chloramphenicol	Gray baby syndrome

SAFe Children Take Really Good Care.

Pathology

"Digressions, objections, delight in mockery, carefree mistrust are signs of health; everything unconditional belongs in pathology."

—Friedrich Nietzsche

"You cannot separate passion from pathology any more than you can separate a person's spirit from his body."

—Richard Selzer

The fundamental principles of pathology are key to understanding diseases in all organ systems. Major topics such as inflammation and neoplasia appear frequently in questions across different organ systems, and such topics are definitely high yield. For example, the concepts of cell injury and inflammation are key to understanding the inflammatory response that follows myocardial infarction, a very common subject of board questions. Similarly, a familiarity with the early cellular changes that culminate in the development of neoplasias—for example, esophageal or colon cancer—is critical. Finally, make sure you recognize the major tumor-associated genes and are comfortable with key cancer concepts such as tumor staging and metastasis.

▶ PATHOLOGY—CELLULAR INJURY

Cellular adaptations	Reversible changes that can be physiologic (eg, uterine enlargement during pregnancy) or pathologic (eg, myocardial hypertrophy 2° to systemic HTN to prevent injury). If stress is excessive or persistent, adaptations can progress to cell injury (eg, significant LV hypertrophy → injury to myofibrils → HF).
Hypertrophy	↑ structural proteins and organelles → ↑ in size of cells.
Hyperplasia	Controlled proliferation of stem cells and differentiated cells → ↑ in number of cells. Excessive stimulation → pathologic hyperplasia (eg, endometrial hyperplasia), which may progress to dysplasia and cancer.
Atrophy	↓ in tissue mass due to ↓ in size (↑ cytoskeleton degradation via ubiquitin-proteasome pathway and autophagy; ↓ protein synthesis) and/or number of cells (apoptosis). Causes include disuse, denervation, loss of blood supply, loss of hormonal stimulation, poor nutrition.
Metaplasia	Reprogramming of stem cells → replacement of one cell type by another that can adapt to a new stress. Usually due to exposure to an irritant, such as gastric acid (→ Barrett esophagus) or cigarette smoke (→ respiratory ciliated columnar epithelium replaced by stratified squamous epithelium). May progress to dysplasia → malignant transformation with persistent insult (eg, Barrett esophagus → esophageal adenocarcinoma). Metaplasia of connective tissue can also occur (eg, myositis ossificans, the formation of bone within muscle after trauma).
Dysplasia	Disordered, precancerous epithelial cell growth. Characterized by loss of uniformity of cell size and shape (pleomorphism); loss of tissue orientation; nuclear changes (eg, ↑ nuclear:cytoplasmic ratio and clumped chromatin). Mild and moderate dysplasias (ie, do not involve entire thickness of epithelium) may regress with alleviation of inciting cause. Severe dysplasia usually becomes irreversible and progresses to carcinoma in situ. Usually preceded by persistent metaplasia or pathologic hyperplasia.

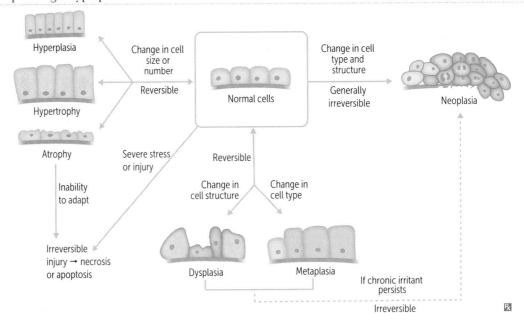

Cell injury

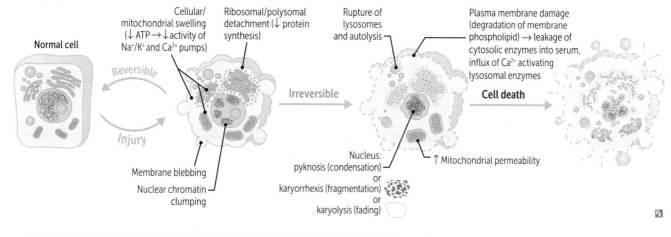

Apoptosis	ATP-dependent programmed cell death. Intrinsic and extrinsic pathways; both pathways activate caspases (cytosolic proteases) → cellular breakdown including cell shrinkage, chromatin condensation, membrane blebbing, and formation of apoptotic bodies, which are then phagocytosed. Characterized by deeply eosinophilic cytoplasm and basophilic nucleus, pyknosis (nuclear shrinkage), and karyorrhexis (fragmentation caused by endonuclease-mediated cleavage). Cell membrane typically remains intact without significant inflammation (unlike necrosis). DNA laddering (fragments in multiples of 180 bp) is a sensitive indicator of apoptosis.
Intrinsic (mitochondrial) pathway	Involved in tissue remodeling in embryogenesis. Occurs when a regulating factor is withdrawn from a proliferating cell population (eg, ↓ IL-2 after a completed immunologic reaction → apoptosis of proliferating effector cells). Also occurs after exposure to injurious stimuli (eg, radiation, toxins, hypoxia). Regulated by Bcl-2 family of proteins. BAX and BAK are proapoptotic, while Bcl-2 and Bcl-xL are antiapoptotic. BAX and BAK form pores in the mitochondrial membrane → release of cytochrome C from inner mitochondrial membrane into the cytoplasm → activation of caspases. Bcl-2 keeps the mitochondrial membrane impermeable, thereby preventing cytochrome C release. Bcl-2 overexpression (eg, follicular lymphoma t[14;18]) → ↓ caspase activation → tumorigenesis.
Extrinsic (death receptor) pathway	2 pathways: 　▪ Ligand receptor interactions (FasL binding to Fas [CD95] or TNF-α binding to its receptor) 　▪ Immune cell (cytotoxic T-cell release of perforin and granzyme B) Fas-FasL interaction is necessary in thymic medullary negative selection. Mutations in Fas ↑ numbers of circulating self-reacting lymphocytes due to failure of clonal deletion. Defective Fas-FasL interactions cause autoimmune lymphoproliferative syndrome.

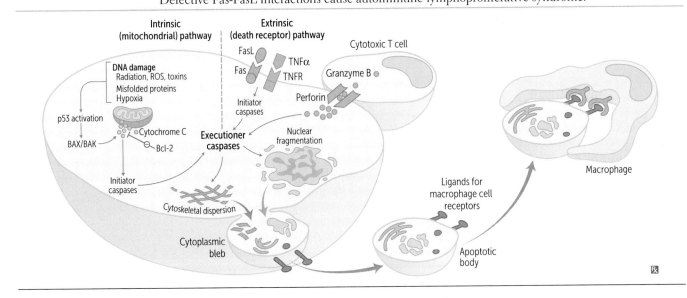

Necrosis

Enzymatic degradation and protein denaturation of cell due to exogenous injury → intracellular components leak. Inflammatory process (unlike apoptosis).

TYPE	SEEN IN	DUE TO	HISTOLOGY
Coagulative	Ischemia/infarcts in most tissues (except brain)	Ischemia or infarction; injury denatures enzymes → proteolysis blocked	Preserved cellular architecture (cell outlines seen), but nuclei disappear; ↑ cytoplasmic binding of eosin stain (→ ↑ eosinophilia; red/pink color) **A**
Liquefactive	Bacterial abscesses, brain infarcts	Neutrophils release lysosomal enzymes that digest the tissue **B**	Early: cellular debris and macrophages Late: cystic spaces and cavitation (brain) Neutrophils and cell debris seen with bacterial infection
Caseous	TB, systemic fungi (eg, *Histoplasma capsulatum*), *Nocardia*	Macrophages wall off the infecting microorganism → granular debris **C**	Fragmented cells and debris surrounded by lymphocytes and macrophages (granuloma)
Fat	Enzymatic: acute pancreatitis (saponification of peripancreatic fat) Nonenzymatic: traumatic (eg, injury to breast tissue)	Damaged cells release lipase, which breaks down triglycerides; liberated fatty acids bind calcium → saponification	Outlines of dead fat cells without peripheral nuclei; saponification of fat (combined with Ca^{2+}) appears dark blue on H&E stain **D**
Fibrinoid	Immune reactions in vessels (eg, polyarteritis nodosa), preeclampsia, hypertensive emergency	Immune complexes combine with fibrin → vessel wall damage (type III hypersensitivity reaction)	Vessel walls are thick and pink **E**
Gangrenous	Distal extremity and GI tract, after chronic ischemia	Dry: ischemia **F**	Coagulative
		Wet: superinfection	Liquefactive superimposed on coagulative

Ischemia

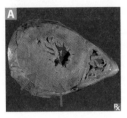

Inadequate blood supply to meet demand. Mechanisms include ↓ arterial perfusion (eg, atherosclerosis), ↓ venous drainage (eg, testicular torsion, Budd-Chiari syndrome), and shock. Regions most vulnerable to hypoxia/ischemia and subsequent infarction:

ORGAN	REGION
Brain	ACA/MCA/PCA boundary areas[a,b]
Heart	Subendocardium (LV)
Kidney	Straight segment of proximal tubule (medulla) Thick ascending limb (medulla)
Liver	Area around central vein (zone III)
Colon	Splenic flexure,[a] rectum[a]

[a]Watershed areas (border zones) receive blood supply from most distal branches of 2 arteries with limited collateral vascularity. These areas are susceptible to ischemia from hypoperfusion.

[b]Neurons most vulnerable to hypoxic-ischemic insults include Purkinje cells of the cerebellum and pyramidal cells of the hippocampus and neocortex (zones 3, 5, 6).

Types of infarcts

Red infarct

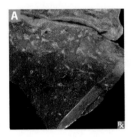

Red (hemorrhagic) infarcts A occur in venous occlusion and tissues with multiple blood supplies, such as liver, lung, intestine, testes; reperfusion (eg, after angioplasty). Reperfusion injury is due to damage by free radicals.

Red = reperfusion.

Pale infarct

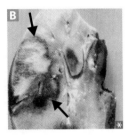

Pale (anemic) infarcts B occur in solid organs with a single (end-arterial) blood supply, such as heart, kidney, and spleen.

Inflammation	Response to eliminate initial cause of cell injury, to remove necrotic cells resulting from the original insult, and to initiate tissue repair. Divided into acute and chronic. The inflammatory response itself can be harmful to the host if the reaction is excessive (eg, septic shock), prolonged (eg, persistent infections such as TB), or inappropriate (eg, autoimmune diseases such as SLE).

Cardinal signs

SIGN	MECHANISM	MEDIATORS
Rubor (redness), calor (warmth)	Vasodilation (relaxation of arteriolar smooth muscle) → ↑ blood flow	Histamine, prostaglandins, bradykinin
Tumor (swelling)	Endothelial contraction/disruption (eg, from tissue damage) → ↑ vascular permeability → leakage of protein-rich fluid from postcapillary venules into interstitial space (exudate) → ↑ oncotic pressure	Endothelial contraction: leukotrienes (C_4, D_4, E_4), histamine, serotonin
Dolor (pain)	Sensitization of sensory nerve endings	Bradykinin, PGE_2
Functio laesa (loss of function)	Cardinal signs above impair function (eg, inability to make fist with hand that has cellulitis)	

Systemic manifestations (acute-phase reaction)

Fever	Pyrogens (eg, LPS) induce macrophages to release IL-1 and TNF → ↑ COX activity in perivascular cells of hypothalamus → ↑ PGE_2 → ↑ temperature set point.	
Leukocytosis	Elevation of WBC count. Type of cell that is predominantly elevated depends on the inciting agent or injury (eg, bacteria → ↑ neutrophils).	Leukemoid reaction—severe elevation in WBC (> 40,000 cells/mm³) caused by some stressors or infections (eg, *Clostridium difficile*).
↑ plasma acute-phase proteins	Factors whose serum concentrations change significantly in response to inflammation. Produced by the liver in both acute and chronic inflammatory states.	Notably induced by IL-6.

Acute phase reactants	More FFiSH in the C (sea).

POSITIVE (UPREGULATED)	
Ferritin	Binds and sequesters iron to inhibit microbial iron scavenging.
Fibrinogen	Coagulation factor; promotes endothelial repair; correlates with ESR.
Serum amyloid A	Prolonged elevation can lead to amyloidosis.
Hepcidin	↓ iron absorption (by degrading ferroportin) and ↓ iron release (from macrophages) → anemia of chronic disease.
C-reactive protein	Opsonin; fixes complement and facilitates phagocytosis. Measured clinically as a nonspecific sign of ongoing inflammation.

NEGATIVE (DOWNREGULATED)	
Albumin	Reduction conserves amino acids for positive reactants.
Transferrin	Internalized by macrophages to sequester iron.

Erythrocyte sedimentation rate

Products of inflammation (eg, fibrinogen) coat RBCs and cause aggregation. The denser RBC aggregates fall at a faster rate within a pipette tube → ↑ ESR. Often co-tested with CRP levels.

↑ ESR	↓ ESR
Most anemias	Sickle cell anemia (altered shape)
Infections	Polycythemia (↑ RBCs "dilute" aggregation factors)
Inflammation (eg, giant cell [temporal] arteritis, polymyalgia rheumatica)	HF
Cancer (eg, metastases, multiple myeloma)	Microcytosis
Renal disease (end-stage or nephrotic syndrome)	Hypofibrinogenemia
Pregnancy	

Acute inflammation

Transient and early response to injury or infection. Characterized by neutrophils in tissue A, often with associated edema. Rapid onset (seconds to minutes) and short duration (minutes to days). Represents a reaction of the innate immune system (ie, less specific response than chronic inflammation).

STIMULI	Infections, trauma, necrosis, foreign bodies.	
MEDIATORS	Toll-like receptors, arachidonic acid metabolites, neutrophils, eosinophils, antibodies (pre-existing), mast cells, basophils, complement, Hageman factor (factor XII).	Inflammasome—Cytoplasmic protein complex that recognizes products of dead cells, microbial products, and crystals (eg, uric acid crystals) → activation of IL-1 and inflammatory response.
COMPONENTS	▪ Vascular: vasodilation (→ ↑ blood flow and stasis) and ↑ endothelial permeability ▪ Cellular: extravasation of leukocytes (mainly neutrophils) from postcapillary venules and accumulation in the focus of injury followed by leukocyte activation	To bring cells and proteins to site of injury or infection. Leukocyte extravasation has 4 steps: margination and rolling, adhesion, transmigration, and migration (chemoattraction).
OUTCOMES	▪ Resolution and healing (IL-10, TGF-β) ▪ Persistent acute inflammation (IL-8) ▪ Abscess (acute inflammation walled off by fibrosis) ▪ Chronic inflammation (antigen presentation by macrophages and other APCs → activation of CD4+ Th cells) ▪ Scarring	Macrophages predominate in the late stages of acute inflammation (peak 2–3 days after onset) and influence the outcome of acute inflammation by secreting cytokines.

Leukocyte extravasation

Extravasation predominantly occurs at postcapillary venules.
WBCs exit from blood vessels at sites of tissue injury and inflammation in 4 steps:

STEP	VASCULATURE/STROMA	LEUKOCYTE
❶ Margination and rolling—defective in leukocyte adhesion deficiency type 2 (↓ Sialyl-Lewis^X)	E-selectin (upregulated by TNF and IL-1)	Sialyl-Lewis^X
	P-selectin (released from Weibel-Palade bodies)	Sialyl-Lewis^X
	GlyCAM-1, CD34	L-selectin
❷ Tight binding (adhesion)—defective in leukocyte adhesion deficiency type 1 (↓ CD18 integrin subunit)	ICAM-1 (CD54)	CD11/18 integrins (LFA-1, Mac-1)
	VCAM-1 (CD106)	VLA-4 integrin
❸ Diapedesis (transmigration)—WBC travels between endothelial cells and exits blood vessel	PECAM-1 (CD31)	PECAM-1 (CD31)
❹ Migration—WBC travels through interstitium to site of injury or infection guided by chemotactic signals	Chemotactic products released in response to bacteria: C5a, IL-8, LTB$_4$, kallikrein, platelet-activating factor	Various

Chronic inflammation	Inflammation of prolonged duration characterized by infiltration of tissue by mononuclear cells (macrophages, lymphocytes, and plasma cells). Tissue destruction and repair (including angiogenesis and fibrosis) occur simultaneously. May or may not be preceded by acute inflammation.
STIMULI	Persistent infections (eg, TB, *T pallidum*, certain fungi and viruses) → type IV hypersensitivity, autoimmune diseases, prolonged exposure to toxic agents (eg, silica) and foreign material.
MEDIATORS	Macrophages are the dominant cells. Chronic inflammation is the result of their interaction with T lymphocytes. ▪ Th1 cells secrete INF-γ → macrophage classical activation (proinflammatory) ▪ Th2 cells secrete IL-4 and IL-13 → macrophage alternative activation (repair and anti-inflammatory)
OUTCOMES	Scarring, amyloidosis and neoplastic transformation (eg, chronic HCV infection → chronic inflammation → hepatocellular carcinoma; *Helicobacter pylori* infection → chronic gastritis → gastric adenocarcinoma).

Granulomatous diseases 	Bacterial: ▪ *Mycobacteria* (tuberculosis, leprosy) ▪ *Bartonella henselae* (cat scratch disease) ▪ *Listeria monocytogenes* (granulomatosis infantiseptica) ▪ *Treponema pallidum* (3° syphilis) Fungal: endemic mycoses (eg, histoplasmosis) Parasitic: schistosomiasis Chronic granulomatous disease Autoinflammatory: ▪ Sarcoidosis ▪ Crohn disease ▪ Primary biliary cholangitis ▪ Subacute (de Quervain/granulomatous) thyroiditis ▪ Granulomatosis with polyangiitis (Wegener) ▪ Eosinophilic granulomatosis with polyangiitis (Churg-Strauss) ▪ Giant cell (temporal) arteritis ▪ Takayasu arteritis Foreign material: berylliosis, talcosis, hypersensitivity pneumonitis	Granulomas (a pattern of chronic inflammation) are composed of epithelioid cells (macrophages with abundant pink cytoplasm) with surrounding multinucleated giant cells and lymphocytes. Th1 cells secrete IFN-γ, activating macrophages. TNF-α from macrophages induces and maintains granuloma formation. Anti-TNF drugs can cause sequestering granulomas to break down → disseminated disease. Always test for latent TB before starting anti-TNF therapy. Associated with hypercalcemia due to calcitriol (1,25-[OH]$_2$ vitamin D$_3$) production. Caseating necrosis is more common with an infectious etiology (eg, TB). Diagnosis of sarcoidosis requires noncaseating granulomas A on biopsy.

Types of calcification

	Dystrophic calcification	Metastatic calcification
CA²⁺ DEPOSITION	In abnormal tissues	In normal tissues
EXTENT	Tends to be localized (eg, calcific aortic stenosis) A shows dystrophic calcification (yellow star), and thick fibrotic wall (red arrows)	Widespread (ie, diffuse, metastatic) B shows metastatic calcifications of alveolar walls in acute pneumonitis (arrows)
ASSOCIATED CONDITIONS	TB (lung and pericardium) and other granulomatous infections, liquefactive necrosis of chronic abscesses, fat necrosis, infarcts, thrombi, schistosomiasis, congenital CMV, toxoplasmosis, rubella, psammoma bodies, CREST syndrome, atherosclerotic plaques can become calcified	Predominantly in interstitial tissues of kidney, lung, and gastric mucosa (these tissues lose acid quickly; ↑ pH favors Ca²⁺ deposition) Nephrocalcinosis of collecting ducts may lead to nephrogenic diabetes insipidus and renal failure
ETIOLOGY	2° to injury or necrosis	2° to hypercalcemia (eg, 1° hyperparathyroidism, sarcoidosis, hypervitaminosis D) or high calcium-phosphate product levels (eg, chronic renal failure with 2° hyperparathyroidism, long-term dialysis, calciphylaxis, multiple myeloma)
SERUM CA²⁺ LEVELS	Patients are usually normocalcemic	Patients usually have abnormal serum Ca²⁺ levels

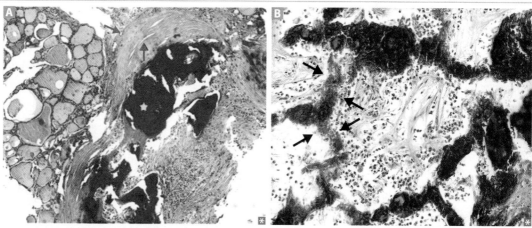

Lipofuscin

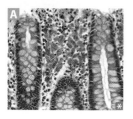

A yellow-brown "wear and tear" pigment A associated with normal aging.
Formed by oxidation and polymerization of autophagocytosed organellar membranes.
Autopsy of elderly person will reveal deposits in heart, colon, liver, kidney, eye, and other organs.

Free radical injury

Free radicals damage cells via membrane lipid peroxidation, protein modification, and DNA breakage.

Initiated via radiation exposure (eg, cancer therapy), metabolism of drugs (phase I), redox reactions, nitric oxide (eg, inflammation), transition metals, WBC (eg, neutrophils, macrophages) oxidative burst.

Free radicals can be eliminated by scavenging enzymes (eg, catalase, superoxide dismutase, glutathione peroxidase), spontaneous decay, antioxidants (eg, vitamins A, C, E), and certain metal carrier proteins (eg, transferrin, ceruloplasmin).

Examples:
- Oxygen toxicity: retinopathy of prematurity (abnormal vascularization), bronchopulmonary dysplasia, reperfusion injury after thrombolytic therapy
- Drug/chemical toxicity: acetaminophen overdose (hepatotoxicity), carbon tetrachloride (converted by cytochrome P-450 into CCl_3 free radical → fatty liver [cell injury → ↓ apolipoprotein synthesis → fatty change], centrilobular necrosis)
- Metal storage diseases: hemochromatosis (iron) and Wilson disease (copper)

Scar formation

Occurs when repair cannot be accomplished by cell regeneration alone. Nonregenerated cells (2° to severe acute or chronic injury) are replaced by connective tissue. 70–80% of tensile strength regained at 3 months; little tensile strength regained thereafter.

SCAR TYPE	Hypertrophic A	Keloid B
COLLAGEN SYNTHESIS	↑ (type III collagen)	↑↑↑ (disorganized types I and III collagen)
COLLAGEN ORGANIZATION	Parallel	Disorganized
EXTENT OF SCAR	Confined to borders of original wound	Extends beyond borders of original wound with "claw-like" projections typically on earlobes, face, upper extremities
RECURRENCE	Infrequent	Frequent
PREDISPOSITION	None	↑ incidence in ethnic groups with darker skin

Wound healing

Tissue mediators

MEDIATOR	ROLE
FGF	Stimulates angiogenesis
TGF-β	Angiogenesis, fibrosis
VEGF	Stimulates angiogenesis
PDGF	Secreted by activated platelets and macrophages Induces vascular remodeling and smooth muscle cell migration Stimulates fibroblast growth for collagen synthesis
Metalloproteinases	Tissue remodeling
EGF	Stimulates cell growth via tyrosine kinases (eg, EGFR/*ErbB1*)

PHASE OF WOUND HEALING	EFFECTOR CELLS	CHARACTERISTICS
Inflammatory (up to 3 days after wound)	Platelets, neutrophils, macrophages	Clot formation, ↑ vessel permeability and neutrophil migration into tissue; macrophages clear debris 2 days later
Proliferative (day 3–weeks after wound)	Fibroblasts, myofibroblasts, endothelial cells, keratinocytes, macrophages	Deposition of granulation tissue and type III collagen, angiogenesis, epithelial cell proliferation, dissolution of clot, and wound contraction (mediated by myofibroblasts) Delayed wound healing in vitamin C deficiency and copper deficiency
Remodeling (1 week–6+ months after wound)	Fibroblasts	Type III collagen replaced by type I collagen, ↑ tensile strength of tissue Collagenases (require zinc to function) break down type III collagen Zinc deficiency → delayed wound healing

Exudate vs transudate

	Exudate	Transudate
	Cellular (cloudy)	Hypocellular (clear)
	↑ protein (> 2.9 g/dL)	↓ protein (< 2.5 g/dL)
	Due to: ▪ Lymphatic obstruction (chylous) ▪ Inflammation/infection ▪ Malignancy	Due to: ▪ ↑ hydrostatic pressure (eg, HF, Na⁺ retention) ▪ ↓ oncotic pressure (eg, cirrhosis, nephrotic syndrome)
Light criteria	Fluid is exudative if ≥ 1 of the following criteria is met: ▪ Pleural effusion protein/serum protein ratio > 0.5 ▪ Pleural effusion LDH/serum LDH ratio > 0.6 ▪ Pleural effusion LDH > ⅔ of the upper limit of normal for serum LDH	

| **Amyloidosis** | Abnormal aggregation of proteins (or their fragments) into β-pleated linear sheets → insoluble fibrils → cellular damage and apoptosis. Amyloid deposits visualized by Congo red stain A, polarized light (apple green birefringence) B, and H&E stain (C shows deposits in glomerular mesangial areas [white arrows], tubular basement membranes [black arrows]). |

COMMON TYPES	FIBRIL PROTEIN	DESCRIPTION	
Systemic			
Primary amyloidosis	AL (from Ig Light chains)	Seen in plasma cell disorders and multiple myeloma	Manifestations include:
Secondary amyloidosis	Serum Amyloid A (AA)	Seen in chronic inflammatory conditions, eg, rheumatoid arthritis, IBD, familial Mediterranean fever, protracted infection	▪ Cardiac (eg, restrictive cardiomyopathy, arrhythmia) ▪ GI (eg, macroglossia, hepatomegaly) ▪ Renal (eg, nephrotic syndrome)
Dialysis-related amyloidosis	β_2-microglobulin	Seen in patients with ESRD and/or on long-term dialysis	▪ Hematologic (eg, easy bruising, splenomegaly) ▪ Neurologic (neuropathy) ▪ Musculoskeletal (carpal tunnel syndrome)
Localized			
Alzheimer disease	β-amyloid protein	Cleaved from amyloid precursor protein (APP)	
Type 2 diabetes mellitus	Islet amyloid polypeptide (IAPP)	Caused by deposition of amylin in pancreatic islets	
Medullary thyroid cancer	Calcitonin (A Cal)		
Isolated atrial amyloidosis	ANP	Common in normal aging ↑ risk of atrial fibrillation	
Systemic senile (age-related) amyloidosis	Normal (wild-type) transthyretin (TTR)	Seen predominantly in cardiac ventricles	Cardiac dysfunction more insidious than in AL amyloidosis
Hereditary			
Familial amyloid cardiomyopathy	Mutated transthyretin (ATTR)	Ventricular endomyocardium deposition → restrictive cardiomyopathy, arrhythmias	5% of African Americans are carriers of mutant allele
Familial amyloid polyneuropathies	Mutated transthyretin (ATTR)	Due to transthyretin gene mutation	

▶ PATHOLOGY—NEOPLASIA

Neoplasia and neoplastic progression	Uncontrolled, clonal proliferation of cells. Can be benign or malignant. Hallmarks of cancer: evasion of apoptosis, growth signal self-sufficiency, anti-growth signal insensitivity, Warburg effect (shift of glucose metabolism away from mitochondria toward glycolysis), sustained angiogenesis, limitless replicative potential, tissue invasion, and metastasis.

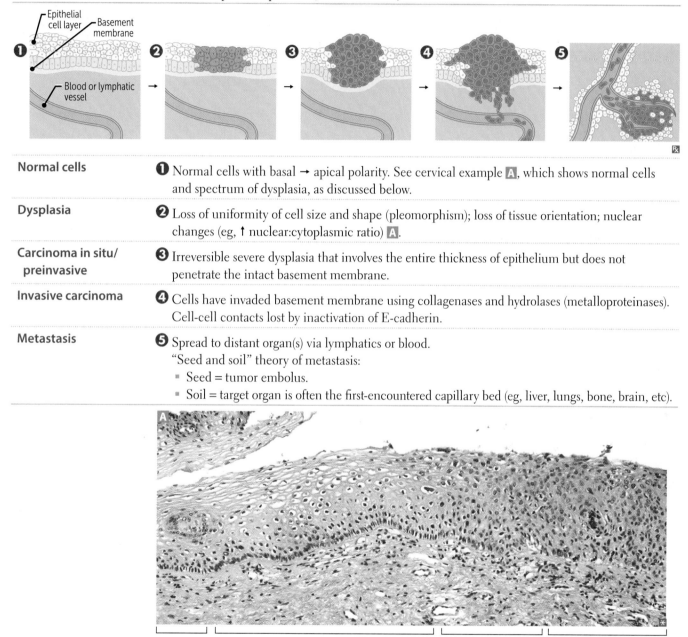

Normal cells	❶ Normal cells with basal → apical polarity. See cervical example **A**, which shows normal cells and spectrum of dysplasia, as discussed below.
Dysplasia	❷ Loss of uniformity of cell size and shape (pleomorphism); loss of tissue orientation; nuclear changes (eg, ↑ nuclear:cytoplasmic ratio) **A**.
Carcinoma in situ/ preinvasive	❸ Irreversible severe dysplasia that involves the entire thickness of epithelium but does not penetrate the intact basement membrane.
Invasive carcinoma	❹ Cells have invaded basement membrane using collagenases and hydrolases (metalloproteinases). Cell-cell contacts lost by inactivation of E-cadherin.
Metastasis	❺ Spread to distant organ(s) via lymphatics or blood. "Seed and soil" theory of metastasis: ▪ Seed = tumor embolus. ▪ Soil = target organ is often the first-encountered capillary bed (eg, liver, lungs, bone, brain, etc).

Normal   Mild dysplasia   Moderate dysplasia   Severe dysplasia/ carcinoma in situ

Tumor nomenclature	**Carcinoma** implies epithelial origin, whereas **sarcoma** denotes mesenchymal origin. Both terms generally imply malignancy.	

Benign tumors are usually well differentiated, well demarcated, low mitotic activity, no metastasis, no necrosis.

Malignant tumors may show poor differentiation, erratic growth, local invasion, metastasis, and ↓ apoptosis. Upregulation of telomerase prevents chromosome shortening and cell death.

Terms for non-neoplastic malformations include hamartoma (disorganized overgrowth of tissues in their native location, eg, Peutz-Jeghers polyps) and choristoma (normal tissue in a foreign location, eg, gastric tissue located in distal ileum in Meckel diverticulum).

CELL TYPE	BENIGN	MALIGNANT
Epithelium	Adenoma, papilloma	Adenocarcinoma, papillary carcinoma
Mesenchyme		
Blood cells		Leukemia, lymphoma
Blood vessels	Hemangioma	Angiosarcoma
Smooth muscle	Leiomyoma	Leiomyosarcoma
Striated muscle	Rhabdomyoma	Rhabdomyosarcoma
Connective tissue	Fibroma	Fibrosarcoma
Bone	Osteoma	Osteosarcoma
Fat	Lipoma	Liposarcoma
Melanocyte	Nevus/mole	Melanoma

Tumor grade vs stage	Differentiation—degree to which a tumor resembles its tissue of origin. Well-differentiated tumors (often less aggressive) closely resemble their tissue of origin, whereas poorly differentiated tumors (often more aggressive) look almost nothing like their tissue of origin.	

Anaplasia—complete lack of differentiation of cells in a malignant neoplasm.

Grade	Degree of cellular differentiation and mitotic activity on histology. Range from low grade (well differentiated) to high grade (poorly differentiated, undifferentiated or anaplastic).	Stage generally has more prognostic value than grade (eg, a high-stage yet low-grade tumor is usually worse than a low-stage yet high-grade tumor). Stage determines Survival.
Stage	Degree of localization/spread based on site and size of 1° lesion, spread to regional lymph nodes, presence of metastases. Based on clinical (c) or pathology (p) findings. Example: cT3N1M0	TNM staging system (Stage = Spread): **T** = Tumor size/invasiveness **N** = Node involvement **M** = Metastases Each TNM factor has independent prognostic value; N and M are often most important.

Paraneoplastic syndromes

MANIFESTATION	DESCRIPTION/MECHANISM	MOST COMMONLY ASSOCIATED TUMOR(S)
Musculoskeletal and cutaneous		
Dermatomyositis	Progressive proximal muscle weakness, Gottron papules, heliotrope rash	Adenocarcinomas, especially ovarian
Acanthosis nigricans	Hyperpigmented velvety plaques in axilla and neck	Gastric adenocarcinoma and other visceral malignancies (but more commonly associated with obesity and insulin resistance)
Sign of Leser-Trélat	Sudden onset of multiple seborrheic keratoses	GI adenocarcinomas and other visceral malignancies
Hypertrophic osteoarthropathy	Abnormal proliferation of skin and bone at distal extremities → clubbing, arthralgia, joint effusions, periostosis of tubular bones	Adenocarcinoma of the lung
Endocrine		
Hypercalcemia	PTHrP	Squamous cell carcinomas of lung, head, and neck; renal, bladder, breast, and ovarian carcinomas
	↑ 1,25-$(OH)_2$ vitamin D_3 (calcitriol)	Lymphoma
Cushing syndrome	↑ ACTH	Small cell lung cancer
Hyponatremia (SIADH)	↑ ADH	
Hematologic		
Polycythemia	↑ Erythropoietin — Paraneoplastic rise to high hematocrit levels	Pheochromocytoma, renal cell carcinoma, HCC, hemangioblastoma, leiomyoma
Pure red cell aplasia	Anemia with low reticulocytes	Thymoma
Good syndrome	Hypogammaglobulinemia	
Trousseau syndrome	Migratory superficial thrombophlebitis	
Nonbacterial thrombotic (marantic) endocarditis	Deposition of sterile platelet thrombi on heart valves	Adenocarcinomas, especially pancreatic
Neuromuscular		
Anti-NMDA receptor encephalitis	Psychiatric disturbance, memory deficits, seizures, dyskinesias, autonomic instability, language dysfunction	Ovarian teratoma
Opsoclonus-myoclonus ataxia syndrome	"Dancing eyes, dancing feet"	Neuroblastoma (children), small cell lung cancer (adults)
Paraneoplastic cerebellar degeneration	Antibodies against antigens in Purkinje cells	Small cell lung cancer (anti-Hu), gynecologic and breast cancers (anti-Yo), and Hodgkin lymphoma (anti-Tr)
Paraneoplastic encephalomyelitis	Antibodies against Hu antigens in neurons	Small cell lung cancer
Lambert-Eaton myasthenic syndrome	Antibodies against presynaptic (P/Q-type) Ca^{2+} channels at NMJ	Small cell lung cancer
Myasthenia gravis	Antibodies against postsynaptic ACh receptors at NMJ	Thymoma

Oncogenes   Gain of function mutation converts proto-oncogene (normal gene) to oncogene → ↑ cancer risk. Need damage to only **one** allele of a proto-oncogene.

GENE	GENE PRODUCT	ASSOCIATED NEOPLASM
ALK	Receptor tyrosine **K**inase	Lung **A**denocarcinoma (Adenocarcinoma of the Lung Kinase)
BCR-ABL	Tyrosine kinase	CML, ALL
BCL-2	Antiapoptotic molecule (inhibits apoptosis)	Follicular and diffuse large **B** cell lymphomas
BRAF	Serine/threonine kinase	Melanoma, non-Hodgkin lymphoma, papillary thyroid carcinoma
c-KIT	Cytokine receptor	Gastrointestinal stromal tumor (GIST)
c-MYC	Transcription factor	Burkitt lymphoma
HER2/neu (c-erbB2)	Receptor tyrosine kinase	Breast and gastric carcinomas
JAK2	Tyrosine kinase	Chronic myeloproliferative disorders
KRAS	GTPase	Colon cancer, lung cancer, pancreatic cancer
MYCL1	Transcription factor	Lung tumor
N-myc (MYCN)	Transcription factor	Neuroblastoma
RET	Receptor tyrosine kinase	MEN 2A and 2B, papillary thyroid carcinoma

Tumor suppressor genes   Loss of function → ↑ cancer risk; both (**two**) alleles of a **t**umor suppressor gene must be lost for expression of disease.

GENE	GENE PRODUCT	ASSOCIATED CONDITION
APC	Negative regulator of β-catenin/WNT pathway	Colorectal cancer (associated with FAP)
BRCA1/BRCA2	DNA repair protein	**B**reast, ovarian, and pancreatic **c**ancer
CDKN2A	p16, blocks $G_1 \to S$ phase	Melanoma, pancreatic cancer
DCC	DCC—**D**eleted in **C**olon **C**ancer	Colon cancer
SMAD4 (DPC4)	DPC—**D**eleted in **P**ancreatic **C**ancer	Pancreatic cancer
MEN1	**Men**in	**M**ultiple **E**ndocrine **N**eoplasia 1
NF1	Neurofibromin (Ras GTPase activating protein)	Neurofibromatosis type **1**
NF2	Merlin (schwannomin) protein	Neurofibromatosis type **2**
PTEN	Negatively regulates PI3k/AKT pathway	Breast, prostate, and endometrial cancer
Rb	Inhibits E2F; blocks $G_1 \to S$ phase	Retinoblastoma, osteosarcoma
TP53	*p*53, activates p21, blocks $G_1 \to S$ phase	Most human cancers, Li-Fraumeni syndrome (multiple malignancies at early age, aka, **SBLA** cancer syndrome: **S**arcoma, **B**reast, **L**eukemia, **A**drenal gland)
TSC1	Hamartin protein	Tuberous sclerosis
TSC2	Tuberin protein	Tuberous sclerosis
VHL	Inhibits hypoxia inducible factor 1a	von Hippel-Lindau disease
WT1	Transcription factor that regulates urogenital development	Wilms tumor (nephroblastoma)

Oncogenic microbes

Microbe	Associated cancer
EBV	Burkitt lymphoma, Hodgkin lymphoma, nasopharyngeal carcinoma, 1° CNS lymphoma (in immunocompromised patients)
HBV, HCV	Hepatocellular carcinoma
HHV-8	Kaposi sarcoma
HPV	Cervical and penile/anal carcinoma (types 16, 18), head and neck cancer
H pylori	Gastric adenocarcinoma and MALT lymphoma
HTLV-1	Adult T-cell leukemia/lymphoma
Liver fluke (*Clonorchis sinensis*)	Cholangiocarcinoma
Schistosoma haematobium	Bladder cancer (squamous cell)

Carcinogens

TOXIN	EXPOSURE	ORGAN	IMPACT
Aflatoxins (*Aspergillus*)	Stored grains and nuts	Liver	Hepatocellular carcinoma
Alkylating agents	Oncologic chemotherapy	Blood	Leukemia/lymphoma
Aromatic amines (eg, benzidine, 2-naphthylamine)	Textile industry (dyes), cigarette smoke (2-naphthylamine)	Bladder	Transitional cell carcinoma
Arsenic	Herbicides (vineyard workers), metal smelting	Liver Lung Skin	Angiosarcoma Lung cancer Squamous cell carcinoma
Asbestos	Old roofing material, shipyard workers	Lung	Bronchogenic carcinoma > mesothelioma
Cigarette smoke		Bladder Cervix Esophagus Kidney Larynx Lung Pancreas	Transitional cell carcinoma Squamous cell carcinoma Squamous cell carcinoma/ adenocarcinoma Renal cell carcinoma Squamous cell carcinoma Squamous cell and small cell carcinoma Pancreatic adenocarcinoma
Ethanol		Esophagus Liver	Squamous cell carcinoma Hepatocellular carcinoma
Ionizing radiation		Thyroid	Papillary thyroid carcinoma
Nitrosamines	Smoked foods	Stomach	Gastric cancer
Radon	By-product of uranium decay, accumulates in basements	Lung	Lung cancer (2nd leading cause after cigarette smoke)
Vinyl chloride	Used to make PVC pipes (plumbers)	Liver	Angiosarcoma

Psammoma bodies

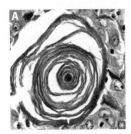

Laminated, concentric spherules with dystrophic calcification **A**, PSaMMoma bodies are seen in:

- Papillary carcinoma of thyroid
- Serous papillary cystadenocarcinoma of ovary
- Meningioma
- Malignant Mesothelioma

Serum tumor markers

Tumor markers should not be used as the 1° tool for cancer diagnosis or screening. They may be used to monitor tumor recurrence and response to therapy, but definitive diagnosis is made via biopsy. Some can be associated with non-neoplastic conditions.

MARKER	IMPORTANT ASSOCIATIONS	NOTES
Alkaline phosphatase	Metastases to bone or liver, Paget disease of bone, seminoma (placental ALP).	Exclude hepatic origin by checking LFTs and GGT levels.
α-fetoprotein	Hepatocellular carcinoma, Endodermal sinus (yolk sac) tumor, Mixed germ cell tumor, Ataxia-telangiectasia, Neural tube defects. (**HE-MAN** is the **alpha** male!)	Normally made by fetus. Transiently elevated in pregnancy. High levels associated with neural tube and abdominal wall defects, low levels associated with Down syndrome.
β-hCG	Hydatidiform moles and Choriocarcinomas (Gestational trophoblastic disease), testicular cancer, mixed germ cell tumor.	Produced by syncytiotrophoblasts of the placenta.
CA 15-3/CA 27-29	Breast cancer.	
CA 19-9	Pancreatic adenocarcinoma.	
CA 125	Ovarian cancer.	
Calcitonin	Medullary thyroid carcinoma (alone and in MEN2A, MEN2B).	
CEA	Major associations: colorectal and pancreatic cancers. Minor associations: gastric, breast, and medullary thyroid carcinomas.	Carcinoembryonic antigen. Very nonspecific.
Chromogranin	Neuroendocrine tumors.	
LDH	Testicular germ cell tumors, ovarian dysgerminoma, other cancers.	Can be used as an indicator of tumor burden.
PSA	Prostate cancer.	Prostate-specific antigen. Can also be elevated in BPH and prostatitis. Questionable risk/benefit for screening. Surveillance marker for recurrent disease after prostatectomy.

Important immunohistochemical stains	Determine primary site of origin for metastatic tumors and characterize tumors that are difficult to classify. Can have prognostic and predictive value.	
STAIN	TARGET	EXAMPLES IDENTIFIED
Vimentin	Mesenchymal tissue (eg, fibroblasts, endothelial cells, macrophages)	Mesenchymal tumors (eg, sarcoma), but also many other tumors (eg, endometrial carcinoma, renal cell carcinoma, meningioma)
S-100	Neural crest cells	Melanoma, schwannoma, Langerhans cell histiocytosis
DesMin	Muscle	Muscle tumors (eg, rhabdomyosarcoma)
Cytokeratin	Epithelial cells	Epithelial tumors (eg, squamous cell carcinoma)
GFAP	NeuroGlia (eg, astrocytes, Schwann cells, oligodendrocytes)	Astrocytoma, Glioblastoma
Neurofilament	Neurons	Neuronal tumors (eg, neuroblastoma)
PSA	Prostatic epithelium	Prostate cancer
TRAP	Tartrate-resistant acid phosphatase	Hairy cell leukemia
Chromogranin and synaptophysin	Neuroendocrine cells	Small cell carcinoma of the lung, carcinoid tumor

P-glycoprotein	Also known as multidrug resistance protein 1 (MDR1). Classically seen in adrenocortical carcinoma but also expressed by other cancer cells (eg, colon, liver). Used to pump out toxins, including chemotherapeutic agents (one mechanism of ↓ responsiveness or resistance to chemotherapy over time).

Cachexia	Weight loss, muscle atrophy, and fatigue that occur in chronic disease (eg, cancer, AIDS, heart failure, COPD). Mediated by TNF, IFN-γ, IL-1, and IL-6.

Cancer epidemiology Skin cancer (basal > squamous >> melanoma) is the most common cancer (not included below).

	MEN	WOMEN	CHILDREN (AGE 0–14)	NOTES
Cancer incidence	1. Prostate 2. Lung 3. Colon/rectum	1. Breast 2. Lung 3. Colon/rectum	1. Leukemia 2. CNS 3. Neuroblastoma	Lung cancer incidence has ↓ in men, but has not changed significantly in women.
Cancer mortality	1. Lung 2. Prostate 3. Colon/rectum	1. Lung 2. Breast 3. Colon/rectum	1. Leukemia 2. CNS 3. Neuroblastoma	Cancer is the 2nd leading cause of death in the United States (heart disease is 1st).

Common metastases Most sarcomas spread hematogenously; most carcinomas spread via lymphatics. However, Four Carcinomas Route Hematogenously: Follicular thyroid carcinoma, Choriocarcinoma, Renal cell carcinoma, and Hepatocellular carcinoma.

SITE OF METASTASIS	1° TUMOR	NOTES
Brain	Lung > breast > melanoma, colon, kidney.	50% of brain tumors are from metastases **A** **B**. Commonly seen as multiple well-circumscribed tumors at gray/white matter junction.
Liver	Colon >> stomach > pancreas.	Liver **C** **D** and lung are the most common sites of metastasis after the regional lymph nodes.
Bone	Prostate, Breast > Kidney, Thyroid, Lung. Lead (**PB**) KeTtLe.	Bone metastasis **E** **F** >> 1° bone tumors (eg, multiple myeloma, lytic). Common mets to bone: breast (mixed), lung (lytic), thyroid (lytic), kidney (lytic), prostate (blastic). Predilection for axial skeleton **G**.

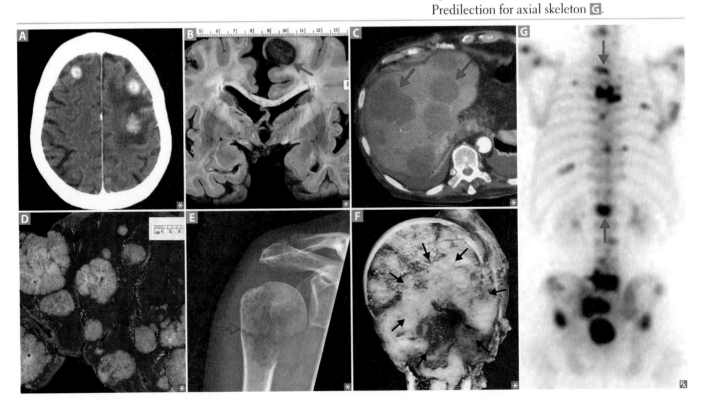

Pharmacology

"Take me, I am the drug; take me, I am hallucinogenic."
— Salvador Dali

"I was under medication when I made the decision not to burn the tapes."
— Richard Nixon

"I wondher why ye can always read a doctor's bill an' ye niver can read his purscription."
— Finley Peter Dunne

"Once you get locked into a serious drug collection, the tendency is to push it as far as you can."
— Hunter S. Thompson

Preparation for pharmacology questions is straightforward. Know all the mechanisms, clinical use, and important adverse effects of key drugs and their major variants. Obscure derivatives are low-yield. Learn their classic and distinguishing toxicities as well as major drug-drug interactions. Reviewing associated biochemistry, physiology, and microbiology concepts can be useful while studying pharmacology. The exam has a strong emphasis on ANS, CNS, antimicrobial, and cardiovascular agents as well as on NSAIDs, which are covered throughout the text. Specific drug dosages or trade names are generally not testable. The exam may use graphs to test various pharmacology content, so make sure you are comfortable interpreting them.

▶ PHARMACOLOGY—PHARMACOKINETICS AND PHARMACODYNAMICS

Enzyme kinetics

Michaelis-Menten kinetics	K_m is inversely related to the affinity of the enzyme for its substrate. V_{max} is directly proportional to the enzyme concentration. Most enzymatic reactions follow a hyperbolic curve (ie, Michaelis-Menten kinetics); however, enzymatic reactions that exhibit a sigmoid curve usually indicate cooperative kinetics (eg, hemoglobin).	[S] = concentration of substrate; V = velocity.

Lineweaver-Burk plot	↑ y-intercept, ↓ V_{max}. The further to the right the x-intercept (ie, closer to zero), the greater the K_m and the lower the affinity. Competitive inhibitors cross each other, whereas **noncompetitive** inhibitors do **not**. **K**ompetitive inhibitors increase K_m.	

	Competitive inhibitors, reversible	Competitive inhibitors, irreversible	Noncompetitive inhibitors
Resemble substrate	Yes	Yes	No
Overcome by ↑ [S]	Yes	No	No
Bind active site	Yes	Yes	No
Effect on V_{max}	Unchanged	↓	↓
Effect on K_m	↑	Unchanged	Unchanged
Pharmacodynamics	↓ potency	↓ efficacy	↓ efficacy

Pharmacokinetics

Bioavailability (F)	Fraction of administered drug reaching systemic circulation unchanged. For an IV dose, F = 100%. Orally: F typically < 100% due to incomplete absorption and first-pass metabolism.
Volume of distribution (V$_d$)	Theoretical volume occupied by the total amount of drug in the body relative to its plasma concentration. Apparent V$_d$ of plasma protein–bound drugs can be altered by liver and kidney disease (↓ protein binding, ↑ V$_d$). Drugs may distribute in more than one compartment.

$$V_d = \frac{\text{amount of drug in the body}}{\text{plasma drug concentration}}$$

V$_d$	COMPARTMENT	DRUG TYPES
Low	Intravascular	Large/charged molecules; plasma protein bound
Medium	ECF	Small hydrophilic molecules
High	All tissues including fat	Small lipophilic molecules, especially if bound to tissue protein

Clearance (CL)	The volume of plasma cleared of drug per unit time. Clearance may be impaired with defects in cardiac, hepatic, or renal function.

$$CL = \frac{\text{rate of elimination of drug}}{\text{plasma drug concentration}} = V_d \times K_e \text{ (elimination constant)}$$

Half-life (t$_{1/2}$)	The time required to change the amount of drug in the body by ½ during elimination. In first-order kinetics, a drug infused at a constant rate takes 4–5 half-lives to reach steady state. It takes 3.3 half-lives to reach 90% of the steady-state level.

$$t_{1/2} = \frac{0.7 \times V_d}{CL} \text{ in first-order elimination}$$

# of half-lives	1	2	3	4
% remaining	50%	25%	12.5%	6.25%

Dosage calculations

$$\text{Loading dose} = \frac{C_p \times V_d}{F}$$

$$\text{Maintenance dose} = \frac{C_p \times CL \times \tau}{F}$$

C_p = target plasma concentration at steady state
τ = dosage interval (time between doses), if not administered continuously

In renal or liver disease, maintenance dose ↓ and loading dose is usually unchanged.
Time to steady state depends primarily on $t_{1/2}$ and is independent of dose and dosing frequency.

Types of drug interactions

TERM	DEFINITION	EXAMPLE
Additive	Effect of substance A and B together is equal to the sum of their individual effects	Aspirin and acetaminophen
Permissive	Presence of substance A is required for the full effects of substance B	Cortisol on catecholamine responsiveness
Synergistic	Effect of substance A and B together is greater than the sum of their individual effects	Clopidogrel with aspirin
Tachyphylactic	Acute decrease in response to a drug after initial/repeated administration	Nitrates, niacin, phenylephrine, LSD, MDMA

Receptor binding

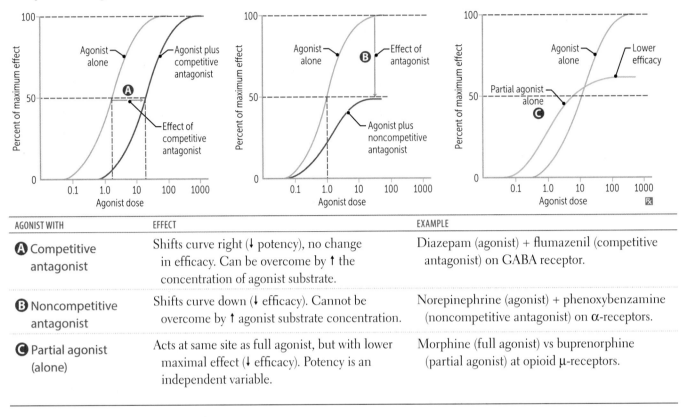

AGONIST WITH	EFFECT	EXAMPLE
Ⓐ Competitive antagonist	Shifts curve right (↓ potency), no change in efficacy. Can be overcome by ↑ the concentration of agonist substrate.	Diazepam (agonist) + flumazenil (competitive antagonist) on GABA receptor.
Ⓑ Noncompetitive antagonist	Shifts curve down (↓ efficacy). Cannot be overcome by ↑ agonist substrate concentration.	Norepinephrine (agonist) + phenoxybenzamine (noncompetitive antagonist) on α-receptors.
Ⓒ Partial agonist (alone)	Acts at same site as full agonist, but with lower maximal effect (↓ efficacy). Potency is an independent variable.	Morphine (full agonist) vs buprenorphine (partial agonist) at opioid μ-receptors.

Elimination of drugs

Zero-order elimination	Rate of elimination is constant regardless of C_p (ie, constant **amount** of drug eliminated per unit time). C_p ↓ linearly with time. Examples of drugs—Phenytoin, Ethanol, and Aspirin (at high or toxic concentrations).	Capacity-limited elimination. PEA (a pea is round, shaped like the "0" in **zero**-order).
First-order elimination	Rate of First-order elimination is directly proportional to the drug concentration (ie, constant Fraction of drug eliminated per unit time). C_p ↓ exponentially with time. Applies to most drugs.	Flow-dependent elimination.

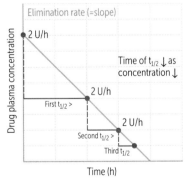

Zero-order elimination

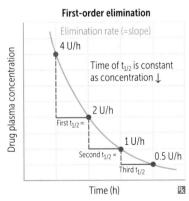

First-order elimination

Urine pH and drug elimination	Ionized species are trapped in urine and cleared quickly. Neutral forms can be reabsorbed.	
Weak acids	Examples: phenobarbital, methotrexate, aspirin (salicylates). Trapped in basic environments. Treat overdose with sodium bicarbonate to alkalinize urine. $$\text{RCOOH} \;\rightleftharpoons\; \text{RCOO}^- + \text{H}^+$$ (lipid soluble) (trapped)	
Weak bases	Example: TCAs, amphetamines. Trapped in acidic environments. Treat overdose with ammonium chloride to acidify urine. $$\text{RNH}_3^+ \;\rightleftharpoons\; \text{RNH}_2 + \text{H}^+$$ (trapped) (lipid soluble) TCA toxicity is generally treated with sodium bicarbonate to overcome the sodium channel-blocking activity of TCAs, but not for accelerating drug elimination.	

Drug metabolism		
Phase I	Reduction, Oxidation, Hydrolysis with cytochrome P-450 usually yield slightly polar, water-soluble metabolites (often still active).	Geriatric patients lose phase I first. **R-OH**
Phase II	Conjugation (Methylation, Glucuronidation, Acetylation, Sulfation) usually yields very polar, inactive metabolites (renally excreted).	Geriatric patients have **More GAS** (phase II). Patients who are slow acetylators have ↑ side effects from certain drugs because of ↓ rate of metabolism.

Efficacy vs potency

Efficacy	Maximal effect a drug can produce. Represented by the y-value (V_{max}). ↑ y-value = ↑ V_{max} = ↑ efficacy. Unrelated to potency (ie, efficacious drugs can have high or low potency). Partial agonists have less efficacy than full agonists.

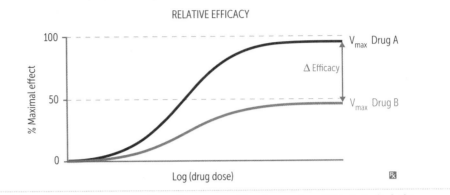

Potency	Amount of drug needed for a given effect. Represented by the x-value (EC_{50}). Left shifting = ↓ EC_{50} = ↑ potency = ↓ drug needed. Unrelated to efficacy (ie, potent drugs can have high or low efficacy).

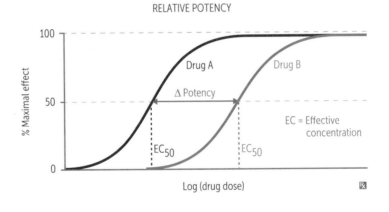

Therapeutic index	Measurement of drug safety. $$\frac{TD_{50}}{ED_{50}} = \frac{\text{median toxic dose}}{\text{median effective dose}}$$ Therapeutic window—dosage range that can safely and effectively treat disease.	TITE: Therapeutic Index = TD_{50} / ED_{50}. Safer drugs have higher TI values. Drugs with lower TI values frequently require monitoring (eg, **W**arfarin, **T**heophylline, **D**igoxin, **L**ithium; **W**arning! **T**hese **D**rugs are **L**ethal!). LD_{50} (lethal median dose) often replaces TD_{50} in animal studies.

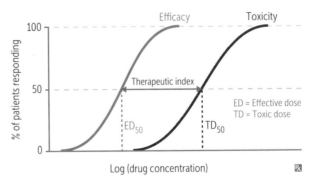

Central and peripheral nervous system

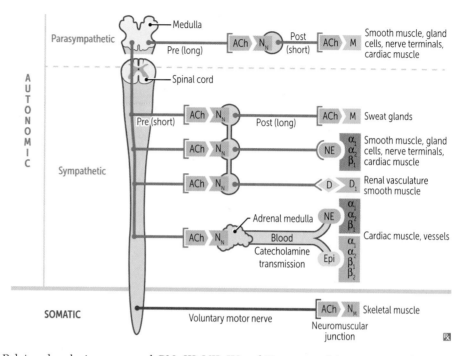

Pelvic splanchnic nerves and CNs III, VII, IX and X are part of the parasympathetic nervous system.
Adrenal medulla is directly innervated by preganglionic sympathetic fibers.
Sweat glands are part of the sympathetic pathway but are innervated by cholinergic fibers.

Acetylcholine receptors	Nicotinic ACh receptors are ligand-gated Na^+/K^+ channels. Two subtypes: N_N (found in autonomic ganglia, adrenal medulla) and N_M (found in neuromuscular junction of skeletal muscle). Muscarinic ACh receptors are G-protein–coupled receptors that usually act through 2nd messengers. 5 subtypes: M_{1-5} found in heart, smooth muscle, brain, exocrine glands, and on sweat glands (cholinergic sympathetic).

G-protein–linked second messengers

RECEPTOR	G-PROTEIN CLASS	MAJOR FUNCTIONS
Sympathetic		
α_1	q	↑ vascular smooth muscle contraction, ↑ pupillary dilator muscle contraction (mydriasis), ↑ intestinal and bladder sphincter muscle contraction
α_2	i	↓ sympathetic (adrenergic) outflow, ↓ insulin release, ↓ lipolysis, ↑ platelet aggregation, ↓ aqueous humor production
β_1	s	↑ heart rate, ↑ contractility (**one heart**), ↑ renin release, ↑ lipolysis
β_2	s	Vasodilation, bronchodilation (**two lungs**), ↑ lipolysis, ↑ insulin release, ↑ glycogenolysis, ↓ uterine tone (tocolysis), ↑ aqueous humor production, ↑ cellular K^+ uptake
β_3	s	↑ lipolysis, ↑ thermogenesis in skeletal muscle, ↑ bladder relaxation
Parasympathetic		
M_1	q	Mediates higher cognitive functions, stimulates enteric nervous system
M_2	i	↓ heart rate and contractility of atria
M_3	q	↑ exocrine gland secretions (eg, lacrimal, sweat, salivary, gastric acid), ↑ gut peristalsis, ↑ bladder contraction, bronchoconstriction, ↑ pupillary sphincter muscle contraction (miosis), ciliary muscle contraction (accommodation), ↑ insulin release
Dopamine		
D_1	s	Relaxes renal vascular smooth muscle, activates direct pathway of striatum
D_2	i	Modulates transmitter release, especially in brain, inhibits indirect pathway of striatum
Histamine		
H_1	q	↑ nasal and bronchial mucus production, ↑ vascular permeability, bronchoconstriction, pruritus, pain
H_2	s	↑ gastric acid secretion
Vasopressin		
V_1	q	↑ vascular smooth muscle contraction
V_2	s	↑ H_2O permeability and reabsorption via upregulating aquaporin-2 in collecting **two**bules (tubules) of kidney

"After **q**isses (kisses), you get a **qiq** (kick) out of **siq** (sick) **sqs** (super **q**inky sex)."

H_1, α_1, V_1, M_1, M_3 Receptor → G_q → Phospholipase C — → DAG → Protein kinase C

HAVe 1 M&M.

Lipids → PIP_2 → IP₃ → ↑ $[Ca^{2+}]_{in}$ → Smooth muscle contraction

β_1, β_2, β_3, D_1, H_2, V_2 Receptor → G_s → Adenylyl cyclase → ATP ↓ cAMP → Protein kinase A → ↑ $[Ca^{2+}]_{in}$ (heart) / Myosin light-chain kinase (smooth muscle)

M_2, α_2, D_2 Receptor → G_i ⊖

MAD 2's.

Autonomic drugs

Release of norepinephrine from a sympathetic nerve ending is modulated by NE itself, acting on presynaptic α_2-autoreceptors → negative feedback.

Amphetamines use the NE transporter (NET) to enter the presynaptic terminal, where they utilize the vesicular monoamine transporter (VMAT) to enter neurosecretory vesicles. This displaces NE from the vesicles. Once NE reaches a concentration threshold within the presynaptic terminal, the action of NET is reversed, and NE is expelled into the synaptic cleft, contributing to the characteristics and effects of ↑ NE observed in patients taking amphetamines.

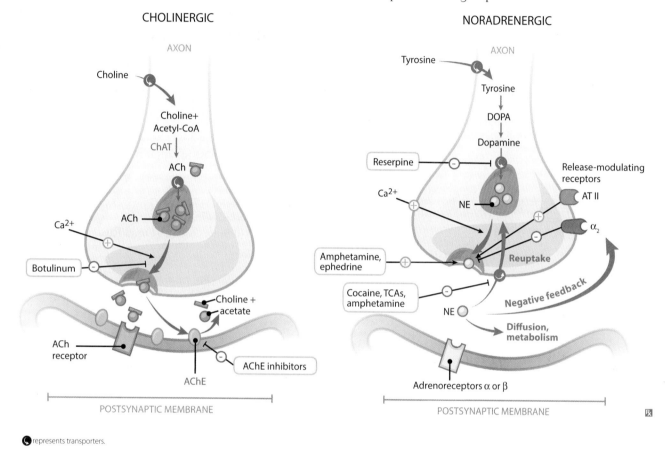

CHOLINERGIC   NORADRENERGIC

🌘 represents transporters.

Cholinomimetic agents	Watch for exacerbation of COPD, asthma, and peptic ulcers in susceptible patients.	
DRUG	ACTION	APPLICATIONS
Direct agonists		
Bethanechol	Activates bowel and bladder smooth muscle; resistant to AChE. No nicotinic activity. "**Bethany, call (bethanechol)** me to activate your bowels and bladder."	Postoperative ileus, neurogenic ileus, urinary retention
Carbachol	**Carb**on copy of acetyl**ch**oline (but resistant to AChE).	Constricts pupil and relieves intraocular pressure in open-angle glaucoma
Methacholine	Stimulates muscarinic receptors in airway when inhaled.	Challenge test for diagnosis of asthma
Pilocarpine	Contracts ciliary muscle of eye (open-angle glaucoma), pupillary sphincter (closed-angle glaucoma); resistant to AChE, can cross blood-brain barrier (tertiary amine). "You **cry**, **drool**, and **sweat** on your '**pilo**.'"	Potent stimulator of sweat, tears, and saliva Open-angle and closed-angle glaucoma, xerostomia (Sjögren syndrome)
Indirect agonists (anticholinesterases)		
Donepezil, rivastigmine, galantamine	↑ ACh.	Alzheimer disease (**Dona Riva** dances at the **gala**).
Edrophonium	↑ ACh.	Historically used to diagnose myasthenia gravis; replaced by anti-AChR Ab (anti-acetylcholine receptor antibody) test.
Neostigmine	↑ ACh. **Neo** CNS = **No** CNS penetration (quaternary amine).	Postoperative and neurogenic ileus and urinary retention, myasthenia gravis, reversal of neuromuscular junction blockade (postoperative).
Physostigmine	↑ ACh. **Ph**reely (freely) crosses blood-brain barrier → CNS (tertiary amine).	Antidote for anticholinergic toxicity; **ph**ysostigmine "**ph**yxes" atropine overdose.
Pyridostigmine	↑ ACh; ↑ muscle strength. **Pyri**dostigmine gets **ri**d of myasthenia gravis.	Myasthenia gravis (long acting); does not penetrate CNS (quaternary amine).

| **Cholinesterase inhibitor poisoning** | Often due to organophosphates, such as parathion, that **irreversibly** inhibit AChE. Causes Diarrhea, Urination, Miosis, Bronchospasm, Bradycardia, Emesis, Lacrimation, Sweating, and Salivation. May lead to respiratory failure if untreated. | DUMBBELSS. Organophosphates are often components of insecticides; poisoning usually seen in farmers. Antidote—atropine (competitive inhibitor) + pralidoxime (regenerates AChE if given early). |

Muscarinic antagonists

DRUGS	ORGAN SYSTEMS	APPLICATIONS
Atropine, homatropine, tropicamide	Eye	Produce mydriasis and cycloplegia.
Benztropine, trihexyphenidyl	CNS	Parkinson disease ("**park** my **Benz**"). Acute dystonia.
Glycopyrrolate	GI, respiratory	Parenteral: preoperative use to reduce airway secretions. Oral: drooling, peptic ulcer.
Hyoscyamine, dicyclomine	GI	Antispasmodics for irritable bowel syndrome.
Ipratropium, tiotropium	Respiratory	COPD, asthma ("**I pray** I can breathe soon!").
Oxybutynin, solifenacin, tolterodine	Genitourinary	Reduce bladder spasms and urge urinary incontinence (overactive bladder).
Scopolamine	CNS	Motion sickness.

Atropine

Muscarinic antagonist. Used to treat bradycardia and for ophthalmic applications.

ORGAN SYSTEM	ACTION	NOTES
Eye	↑ pupil dilation, cycloplegia	Blocks **DUMBBeLSS** in cholinesterase inhibitor poisoning. Does not block excitation of skeletal muscle and CNS (mediated by nicotinic receptors).
Airway	Bronchodilation, ↓ secretions	
Stomach	↓ acid secretion	
Gut	↓ motility	
Bladder	↓ urgency in cystitis	
ADVERSE EFFECTS	↑ body **temperature** (due to ↓ sweating); rapid pulse; dry mouth; **dry, flushed skin**; **cycloplegia**; constipation; **disorientation** Can cause acute angle-closure glaucoma in elderly (due to mydriasis), **urinary retention** in men with prostatic hyperplasia, and hyperthermia in infants.	Side effects: **Hot** as a hare **Dry** as a bone **Red** as a beet **Blind** as a bat **Mad** as a hatter **Full** as a flask Jimson weed (*Datura*) → gardener's pupil (mydriasis due to plant alkaloids)

Sympathomimetics

DRUG	ACTION	APPLICATIONS
Direct sympathomimetics		
Albuterol, salmeterol, terbutaline	$\beta_2 > \beta_1$	Albuterol for acute asthma or COPD. Salmeterol for long-term asthma or COPD management. Terbutaline for acute bronchospasm in asthma and tocolysis.
Dobutamine	$\beta_1 > \beta_2, \alpha$	Heart failure (HF), cardiogenic shock (inotropic > chronotropic), cardiac stress testing.
Dopamine	$D_1 = D_2 > \beta > \alpha$	Unstable bradycardia, HF, shock; inotropic and chronotropic effects at lower doses due to β effects; vasoconstriction at high doses due to α effects.
Epinephrine	$\beta > \alpha$	Anaphylaxis, asthma, open-angle glaucoma; α effects predominate at high doses. Significantly stronger effect at β_2-receptor than norepinephrine.
Fenoldopam	D_1	Postoperative hypertension, hypertensive crisis. Vasodilator (coronary, peripheral, renal, and splanchnic). Promotes natriuresis. Can cause hypotension and tachycardia.
Isoproterenol	$\beta_1 = \beta_2$	Electrophysiologic evaluation of tachyarrhythmias. Can worsen ischemia. Has negligible α effect.
Midodrine	α_1	Autonomic insufficiency and postural hypotension. May exacerbate supine hypertension.
Mirabegron	β_3	Urinary urge incontinence or overactive bladder.
Norepinephrine	$\alpha_1 > \alpha_2 > \beta_1$	Hypotension, septic shock.
Phenylephrine	$\alpha_1 > \alpha_2$	Hypotension (vasoconstrictor), ocular procedures (mydriatic), rhinitis (decongestant), ischemic priapism.
Indirect sympathomimetics		
Amphetamine	Indirect general agonist, reuptake inhibitor, also releases stored catecholamines	Narcolepsy, obesity, ADHD.
Cocaine	Indirect general agonist, reuptake inhibitor	Causes vasoconstriction and local anesthesia. Caution when giving β-blockers if cocaine intoxication is suspected (can lead to unopposed α_1 activation, activation → extreme hypertension, coronary vasospasm).
Ephedrine	Indirect general agonist, releases stored catecholamines	Nasal decongestion (pseudoephedrine), urinary incontinence, hypotension.

Norepinephrine vs isoproterenol

NE ↑ systolic and diastolic pressures as a result of α_1-mediated vasoconstriction → ↑ mean arterial pressure → reflex bradycardia. However, isoproterenol (rarely used) has little α effect but causes β_2-mediated vasodilation, resulting in ↓ mean arterial pressure and ↑ heart rate through β_1 and reflex activity.

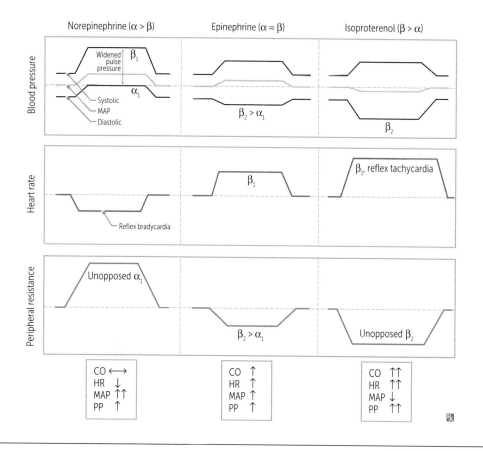

Sympatholytics (α_2-agonists)

DRUG	APPLICATIONS	ADVERSE EFFECTS
Clonidine, guanfacine	Hypertensive urgency (limited situations), ADHD, Tourette syndrome, symptom control in opioid withdrawal	CNS depression, bradycardia, hypotension, respiratory depression, miosis, rebound hypertension with abrupt cessation
α-methyldopa	Hypertension in pregnancy	Direct Coombs ⊕ hemolysis, drug-induced lupus
Tizanidine	Relief of spasticity	Hypotension, weakness, xerostomia

α-blockers

DRUG	APPLICATIONS	ADVERSE EFFECTS
Nonselective		
Phenoxybenzamine	Irreversible. Pheochromocytoma (used preoperatively) to prevent catecholamine (hypertensive) crisis	Orthostatic hypotension, reflex tachycardia
Phentolamine	Reversible. Give to patients on MAO inhibitors who eat tyramine-containing foods and for severe cocaine-induced hypertension (2nd line)	
α_1 selective (-osin ending)		
Prazosin, terazosin, doxazosin, tamsulosin	Urinary symptoms of BPH; PTSD (prazosin); hypertension (except tamsulosin)	1st-dose orthostatic hypotension, dizziness, headache
α_2 selective		
Mirtazapine	Depression	Sedation, ↑ serum cholesterol, ↑ appetite

Effects of α-blocker (eg, phentolamine) on BP responses to epinephrine and phenylephrine

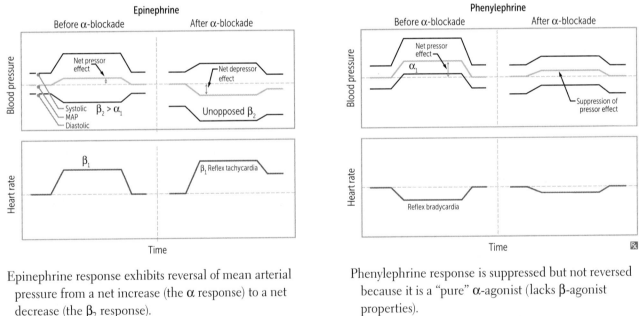

Epinephrine response exhibits reversal of mean arterial pressure from a net increase (the α response) to a net decrease (the β_2 response).

Phenylephrine response is suppressed but not reversed because it is a "pure" α-agonist (lacks β-agonist properties).

β-blockers

Acebutolol, atenolol, betaxolol, bisoprolol, carvedilol, esmolol, labetalol, metoprolol, nadolol, nebivolol, pindolol, propranolol, timolol.

APPLICATION	ACTIONS	NOTES/EXAMPLES
Angina pectoris	↓ heart rate and contractility, resulting in ↓ O_2 consumption	
Glaucoma	↓ production of aqueous humor	Timolol
Heart failure	↓ mortality	Bisoprolol, carvedilol, metoprolol
Hypertension	↓ cardiac output, ↓ renin secretion (due to β_1-receptor blockade on JGA cells)	
Hyperthyroidism	Symptom control (↓ heart rate, ↓ tremor), thyroid storm	Propranolol
Hypertrophic cardiomyopathy	↓ heart rate → ↑ filling time, relieving obstruction	
Myocardial infarction	↓ mortality	
Supraventricular tachycardia	↓ AV conduction velocity (class II antiarrhythmic)	Metoprolol, esmolol
Variceal bleeding	↓ hepatic venous pressure gradient and portal hypertension (prophylactic use)	Nadolol, propranolol, carvedilol
ADVERSE EFFECTS	Erectile dysfunction, cardiovascular (bradycardia, AV block, HF), CNS (seizures, sleep alterations), dyslipidemia (metoprolol), and asthma/COPD exacerbations	Use with caution in cocaine users due to risk of unopposed α-adrenergic receptor agonist activity
SELECTIVITY	β_1-selective antagonists ($\beta_1 > \beta_2$)—acebutolol (partial agonist), atenolol, betaxolol, bisoprolol, esmolol, metoprolol	Selective antagonists mostly go from **A** to **M** (β_1 with 1st half of alphabet)
	Nonselective antagonists ($\beta_1 = \beta_2$)—nadolol, pindolol (partial agonist), propranolol, timolol	Nonselective antagonists mostly go from **N** to **Z** (β_2 with 2nd half of alphabet)
	Nonselective α- and β-antagonists—carve**dilol**, labeta**lol**	Nonselective α- and β-antagonists have **modified** **suffixes** (instead of "-olol")
	Nebivolol combines cardiac-selective β_1-adrenergic blockade with stimulation of β_3-receptors (activate nitric oxide synthase in the vasculature and ↓ SVR)	Nebivolol increases **NO**

Ingested seafood toxins Toxin actions include Histamine release, Total block of Na$^+$ channels, or opening of Na$^+$ channels to Cause depolarization.

TOXIN	SOURCE	ACTION	SYMPTOMS	TREATMENT
Histamine (scombroid poisoning)	Spoiled dark-meat fish such as tuna, mahi-mahi, mackerel, and bonito.	Bacterial histidine decarboxylase converts histidine to histamine. Frequently misdiagnosed as fish allergy.	Mimics anaphylaxis: acute burning sensation of mouth, flushing of face, erythema, urticaria, itching. May progress to bronchospasm, angioedema, hypotension.	Antihistamines. Albuterol and epinephrine if needed.
Tetrodotoxin	Pufferfish.	Highly potent toxin; binds fast voltage-gated Na$^+$ channels in cardiac/nerve tissue, preventing depolarization.	Nausea, diarrhea, paresthesias, weakness, dizziness, loss of reflexes.	Supportive.
Ciguatoxin	Reef fish such as barracuda, snapper, and moray eel.	Opens Na$^+$ channels, causing depolarization.	Nausea, vomiting, diarrhea; perioral numbness; reversal of hot and cold sensations; bradycardia, heart block, hypotension.	Supportive.

Beers criteria Widely used criteria developed to reduce potentially inappropriate prescribing and harmful polypharmacy in the geriatric population. Includes > 50 medications that should be avoided in elderly patients due to ↓ efficacy and/or ↑ risk of adverse events. Examples include:

- α-blockers (↑ risk of hypotension)
- Anticholinergics, antidepressants, antihistamines, opioids (↑ risk of delirium, sedation, falls, constipation, urinary retention)
- Benzodiazepines (↑ risk of delirium, sedation, falls)
- NSAIDs (↑ risk of GI bleeding, especially with concomitant anticoagulation)
- PPIs (↑ risk of *C difficile* infection)

▶ PHARMACOLOGY—TOXICITIES AND SIDE EFFECTS

Specific toxicity treatments

TOXIN	TREATMENT
Acetaminophen	N-acetylcysteine (replenishes glutathione)
AChE inhibitors, organophosphates	Atropine > pralidoxime
Antimuscarinic, anticholinergic agents	Physostigmine, control hyperthermia
Arsenic	Dimercaprol, succimer
Benzodiazepines	Flumazenil
β-blockers	Atropine, glucagon
Carbon monoxide	100% O_2, hyperbaric O_2
Copper	**Penicillamine, trientine (Copper penny)**
Cyanide	Nitrite + thiosulfate, hydroxocobalamin
Digitalis (digoxin)	Anti-dig Fab fragments
Heparin	Protamine sulfate
Iron	Deferoxamine, deferasirox, deferiprone
Lead	EDTA, dimercaprol, succimer, penicillamine
Mercury	Dimercaprol, succimer
Methanol, ethylene glycol (antifreeze)	Fomepizole > ethanol, dialysis
Methemoglobin	**Methylene blue, vitamin C (reducing agent)**
OpiOids	NalOxOne
Salicylates	$NaHCO_3$ (alkalinize urine), dialysis
TCAs	$NaHCO_3$ (stabilizes cardiac cell membrane)
Warfarin	Vitamin K (delayed effect), fresh frozen plasma (immediate)

Drug reactions—cardiovascular

DRUG REACTION	CAUSAL AGENTS
Coronary vasospasm	Cocaine, Amphetamines, Sumatriptan, Ergot alkaloids (**CASE**)
Cutaneous flushing	Vancomycin, Adenosine, Niacin, Ca^{2+} channel blockers, Echinocandins, Nitrates (flushed from **VANCEN** [dancing]) Red man syndrome—rate-dependent infusion reaction to vancomycin causing widespread pruritic erythema. Manage with diphenhydramine, slower infusion rate.
Dilated cardiomyopathy	Anthracyclines (eg, Doxorubicin, Daunorubicin); prevent with Dexrazoxane
Torsades de pointes	Agents that prolong QT interval: antiArrhythmics (class IA, III), antiBiotics (eg, macrolides), anti"C"ychotics (eg, haloperidol), antiDepressants (eg, TCAs), antiEmetics (eg, ondansetron) (**ABCDE**)

Drug reactions—endocrine/reproductive

DRUG REACTION	CAUSAL AGENTS	NOTES
Adrenocortical insufficiency	HPA suppression 2° to glucocorticoid withdrawal	
Diabetes insipidus	Lithium, demeclocycline	
Hot flashes	SERMs (eg, tamoxifen, clomiphene, raloxifene)	
Hyperglycemia	Tacrolimus, Protease inhibitors, Niacin, HCTZ, Corticosteroids	The People Need Hard Candies
Hyperprolactinemia	Typical antipsychotics (eg, haloperidol), atypical antipsychotics (eg, quetiapine), metoclopramide, methyldopa	Presents with hypogonadism (eg, infertility, amenorrhea, erectile dysfunction) and galactorrhea (more common in men)
Hyperthyroidism	Lithium, amiodarone	
Hypothyroidism	AMiodarone, SUlfonamides, Lithium	I AM SUddenly Lethargic
SIADH	Carbamazepine, Cyclophosphamide, SSRIs	Can't Concentrate Serum Sodium

Drug reactions—gastrointestinal

DRUG REACTION	CAUSAL AGENTS	NOTES
Acute cholestatic hepatitis, jaundice	Macrolides (eg, erythromycin)	
Diarrhea	Acamprosate, antidiabetic agents (acarbose, metformin, pramlintide), colchicine, cholinesterase inhibitors, lipid-lowering agents (eg, ezetimibe, orlistat), macrolides (eg, erythromycin), quinidine, SSRIs	
Focal to massive hepatic necrosis	Halothane, *Amanita phalloides* (death cap mushroom), Valproic acid, Acetaminophen	Liver "HAVAc"
Hepatitis	Rifampin, isoniazid, pyrazinamide, statins, fibrates	
Pancreatitis	Didanosine, Corticosteroids, Alcohol, Valproic acid, Azathioprine, Diuretics (furosemide, HCTZ)	Drugs Causing A Violent Abdominal Distress
Pill-induced esophagitis	Bisphosphonates, ferrous sulfate, NSAIDs, potassium chloride, tetracyclines	Caustic effect minimized with upright posture and adequate water ingestion.
Pseudomembranous colitis	Ampicillin, cephalosporins, clindamycin, fluoroquinolones	Antibiotics predispose to superinfection by resistant *C difficile*

Drug reactions—hematologic

DRUG REACTION	CAUSAL AGENTS	NOTES
Agranulocytosis	Clozapine, Carbamazepine, Propylthiouracil, Methimazole, Colchicine, Ganciclovir	Can Cause Pretty Major Collapse of Granulocytes
Aplastic anemia	Carbamazepine, Methimazole, NSAIDs, Benzene, Chloramphenicol, Propylthiouracil	Can't Make New Blood Cells Properly
Direct Coombs-positive hemolytic anemia	Penicillin, methylDopa, Cephalosporins	P Diddy Coombs
Drug reaction with eosinophilia and systemic symptoms	Allopurinol, anticonvulsants, antibiotics, sulfa drugs	DRESS is a potentially fatal delayed hypersensitivity reaction. Latency period (2–8 weeks) followed by fever, morbilliform skin rash, and frequent multiorgan involvement. Treatment: withdrawal of offending drug, corticosteroids.
Gray baby syndrome	Chloramphenicol	
Hemolysis in G6PD deficiency	Isoniazid, Sulfonamides, Dapsone, Primaquine, Aspirin, Ibuprofen, Nitrofurantoin	Hemolysis IS D PAIN
Megaloblastic anemia	Hydroxyurea, Phenytoin, Methotrexate, Sulfa drugs	You're having a **mega** blast with **PMS**
Thrombocytopenia	Heparin, Vancomycin, Linezolid	Help! Very Low platelets
Thrombotic complications	Combined oral contraceptives, hormone replacement therapy, SERMs (eg, tamoxifen, raloxifene, clomiphene)	Estrogen-mediated side effect

Drug reactions—musculoskeletal/skin/connective tissue

DRUG REACTION	CAUSAL AGENTS	NOTES
Drug-induced lupus	Methyldopa, Sulfa drugs, Hydralazine, Isoniazid, Procainamide, Phenytoin, Etanercept	Having lupus is Mega "SHIPP-E"
Fat redistribution	Protease inhibitors, Glucocorticoids	Fat PiG
Gingival hyperplasia	Cyclosporine, Ca^{2+} channel blockers, Phenytoin	Can Cause Puffy gums
Hyperuricemia (gout)	Pyrazinamide, Thiazides, Furosemide, Niacin, Cyclosporine	Painful Tophi and Feet Need Care
Myopathy	Statins, fibrates, niacin, colchicine, daptomycin, hydroxychloroquine, interferon-α, penicillamine, glucocorticoids	
Osteoporosis	Corticosteroids, depot medroxyprogesterone acetate, GnRH agonists, aromatase inhibitors, anticonvulsants, heparin, PPIs	
Photosensitivity	Sulfonamides, Amiodarone, Tetracyclines, 5-FU	SAT For Photo
Rash (Stevens-Johnson syndrome)	Anti-epileptic drugs (especially lamotrigine), allopurinol, sulfa drugs, penicillin	Steven Johnson has epileptic allergy to sulfa drugs and penicillin
Teeth discoloration	Tetracyclines	Teethracyclines
Tendon and cartilage damage	Fluoroquinolones	

Drug reactions—neurologic

DRUG REACTION	CAUSAL AGENTS	NOTES
Cinchonism	Quinidine, quinine	Can present with tinnitus, hearing/vision loss, psychosis, and cognitive impairment
Parkinson-like syndrome	Antipsychotics, Reserpine, Metoclopramide	Cogwheel rigidity of **ARM**
Peripheral neuropathy	Phenytoin, vincristine	
Pseudotumor cerebri	Growth hormones, tetracyclines, vitamin A	
Seizures	Isoniazid (vitamin B_6 deficiency), Bupropion, Imipenem/cilastatin, Tramadol, Enflurane	With seizures, I BITE my tongue
Tardive dyskinesia	Antipsychotics, metoclopramide	
Visual disturbance	Topiramate (blurred vision/diplopia, haloes), Digoxin (yellow-tinged vision), Isoniazid (optic neuropathy/color vision changes), Vigabatrin (bilateral visual field defects), PDE-5 inhibitors (blue-tinged vision), Ethambutol (color vision changes)	These Drugs Irritate Very Precious Eyes

Drug reactions—renal/genitourinary

DRUG REACTION	CAUSAL AGENTS	NOTES
Fanconi syndrome	Cisplatin, ifosfamide, expired tetracyclines, tenofovir	
Hemorrhagic cystitis	Cyclophosphamide, ifosfamide	Prevent by coadministering with mesna
Interstitial nephritis	Penicillins, furosemide, NSAIDs, proton pump inhibitors, sulfa drugs	

Drug reactions—respiratory

DRUG REACTION	CAUSAL AGENTS	NOTES
Dry cough	ACE inhibitors	
Pulmonary fibrosis	Methotrexate, Nitrofurantoin, Carmustine, Bleomycin, Busulfan, Amiodarone	My Nose Cannot Breathe Bad Air

Drug reactions—multiorgan

DRUG REACTION	CAUSAL AGENTS	NOTES
Antimuscarinic	Atropine, TCAs, H_1-blockers, antipsychotics	
Disulfiram-like reaction	1st-generation Sulfonylureas, Procarbazine, certain Cephalosporins, Griseofulvin, Metronidazole	Sorry Pals, Can't Go Mingle.
Nephrotoxicity/ ototoxicity	Loop diuretics, Aminoglycosides, cisPlatin, Vancomycin, amphoTERicin B	Listen And Pee Very TERriBly. Cisplatin toxicity may respond to amifostine.

Drugs affecting pupil size

↑ pupil size	↓ pupil size
Anticholinergics (atropine, TCA, tropicamide, scopolamine, antihistamines)	Antipsychotics (haloperidol, risperidone, olanzapine)
Drugs of abuse (amphetamines, cocaine, LSD)	Drugs of abuse (eg, heroin/opioids)
Sympathomimetics	Parasympathomimetics (pilocarpine), organophosphates

Cytochrome P-450 interactions (selected)

Inducers (+)	Substrates	Inhibitors (–)
Modafinil	Anti-epileptics	Sodium valproate
Chronic alcohol use	Theophylline	Isoniazid
St. John's wort	Warfarin	Cimetidine
Phenytoin	OCPs	Ketoconazole
Phenobarbital		Fluconazole
Nevirapine		Acute alcohol abuse
Rifampin		Chloramphenicol
Griseofulvin		Erythromycin/clarithromycin
Carbamazepine		Sulfonamides
		Ciprofloxacin
		Omeprazole
		Metronidazole
		Amiodarone
		Grapefruit juice
Most chronic alcoholics Steal Phen-Phen and Never Refuse Greasy Carbs	Always Think When Outdoors	SICKFACES.COM (when I Am drinking Grapefruit juice)

Sulfa drugs — Sulfonamide antibiotics, Sulfasalazine, Probenecid, Furosemide, Acetazolamide, Celecoxib, Thiazides, Sulfonylureas. Patients with sulfa allergies may develop fever, urinary tract infection, Stevens-Johnson syndrome, hemolytic anemia, thrombocytopenia, agranulocytosis, acute interstitial nephritis, and urticaria (hives). Symptoms range from mild to life threatening.

Scary Sulfa Pharm FACTS

▶ PHARMACOLOGY—MISCELLANEOUS

Drug names

ENDING	CATEGORY	EXAMPLE
Antimicrobial		
-azole	Ergosterol synthesis inhibitor	Ketoconazole
-bendazole	Antiparasitic/antihelminthic	Mebendazole
-cillin	Transpeptidase (penicillin-binding protein)	Ampicillin
-cycline	Protein synthesis inhibitor	Tetracycline
-ivir	Neuraminidase inhibitor	Oseltamivir
-navir	Protease inhibitor	Ritonavir
-ovir	DNA polymerase inhibitor	Acyclovir
-thromycin	Macrolide antibiotic	Azithromycin
CNS		
-ane	Inhalational general anesthetic	Halothane
-azine	Typical antipsychotic	Thioridazine
-barbital	Barbiturate	Phenobarbital
-caine	Local anesthetic	Lidocaine
-ipramine, -triptyline	TCA	Imipramine, amitriptyline
-triptan	$5\text{-HT}_{1B/1D}$ agonist	Sumatriptan
-zepam, -zolam	Benzodiazepine	Diazepam, alprazolam
Autonomic		
-chol	Cholinergic agonist	Bethanechol, carbachol
-curium, -curonium	Nondepolarizing paralytic	Atracurium, vecuronium
-olol	β-blocker	Propranolol
-stigmine	AChE inhibitor	Neostigmine
-terol	β_2-agonist	Albuterol
-zosin	α_1-antagonist	Prazosin
Cardiovascular		
-afil	PDE-5 inhibitor	Sildenafil
-dipine	Dihydropyridine Ca^{2+} channel blocker	Amlodipine
-pril	ACE inhibitor	Captopril
-sartan	Angiotensin-II receptor blocker	Losartan
-xaban	Direct factor Xa inhibitor	Apixaban, edoxaban, rivaroxaban
Other		
-dronate	Bisphosphonate	Alendronate
-gliptin	DPP-4 inhibitors	Sitagliptin
-glitazone	PPAR-γ activator	Rosiglitazone
-limus	Calcineurin inhibitor	Everolimus, tacrolimus
-prazole	Proton pump inhibitor	Omeprazole
-prost	Prostaglandin analog	Latanoprost
-sentan	Endothelin receptor antagonist	Bosentan
-tidine	H_2-antagonist	Cimetidine
-tropin	Pituitary hormone	Somatotropin

Biologic agents

ENDING	CATEGORY	EXAMPLE
Monoclonal antibodies (-mab)—target overexpressed cell surface receptors		
-ximab	Chimeric human-mouse monoclonal Ab	Rituximab
-zumab	Humanized mouse monoclonal Ab	Bevacizumab
-mumab	Human monoclonal Ab	Ipilimumab
Small molecule inhibitors (-ib)—target intracellular molecules		
-tinib	Tyrosine kinase inhibitor	Imatinib
-zomib	Proteasome inhibitor	Bortezomib
-ciclib	Cyclin-dependent kinase inhibitor	Palbociclib
Receptor fusion proteins (-cept)		
-cept	TNF-α antagonist	Etanercept
Interleukin receptor modulators (-kin)—agonists and antagonists of interleukin receptors		
-leukin	IL-2 agonist/analog	Aldesleukin
-kinra	Interleukin receptor antagonist	Anakinra

▶ NOTES

Public Health Sciences

"It is a mathematical fact that fifty percent of all doctors graduate in the bottom half of their class."

—Unknown

"There are two kinds of statistics: the kind you look up and the kind you make up."

—Rex Stout

"On a long enough timeline, the survival rate for everyone drops to zero."
—Chuck Palahniuk

"There are three kinds of lies: lies, damned lies, and statistics."
—Mark Twain

A heterogenous mix of epidemiology, biostatistics, ethics, law, healthcare delivery, patient safety, quality improvement, and more falls under the heading of public health sciences. Biostatistics and epidemiology are the foundations of evidence-based medicine and are very high yield. Make sure you can quickly apply biostatistical equations such as sensitivity, specificity, and predictive values in a problem-solving format. Also, know how to set up your own 2×2 tables. Quality improvement and patient safety topics were introduced a few years ago on the exam and represent trends in health system science. Medical ethics questions often require application of principles. Typically, you are presented with a patient scenario and then asked how you would respond.

▶ PUBLIC HEALTH SCIENCES—EPIDEMIOLOGY AND BIOSTATISTICS

Observational studies

STUDY TYPE	DESIGN	MEASURES/EXAMPLE
Cross-sectional study	Frequency of disease and frequency of risk-related factors are assessed in the present. Asks, "What is happening?"	Disease prevalence. Can show risk factor association with disease, but does not establish causality.
Case-control study	Compares a group of people with disease to a group without disease. Looks to see if odds of prior exposure or risk factor differs by disease state. Asks, "What happened?"	Odds ratio (OR). Patients with COPD had higher odds of a smoking history than those without COPD.
Cohort study	Compares a group with a given exposure or risk factor to a group without such exposure. Looks to see if exposure or risk factor is associated with later development of disease. Can be prospective (asks, "Who will develop disease?") or retrospective (asks, "Who developed the disease [exposed vs nonexposed]?").	Relative risk (RR). Smokers had a higher risk of developing COPD than nonsmokers.
Twin concordance study	Compares the frequency with which both monozygotic twins vs both dizygotic twins develop the same disease.	Measures heritability and influence of environmental factors ("nature vs nurture").
Adoption study	Compares siblings raised by biological vs adoptive parents.	Measures heritability and influence of environmental factors.

Clinical trial	Experimental study involving humans. Compares therapeutic benefits of 2 or more treatments, or of treatment and placebo. Study quality improves when study is randomized, controlled, and double-blinded (ie, neither patient nor doctor knows whether the patient is in the treatment or control group). Triple-blind refers to the additional blinding of the researchers analyzing the data. Four phases ("Does the drug **SWIM**?").

DRUG TRIALS	TYPICAL STUDY SAMPLE	PURPOSE
Phase I	Small number of healthy volunteers or patients with disease of interest.	"Is it **S**afe?" Assesses safety, toxicity, pharmacokinetics, and pharmacodynamics.
Phase II	Moderate number of patients with disease of interest.	"Does it **W**ork?" Assesses treatment efficacy, optimal dosing, and adverse effects.
Phase III	Large number of patients randomly assigned either to the treatment under investigation or to the best available treatment (or placebo).	"Is it as good or better?" Compares the new treatment to the current standard of care (any **I**mprovement?).
Phase IV	Postmarketing surveillance of patients after treatment is approved.	"Can it stay?" Detects rare or long-term adverse effects. Can result in treatment being withdrawn from **M**arket.

Evaluation of diagnostic tests

Uses 2 × 2 table comparing test results with the actual presence of disease.

Sensitivity and specificity are fixed properties of a test. PPV and NPV vary depending on disease prevalence in population being tested.

		Disease ⊕	Disease ⊖	
Test	⊕	TP	FP	PPV $= TP/(TP + FP)$
	⊖	FN	TN	NPV $= TN/(TN + FN)$
		Sensitivity $= TP/(TP + FN)$	Specificity $= TN/(TN + FP)$	Prevalence $\frac{TP + FN}{(TP + FN + FP + TN)}$

Sensitivity (true-positive rate)

Proportion of all people with disease who test positive, or the probability that when the disease is present, the test is positive.

Value approaching 100% is desirable for **ruling out** disease and indicates a **low false-negative rate**. High sensitivity test used for screening in diseases with low prevalence.

$= TP / (TP + FN)$

$= 1 - FN$ rate

SN-N-OUT = highly **SeN**sitive test, when Negative, rules **OUT** disease

If sensitivity is 100%, then FN is zero. So, all negatives must be TNs.

Specificity (true-negative rate)

Proportion of all people without disease who test negative, or the probability that when the disease is absent, the test is negative.

Value approaching 100% is desirable for **ruling in** disease and indicates a **low false-positive rate**. High specificity test used for confirmation after a positive screening test.

$= TN / (TN + FP)$

$= 1 - FP$ rate

SP-P-IN = highly **SP**ecific test, when **P**ositive, rules **IN** disease

If specificity is 100%, then FP is zero. So, all positives must be TPs.

Positive predictive value

Probability that a person who has a positive test result actually has the disease.

$PPV = TP / (TP + FP)$

PPV varies directly with pretest probability (baseline risk, such as prevalence of disease): high pretest probability → high PPV

Negative predictive value

Probability that a person with a negative test result actually does not have the disease.

$NPV = TN / (TN + FN)$

NPV varies inversely with prevalence or pretest probability

POSSIBLE CUTOFF VALUES
A = 100% sensitivity cutoff value
B = practical compromise between specificity and sensitivity
C = 100% specificity cutoff value

Lowering the cutoff point: B → A (↑ FP ↓ FN)	↑ Sensitivity ↑ NPV ↓ Specificity ↓ PPV
Raising the cutoff point: B → C (↑ FN ↓ FP)	↑ Specificity ↑ PPV ↓ Sensitivity ↓ NPV

Likelihood ratio

Likelihood that a given test result would be expected in a patient with the target disorder compared to the likelihood that the same result would be expected in a patient without the target disorder.

$LR^+ > 10$ and/or $LR^- < 0.1$ indicate a very useful diagnostic test.

LRs can be multiplied with pretest odds of disease to estimate posttest odds.

$$LR^+ = \frac{sensitivity}{1 - specificity} = \frac{TP \ rate}{FP \ rate}$$

$$LR^- = \frac{1 - sensitivity}{specificity} = \frac{FN \ rate}{TN \ rate}$$

Quantifying risk	Definitions and formulas are based on the classic 2×2 or contingency table.	

Disease

	⊕	⊖
Risk factor or intervention ⊕	a	b
⊖	c	d

Odds ratio	Typically used in case-control studies. OR depicts the odds of a certain exposure given an event (eg, disease; a/c) vs the odds of exposure in the absence of that event (eg, no disease; b/d).	$OR = \dfrac{a/c}{b/d} = \dfrac{ad}{bc}$
Relative risk	Typically used in cohort studies. Risk of developing disease in the exposed group divided by risk in the unexposed group (eg, if 5/10 people exposed to radiation get cancer, and 1/10 people not exposed to radiation get cancer, the relative risk is 5, indicating a 5 times greater risk of cancer in the exposed than unexposed). For rare diseases (low prevalence), OR approximates RR. RR = 1 → no association between exposure and disease. RR > 1 → exposure associated with ↑ disease occurrence. RR < 1 → exposure associated with ↓ disease occurrence.	$RR = \dfrac{a/(a + b)}{c/(c + d)}$
Attributable risk	The difference in risk between exposed and unexposed groups (eg, if risk of lung cancer in smokers is 21% and risk in nonsmokers is 1%, then the attributable risk is 20%).	$AR = \dfrac{a}{a + b} - \dfrac{c}{c + d}$
Relative risk reduction	The proportion of risk reduction attributable to the intervention as compared to a control (eg, if 2% of patients who receive a flu shot develop the flu, while 8% of unvaccinated patients develop the flu, then RR = 2/8 = 0.25, and RRR = 0.75).	$RRR = 1 - RR$
Absolute risk reduction	The difference in risk (not the proportion) attributable to the intervention as compared to a control (eg, if 8% of people who receive a placebo vaccine develop the flu vs 2% of people who receive a flu vaccine, then ARR = 8% − 2% = 6% = .06).	$ARR = \dfrac{c}{c + d} - \dfrac{a}{a + b}$
Number needed to treat	Number of patients who need to be treated for 1 patient to benefit. Lower number = better treatment.	$NNT = 1/ARR$
Number needed to harm	Number of patients who need to be exposed to a risk factor for 1 patient to be harmed. Higher number = safer exposure.	$NNH = 1/AR$

Incidence vs prevalence	$\text{Incidence} = \dfrac{\text{\# of new cases}}{\text{\# of people at risk}}$ (during a specified time period)	Incidence looks at new cases (**incidents**).

$\text{Prevalence} = \dfrac{\text{\# of existing cases}}{\text{Total \# of people in a population}}$ (at a point in time)

Prevalence looks at **all** current cases.

$\dfrac{\text{Prevalence}}{1-\text{prevalence}} = \text{Incidence rate} \times \dfrac{\text{average duration}}{\text{of disease}}$

Prevalence ≈ incidence for short duration disease (eg, common cold).
Prevalence > incidence for chronic diseases, due to large # of existing cases (eg, diabetes).

Prevalence ~ pretest probability.
↑ prevalence → ↑ PPV and ↓ NPV.

Precision vs accuracy

Precision (reliability)	The consistency and reproducibility of a test. The absence of random variation in a test.	Random error ↓ precision in a test. ↑ precision → ↓ standard deviation. ↑ precision → ↑ statistical power $(1-\beta)$.
Accuracy (validity)	The trueness of test measurements. The absence of systematic error or bias in a test.	Systematic error ↓ accuracy in a test.

Bias and study errors

TYPE	DEFINITION	EXAMPLES	STRATEGIES TO REDUCE BIAS
Recruiting participants			
Selection bias	Nonrandom sampling or treatment allocation of subjects such that study population is not representative of target population. Most commonly a sampling bias.	Berkson bias—study population selected from hospital is less healthy than general population Non-response bias—participating subjects differ from nonrespondents in meaningful ways	Randomization Ensure the choice of the right comparison/reference group
Performing study			
Recall bias	Awareness of disorder alters recall by subjects; common in retrospective studies.	Patients with disease recall exposure after learning of similar cases	Decrease time from exposure to follow-up
Measurement bias	Information is gathered in a systemically distorted manner.	Association between HTN and MI not observed when using faulty automatic sphygmomanometer Hawthorne effect—participants change behavior upon awareness of being observed	Use objective, standardized, and previously tested methods of data collection that are planned ahead of time Use placebo group
Procedure bias	Subjects in different groups are not treated the same.	Patients in treatment group spend more time in highly specialized hospital units	Blinding and use of placebo reduce influence of participants and researchers on procedures and interpretation of outcomes as neither are aware of group allocation
Observer-expectancy bias	Researcher's belief in the efficacy of a treatment changes the outcome of that treatment (aka, Pygmalion effect).	An observer expecting treatment group to show signs of recovery is more likely to document positive outcomes	
Interpreting results			
Confounding bias	When a factor is related to both the exposure and outcome, but not on the causal pathway, it distorts or confuses effect of exposure on outcome. Contrast with effect modification.	Pulmonary disease is more common in coal workers than the general population; however, people who work in coal mines also smoke more frequently than the general population	Multiple/repeated studies Crossover studies (subjects act as their own controls) Matching (patients with similar characteristics in both treatment and control groups)
Lead-time bias	Early detection is confused with ↑ survival.	Early detection makes it seem like survival has increased, but the disease's natural history has not changed	Measure "back-end" survival (adjust survival according to the severity of disease at the time of diagnosis)
Length-time bias	Screening test detects diseases with long latency period, while those with shorter latency period become symptomatic earlier.	A slowly progressive cancer is more likely detected by a screening test than a rapidly progressive cancer	A randomized controlled trial assigning subjects to the screening program or to no screening

Statistical distribution

Measures of central tendency	Mean = (sum of values)/(total number of values).	Most affected by outliers (extreme values).
	Median = middle value of a list of data sorted from least to greatest.	If there is an even number of values, the median will be the average of the middle two values.
	Mode = most common value.	Least affected by outliers.
Measures of dispersion	Standard deviation = how much variability exists in a set of values, around the mean of these values. Standard error = an estimate of how much variability exists in a (theoretical) set of sample means around the true population mean.	σ = SD; n = sample size. Variance = $(SD)^2$. SE = $\sigma/\sqrt{n}$. SE ↓ as n ↑.
Normal distribution	Gaussian, also called bell-shaped. Mean = median = mode.	

Nonnormal distributions

Bimodal	Suggests two different populations (eg, metabolic polymorphism such as fast vs slow acetylators; age at onset of Hodgkin lymphoma; suicide rate by age).	
Positive skew	Typically, mean > median > mode. Asymmetry with longer tail on right.	
Negative skew	Typically, mean < median < mode. Asymmetry with longer tail on left.	

Statistical hypotheses

Null (H_0)	Hypothesis of no difference or relationship (eg, there is no association between the disease and the risk factor in the population).
Alternative (H_1)	Hypothesis of some difference or relationship (eg, there is some association between the disease and the risk factor in the population).

Outcomes of statistical hypothesis testing

Correct result	Stating that there is an effect or difference when one exists (null hypothesis rejected in favor of alternative hypothesis). Stating that there is no effect or difference when none exists (null hypothesis not rejected).	

	Reality	
	H_1	H_0
Study rejects H_0	Power $(1 - \beta)$	α Type I error
Study does not reject H_0	β Type II error	Correct

Incorrect result

Type I error (α)	Stating that there is an effect or difference when none exists (null hypothesis incorrectly rejected in favor of alternative hypothesis). α is the probability of making a type I error. p is judged against a preset α level of significance (usually 0.05). If $p < 0.05$, then there is less than a 5% chance that the data will show something that is not really there.	Also known as false-positive error. α = you accused an innocent man. You can never "prove" the alternate hypothesis, but you can reject the null hypothesis as being very unlikely.
Type II error (β)	Stating that there is not an effect or difference when one exists (null hypothesis is not rejected when it is in fact false). β is the probability of making a type II error. β is related to statistical power $(1 - \beta)$, which is the probability of rejecting the null hypothesis when it is false. ↑ power and ↓ β by: ▪ ↑ sample size ▪ ↑ expected effect size ▪ ↑ precision of measurement	Also known as false-negative error. β = you blindly let the guilty man go free. If you ↑ sample size, you ↑ power. There is **power in numbers**.
Confidence interval	Range of values within which the true mean of the population is expected to fall, with a specified probability. CI for sample mean = $\bar{x} \pm Z(SE)$ The 95% CI (corresponding to $\alpha = .05$) is often used. For the 95% CI, $Z = 1.96$. For the 99% CI, $Z = 2.58$.	If the 95% CI for a mean difference between 2 variables includes 0, then there is no significant difference and H_0 is not rejected. If the 95% CI for odds ratio or relative risk includes 1, H_0 is not rejected. If the CIs between 2 groups do not overlap → statistically significant difference exists. If the CIs between 2 groups overlap → usually no significant difference exists.

Meta-analysis A method of statistical analysis that pools summary data (eg, means, RRs) from multiple studies for a more precise estimate of the size of an effect. Also estimates heterogeneity of effect sizes between studies.

Improves strength of evidence and generalizability of study findings. Limited by quality of individual studies and bias in study selection.

Common statistical tests

t-test	Checks differences between **means** of 2 groups.	Tea is meant for 2. Example: comparing the mean blood pressure between men and women.
ANOVA	Checks differences between means of 3 or more groups.	3 words: **AN**alysis **O**f **VA**riance. Example: comparing the mean blood pressure between members of 3 different ethnic groups.
Chi-square (χ^2)	Checks differences between 2 or more percentages or proportions of **categorical** outcomes (not mean values).	Pronounce **Chi-tegorical.** Example: comparing the percentage of members of 3 different ethnic groups who have essential hypertension.

Pearson correlation coefficient

r is always between −1 and +1. The closer the absolute value of r is to 1, the stronger the linear correlation between the 2 variables.

Positive r value → positive correlation (as one variable ↑, the other variable ↑).

Negative r value → negative correlation (as one variable ↑, the other variable ↓).

Coefficient of determination = r^2 (amount of variance in one variable that can be explained by variance in another variable).

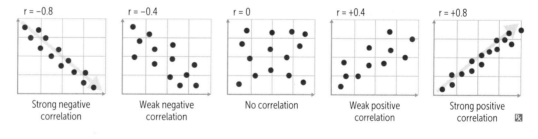

$r = -0.8$	$r = -0.4$	$r = 0$	$r = +0.4$	$r = +0.8$
Strong negative correlation	Weak negative correlation	No correlation	Weak positive correlation	Strong positive correlation

▶ BEHAVIORAL SCIENCE—ETHICS

Core ethical principles

Autonomy	Obligation to respect patients as individuals (truth-telling, confidentiality), to create conditions necessary for autonomous choice (informed consent), and to honor their preference in accepting or not accepting medical care.
Beneficence	Physicians have a special ethical (fiduciary) duty to act in the patient's best interest. May conflict with autonomy (an informed patient has the right to decide) or what is best for society (eg, mandatory TB treatment). Traditionally, patient interest supersedes.
Nonmaleficence	"Do no harm." Must be balanced against beneficence; if the benefits outweigh the risks, a patient may make an informed decision to proceed (most surgeries and medications fall into this category).
Justice	To treat persons fairly and equitably. This does not always imply equally (eg, triage).

Informed consent

A process (not just a document/signature) that requires:
- Disclosure: discussion of pertinent information
- Understanding: ability to comprehend
- Capacity: ability to reason and make one's own decisions (distinct from competence, a legal determination)
- Voluntariness: freedom from coercion and manipulation

Patients must have an intelligent understanding of their diagnosis and the risks/benefits of proposed treatment and alternative options, including no treatment.

Patient must be informed that he or she can revoke written consent at any time, even orally.

Exceptions to informed consent (**WIPE** it away):
- **W**aiver—patient explicitly waives the right of informed consent
- **L**egally **I**ncompetent—patient lacks decision-making capacity (obtain consent from legal surrogate)
- **T**herapeutic **P**rivilege—withholding information when disclosure would severely harm the patient or undermine informed decision-making capacity
- **E**mergency situation—implied consent may apply

Consent for minors

A minor is generally any person < 18 years old. Parental consent laws in relation to healthcare vary by state. In general, parental consent should be obtained, but exceptions exist for emergency treatment (eg, blood transfusions) or if minor is legally emancipated (eg, married, self supporting, or in the military).

Situations in which parental consent is usually not required:
- **Sex** (contraception, STIs, pregnancy)
- **Drugs** (substance abuse)
- **Rock and roll** (emergency/trauma)

Physicians should always encourage healthy minor-guardian communication.

Physician should seek a minor's assent even if their consent is not required.

Decision-making capacity	Physician must determine whether the patient is psychologically and legally capable of making a particular healthcare decision. Note that decisions made with capacity cannot be revoked simply if the patient later loses capacity. Capacity is determined by a physician for a specific healthcare-related decision (eg, to refuse medical care). Competency is determined by a judge and usually refers to more global categories of decision making (eg, legally unable to make any healthcare-related decision). Components (think **GIEMSA**): ▪ Decision is consistent with patient's values and **G**oals ▪ Patient is **I**nformed (knows and understands) ▪ Patient **E**xpresses a choice ▪ Decision is not a result of altered **M**ental status (eg, delirium, psychosis, intoxication), Mood disorder ▪ Decision remains **S**table over time ▪ Patient is ≥ 18 years of **A**ge or otherwise legally emancipated

Advance directives	Instructions given by a patient in anticipation of the need for a medical decision. Details vary per state law.
Oral advance directive	Incapacitated patient's prior oral statements commonly used as guide. Problems arise from variance in interpretation. If patient was informed, directive was specific, patient made a choice, and decision was repeated over time to multiple people, then the oral directive is more valid.
Written advance directive	Specifies specific healthcare interventions that a patient anticipates he or she would accept or reject during treatment for a critical or life-threatening illness. A living will is an example.
Medical power of attorney	Patient designates an agent to make medical decisions in the event that he/she loses decision-making capacity. Patient may also specify decisions in clinical situations. Can be revoked by patient if decision-making capacity is intact. More flexible than a living will.
Do not resuscitate order	DNR order prohibits cardiopulmonary resuscitation (CPR). Other resuscitative measures that may follow (eg, intubation) are also typically avoided.

Surrogate decision-maker	If a patient loses decision-making capacity and has not prepared an advance directive, individuals (surrogates) who know the patient must determine what the patient would have done. Priority of surrogates: spouse → adult **Ch**ildren → **P**arents → **S**iblings → other relatives (the spouse **ChiPS** in).

Ethical situations

SITUATION	APPROPRIATE RESPONSE
Patient is not adherent.	Attempt to identify the reason for nonadherence and determine his/her willingness to change; do not coerce the patient into adhering and do not refer him/her to another physician.
Patient desires an unnecessary procedure.	Attempt to understand why the patient wants the procedure and address underlying concerns. Do not refuse to see the patient and do not refer him/her to another physician. Avoid performing unnecessary procedures.
Patient has difficulty taking medications.	Provide written instructions; attempt to simplify treatment regimens; use teach-back method (ask patient to repeat regimen back to physician) to ensure comprehension.
Family members ask for information about patient's prognosis.	Avoid discussing issues with relatives without the patient's permission.
A patient's family member asks you not to disclose the results of a test if the prognosis is poor because the patient will be "unable to handle it."	Attempt to identify why the family member believes such information would be detrimental to the patient's condition. Explain that as long as the patient has decision-making capacity and does not indicate otherwise, communication of information concerning his/her care will not be withheld. However, if you believe the patient might seriously harm himself or others if informed, then you may invoke therapeutic privilege and withhold the information.
A 17-year-old girl is pregnant and requests an abortion.	Many states require parental notification or consent for minors for an abortion. Unless there are specific medical risks associated with pregnancy, a physician should not sway the patient's decision for, or against, an elective abortion (regardless of maternal age or fetal condition).
A 15-year-old girl is pregnant and wants to keep the child. Her parents want you to tell her to give the child up for adoption.	The patient retains the right to make decisions regarding her child, even if her parents disagree. Provide information to the teenager about the practical issues of caring for a baby. Discuss the options, if requested. Encourage discussion between the teenager and her parents to reach the best decision.
A terminally ill patient requests physician assistance in ending his/her own life.	In the overwhelming majority of states, refuse involvement in any form of physician-assisted suicide. Physicians may, however, prescribe medically appropriate analgesics that coincidentally shorten the patient's life.
Patient is suicidal.	Assess the seriousness of the threat. If it is serious, suggest that the patient remain in the hospital voluntarily; patient can be hospitalized involuntarily if he/she refuses.
Patient states that he/she finds you attractive.	Ask direct, closed-ended questions and use a chaperone if necessary. Romantic relationships with patients are never appropriate. It may be necessary to transition care to another physician.
A woman who had a mastectomy says she now feels "ugly."	Find out why the patient feels this way. Do not offer falsely reassuring statements (eg, "You still look good").
Patient is angry about the long time he/she spent in the waiting room.	Acknowledge the patient's anger, but do not take a patient's anger personally. Apologize for any inconvenience. Stay away from efforts to explain the delay.
Patient is upset with the way he/she was treated by another doctor.	Suggest that the patient speak directly to that physician regarding his/her concerns. If the problem is with a member of the office staff, tell the patient you will speak to that person.
An invasive test is performed on the wrong patient.	Regardless of the outcome, a physician is ethically obligated to inform a patient that a mistake has been made.
A patient requires a treatment not covered by his/her insurance.	Never limit or deny care because of the expense in time or money. Discuss all treatment options with patients, even if some are not covered by their insurance companies.

Ethical situations *(continued)*

SITUATION	APPROPRIATE RESPONSE
A 7-year-old boy loses a sister to cancer and now feels responsible.	At ages 5–7, children begin to understand that death is permanent, that all life functions end completely at death, and that everything that is alive eventually dies. Provide a direct, concrete description of his sister's death. Avoid clichés and euphemisms. Reassure the boy that he is not responsible. Identify and normalize fears and feelings. Encourage play and healthy coping behaviors (eg, remembering her in his own way).
Patient is victim of intimate partner violence.	Ask if patient is safe and has an emergency plan. Do not necessarily pressure patient to leave his or her partner, or disclose the incident to the authorities (unless required by state law).
Patient wants to try alternative or holistic medicine.	Find out why and allow patient to do so as long as there are no contraindications, medication interactions, or adverse effects to the new treatment.
Physician colleague presents to work impaired.	If impaired or incompetent, colleague is a threat to patient safety. Report the situation to local supervisory personnel. Should the organization fail to take action, alert the state licensing board.
Patient is officially determined to suffer brain death. Patient's family insists on maintaining life support indefinitely because patient is still moving when touched.	Gently explain to family that there is no chance of recovery, and that brain death is equivalent to death. Movement is due to spinal arc reflex and is not voluntary. Bring case to appropriate ethics board regarding futility of care and withdrawal of life support.
A pharmaceutical company offers you a sponsorship in exchange for advertising its new drug.	Reject this offer. Generally, decline gifts and sponsorships to avoid any appearance of conflict of interest. The AMA Code of Ethics does make exceptions for gifts directly benefitting patients; gifts of minimal value; special funding for medical education of students, residents, fellows; grants whose recipients are chosen by independent institutional criteria; and funds that are distributed without attribution to sponsors.
An adult refuses care because it is against his/her religious beliefs.	Work with the patient by either explaining the treatment or pursuing alternative treatments. However, a physician should never force a competent adult to receive care if it is contrary to the patient's religious beliefs.
Mother and 15-year-old daughter are unresponsive following a car accident and are bleeding internally. Father says do not transfuse because they are Jehovah's Witnesses.	Transfuse daughter, but do not transfuse mother. Emergent care can be refused by the healthcare proxy for an adult, particularly when patient preferences are known or reasonably inferred, but not for a minor based solely on faith.
A 2-year-old girl presents with injuries inconsistent with parental story.	Contact child protective services and ensure child is in a safe location. Physicians are required by law to report any reasonable suspicion of child abuse or endangerment.

Confidentiality

Confidentiality respects patient privacy and autonomy. If the patient is incapacitated or the situation is emergent, disclosing information to family and friends should be guided by professional judgment of patient's best interest. The patient may voluntarily waive the right to confidentiality (eg, insurance company request).

General principles for exceptions to confidentiality:
- Potential physical harm to others is serious and imminent
- Likelihood of harm to self is great
- No alternative means exist to warn or to protect those at risk
- Physicians can take steps to prevent harm

Examples of exceptions to patient confidentiality (many are state-specific) include the following ("The physician's good judgment **SAVED** the day"):
- **S**uicidal/homicidal patients
- **A**buse (children, elderly, and/or prisoners)
- Duty to protect—State-specific laws that sometimes allow physician to inform or somehow protect potential **V**ictim from harm.
- **E**pileptic patients and other impaired automobile drivers.
- Reportable **D**iseases (eg, STIs, hepatitis, food poisoning); physicians may have a duty to warn public officials, who will then notify people at risk. Dangerous communicable diseases, such as TB or Ebola, may require involuntary treatment.

▶ PUBLIC HEALTH SCIENCES—THE WELL PATIENT

Car seats for children

Children should ride in rear-facing car seats until they are 2 years old and in car seats with a harness until they are 4 years. Older children should use a booster seat until they are 8 years old or until the seat belt fits properly. Children < 12 years old should not ride in a seat with a front-facing airbag.

Changes in the elderly

Sexual changes:
- Men—slower erection/ejaculation, longer refractory period.
- Women—vaginal shortening, thinning, and dryness.

Sleep patterns: ↓ REM and slow-wave sleep; ↑ sleep onset latency; ↑ early awakenings.

↑ suicide rate.

↓ vision and hearing.

↓ immune response.

↓ renal, pulmonary, and GI function.

↓ muscle mass, ↑ fat.

Intelligence does not decrease.

▶ PUBLIC HEALTH SCIENCES—HEALTHCARE DELIVERY

Disease prevention

Primary disease prevention	Prevent disease before it occurs (eg, HPV vaccination)
Secondary disease prevention	Screen early for and manage existing but asymptomatic disease (eg, Pap smear for cervical cancer)
Tertiary disease prevention	Treatment to reduce complications from disease that is ongoing or has long-term effects (eg, chemotherapy)
Quaternary disease prevention	Identifying patients at risk of unnecessary treatment, protecting from the harm of new interventions (eg, electronic sharing of patient records to avoid duplicating recent imaging studies)

Major medical insurance plans

PLAN	PROVIDERS	PAYMENTS	SPECIALIST CARE
Exclusive provider organization	Restricted to limited panel (except emergencies)		No referral required
Health maintenance organization	Restricted to limited panel (except emergencies)	Denied for any service that does not meet established, evidence-based guidelines	Requires referral from primary care provider
Point of service	Patient can see providers outside network	Higher copays and deductibles for out-of-network services	Requires referral from primary care provider
Preferred provider organization	Patient can see providers outside network	Higher copays and deductibles for all services	No referral required

Healthcare payment models

Bundled payment	Healthcare organization receives a set amount per service, regardless of ultimate cost, to be divided among all providers and facilities involved.
Capitation	Physicians receive a set amount per patient assigned to them per period of time, regardless of how much the patient uses the healthcare system. Used by some HMOs.
Discounted fee-for-service	Patient pays for each individual service at a discounted rate predetermined by providers and payers (eg, PPOs).
Fee-for-service	Patient pays for each individual service.
Global payment	Patient pays for all expenses associated with a single incident of care with a single payment. Most commonly used during elective surgeries, as it covers the cost of surgery as well as the necessary pre- and postoperative visits.

Medicare and Medicaid	Medicare and Medicaid—federal social healthcare programs that originated from amendments to the Social Security Act. Medicare is available to patients ≥ 65 years old, < 65 with certain disabilities, and those with end-stage renal disease. Medicaid is joint federal and state health assistance for people with limited income and/or resources.	MedicarE is for Elderly. MedicaiD is for Destitute. The 4 parts of Medicare: ▪ Part A: HospitAl insurance, home hospice care ▪ Part B: Basic medical Bills (eg, doctor's fees, diagnostic testing) ▪ Part C: (parts A + B = Combo) delivered by approved private companies ▪ Part D: Prescription Drugs
Hospice care	Medical care focused on providing comfort and palliation instead of definitive cure. Available to patients on Medicare or Medicaid and in most private insurance plans whose life expectancy is < 6 months. During end-of-life care, priority is given to improving the patient's comfort and relieving pain (often includes opioid, sedative, or anxiolytic medications). Facilitating comfort is prioritized over potential side effects (eg, respiratory depression). This prioritization of positive effects over negative effects is known as the **principle of double effect**.	

Common causes of death (US) by age

	< 1 YR	1–14 YR	15–34 YR	35–44 YR	45–64 YR	65+ YR
#1	Congenital malformations	Unintentional injury	Unintentional injury	Unintentional injury	Cancer	Heart disease
#2	Preterm birth	Cancer	Suicide	Cancer	Heart disease	Cancer
#3	SIDS	Congenital malformations	Homicide	Heart disease	Unintentional injury	Chronic respiratory disease

Hospitalized conditions with frequent readmissions	Defined as readmission for any reason within 30 days of discharge from original admission. Readmissions may be reduced by discharge planning and outpatient follow-up appointments.

	MEDICARE	MEDICAID	PRIVATE INSURANCE	UNINSURED
#1	Congestive HF	Mood disorders	Maintenance of chemotherapy or radiotherapy	Mood disorders
#2	Septicemia	Schizophrenia/psychotic disorders	Mood disorders	Alcohol-related disorders
#3	Pneumonia	Diabetes mellitus with complications	Complications of surgical procedures or medical care	Diabetes mellitus with complications

▸ PUBLIC HEALTH SCIENCES—QUALITY AND SAFETY

Safety culture	Organizational environment in which everyone can freely bring up safety concerns without fear of censure. Facilitates error identification.	Event reporting systems collect data on errors for internal and external monitoring.
Human factors design	Forcing functions (those that prevent undesirable actions [eg, connecting feeding syringe to IV tubing]) are the most effective. Standardization improves process reliability (eg, clinical pathways, guidelines, checklists). Simplification reduces wasteful activities (eg, consolidating electronic medical records).	Deficient designs hinder workflow and lead to staff workarounds that bypass safety features (eg, patient ID barcodes affixed to computers due to unreadable wristbands).

PDSA cycle

Process improvement model to test changes in real clinical setting. Impact on patients:

- Plan—define problem and solution
- Do—test new process
- Study—measure and analyze data
- Act—integrate new process into regular workflow

Quality measurements

	MEASURE	EXAMPLE
Structural	Physical equipment, resources, facilities	Number of diabetes educators
Process	Performance of system as planned	Percentage of diabetic patients whose HbA_{1c} was measured in the past 6 months
Outcome	Impact on patients	Average HbA_{1c} of patients with diabetes
Balancing	Impact on other systems/outcomes	Incidence of hypoglycemia among patients who tried an intervention to lower HbA_{1c}

Swiss cheese model

Focuses on systems and conditions rather than an individual's error. The risk of a threat becoming a reality is mitigated by differing layers and types of defenses. Patient harm can occur despite multiple safeguards when "the holes in the cheese line up."

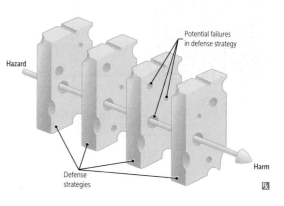

Types of medical errors	May involve patient identification, diagnosis, monitoring, nosocomial infection, medications, procedures, devices, documentation, handoffs. Medical errors should be disclosed to patients, independent of immediate outcome (harmful or not).	
Active error	Occurs at level of frontline operator (eg, wrong IV pump dose programmed).	Immediate impact.
Latent error	Occurs in processes indirect from operator but impacts patient care (eg, different types of IV pumps used within same hospital).	Accident waiting to happen.

Medical error analysis

	DESIGN	METHODS
Root cause analysis	Retrospective approach. Applied after failure event to prevent recurrence.	Uses records and participant interviews to identify all the underlying problems (eg, process, people, environment, equipment, materials, management) that led to an error.
Failure mode and effects analysis	Forward-looking approach. Applied before process implementation to prevent failure occurrence.	Uses inductive reasoning to identify all the ways a process might fail and prioritizes them by their probability of occurrence and impact on patients.

SECTION III

High-Yield
Organ Systems

"Symptoms, then, are in reality nothing but the cry from suffering organs."
—Jean-Martin Charcot

"Man is an intelligence in servitude to his organs."
—Aldous Huxley

"When every part of the machine is correctly adjusted and in perfect harmony, health will hold dominion over the human organism by laws as natural and immutable as the laws of gravity."
—Andrew T. Still

▶ APPROACHING THE ORGAN SYSTEMS

In this section, we have divided the High-Yield Facts into the major **Organ Systems**. Within each Organ System are several subsections, including **Embryology, Anatomy, Physiology, Pathology**, and **Pharmacology**. As you progress through each Organ System, refer back to information in the previous subsections to organize these basic science subsections into a "vertically integrated" framework for learning. Below is some general advice for studying the organ systems by these subsections.

Embryology

Relevant embryology is included in each organ system subsection. Embryology tends to correspond well with the relevant anatomy, especially with regard to congenital malformations.

Anatomy

Several topics fall under this heading, including gross anatomy, histology, and neuroanatomy. Do not memorize all the small details; however, do not ignore anatomy altogether. Review what you have already learned and what you wish you had learned. Many questions require two or more steps. The first step is to identify a structure on anatomic cross section, electron micrograph, or photomicrograph. The second step may require an understanding of the clinical significance of the structure.

When studying, stress clinically important material. For example, be familiar with gross anatomy and radiologic anatomy related to specific diseases (eg, Pancoast tumor, Horner syndrome), traumatic injuries (eg, fractures, sensory and motor nerve deficits), procedures (eg, lumbar puncture), and common surgeries (eg, cholecystectomy). There are also many questions on the exam involving x-rays, CT scans, and neuro MRI scans. Many students suggest browsing through a general radiology atlas, pathology atlas, and histology atlas. Focus on learning basic anatomy at key levels in the body (eg, sagittal brain MRI; axial CT of the midthorax, abdomen, and pelvis). Basic neuroanatomy (especially pathways, blood supply, and functional anatomy), associated neuropathology, and neurophysiology have good yield. Please note that many of the photographic images in this book are for illustrative purposes and are not necessarily reflective of Step 1 emphasis.

Physiology

The portion of the examination dealing with physiology is broad and concept oriented and thus does not lend itself as well to fact-based review. Diagrams are often the best study aids, especially given the increasing number of questions requiring the interpretation of diagrams. Learn to apply basic physiologic relationships in a variety of ways (eg, the Fick equation, clearance equations). You are seldom asked to perform complex calculations. Hormones are the focus of many questions, so learn their sites of production and action as well as their regulatory mechanisms.

A large portion of the physiology tested on the USMLE Step 1 is clinically relevant and involves understanding physiologic changes associated with pathologic processes (eg, changes in pulmonary function with COPD). Thus, it is worthwhile to review the physiologic changes that are found with common pathologies of the major organ systems (eg, heart, lungs, kidneys, GI tract) and endocrine glands.

Pathology

Questions dealing with this discipline are difficult to prepare for because of the sheer volume of material involved. Review the basic principles and hallmark characteristics of the key diseases. Given the clinical orientation of Step 1, it is no longer sufficient to know only the "buzzword" associations of certain diseases (eg, café-au-lait macules and neurofibromatosis); you must also know the clinical descriptions of these findings.

Given the clinical slant of the USMLE Step 1, it is also important to review the classic presenting signs and symptoms of diseases as well as their associated laboratory findings. Delve into the signs, symptoms, and pathophysiology of major diseases that have a high prevalence in the United States (eg, alcoholism, diabetes, hypertension, heart failure, ischemic heart disease, infectious disease). Be prepared to think one step beyond the simple diagnosis to treatment or complications.

The examination includes a number of color photomicrographs and photographs of gross specimens that are presented in the setting of a brief clinical history. However, read the question and the choices carefully before looking at the illustration, because the history will help you identify the pathologic process. Flip through an illustrated pathology textbook, color atlases, and appropriate Web sites in order to look at the pictures in the days before the exam. Pay attention to potential clues such as age, sex, ethnicity, occupation, recent activities and exposures, and specialized lab tests.

Pharmacology

Preparation for questions on pharmacology is straightforward. Memorizing all the key drugs and their characteristics (eg, mechanisms, clinical use, and important side effects) is high yield. Focus on understanding the prototype drugs in each class. Avoid memorizing obscure derivatives. Learn the "classic" and distinguishing toxicities of the major drugs. Do not bother with drug dosages or trade names. Reviewing associated biochemistry, physiology, and microbiology can be useful while studying pharmacology. There is a strong emphasis on ANS, CNS, antimicrobial, and cardiovascular agents as well as NSAIDs. Much of the material is clinically relevant. Newer drugs on the market are also fair game.

Cardiovascular

"As for me, except for an occasional heart attack, I feel as young as I ever did."

—Robert Benchley

"Hearts will never be practical until they are made unbreakable."
—The Wizard of Oz

"As the arteries grow hard, the heart grows soft."

—H. L. Mencken

"Nobody has ever measured, not even poets, how much the heart can hold."

—Zelda Fitzgerald

"Only from the heart can you touch the sky."

—Rumi

"It is not the size of the man but the size of his heart that matters."
—Evander Holyfield

The cardiovascular system is one of the highest yield areas for the boards and, for some students, may be the most challenging. Focusing on understanding the mechanisms instead of memorizing the details can make a big difference, especially for this topic. Pathophysiology of atherosclerosis and heart failure, MOA of drugs (particular physiology interactions) and their adverse effects, ECGs of heart blocks, the cardiac cycle, and the Starling curve are some of the more high-yield topics. Differentiating between systolic and diastolic dysfunction is also very important. Heart murmurs and maneuvers that affect these murmurs have also been high yield.

▶ CARDIOVASCULAR—EMBRYOLOGY

Heart embryology

EMBRYONIC STRUCTURE	GIVES RISE TO
Truncus arteriosus	Ascending aorta and pulmonary trunk
Bulbus cordis	Smooth parts (outflow tract) of left and right ventricles
Endocardial cushion	Atrial septum, membranous interventricular septum; AV and semilunar valves
Primitive atrium	Trabeculated part of left and right atria
Primitive ventricle	Trabeculated part of left and right ventricles
Primitive pulmonary vein	Smooth part of left atrium
Left horn of sinus venosus	Coronary sinus
Right horn of sinus venosus	Smooth part of right atrium (sinus venarum)
Right common cardinal vein and right anterior cardinal vein	Superior vena cava (SVC)

Heart morphogenesis   First functional organ in vertebrate embryos; beats spontaneously by week 4 of development.

Cardiac looping   Primary heart tube loops to establish left-right polarity; begins in week 4 of gestation.   Defect in left-right Dynein (involved in L/R asymmetry) can lead to Dextrocardia, as seen in Kartagener syndrome (1° ciliary Dyskinesia).

Septation of the chambers

Atria

❶ Septum primum grows toward endocardial cushions, narrowing foramen primum.
❷ Foramen secundum forms in septum primum (foramen primum disappears).
❸ Septum secundum develops as foramen secundum maintains right-to-left shunt.
❹ Septum secundum expands and covers most of the foramen secundum. The residual foramen is the foramen ovale.
❺ Remaining portion of septum primum forms valve of foramen ovale.

6. (Not shown) Septum secundum and septum primum fuse to form the atrial septum.
7. (Not shown) Foramen ovale usually closes soon after birth because of ↑ LA pressure.

Patent foramen ovale—caused by failure of septum primum and septum secundum to fuse after birth; most are left untreated. Can lead to paradoxical emboli (venous thromboemboli that enter systemic arterial circulation), similar to those resulting from an ASD.

Heart morphogenesis *(continued)*

Ventricles	
❶ Muscular interventricular septum forms. Opening is called interventricular foramen. ❷ Aorticopulmonary septum rotates and fuses with muscular ventricular septum to form membranous interventricular septum, closing interventricular foramen. ❸ Growth of endocardial cushions separates atria from ventricles and contributes to both atrial septation and membranous portion of the interventricular septum.	Ventricular septal defect—most common congenital cardiac anomaly, usually occurs in membranous septum.

Outflow tract formation	Neural crest and endocardial cell migrations → truncal and bulbar ridges that spiral and fuse to form aorticopulmonary septum → ascending aorta and pulmonary trunk.	Conotruncal abnormalities associated with failure of neural crest cells to migrate: ▪ Transposition of great vessels. ▪ Tetralogy of Fallot. ▪ Persistent truncus arteriosus.
Valve development	Aortic/pulmonary: derived from endocardial cushions of outflow tract. Mitral/tricuspid: derived from fused endocardial cushions of the AV canal.	Valvular anomalies may be stenotic, regurgitant, atretic (eg, tricuspid atresia), or displaced (eg, Ebstein anomaly).

Fetal circulation

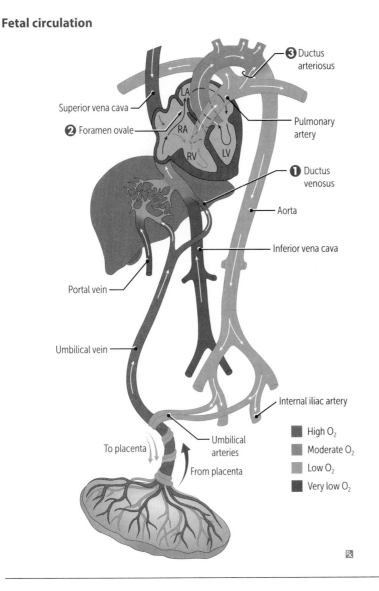

Superior vena cava

❷ Foramen ovale

Portal vein

Umbilical vein

To placenta

From placenta

Umbilical arteries

❸ Ductus arteriosus

Pulmonary artery

❶ Ductus venosus

Aorta

Inferior vena cava

Internal iliac artery

- ■ High O_2
- ■ Moderate O_2
- ■ Low O_2
- ■ Very low O_2

Blood in umbilical vein has a Po_2 of ≈ 30 mm Hg and is ≈ 80% saturated with O_2. Umbilical arteries have low O_2 saturation.

3 important shunts:

❶ Blood entering fetus through the umbilical vein is conducted via the **ductus venosus** into the IVC, bypassing hepatic circulation.

❷ Most of the highly Oxygenated blood reaching the heart via the IVC is directed through the **foramen Ovale** and pumped into the aorta to supply the head and body.

❸ Deoxygenated blood from the SVC passes through the RA → RV → main pulmonary artery → **Ductus arteriosus** → Descending aorta; shunt is due to high fetal pulmonary artery resistance (due partly to low O_2 tension).

At birth, infant takes a breath → ↓ resistance in pulmonary vasculature → ↑ left atrial pressure vs right atrial pressure → foramen ovale closes (now called fossa ovalis); ↑ in O_2 (from respiration) and ↓ in prostaglandins (from placental separation) → closure of ductus arteriosus.

Indomethacin helps close PDA → ligamentum arteriosum (remnant of ductus arteriosus).

Prostaglandins E_1 and E_2 kEEp PDA open.

Fetal-postnatal derivatives

FETAL STRUCTURE	POSTNATAL DERIVATIVE	NOTES
AllaNtois → urachus	MediaN umbilical ligament	Urachus is part of allantoic duct between bladder and umbilicus.
Ductus arteriosus	Ligamentum arteriosum	
Ductus venosus	Ligamentum venosum	
Foramen ovale	Fossa ovalis	
Notochord	Nucleus pulposus	
UmbiLical arteries	MediaL umbilical ligaments	
Umbilical vein	Ligamentum teres hepatis (round ligament)	Contained in falciform ligament.

▶ CARDIOVASCULAR—ANATOMY

Anatomy of the heart

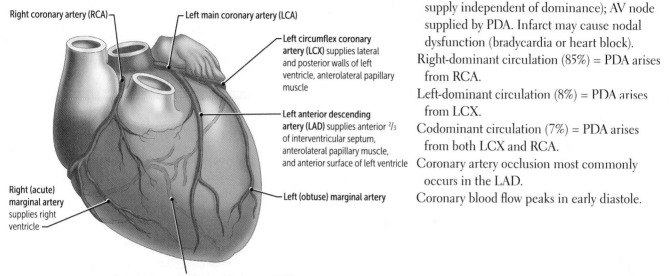

Right coronary artery (RCA)

Left main coronary artery (LCA)

Left circumflex coronary artery (LCX) supplies lateral and posterior walls of left ventricle, anterolateral papillary muscle

Left anterior descending artery (LAD) supplies anterior $^2/_3$ of interventricular septum, anterolateral papillary muscle, and anterior surface of left ventricle

Left (obtuse) marginal artery

Right (acute) marginal artery supplies right ventricle

Posterior descending/interventricular artery (PDA) supplies AV node, posterior $^1/_3$ of interventricular septum, posterior $^2/_3$ walls of ventricles, and posteromedial papillary muscle

SA node commonly supplied by RCA (blood supply independent of dominance); AV node supplied by PDA. Infarct may cause nodal dysfunction (bradycardia or heart block).

Right-dominant circulation (85%) = PDA arises from RCA.

Left-dominant circulation (8%) = PDA arises from LCX.

Codominant circulation (7%) = PDA arises from both LCX and RCA.

Coronary artery occlusion most commonly occurs in the LAD.

Coronary blood flow peaks in early diastole.

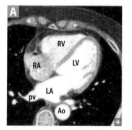

The most posterior part of the heart is the left atrium **A**; enlargement can cause dysphagia (due to compression of the esophagus) or hoarseness (due to compression of the left recurrent laryngeal nerve, a branch of the vagus nerve).

Pericardium consists of 3 layers (from outer to inner):
- Fibrous pericardium
- Parietal layer of serous pericardium
- Visceral layer of serous pericardium

Pericardial cavity lies between parietal and visceral layers.

Pericardium innervated by phrenic nerve. Pericarditis can cause referred pain to the shoulder.

▶ CARDIOVASCULAR—PHYSIOLOGY

Cardiac output	$CO = $ stroke volume $(SV) \times$ heart rate (HR) Fick principle: $$CO = \frac{\text{rate of } O_2 \text{ consumption}}{\text{arterial } O_2 \text{ content} - \text{venous } O_2 \text{ content}}$$ Mean arterial pressure $(MAP) = CO \times$ total peripheral resistance (TPR) MAP (at resting HR) $= \frac{2}{3}$ diastolic pressure $+ \frac{1}{3}$ systolic pressure Pulse pressure = systolic pressure – diastolic pressure Pulse pressure is proportional to SV, inversely proportional to arterial compliance. SV = end-diastolic volume (EDV) – end-systolic volume (ESV)	During the early stages of exercise, CO is maintained by ↑ HR and ↑ SV. During the late stages of exercise, CO is maintained by ↑ HR only (SV plateaus). Diastole is preferentially shortened with ↑ HR; less filling time → ↓ CO (eg, ventricular tachycardia). ↑ pulse pressure in hyperthyroidism, aortic regurgitation, aortic stiffening (isolated systolic hypertension in elderly), obstructive sleep apnea (↑ sympathetic tone), anemia, exercise (transient). ↓ pulse pressure in aortic stenosis, cardiogenic shock, cardiac tamponade, advanced heart failure (HF).

Cardiac output variables

Stroke volume	Stroke Volume affected by Contractility, Afterload, and Preload. ↑ SV with: • ↑ Contractility (eg, anxiety, exercise) • ↑ Preload (eg, early pregnancy) • ↓ Afterload	SV CAP. A failing heart has ↓ SV (systolic and/or diastolic dysfunction)

Contractility	Contractility (and SV) ↑ with:
	• Catecholamine stimulation via β_1 receptor:
	  • Ca^{2+} channels phosphorylated → ↑ Ca^{2+} entry → ↑ Ca^{2+}-induced Ca^{2+} release and ↑ Ca^{2+} storage in sarcoplasmic reticulum
	  • Phospholamban phosphorylation → active Ca^{2+} ATPase → ↑ Ca^{2+} storage in sarcoplasmic reticulum
	• ↑ intracellular Ca^{2+}
	• ↓ extracellular Na^+ (↓ activity of Na^+/Ca^{2+} exchanger)
	• Digitalis (blocks Na^+/K^+ pump → ↑ intracellular Na^+ → ↓ Na^+/Ca^{2+} exchanger activity → ↑ intracellular Ca^{2+})
		Contractility (and SV) ↓ with:
		• β_1-blockade (↓ cAMP)
		• HF with systolic dysfunction
		• Acidosis
		• Hypoxia/hypercapnia (↓ Po_2/↑ Pco_2)
		• Non-dihydropyridine Ca^{2+} channel blockers

Preload	Preload approximated by ventricular EDV; depends on venous tone and circulating blood volume.	VEnous vasodilators (eg, nitroglycerin) ↓ prEload.
Afterload	Afterload approximated by MAP. ↑ afterload → ↑ pressure → ↑ wall tension per Laplace's law. LV compensates for ↑ afterload by thickening (hypertrophy) in order to ↓ wall tension.	Arterial vasodilators (eg, hydrAlAzine) ↓ Afterload. ACE inhibitors and ARBs ↓ both preload and afterload. Chronic hypertension (↑ MAP) → LV hypertrophy.
Myocardial oxygen demand	MyoCARDial O_2 demand is ↑ by: • ↑ Contractility • ↑ Afterload (proportional to arterial pressure) • ↑ heart Rate • ↑ Diameter of ventricle (↑ wall tension)	Wall tension follows Laplace's law: Wall tension = pressure × radius $$\text{Wall stress} = \frac{\text{pressure} \times \text{radius}}{2 \times \text{wall thickness}}$$
Ejection fraction	$$EF = \frac{SV}{EDV} = \frac{EDV - ESV}{EDV}$$ Left ventricular EF is an index of ventricular contractility.	EF ↓ in systolic HF. EF normal in HF with preserved ejection fraction.

Starling curve

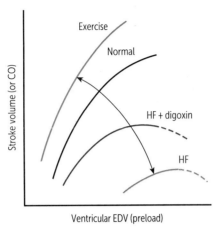

Force of contraction is proportional to end-diastolic length of cardiac muscle fiber (preload).

↑ contractility with catecholamines, positive inotropes (eg, digoxin).

↓ contractility with loss of myocardium (eg, MI), β-blockers (acutely), non-dihydropyridine Ca^{2+} channel blockers, dilated cardiomyopathy.

Resistance, pressure, flow

$\Delta P = Q \times R$

Similar to Ohm's law: $\Delta V = IR$

Volumetric flow rate (Q) = flow velocity (v) × cross-sectional area (A)

Resistance

$$= \frac{\text{driving pressure } (\Delta P)}{\text{flow } (Q)} = \frac{8\eta \, (\text{viscosity}) \times \text{length}}{\pi r^4}$$

Total resistance of vessels in series:

$R_T = R_1 + R_2 + R_3 \ldots$

Total resistance of vessels in parallel:

$$\frac{1}{R_T} = \frac{1}{R_1} + \frac{1}{R_2} + \frac{1}{R_3} \ldots$$

Capillaries have highest total cross-sectional area and lowest flow velocity.

Pressure gradient drives flow from high pressure to low pressure.

Arterioles account for most of TPR. Veins provide most of blood storage capacity.

Viscosity depends mostly on hematocrit.

Viscosity ↑ in hyperproteinemic states (eg, multiple myeloma), polycythemia.

Viscosity ↓ in anemia.

Compliance = $\Delta V/\Delta P$.

Cardiac and vascular function curves

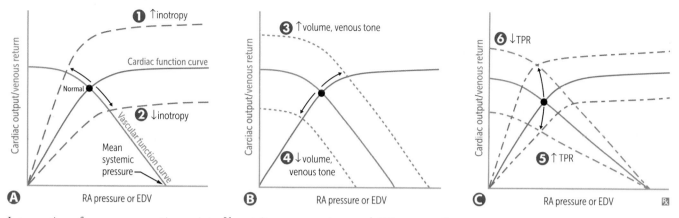

Intersection of curves = operating point of heart (ie, venous return and CO are equal).

GRAPH	EFFECT	EXAMPLES
A Inotropy	Changes in contractility → altered CO for a given RA pressure (preload).	**1** Catecholamines, digoxin ⊕, exercise **2** HF with reduced EF, narcotic overdose, sympathetic inhibition ⊖
B Venous return	Changes in circulating volume or venous tone → altered RA pressure for a given CO. Mean systemic pressure (x-intercept) changes with volume/venous tone.	**3** Fluid infusion, sympathetic activity ⊕ **4** Acute hemorrhage, spinal anesthesia ⊖
C Total peripheral resistance	At a given mean systemic pressure (x-intercept) and RA pressure, changes in TPR → altered CO.	**5** Vasopressors ⊕ **6** Exercise, AV shunt ⊖

Changes often occur in tandem, and may be reinforcing (eg, exercise ↑ inotropy and ↓ TPR to maximize CO) or compensatory (eg, HF ↓ inotropy → fluid retention to ↑ preload to maintain CO).

Pressure-volume loops and cardiac cycle

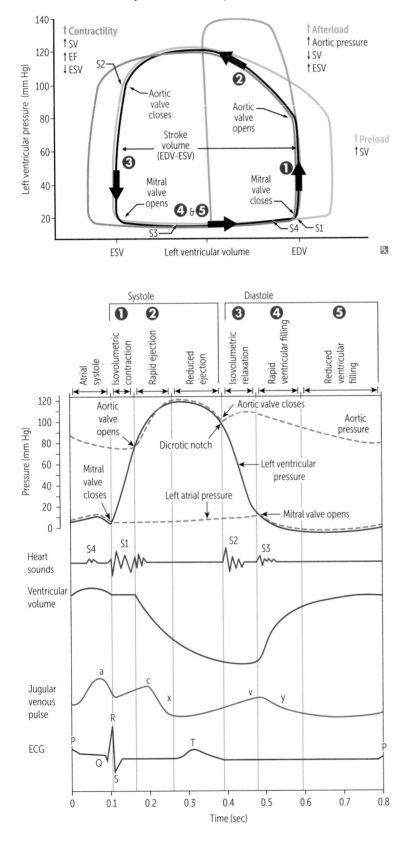

The black loop represents normal cardiac physiology.

Phases—left ventricle:
1. Isovolumetric contraction—period between mitral valve closing and aortic valve opening; period of highest O_2 consumption
2. Systolic ejection—period between aortic valve opening and closing
3. Isovolumetric relaxation—period between aortic valve closing and mitral valve opening
4. Rapid filling—period just after mitral valve opening
5. Reduced filling—period just before mitral valve closing

Heart sounds:
S1—mitral and tricuspid valve closure. Loudest at mitral area.
S2—aortic and pulmonary valve closure. Loudest at left upper sternal border.
S3—in early diastole during rapid ventricular filling phase. Associated with ↑ filling pressures (eg, mitral regurgitation, HF) and more common in dilated ventricles (but can be normal in children, young adults, and pregnant women).
S4—in late diastole ("atrial kick"). Best heard at apex with patient in left lateral decubitus position. High atrial pressure. Associated with ventricular noncompliance (eg, hypertrophy). Left atrium must push against stiff LV wall. Consider abnormal, regardless of patient age.

Jugular venous pulse (JVP):
a wave—atrial contraction. Absent in atrial fibrillation (AF).
c wave—RV contraction (closed tricuspid valve bulging into atrium).
x descent—downward displacement of closed tricuspid valve during rapid ventricular ejection phase. Reduced or absent in tricuspid regurgitation and right HF because pressure gradients are reduced.
v wave—↑ right atrial pressure due to filling ("villing") against closed tricuspid valve.
y descent—RA emptying into RV. Prominent in constrictive pericarditis, absent in cardiac tamponade.

Splitting

Normal splitting	Inspiration → drop in intrathoracic pressure → ↑ venous return → ↑ RV filling → ↑ RV stroke volume → ↑ RV ejection time → delayed closure of pulmonic valve. ↓ pulmonary impedance (↑ capacity of the pulmonary circulation) also occurs during inspiration, which contributes to delayed closure of pulmonic valve.	E — S1 · A2 P2 I — S1 · A2 P2 Normal delay
Wide splitting	Seen in conditions that delay RV emptying (eg, pulmonic stenosis, right bundle branch block). Causes delayed pulmonic sound (especially on inspiration). An exaggeration of normal splitting.	E — S1 · A2 P2 I — S1 · A2 P2 Abnormal delay
Fixed splitting	Heard in ASD. ASD → left-to-right shunt → ↑ RA and RV volumes → ↑ flow through pulmonic valve such that, regardless of breath, pulmonic closure is greatly delayed.	E — S1 · A2 P2 (=) I — S1 · A2 P2 (=)
Paradoxical splitting	Heard in conditions that delay aortic valve closure (eg, aortic stenosis, left bundle branch block). Normal order of valve closure is reversed so that P2 sound occurs before delayed A2 sound. Therefore on inspiration, P2 closes later and moves closer to A2, thereby "paradoxically" eliminating the split (usually heard in expiration).	E — S1 · P2 A2 I — S1 · P2 A2 Rx E = Expiration I = Inspiration

Auscultation of the heart

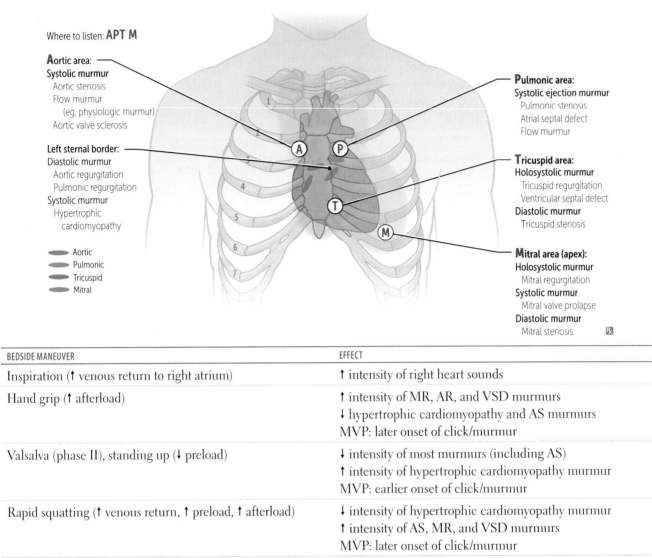

Where to listen: **APT M**

Aortic area:
Systolic murmur
　Aortic stenosis
　Flow murmur
　　(eg, physiologic murmur)
　Aortic valve sclerosis

Left sternal border:
Diastolic murmur
　Aortic regurgitation
　Pulmonic regurgitation
Systolic murmur
　Hypertrophic
　　cardiomyopathy

　Aortic
　Pulmonic
　Tricuspid
　Mitral

Pulmonic area:
Systolic ejection murmur
　Pulmonic stenosis
　Atrial septal defect
　Flow murmur

Tricuspid area:
Holosystolic murmur
　Tricuspid regurgitation
　Ventricular septal defect
Diastolic murmur
　Tricuspid stenosis

Mitral area (apex):
Holosystolic murmur
　Mitral regurgitation
Systolic murmur
　Mitral valve prolapse
Diastolic murmur
　Mitral stenosis

BEDSIDE MANEUVER	EFFECT
Inspiration (↑ venous return to right atrium)	↑ intensity of right heart sounds
Hand grip (↑ afterload)	↑ intensity of MR, AR, and VSD murmurs ↓ hypertrophic cardiomyopathy and AS murmurs MVP: later onset of click/murmur
Valsalva (phase II), standing up (↓ preload)	↓ intensity of most murmurs (including AS) ↑ intensity of hypertrophic cardiomyopathy murmur MVP: earlier onset of click/murmur
Rapid squatting (↑ venous return, ↑ preload, ↑ afterload)	↓ intensity of hypertrophic cardiomyopathy murmur ↑ intensity of AS, MR, and VSD murmurs MVP: later onset of click/murmur

Systolic heart sounds include the murmurs of aortic/pulmonic stenosis, mitral/tricuspid regurgitation, VSD, MVP, hypertrophic cardiomyopathy.

Diastolic heart sounds include the murmurs of aortic/pulmonic regurgitation, mitral/tricuspid stenosis.

Heart murmurs

Systolic

Aortic stenosis

S1   S2

Crescendo-decrescendo systolic ejection murmur and soft S2 (ejection click may be present). LV >> aortic pressure during systole. Loudest at heart base; radiates to carotids. "Pulsus parvus et tardus"—pulses are weak with a delayed peak. Can lead to Syncope, Angina, and Dyspnea on exertion (SAD). Most commonly due to age-related calcification in older patients (> 60 years old) or in younger patients with early-onset calcification of bicuspid aortic valve.

Mitral/tricuspid regurgitation

S1   S2

Holosystolic, high-pitched "blowing murmur."
Mitral—loudest at apex and radiates toward axilla. MR is often due to ischemic heart disease (post-MI), MVP, LV dilatation.
Tricuspid—loudest at tricuspid area. TR commonly caused by RV dilatation.
Rheumatic fever and infective endocarditis can cause either MR or TR.

Mitral valve prolapse

S1   MC   S2

Late systolic crescendo murmur with midsystolic click (MC; due to sudden tensing of chordae tendineae). Most frequent valvular lesion. Best heard over apex. Loudest just before S2. Usually benign. Can predispose to infective endocarditis. Can be caused by myxomatous degeneration (1° or 2° to connective tissue disease such as Marfan or Ehlers-Danlos syndrome), rheumatic fever, chordae rupture.

Ventricular septal defect

S1   S2

Holosystolic, harsh-sounding murmur. Loudest at tricuspid area.

Diastolic

Aortic regurgitation

S1   S2

High-pitched "blowing" early diastolic decrescendo murmur. Long diastolic murmur, hyperdynamic pulse, and head bobbing when severe and chronic. Wide pulse pressure. Often due to aortic root dilation, bicuspid aortic valve, endocarditis, rheumatic fever. Progresses to left HF.

Mitral stenosis

S1   S2 OS

Follows opening snap (OS; due to abrupt halt in leaflet motion in diastole, after rapid opening due to fusion at leaflet tips). Delayed rumbling mid-to-late diastolic murmur (↓ interval between S2 and OS correlates with ↑ severity). LA >> LV pressure during diastole.
Often a late (and highly specific) sequela of rheumatic fever. Chronic MS can result in LA dilatation → dysphagia/hoarseness via compression of esophagus/left recurrent laryngeal nerve, respectively.

Continuous

Patent ductus arteriosus

S1   S2

Continuous machine-like murmur. Best heard at left infraclavicular area. Loudest at S2. Often due to congenital rubella or prematurity.
"PDA's (Public Displays of Affection) are continuously annoying."

Myocardial action potential

Also occurs in bundle of His and Purkinje fibers.

Phase 0 = rapid upstroke and depolarization—voltage-gated Na^+ channels open.

Phase 1 = initial repolarization—inactivation of voltage-gated Na^+ channels. Voltage-gated K^+ channels begin to open.

Phase 2 = plateau—Ca^{2+} influx through voltage-gated Ca^{2+} channels balances K^+ efflux. Ca^{2+} influx triggers Ca^{2+} release from sarcoplasmic reticulum and myocyte contraction.

Phase 3 = rapid repolarization—massive K^+ efflux due to opening of voltage-gated slow K^+ channels and closure of voltage-gated Ca^{2+} channels.

Phase 4 = resting potential—high K^+ permeability through K^+ channels.

In contrast to skeletal muscle:
- Cardiac muscle action potential has a plateau, which is due to Ca^{2+} influx and K^+ efflux.
- Cardiac muscle contraction requires Ca^{2+} influx from ECF to induce Ca^{2+} release from sarcoplasmic reticulum (Ca^{2+}-induced Ca^{2+} release).
- Cardiac myocytes are electrically coupled to each other by gap junctions.

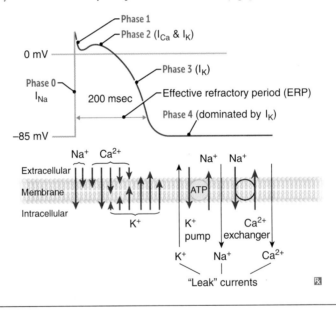

Pacemaker action potential

Occurs in the SA and AV nodes. Key differences from the ventricular action potential include:

Phase 0 = upstroke—opening of voltage-gated Ca^{2+} channels. Fast voltage-gated Na^+ channels are permanently inactivated because of the less negative resting potential of these cells. Results in a slow conduction velocity that is used by the AV node to prolong transmission from the atria to ventricles.

Phases 1 and 2 are absent.

Phase 3 = repolarization—inactivation of the Ca^{2+} channels and ↑ activation of K^+ channels → ↑ K^+ efflux.

Phase 4 = slow spontaneous diastolic depolarization due to I_f ("funny current"). I_f channels responsible for a slow, mixed Na^+/K^+ inward current; different from I_{Na} in phase 0 of ventricular action potential. Accounts for automaticity of SA and AV nodes. The slope of phase 4 in the SA node determines HR. ACh/adenosine ↓ the rate of diastolic depolarization and ↓ HR, while catecholamines ↑ depolarization and ↑ HR. Sympathetic stimulation ↑ the chance that I_f channels are open and thus ↑ HR.

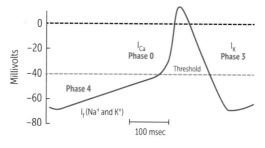

Electrocardiogram

Conduction pathway: SA node → atria → AV node → bundle of His → right and left bundle branches → Purkinje fibers → ventricles; left bundle branch divides into left anterior and posterior fascicles.

SA node "pacemaker" inherent dominance with slow phase of upstroke.

AV node—located in posteroinferior part of interatrial septum. Blood supply usually from RCA. 100-msec delay allows time for ventricular filling.

Pacemaker rates—SA > AV > bundle of His/ Purkinje/ventricles.

Speed of conduction—Purkinje > atria > ventricles > AV node.

P wave—atrial depolarization. Atrial repolarization is masked by QRS complex.

PR interval—time from start of atrial depolarization to start of ventricular depolarization (normally < 200 msec).

QRS complex—ventricular depolarization (normally < 120 msec).

QT interval—ventricular depolarization, mechanical contraction of the ventricles, ventricular repolarization.

T wave—ventricular repolarization. T-wave inversion may indicate ischemia or recent MI.

J point—junction between end of QRS complex and start of ST segment.

ST segment—isoelectric, ventricles depolarized.

U wave—prominent in hypokalemia (think hyp"U"kalemia), bradycardia.

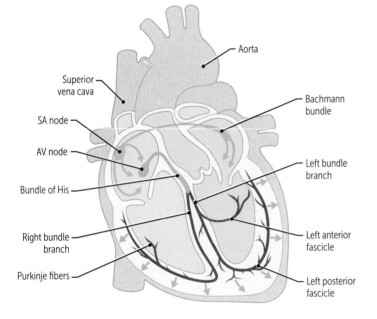

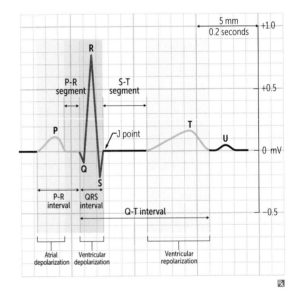

Torsades de pointes	Polymorphic ventricular tachycardia, characterized by shifting sinusoidal waveforms on ECG; can progress to ventricular fibrillation (VF). Long QT interval predisposes to torsades de pointes. Caused by drugs, ↓ K$^+$, ↓ Mg^{2+}, congenital abnormalities. Treatment includes magnesium sulfate.	Drug-induced long QT (**ABCDE**): **A**nti**A**rrhythmics (class IA, III) **A**nti**B**iotics (eg, macrolides) **A**nti"**C**"ychotics (eg, haloperidol) **A**nti**D**epressants (eg, TCAs) **A**nti**E**metics (eg, ondansetron) Torsades de pointes = twisting of the points
Congenital long QT syndrome	Inherited disorder of myocardial repolarization, typically due to ion channel defects; ↑ risk of sudden cardiac death (SCD) due to torsades de pointes. Includes: ▪ Romano-Ward syndrome—autosomal dominant, pure cardiac phenotype (no deafness). ▪ Jervell and Lange-Nielsen syndrome—autosomal recessive, sensorineural deafness.	
Brugada syndrome	Autosomal dominant disorder most common in Asian males. ECG pattern of pseudo-right bundle branch block and ST elevations in V$_1$-V$_3$. ↑ risk of ventricular tachyarrhythmias and SCD. Prevent SCD with implantable cardioverter-defibrillator (ICD).	
Wolff-Parkinson-White syndrome	Most common type of ventricular pre-excitation syndrome. Abnormal fast accessory conduction pathway from atria to ventricle (bundle of Kent) bypasses the rate-slowing AV node → ventricles begin to partially depolarize earlier → characteristic delta wave with widened QRS complex and shortened PR interval on ECG. May result in reentry circuit → supraventricular tachycardia.	

ECG tracings

RHYTHM	DESCRIPTION	EXAMPLE
Atrial fibrillation	Chaotic and erratic baseline with no discrete P waves in between irregularly spaced QRS complexes. Irregularly irregular heartbeat. Most common risk factors include hypertension and coronary artery disease (CAD). Can lead to thromboembolic events, particularly stroke. Treatment includes anticoagulation, rate control, rhythm control, and/or cardioversion.	$RR_1 \neq RR_2 \neq RR_3 \neq RR_4$ Irregular baseline (absent P waves)
Atrial flutter	A rapid succession of identical, back-to-back atrial depolarization waves. The identical appearance accounts for the "sawtooth" appearance of the flutter waves. Treat like atrial fibrillation. Definitive treatment is catheter ablation.	$RR_1 = RR_2 = RR_3$ 4:1 sawtooth pattern
Ventricular fibrillation	A completely erratic rhythm with no identifiable waves. Fatal arrhythmia without immediate CPR and defibrillation.	No discernible rhythm

AV block

RHYTHM	DESCRIPTION	EXAMPLE
First-degree AV block	The PR interval is prolonged (> 200 msec). Benign and asymptomatic. No treatment required.	$PR_1 = PR_2 = PR_3 = PR_4$
Second-degree AV block		
Mobitz type I (Wenckebach)	Progressive lengthening of PR interval until a beat is "dropped" (a P wave not followed by a QRS complex). Usually asymptomatic. Variable RR interval with a pattern (regularly irregular).	$PR_1 < PR_2 < PR_3$ P wave, absent QRS
Mobitz type II	Dropped beats that are not preceded by a change in the length of the PR interval (as in type I). May progress to 3rd-degree block. Often treated with pacemaker.	$PR_1 = PR_2$ P wave, absent QRS
Third-degree (complete) AV block	The atria and ventricles beat independently of each other. P waves and QRS complexes not rhythmically associated. Atrial rate > ventricular rate. Usually treated with pacemaker. Can be caused by Lyme disease.	$RR_1 = RR_2$ P wave on QRS complex P wave on T wave $PP_1 = PP_2 = PP_3 = PP_4$

Atrial natriuretic peptide	Released from **atrial myocytes** in response to ↑ blood volume and atrial pressure. Acts via cGMP. Causes vasodilation and ↓ Na^+ reabsorption at the renal collecting tubule. Dilates afferent renal arterioles and constricts efferent arterioles, promoting diuresis and contributing to "aldosterone escape" mechanism.
B-type (brain) natriuretic peptide	Released from **ventricular myocytes** in response to ↑ tension. Similar physiologic action to ANP, with longer half-life. BNP blood test used for diagnosing HF (very good negative predictive value). Available in recombinant form (nesiritide) for treatment of HF.

Baroreceptors and chemoreceptors

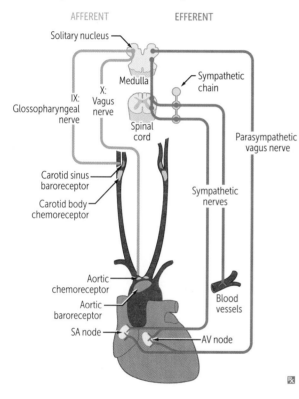

Receptors:

- Aortic arch transmits via vagus nerve to solitary nucleus of medulla (responds to ↓ and ↑ in BP).
- Carotid sinus (dilated region at carotid bifurcation) transmits via glossopharyngeal nerve to solitary nucleus of medulla (responds to ↓ and ↑ in BP).

Baroreceptors:

- Hypotension—↓ arterial pressure → ↓ stretch → ↓ afferent baroreceptor firing → ↑ efferent sympathetic firing and ↓ efferent parasympathetic stimulation → vasoconstriction, ↑ HR, ↑ contractility, ↑ BP. Important in the response to severe hemorrhage.
- Carotid massage—↑ pressure on carotid sinus → ↑ stretch → ↑ afferent baroreceptor firing → ↑ AV node refractory period → ↓ HR.
- Component of Cushing reflex (triad of hypertension, bradycardia, and respiratory depression)—↑ intracranial pressure constricts arterioles → cerebral ischemia → ↑ pCO_2 and ↓ pH → central reflex sympathetic ↑ in perfusion pressure (hypertension) → ↑ stretch → peripheral reflex baroreceptor–induced bradycardia.

Chemoreceptors:

- Peripheral—carotid and aortic bodies are stimulated by ↓ Po_2 (< 60 mm Hg), ↑ Pco_2, and ↓ pH of blood.
- Central—are stimulated by changes in pH and Pco_2 of brain interstitial fluid, which in turn are influenced by arterial CO_2. Do not directly respond to Po_2.

Normal cardiac pressures

Pulmonary capillary wedge pressure (PCWP; in mm Hg) is a good approximation of left atrial pressure. In mitral stenosis, PCWP > LV end diastolic pressure. PCWP is measured with pulmonary artery catheter (Swan-Ganz catheter).

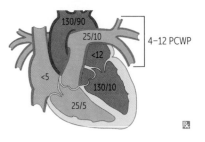

Autoregulation

How blood flow to an organ remains constant over a wide range of perfusion pressures.

ORGAN	FACTORS DETERMINING AUTOREGULATION	
Heart	Local metabolites (vasodilatory): adenosine, NO, CO_2, ↓ O_2	The pulmonary vasculature is unique in that alveolar hypoxia causes vasoconstriction so that only well-ventilated areas are perfused. In other organs, hypoxia causes vasodilation.
Brain	Local metabolites (vasodilatory): CO_2 (pH)	
Kidneys	Myogenic and tubuloglomerular feedback	
Lungs	Hypoxia causes vasoconstriction	
Skeletal muscle	Local metabolites during exercise: CO_2, H^+, Adenosine, Lactate, K^+ At rest: sympathetic tone	CHALK.
Skin	Sympathetic stimulation most important mechanism for temperature control	

Capillary fluid exchange

Starling forces determine fluid movement through capillary membranes:

- P_c = capillary pressure—pushes fluid out of capillary
- P_i = interstitial fluid pressure—pushes fluid into capillary
- π_c = plasma colloid osmotic (oncotic) pressure—pulls fluid into capillary
- π_i = interstitial fluid colloid osmotic pressure—pulls fluid out of capillary

J_v = net fluid flow = $K_f [(P_c - P_i) - \sigma(\pi_c - \pi_i)]$

K_f = capillary permeability to fluid

σ = reflection coefficient (measure of capillary permeability to protein)

Edema—excess fluid outflow into interstitium commonly caused by:

- ↑ capillary pressure (↑ P_c; eg, HF)
- ↓ plasma proteins (↓ π_c; eg, nephrotic syndrome, liver failure, protein malnutrition)
- ↑ capillary permeability (↑ K_f; eg, toxins, infections, burns)
- ↑ interstitial fluid colloid osmotic pressure (↑ π_i; eg, lymphatic blockage)

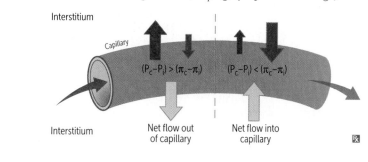

Interstitium

Capillary

$(P_c - P_i) > (\pi_c - \pi_i)$ $(P_c - P_i) < (\pi_c - \pi_i)$

Interstitium

Net flow out of capillary   Net flow into capillary

▶ CARDIOVASCULAR—PATHOLOGY

Congenital heart diseases

RIGHT-TO-LEFT SHUNTS	Early cyanosis—"blue babies." Often diagnosed prenatally or become evident immediately after birth. Usually require urgent surgical treatment and/or maintenance of a PDA.	The 5 Ts: 1. Truncus arteriosus (1 vessel) 2. Transposition (2 switched vessels) 3. Tricuspid atresia (3 = Tri) 4. Tetralogy of Fallot (4 = Tetra) 5. TAPVR (5 letters in the name)
Persistent truncus arteriosus	Truncus arteriosus fails to divide into pulmonary trunk and aorta due to lack of aorticopulmonary septum formation; most patients have accompanying VSD.	
D-transposition of great vessels	Aorta leaves RV (anterior) and pulmonary trunk leaves LV (posterior) → separation of systemic and pulmonary circulations. Not compatible with life unless a shunt is present to allow mixing of blood (eg, VSD, PDA, or patent foramen ovale). Due to failure of the aorticopulmonary septum to spiral. Without surgical intervention, most infants die within the first few months of life.	
Tricuspid atresia	Absence of tricuspid valve and hypoplastic RV; requires both ASD and VSD for viability.	
Tetralogy of Fallot	Caused by anterosuperior displacement of the infundibular septum. Most common cause of early childhood cyanosis. ❶ Pulmonary infundibular stenosis (most important determinant for prognosis) ❷ Right ventricular hypertrophy (RVH)—boot-shaped heart on CXR **A** ❸ Overriding aorta ❹ VSD Pulmonary stenosis forces right-to-left flow across VSD → RVH, "tet spells" (often caused by crying, fever, and exercise due to exacerbation of RV outflow obstruction).	PROVe. Squatting: ↑ SVR, ↓ right-to-left shunt, improves cyanosis. Treatment: early surgical correction.
Total anomalous pulmonary venous return	Pulmonary veins drain into right heart circulation (SVC, coronary sinus, etc); associated with ASD and sometimes PDA to allow for right-to-left shunting to maintain CO.	
Ebstein anomaly	Characterized by displacement of tricuspid valve leaflets downward into RV, artificially "atrializing" the ventricle. Associated with tricuspid regurgitation, accessory conduction pathways, and right-sided HF. Can be caused by lithium exposure in utero.	

Congenital heart diseases (continued)

LEFT-TO-RIGHT SHUNTS	Acyanotic at presentation; cyanosis may occur years later.	Right-to-Left shunts: ea**RL**y cyanosis. Left-to-**R**ight shunts: "Late**R**" cyanosis.
Ventricular septal defect 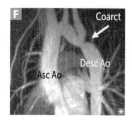	Most common congenital cardiac defect. Asymptomatic at birth, may manifest weeks later or remain asymptomatic throughout life. Most self resolve; larger lesions may lead to LV overload and HF.	O_2 saturation ↑ in RV and pulmonary artery. Frequency: VSD > ASD > PDA.
Atrial septal defect	Defect in interatrial septum **C**; wide, fixed split S2. Ostium secundum defects most common and usually an isolated finding; ostium primum defects rarer and usually occur with other cardiac anomalies. Symptoms range from none to HF. Distinct from patent foramen ovale in that septa are missing tissue rather than unfused.	O_2 saturation ↑ in RA, RV, and pulmonary artery. May lead to paradoxical emboli (systemic venous emboli use ASD to bypass lungs and become systemic arterial emboli).
Patent ductus arteriosus	In fetal period, shunt is right to left (normal). In neonatal period, ↓ pulmonary vascular resistance → shunt becomes left to right → progressive RVH and/or LVH and HF. Associated with a continuous, "machine-like" murmur. Patency is maintained by PGE synthesis and low O_2 tension. Uncorrected PDA **D** can eventually result in late cyanosis in the lower extremities (differential cyanosis).	"**End**omethacin" (indomethacin) **ends** patency of PDA; PGE keeps ductus **G**oing (may be necessary to sustain life in conditions such as transposition of the great vessels). PDA is normal in utero and normally closes only after birth.
Eisenmenger syndrome	Uncorrected left-to-right shunt (VSD, ASD, PDA) → ↑ pulmonary blood flow → pathologic remodeling of vasculature → pulmonary arterial hypertension. RVH occurs to compensate → shunt becomes right to left. Causes late cyanosis, clubbing **E**, and polycythemia. Age of onset varies.	

OTHER ANOMALIES		
Coarctation of the aorta	Aortic narrowing **F** near insertion of ductus arteriosus ("juxtaductal"). Associated with bicuspid aortic valve, other heart defects, and Turner syndrome. Hypertension in upper extremities and weak, delayed pulse in lower extremities (brachial-femoral delay). With age, intercostal arteries enlarge due to collateral circulation; arteries erode ribs → notched appearance on CXR. Complications include HF, ↑ risk of cerebral hemorrhage (berry aneurysms), aortic rupture, and possible endocarditis.	

Congenital cardiac defect associations

DISORDER	DEFECT
Alcohol exposure in utero (fetal alcohol syndrome)	VSD, PDA, ASD, tetralogy of Fallot
Congenital rubella	PDA, pulmonary artery stenosis, septal defects
Down syndrome	AV septal defect (endocardial cushion defect), VSD, ASD
Infant of diabetic mother	Transposition of great vessels, VSD
Marfan syndrome	MVP, thoracic aortic aneurysm and dissection, aortic regurgitation
Prenatal lithium exposure	Ebstein anomaly
Turner syndrome	Bicuspid aortic valve, coarctation of aorta
Williams syndrome	Supravalvular aortic stenosis
22q11 syndromes	Truncus arteriosus, tetralogy of Fallot

Hypertension

Defined as persistent systolic BP ≥ 140 mm Hg and/or diastolic BP ≥ 90 mm Hg

RISK FACTORS

↑ age, obesity, diabetes, physical inactivity, excess salt intake, excess alcohol intake, cigarette smoking, family history; African American > Caucasian > Asian.

FEATURES

90% of hypertension is 1° (essential) and related to ↑ CO or ↑ TPR. Remaining 10% mostly 2° to renal/renovascular diseases such as fibromuscular dysplasia (characteristic "string of beads" appearance of renal artery **A**) and atherosclerotic renal artery stenosis or to 1° hyperaldosteronism.

Hypertensive urgency—severe (≥ 180/≥ 120 mm Hg) hypertension without acute end-organ damage.

Hypertensive emergency—severe hypertension with evidence of acute end-organ damage (eg, encephalopathy, stroke, retinal hemorrhages and exudates, papilledema, MI, HF, aortic dissection, kidney injury, microangiopathic hemolytic anemia, eclampsia).

PREDISPOSES TO

CAD, LVH, HF, atrial fibrillation; aortic dissection, aortic aneurysm; stroke; chronic kidney disease (hypertensive nephropathy); retinopathy.

Hyperlipidemia signs

Xanthomas	Plaques or nodules composed of lipid-laden histiocytes in skin **A**, especially the eyelids (xanthelasma **B**).
Tendinous xanthoma	Lipid deposit in tendon **C**, especially Achilles.
Corneal arcus	Lipid deposit in cornea. Common in elderly (arcus senilis **D**), but appears earlier in life with hypercholesterolemia.

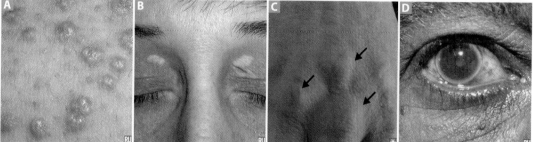

Arteriosclerosis

Hardening of arteries, with arterial wall thickening and loss of elasticity.

Arteriolosclerosis	Common. Affects small arteries and arterioles. Two types: hyaline (thickening of vessel walls in essential hypertension or diabetes mellitus **A**) and hyperplastic ("onion skinning" in severe hypertension **B** with proliferation of smooth muscle cells).
Mönckeberg sclerosis (medial calcific sclerosis)	Uncommon. Affects medium-sized arteries. Calcification of internal elastic lamina and media of arteries → vascular stiffening without obstruction. "Pipestem" appearance on x-ray **C**. Does not obstruct blood flow; intima not involved.

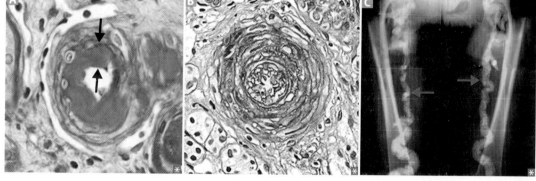

Atherosclerosis	Very common. Disease of elastic arteries and large- and medium-sized muscular arteries; a form of arteriosclerosis caused by buildup of cholesterol plaques.
LOCATION	Abdominal aorta > coronary artery > popliteal artery > carotid artery **A**. "After I workout my **abs**, I grab a **Corona** and **pop** my collar up to my **carotid**."
RISK FACTORS	Modifiable: smoking, hypertension, dyslipidemia ($\uparrow$ LDL, $\downarrow$ HDL), diabetes. Non-modifiable: age, sex ($\uparrow$ in men and postmenopausal women), family history.
SYMPTOMS	Angina, claudication, but can be asymptomatic.
PROGRESSION	Inflammation important in pathogenesis: endothelial cell dysfunction → macrophage and LDL accumulation → foam cell formation → fatty streaks → smooth muscle cell migration (involves PDGF and FGF), proliferation, and extracellular matrix deposition → fibrous plaque → complex atheromas **B**.
COMPLICATIONS	Aneurysms, ischemia, infarcts, peripheral vascular disease, thrombus, emboli.

Aortic aneurysm	Localized pathologic dilatation of the aorta. May cause abdominal and/or back pain, which is a sign of leaking, dissection, or imminent rupture.
Abdominal aortic aneurysm	Associated with atherosclerosis. Risk factors include history of tobacco use, $\uparrow$ age, male sex, family history. May present as palpable pulsatile abdominal mass (arrows in **A** point to outer dilated calcified aortic wall, with partial crescent-shaped non-opacification of aorta due to flap/clot). Most often infrarenal (distal to origin of renal arteries).
Thoracic aortic aneurysm	Associated with cystic medial degeneration. Risk factors include hypertension, bicuspid aortic valve, connective tissue disease (eg, Marfan syndrome). Also associated with 3° syphilis (obliterative endarteritis of the vasa vasorum). Aortic root dilatation may lead to aortic valve regurgitation.
Traumatic aortic rupture	Due to trauma and/or deceleration injury, most commonly at aortic isthmus (proximal descending aorta just distal to origin of left subclavian artery).

Aortic dissection

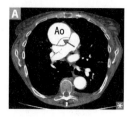

Longitudinal intimal tear forming a false lumen. Associated with hypertension, bicuspid aortic valve, inherited connective tissue disorders (eg, Marfan syndrome). Can present with tearing, sudden-onset chest pain radiating to the back +/– markedly unequal BP in arms. CXR shows mediastinal widening. Can result in organ ischemia, aortic rupture, death. Two types:
- Stanford type **A** (proximal): involves **A**scending aorta **A**. May extend to aortic arch or descending aorta. May result in acute aortic regurgitation or cardiac tamponade. Treatment: surgery.
- Stanford type **B** (distal): involves only descending aorta (**B**elow ligamentum arteriosum). Treat medically with β-blockers, then vasodilators.

Ischemic heart disease manifestations

Angina	Chest pain due to ischemic myocardium 2° to coronary artery narrowing or spasm; no myocyte necrosis. • Stable—usually 2° to atherosclerosis (≥ 70% occlusion); exertional chest pain in classic distribution (usually with ST depression on ECG), resolving with rest or nitroglycerin. • Vasospastic (also known as Prinzmetal or Variant)—occurs at rest 2° to coronary artery spasm; transient ST elevation on ECG. Smoking is a risk factor; hypertension and hypercholesterolemia are not. Triggers include cocaine, alcohol, and triptans. Treat with Ca^{2+} channel blockers, nitrates, and smoking cessation (if applicable). • Unstable—thrombosis with incomplete coronary artery occlusion; +/– ST depression and/or T-wave inversion on ECG but no cardiac biomarker elevation (unlike NSTEMI); ↑ in frequency or intensity of chest pain or any chest pain at rest.
Coronary steal syndrome	Distal to coronary stenosis, vessels are maximally dilated at baseline. Administration of vasodilators (eg, dipyridamole, regadenoson) dilates normal vessels → blood is shunted toward well-perfused areas → ischemia in myocardium perfused by stenosed vessels. Principle behind pharmacologic stress tests with coronary vasodilators.
Sudden cardiac death	Death from cardiac causes within 1 hour of onset of symptoms, most commonly due to a lethal arrhythmia (eg, VF). Associated with CAD (up to 70% of cases), cardiomyopathy (hypertrophic, dilated), and hereditary ion channelopathies (eg, long QT syndrome, Brugada syndrome). Prevent with ICD.
Chronic ischemic heart disease	Progressive onset of HF over many years due to chronic ischemic myocardial damage.
Myocardial infarction	Most often due to rupture of coronary artery atherosclerotic plaque → acute thrombosis. ↑ cardiac biomarkers (CK-MB, troponins) are diagnostic.

ST-segment elevation MI (STEMI)	**Non–ST-segment elevation MI (NSTEMI)**
Transmural infarcts	Subendocardial infarcts
Full thickness of myocardial wall involved	Subendocardium (inner ⅓) especially
ST elevation on ECG, Q waves	vulnerable to ischemia
	ST depression on ECG

Evolution of myocardial infarction

Commonly occluded coronary arteries: LAD > RCA > circumflex.

Symptoms: diaphoresis, nausea, vomiting, severe retrosternal pain, pain in left arm and/or jaw, shortness of breath, fatigue.

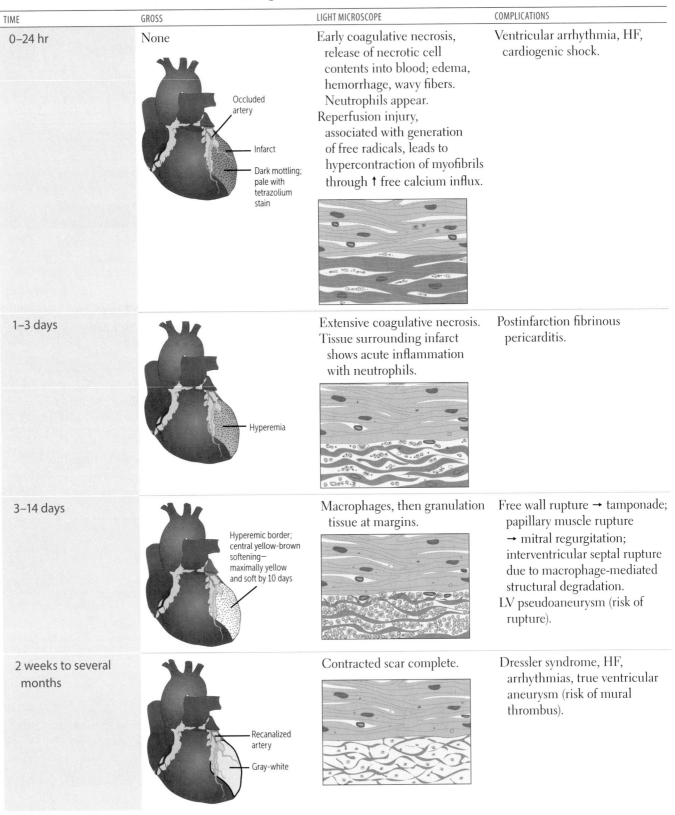

TIME	GROSS	LIGHT MICROSCOPE	COMPLICATIONS
0–24 hr	None Occluded artery Infarct Dark mottling; pale with tetrazolium stain	Early coagulative necrosis, release of necrotic cell contents into blood; edema, hemorrhage, wavy fibers. Neutrophils appear. Reperfusion injury, associated with generation of free radicals, leads to hypercontraction of myofibrils through ↑ free calcium influx.	Ventricular arrhythmia, HF, cardiogenic shock.
1–3 days	Hyperemia	Extensive coagulative necrosis. Tissue surrounding infarct shows acute inflammation with neutrophils.	Postinfarction fibrinous pericarditis.
3–14 days	Hyperemic border; central yellow-brown softening— maximally yellow and soft by 10 days	Macrophages, then granulation tissue at margins.	Free wall rupture → tamponade; papillary muscle rupture → mitral regurgitation; interventricular septal rupture due to macrophage-mediated structural degradation. LV pseudoaneurysm (risk of rupture).
2 weeks to several months	Recanalized artery Gray-white	Contracted scar complete.	Dressler syndrome, HF, arrhythmias, true ventricular aneurysm (risk of mural thrombus).

Diagnosis of myocardial infarction

In the first 6 hours, ECG is the gold standard. Cardiac troponin I rises after 4 hours (peaks at 24 hr) and is ↑ for 7–10 days; more specific than other protein markers.

CK-MB rises after 6–12 hours (peaks at 16–24 hr) and is predominantly found in myocardium but can also be released from skeletal muscle. Useful in diagnosing reinfarction following acute MI because levels return to normal after 48 hours.

Large MIs lead to greater elevations in troponin I and CK-MB. Exact curves vary with testing procedure.

ECG changes can include ST elevation (STEMI, transmural infarct), ST depression (NSTEMI, subendocardial infarct), hyperacute (peaked) T waves, T-wave inversion, new left bundle branch block, and pathologic Q waves or poor R wave progression (evolving or old transmural infarct).

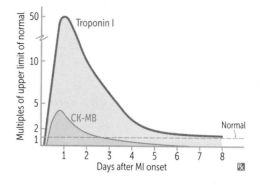

ECG localization of STEMI

INFARCT LOCATION	LEADS WITH ST ELEVATIONS OR Q WAVES
Anteroseptal (LAD)	V_1–V_2
Anteroapical (distal LAD)	V_3–V_4
Anterolateral (LAD or LCX)	V_5–V_6
Lateral (LCX)	I, aVL
InFerior (RCA)	II, III, aVF
Posterior (PDA)	V_7–V_9, ST depression in V_1–V_3 with tall R waves

Myocardial infarction complications

Cardiac arrhythmia	Occurs within the first few days after MI. Important cause of death before reaching the hospital and within the first 24 hours post-MI.
Postinfarction fibrinous pericarditis	Occurs 1–3 days after MI. Friction rub.
Papillary muscle rupture	Occurs 2–7 days after MI. Posteromedial papillary muscle rupture **A** ↑ risk due to single blood supply from posterior descending artery. Can result in severe mitral regurgitation.
Interventricular septal rupture	Occurs 3–5 days after MI. Macrophage-mediated degradation → VSD → ↑ O_2 saturation and pressure in RV.
Ventricular pseudoaneurysm formation	Occurs 3–14 days after MI. Contained free wall rupture **B**; ↓ CO, risk of arrhythmia, embolus from mural thrombus.
Ventricular free wall rupture	Occurs 5–14 days after MI. Free wall rupture **C** → cardiac tamponade. LV hypertrophy and previous MI protect against free wall rupture. Acute form usually leads to sudden death.
True ventricular aneurysm	Occurs 2 weeks to several months after MI. Outward bulge with contraction ("dyskinesia"), associated with fibrosis.
Dressler syndrome	Occurs several weeks after MI. Autoimmune phenomenon resulting in fibrinous pericarditis.
LV failure and pulmonary edema	Can occur 2° to LV infarction, VSD, free wall rupture, papillary muscle rupture with mitral regurgitation.

Acute coronary syndrome treatments	**Unstable angina/NSTEMI**—Anticoagulation (eg, heparin), antiplatelet therapy (eg, aspirin) + ADP receptor inhibitors (eg, clopidogrel), β-blockers, ACE inhibitors, statins. Symptom control with nitroglycerin and morphine. **STEMI**—In addition to above, reperfusion therapy most important (percutaneous coronary intervention preferred over fibrinolysis).

Cardiomyopathies

Dilated cardiomyopathy 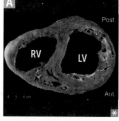	Most common cardiomyopathy (90% of cases). Often idiopathic or familial. Other etiologies include chronic **A**lcohol abuse, wet **B**eriberi, **C**oxsackie B viral myocarditis, chronic **C**ocaine use, **C**hagas disease, **D**oxorubicin toxicity, hemochromatosis, sarcoidosis, thyrotoxicosis, peripartum cardiomyopathy. Findings: HF, S3, systolic regurgitant murmur, dilated heart on echocardiogram, balloon appearance of heart on CXR. Treatment: Na⁺ restriction, ACE inhibitors, β-blockers, diuretics, digoxin, ICD, heart transplant.	Leads to systolic dysfunction. Dilated cardiomyopathy displays eccentric hypertrophy **A** (sarcomeres added in series). ABCCCD. Takotsubo cardiomyopathy: broken heart syndrome—ventricular apical ballooning likely due to increased sympathetic stimulation (eg, stressful situations).
Hypertrophic obstructive cardiomyopathy 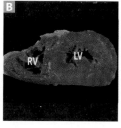	60–70% of cases are familial, autosomal dominant (most commonly due to mutations in genes encoding sarcomeric proteins, such as myosin binding protein C and β-myosin heavy chain). Causes syncope during exercise and may lead to sudden death (eg, in young athletes) due to ventricular arrhythmia. Findings: S4, systolic murmur. May see mitral regurgitation due to impaired mitral valve closure. Treatment: cessation of high-intensity athletics, use of β-blocker or non-dihydropyridine Ca²⁺ channel blockers (eg, verapamil). ICD if patient is high risk.	Diastolic dysfunction ensues. Marked ventricular concentric hypertrophy (sarcomeres added in parallel) **B**, often septal predominance. Myofibrillar disarray and fibrosis. Physiology of HOCM—asymmetric septal hypertrophy and systolic anterior motion of mitral valve → outflow obstruction → dyspnea, possible syncope. Other causes of concentric LV hypertrophy: chronic HTN, Friedreich ataxia.
Restrictive/infiltrative cardiomyopathy	Postradiation fibrosis, **L**öffler endocarditis, **E**ndocardial fibroelastosis (thick fibroelastic tissue in endocardium of young children), **A**myloidosis, **S**arcoidosis, **H**emochromatosis (although dilated cardiomyopathy is more common) (Puppy **LEASH**).	Diastolic dysfunction ensues. Can have low-voltage ECG despite thick myocardium (especially in amyloidosis). Löffler endocarditis—associated with hypereosinophilic syndrome; histology shows eosinophilic infiltrates in myocardium.

Heart failure 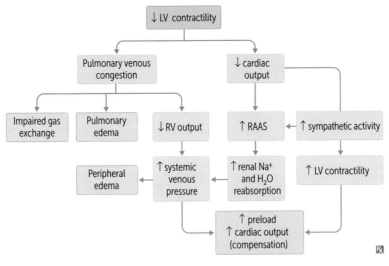	Clinical syndrome of cardiac pump dysfunction → congestion and low perfusion. Symptoms include dyspnea, orthopnea, fatigue; signs include S3 heart sound, rales, jugular venous distention (JVD), pitting edema **A**. Systolic dysfunction—reduced EF, ↑ EDV; ↓ contractility often 2° to ischemia/MI or dilated cardiomyopathy. Diastolic dysfunction—preserved EF, normal EDV; ↓ compliance (↑ EDP) often 2° to myocardial hypertrophy. Right HF most often results from left HF. Cor pulmonale refers to isolated right HF due to pulmonary cause. ACE inhibitors or angiotensin II receptor blockers, β-blockers (except in acute decompensated HF), and spironolactone ↓ mortality. Thiazide or loop diuretics are used mainly for symptomatic relief. Hydralazine with nitrate therapy improves both symptoms and mortality in select patients.

Left heart failure

Orthopnea	Shortness of breath when supine: ↑ venous return from redistribution of blood (immediate gravity effect) exacerbates pulmonary vascular congestion.
Paroxysmal nocturnal dyspnea	Breathless awakening from sleep: ↑ venous return from redistribution of blood, reabsorption of peripheral edema, etc.
Pulmonary edema	↑ pulmonary venous pressure → pulmonary venous distention and transudation of fluid. Presence of hemosiderin-laden macrophages ("HF" cells) in lungs.

Right heart failure

Hepatomegaly (nutmeg liver)	↑ central venous pressure → ↑ resistance to portal flow. Rarely, leads to "cardiac cirrhosis."
Jugular venous distention	↑ venous pressure.
Peripheral edema	↑ venous pressure → fluid transudation.

Shock

Inadequate organ perfusion and delivery of nutrients necessary for normal tissue and cellular function. Initially may be reversible but life threatening if not treated promptly.

	CAUSED BY	SKIN	PCWP (PRELOAD)	CO	SVR (AFTERLOAD)	TREATMENT
Hypovolemic shock	Hemorrhage, dehydration, burns	Cold, clammy	↓↓	↓	↑	IV fluids
Cardiogenic shock	Acute MI, HF, valvular dysfunction, arrhythmia	Cold, clammy	↑ or ↓	↓↓	↑	Inotropes, diuresis
Obstructive shock	Cardiac tamponade, pulmonary embolism, tension pneumothorax					Relieve obstruction
Distributive shock	Sepsis, anaphylaxis CNS injury	Warm Dry	↓ ↓	↑ ↓	↓↓ ↓↓	IV fluids, pressors, epinephrine (anaphylaxis)

Bacterial endocarditis

Acute—*S aureus* (high virulence). Large vegetations on previously normal valves A. Rapid onset.

Subacute—viridans streptococci (low virulence). Smaller vegetations on congenitally abnormal or diseased valves. Sequela of dental procedures. Gradual onset.

Symptoms: fever (most common), new murmur, Roth spots (round white spots on retina surrounded by hemorrhage B), Osler nodes (tender raised lesions on finger or toe pads C due to immune complex deposition), Janeway lesions (small, painless, erythematous lesions on palm or sole) D, splinter hemorrhages E on nail bed.

Associated with glomerulonephritis, septic arterial or pulmonary emboli.

May be nonbacterial (marantic/thrombotic) 2° to malignancy, hypercoagulable state, or lupus.

♥ Bacteria **FROM JANE** ♥:
Fever
Roth spots
Osler nodes
Murmur
Janeway lesions
Anemia
Nail-bed hemorrhage
Emboli

Requires multiple blood cultures for diagnosis.

If culture ⊖, most likely *Coxiella burnetti*, *Bartonella* spp, HACEK (*Haemophilus*, *Aggregatibacter* [formerly *Actinobacillus*], *Cardiobacterium*, *Eikenella*, *Kingella*).

Mitral valve is most frequently involved.

Tricuspid valve endocarditis is associated with IV drug abuse (don't "tri" drugs). Associated with *S aureus*, *Pseudomonas*, and *Candida*.

S bovis (*gallolyticus*) is present in colon cancer, *S epidermidis* on prosthetic valves.

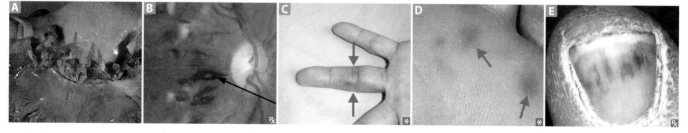

Rheumatic fever

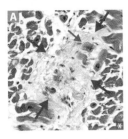

A consequence of pharyngeal infection with group A β-hemolytic streptococci. Late sequelae include rheumatic heart disease, which affects heart valves—mitral > aortic >> tricuspid (high-pressure valves affected most). Early lesion is mitral valve regurgitation; late lesion is mitral stenosis.

Associated with Aschoff bodies (granuloma with giant cells [blue arrows in]), Anitschkow cells (enlarged macrophages with ovoid, wavy, rod-like nucleus [red arrow in]), ↑ anti-streptolysin O (ASO) titers.

Immune mediated (type II hypersensitivity); not a direct effect of bacteria. Antibodies to M protein cross-react with self antigens (molecular mimicry).

Treatment/prophylaxis: penicillin.

J♥NES (major criteria):
Joint (migratory polyarthritis)
♥ (carditis)
Nodules in skin (subcutaneous)
Erythema marginatum (evanescent rash with ring margin)
Sydenham chorea

Acute pericarditis

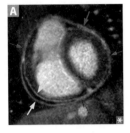

Inflammation of the pericardium [, red arrows]. Commonly presents with sharp pain, aggravated by inspiration, and relieved by sitting up and leaning forward. Often complicated by pericardial effusion [between yellow arrows in]. Presents with friction rub. ECG changes include widespread ST-segment elevation and/or PR depression.

Causes include idiopathic (most common; presumed viral), confirmed infection (eg, coxsackievirus B), neoplasia, autoimmune (eg, SLE, rheumatoid arthritis), uremia, cardiovascular (acute STEMI or Dressler syndrome), radiation therapy.

Myocarditis	Inflammation of myocardium → global enlargement of heart and dilation of all chambers. Major cause of SCD in adults < 40 years old.
	Presentation highly variable, can include dyspnea, chest pain, fever, arrhythmias (persistent tachycardia out of proportion to fever is characteristic).
	Multiple causes:
	  ▪ Viral (eg, adenovirus, coxsackie B, parvovirus B19, HIV, HHV-6); lymphocytic infiltrate with focal necrosis highly indicative of viral myocarditis.
	  ▪ Parasitic (eg, *Trypanosoma cruzi, Toxoplasma gondii*)
	  ▪ Bacterial (eg, *Borrelia burgdorferi, Mycoplasma pneumoniae*)
	  ▪ Toxins (eg, carbon monoxide, black widow venom)
	  ▪ Rheumatic fever
	  ▪ Drugs (eg, doxorubicin, cocaine)
	  ▪ Autoimmune (eg, Kawasaki disease, sarcoidosis, SLE, polymyositis/dermatomyositis)
	Complications include sudden death, arrhythmias, heart block, dilated cardiomyopathy, HF, mural thrombus with systemic emboli.

Cardiac tamponade 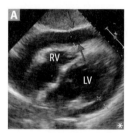	Compression of the heart by fluid (eg, blood, effusions [arrows in **A**] in pericardial space) → ↓ CO. Equilibration of diastolic pressures in all 4 chambers. Findings: Beck triad (hypotension, distended neck veins, distant heart sounds), ↑ HR, pulsus paradoxus. ECG shows low-voltage QRS and electrical alternans (due to "swinging" movement of heart in large effusion). **Pulsus paradoxus**—↓ in amplitude of systolic BP by > 10 mm Hg during inspiration. Seen in cardiac tamponade, asthma, obstructive sleep apnea, pericarditis, croup.

Syphilitic heart disease	3° syphilis disrupts the vasa vasorum of the aorta with consequent atrophy of vessel wall and dilatation of aorta and valve ring. May see calcification of aortic root, ascending aortic arch, and thoracic aorta. Leads to "tree bark" appearance of aorta.	Can result in aneurysm of ascending aorta or aortic arch, aortic insufficiency.

Vasculitides

	EPIDEMIOLOGY/PRESENTATION	PATHOLOGY/LABS
Large-vessel vasculitis		
Giant cell (temporal) arteritis	Usually elderly females. Unilateral headache (temporal artery), jaw claudication. May lead to irreversible blindness due to ophthalmic artery occlusion. Associated with polymyalgia rheumatica.	Most commonly affects branches of carotid artery. Focal granulomatous inflammation **A**. ↑ ESR. Treat with high-dose corticosteroids prior to temporal artery biopsy to prevent blindness.
Takayasu arteritis	Usually Asian females < 40 years old. "Pulseless disease" (weak upper extremity pulses), fever, night sweats, arthritis, myalgias, skin nodules, ocular disturbances.	Granulomatous thickening and narrowing of aortic arch and proximal great vessels **B**. ↑ ESR. Treat with corticosteroids.
Medium-vessel vasculitis		
Polyarteritis nodosa	Usually middle-aged men. Hepatitis B seropositivity in 30% of patients. Fever, weight loss, malaise, headache. GI: abdominal pain, melena. Hypertension, neurologic dysfunction, cutaneous eruptions, renal damage.	Typically involves renal and visceral vessels, not pulmonary arteries. Transmural inflammation of the arterial wall with fibrinoid necrosis. Different stages of inflammation may coexist in different vessels. Innumerable renal microaneurysms **C** and spasms on arteriogram. Treat with corticosteroids, cyclophosphamide.
Kawasaki disease (mucocutaneous lymph node syndrome)	Asian children < 4 years old. Conjunctival injection, Rash (polymorphous → desquamating), Adenopathy (cervical), Strawberry tongue (oral mucositis) **D**, Hand-foot changes (edema, erythema), fever.	**CRASH** and burn. May develop coronary artery aneurysms **E**; thrombosis or rupture can cause death. Treat with IV immunoglobulin and aspirin.
Buerger disease (thromboangiitis obliterans)	Heavy smokers, males < 40 years old. Intermittent claudication may lead to gangrene **F**, autoamputation of digits, superficial nodular phlebitis. Raynaud phenomenon is often present.	Segmental thrombosing vasculitis with vein and nerve involvement. Treat with smoking cessation.
Small-vessel vasculitis		
Granulomatosis with polyangiitis (Wegener)	Upper respiratory tract: perforation of nasal septum, chronic sinusitis, otitis media, mastoiditis. Lower respiratory tract: hemoptysis, cough, dyspnea. Renal: hematuria, red cell casts.	Triad: ▪ Focal necrotizing vasculitis ▪ Necrotizing granulomas in the lung and upper airway ▪ Necrotizing glomerulonephritis PR3-ANCA/c-ANCA **G** (anti-proteinase 3). CXR: large nodular densities. Treat with cyclophosphamide, corticosteroids.
Microscopic polyangiitis	Necrotizing vasculitis commonly involving lung, kidneys, and skin with pauci-immune glomerulonephritis and palpable purpura. Presentation similar to granulomatosis with polyangiitis but without nasopharyngeal involvement.	No granulomas. MPO-ANCA/p-ANCA **H** (anti-myeloperoxidase). Treat with cyclophosphamide, corticosteroids.

Vasculitides (continued)

	EPIDEMIOLOGY/PRESENTATION	PATHOLOGY/LABS
Small-vessel vasculitis (continued)		
Behçet syndrome	High incidence in Turkish and eastern Mediterranean descent. Recurrent aphthous ulcers, genital ulcerations, uveitis, erythema nodosum. Can be precipitated by HSV or parvovirus. Flares last 1–4 weeks.	Immune complex vasculitis. Associated with HLA-B51.
Eosinophilic granulomatosis with polyangiitis (Churg-Strauss)	Asthma, sinusitis, skin nodules or purpura, peripheral neuropathy (eg, wrist/foot drop). Can also involve heart, GI, kidneys (pauci-immune glomerulonephritis).	Granulomatous, necrotizing vasculitis with eosinophilia **I**. MPO-ANCA/p-ANCA, ↑ IgE level.
Immunoglobulin A vasculitis	Also known as Henoch-Schönlein purpura. Most common childhood systemic vasculitis. Often follows URI. Classic triad: <ul><li>Skin: palpable purpura on buttocks/legs **J**</li><li>Arthralgias</li><li>GI: abdominal pain (associated with intussusception)</li></ul>	Vasculitis 2° to IgA immune complex deposition. Associated with IgA nephropathy (Berger disease).

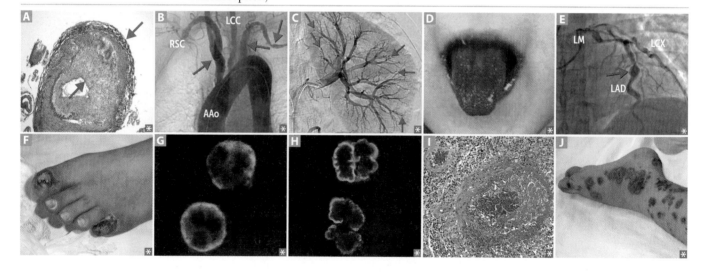

Cardiac tumors

Most common heart tumor is a metastasis (eg, melanoma).

Myxomas

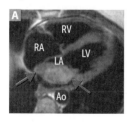

Most common 1° cardiac tumor in adults (arrows in **A**). 90% occur in the atria (mostly left atrium). Myxomas are usually described as a "ball valve" obstruction in the left atrium (associated with multiple syncopal episodes). May auscultate early diastolic "tumor plop" sound. Histology: gelatinous material, myxoma cells immersed in glycosaminoglycans.

Rhabdomyomas

Most frequent 1° cardiac tumor in children (associated with tuberous sclerosis). Histology: hamartomatous growths.

Kussmaul sign	↑ in JVP on inspiration instead of a normal ↓. Inspiration → negative intrathoracic pressure not transmitted to heart → impaired filling of right ventricle → blood backs up into vena cava → JVD. May be seen with constrictive pericarditis, restrictive cardiomyopathies, right atrial or ventricular tumors.
Hereditary hemorrhagic telangiectasia	Also known as Osler-Weber-Rendu syndrome. Inherited disorder of blood vessels. Findings: blanching lesions (telangiectasias) on skin and mucous membranes, recurrent epistaxis, skin discolorations, arteriovenous malformations (AVMs), GI bleeding, hematuria.

▶ CARDIOVASCULAR—PHARMACOLOGY

Hypertension treatment

Primary (essential) hypertension	Thiazide diuretics, ACE inhibitors, angiotensin II receptor blockers (ARBs), dihydropyridine Ca^{2+} channel blockers.	
Hypertension with heart failure	Diuretics, ACE inhibitors/ARBs, β-blockers (compensated HF), aldosterone antagonists.	β-blockers must be used cautiously in decompensated HF and are contraindicated in cardiogenic shock. In HF, ARBs may be combined with the neprilysin inhibitor sacubitril.
Hypertension with diabetes mellitus	ACE inhibitors/ARBs, Ca^{2+} channel blockers, thiazide diuretics, β-blockers.	ACE inhibitors/ARBs are protective against diabetic nephropathy.
Hypertension in asthma	ARBs, Ca^{2+} channel blockers, thiazide diuretics, selective β-blockers.	Avoid nonselective β-blockers to prevent $β_2$-receptor–induced bronchoconstriction. Avoid ACE inhibitors to prevent confusion between drug or asthma-related cough.
Hypertension in pregnancy	Hydralazine, labetalol, methyldopa, nifedipine.	"He likes my neonate."

Calcium channel blockers	Amlodipine, clevidipine, nicardipine, nifedipine, nimodipine (dihydropyridines, act on vascular smooth muscle); diltiazem, verapamil (non-dihydropyridines, act on heart).
MECHANISM	Block voltage-dependent L-type calcium channels of cardiac and smooth muscle → ↓ muscle contractility. Vascular smooth muscle—amlodipine = nifedipine > diltiazem > verapamil. Heart—verapamil > diltiazem > amlodipine = nifedipine (verapamil = ventricle).
CLINICAL USE	Dihydropyridines (except nimodipine): hypertension, angina (including Prinzmetal), Raynaud phenomenon. Nimodipine: subarachnoid hemorrhage (prevents cerebral vasospasm). Nicardipine, clevidipine: hypertensive urgency or emergency. Non-dihydropyridines: hypertension, angina, atrial fibrillation/flutter.
ADVERSE EFFECTS	Non-dihydropyridine: cardiac depression, AV block, hyperprolactinemia, constipation, gingival hyperplasia. Dihydropyridine: peripheral edema, flushing, dizziness.

Hydralazine	
MECHANISM	↑ cGMP → smooth muscle relaxation. Vasodilates arterioles > veins; afterload reduction.
CLINICAL USE	Severe hypertension (particularly acute), HF (with organic nitrate). Safe to use during pregnancy. Frequently coadministered with a β-blocker to prevent reflex tachycardia.
ADVERSE EFFECTS	Compensatory tachycardia (contraindicated in angina/CAD), fluid retention, headache, angina. SLE-like syndrome.

Hypertensive emergency	Treat with clevidipine, fenoldopam, labetalol, nicardipine, or nitroprusside.
Nitroprusside	Short acting; ↑ cGMP via direct release of NO. Can cause cyanide toxicity (releases cyanide).
Fenoldopam	Dopamine D_1 receptor agonist—coronary, peripheral, renal, and splanchnic vasodilation. ↓ BP, ↑ natriuresis. Also used postoperatively as an antihypertensive. Can cause hypotension and tachycardia.

Nitrates	Nitroglycerin, isosorbide dinitrate, isosorbide mononitrate.
MECHANISM	Vasodilate by ↑ NO in vascular smooth muscle → ↑ in cGMP and smooth muscle relaxation. Dilate veins >> arteries. ↓ preload.
CLINICAL USE	Angina, acute coronary syndrome, pulmonary edema.
ADVERSE EFFECTS	Reflex tachycardia (treat with β-blockers), hypotension, flushing, headache, "Monday disease" in industrial exposure: development of tolerance for the vasodilating action during the work week and loss of tolerance over the weekend → tachycardia, dizziness, headache upon reexposure. Contraindicated in right ventricular infarction.

Antianginal therapy   Goal is reduction of myocardial O_2 consumption (MVO_2) by ↓ 1 or more of the determinants of MVO_2: end-diastolic volume, BP, HR, contractility.

COMPONENT	NITRATES	β-BLOCKERS	NITRATES + β-BLOCKERS
End-diastolic volume	↓	No effect or ↑	No effect or ↓
Blood pressure	↓	↓	↓
Contractility	No effect	↓	Little/no effect
Heart rate	↑ (reflex response)	↓	No effect or ↓
Ejection time	↓	↑	Little/no effect
MVO_2	↓	↓	↓↓

Verapamil is similar to β-blockers in effect.
Pindolol and acebutolol are partial β-agonists that should be used with caution in angina.

Ranolazine

MECHANISM	Inhibits the late phase of sodium current thereby reducing diastolic wall tension and oxygen consumption. Does not affect heart rate or contractility.
CLINICAL USE	Angina refractory to other medical therapies.
ADVERSE EFFECTS	Constipation, dizziness, headache, nausea, QT prolongation.

Milrinone

MECHANISM	Selective PDE-3 inhibitor. In cardiomyocytes: ↑ cAMP accumulation → ↑ Ca^{2+} influx → ↑ inotropy and chronotropy. In vascular smooth muscle: ↑ cAMP accumulation → inhibition of MLCK activity → general vasodilation.
CLINICAL USE	Short-term use in acute decompensated HF.
ADVERSE EFFECTS	Arrhythmias, hypotension.

Lipid-lowering agents

DRUG	LDL	HDL	TRIGLYCERIDES	MECHANISMS OF ACTION	ADVERSE EFFECTS/PROBLEMS
HMG-CoA reductase inhibitors (eg, lovastatin, pravastatin)	↓↓↓	↑	↓	Inhibit conversion of HMG-CoA to mevalonate, a cholesterol precursor; ↓ mortality in CAD patients	Hepatotoxicity (↑ LFTs), myopathy (esp. when used with fibrates or niacin)
Bile acid resins Cholestyramine, colestipol, colesevelam	↓↓	Slightly ↑	Slightly ↑	Prevent intestinal reabsorption of bile acids; liver must use cholesterol to make more	GI upset, ↓ absorption of other drugs and fat-soluble vitamins
Ezetimibe	↓↓	↑/—	↓/—	Prevent cholesterol absorption at small intestine brush border	Rare ↑ LFTs, diarrhea
Fibrates Gemfibrozil, bezafibrate, fenofibrate	↓	↑	↓↓↓	Upregulate LPL → ↑ TG clearance; Activates PPAR-α to induce HDL synthesis	Myopathy (↑ risk with statins), cholesterol gallstones (via inhibition of cholesterol 7α-hydroxylase)
Niacin (vitamin B_3)	↓↓	↑↑	↓	Inhibits lipolysis (hormone-sensitive lipase) in adipose tissue; reduces hepatic VLDL synthesis	Red, flushed face, which is ↓ by NSAIDs or long-term use; Hyperglycemia; Hyperuricemia
PCSK9 inhibitors Alirocumab, evolocumab	↓↓↓	↑	↓	Inactivation of LDL-receptor degradation, increasing amount of LDL removed from bloodstream	Myalgias, delirium, dementia, other neurocognitive effects

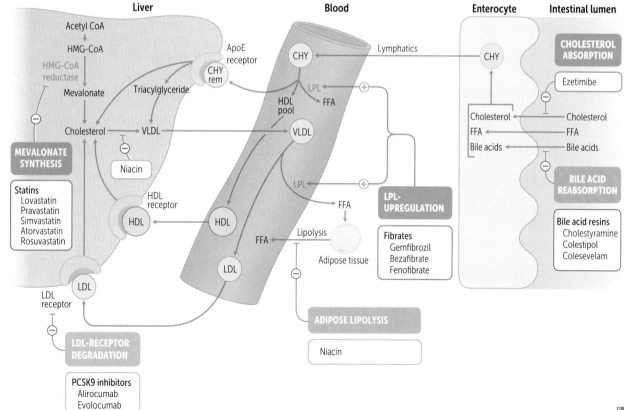

Cardiac glycosides	Digoxin.
MECHANISM	Direct inhibition of Na^+/K^+ ATPase → indirect inhibition of Na^+/Ca^{2+} exchanger. ↑ $[Ca^{2+}]_i$ → positive inotropy. Stimulates vagus nerve → ↓ HR.

CLINICAL USE	HF (↑ contractility); atrial fibrillation (↓ conduction at AV node and depression of SA node).
ADVERSE EFFECTS	Cholinergic—nausea, vomiting, diarrhea, blurry yellow vision (think van Gogh), arrhythmias, AV block. Can lead to hyperkalemia, which indicates poor prognosis. Factors predisposing to toxicity: renal failure (↓ excretion), hypokalemia (permissive for digoxin binding at K^+-binding site on Na^+/K^+ ATPase), drugs that displace digoxin from tissue-binding sites, and ↓ clearance (eg, verapamil, amiodarone, quinidine).
ANTIDOTE	Slowly normalize K^+, cardiac pacer, anti-digoxin Fab fragments, Mg^{2+}.

Antiarrhythmics— sodium channel blockers (class I)	Slow or block (↓) conduction (especially in depolarized cells). ↓ slope of phase 0 depolarization. Are state dependent (selectively depress tissue that is frequently depolarized [eg, tachycardia]).	

Class IA	Quinidine, Procainamide, Disopyramide. "The Queen Proclaims Diso's pyramid."	**Class IA**
MECHANISM	↑ AP duration, ↑ effective refractory period (ERP) in ventricular action potential, ↑ QT interval, some potassium channel blocking effects.	0 mV ⎯⎯⎯ Slope of phase 0 I_{Na}
CLINICAL USE	Both atrial and ventricular arrhythmias, especially re-entrant and ectopic SVT and VT.	
ADVERSE EFFECTS	Cinchonism (headache, tinnitus with quinidine), reversible SLE-like syndrome (procainamide), HF (disopyramide), thrombocytopenia, torsades de pointes due to ↑ QT interval.	
Class IB	Lidocaine, MexileTine. "I'd Buy Liddy's Mexican Tacos."	**Class IB**
MECHANISM	↓ AP duration. Preferentially affect ischemic or depolarized Purkinje and ventricular tissue. Phenytoin can also fall into the IB category.	0 mV ⎯⎯⎯ Slope of phase 0 I_{Na}
CLINICAL USE	Acute ventricular arrhythmias (especially post-MI), digitalis-induced arrhythmias. IB is Best post-MI.	
ADVERSE EFFECTS	CNS stimulation/depression, cardiovascular depression.	
Class IC	Flecainide, Propafenone. "Can I have Fries, Please."	**Class IC**
MECHANISM	Significantly prolongs ERP in AV node and accessory bypass tracts. No effect on ERP in Purkinje and ventricular tissue. Minimal effect on AP duration.	0 mV ⎯⎯⎯ Slope of phase 0 I_{Na}
CLINICAL USE	SVTs, including atrial fibrillation. Only as a last resort in refractory VT.	
ADVERSE EFFECTS	Proarrhythmic, especially post-MI (contraindicated). IC is Contraindicated in structural and ischemic heart disease.	

Antiarrhythmics— β-blockers (class II)	Metoprolol, propranolol, esmolol, atenolol, timolol, carvedilol.
MECHANISM	Decrease SA and AV nodal activity by ↓ cAMP, ↓ Ca^{2+} currents. Suppress abnormal pacemakers by ↓ slope of phase 4. AV node particularly sensitive—↑ PR interval. Esmolol very short acting.
CLINICAL USE	SVT, ventricular rate control for atrial fibrillation and atrial flutter.
ADVERSE EFFECTS	Impotence, exacerbation of COPD and asthma, cardiovascular effects (bradycardia, AV block, HF), CNS effects (sedation, sleep alterations). May mask the signs of hypoglycemia. Metoprolol can cause dyslipidemia. Propranolol can exacerbate vasospasm in Prinzmetal angina. β-blockers (except the nonselective α- and β-antagonists carvedilol and labetalol) cause unopposed $α_1$-agonism if given alone for pheochromocytoma or cocaine toxicity. Treat β-blocker overdose with saline, atropine, glucagon.

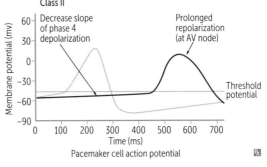

Pacemaker cell action potential

Antiarrhythmics— potassium channel blockers (class III)	Amiodarone, Ibutilide, Dofetilide, Sotalol.	AIDS.
MECHANISM	↑ AP duration, ↑ ERP, ↑ QT interval.	
CLINICAL USE	Atrial fibrillation, atrial flutter; ventricular tachycardia (amiodarone, sotalol).	
ADVERSE EFFECTS	Sotalol—torsades de pointes, excessive β blockade. Ibutilide—torsades de pointes. Amiodarone—pulmonary fibrosis, hepatotoxicity, hypothyroidism or hyperthyroidism (amiodarone is 40% iodine by weight), acts as hapten (corneal deposits, blue/gray skin deposits resulting in photodermatitis), neurologic effects, constipation, cardiovascular effects (bradycardia, heart block, HF).	Remember to check PFTs, LFTs, and TFTs when using amiodarone. Amiodarone is lipophilic and has class I, II, III, and IV effects.

Class III

0 mV

Markedly prolonged repolarization (I_K)

−85 mV

Cell action potential

Antiarrhythmics— calcium channel blockers (class IV)	Verapamil, diltiazem.
MECHANISM	↓ conduction velocity, ↑ ERP, ↑ PR interval.
CLINICAL USE	Prevention of nodal arrhythmias (eg, SVT), rate control in atrial fibrillation.
ADVERSE EFFECTS	Constipation, flushing, edema, cardiovascular effects (HF, AV block, sinus node depression).

Other antiarrhythmics

Adenosine	↑ K⁺ out of cells → hyperpolarizing the cell and ↓ I_{Ca}, decreasing AV node conduction. Drug of choice in diagnosing/terminating certain forms of SVT. Very short acting (~ 15 sec). Effects blunted by theophylline and caffeine (both are adenosine receptor antagonists). Adverse effects include flushing, hypotension, chest pain, sense of impending doom, bronchospasm.
Mg^{2+}	Effective in torsades de pointes and digoxin toxicity.

Ivabradine

MECHANISM	Selective inhibition of funny sodium channels (I_f), prolonging slow depolarization phase (phase 4). ↓ SA node firing; negative chronotropic effect without inotropy. Reduces cardiac O_2 requirement.
CLINICAL USE	Chronic stable angina in patients who cannot take β-blockers. Chronic HF with reduced ejection fraction.
ADVERSE EFFECTS	Luminous phenomena/visual brightness, hypertension, bradycardia.

▶ NOTES

Endocrine

"If you skew the endocrine system, you lose the pathways to self."
—Hilary Mantel

"We have learned that there is an endocrinology of elation and despair, a chemistry of mystical insight, and, in relation to the autonomic nervous system, a meteorology and even . . . an astro-physics of changing moods."
—Aldous (Leonard) Huxley

"Chocolate causes certain endocrine glands to secrete hormones that affect your feelings and behavior by making you happy."
—Elaine Sherman, *Book of Divine Indulgences*

The endocrine system comprises widely distributed organs that work in a highly integrated manner to orchestrate a state of hormonal equilibrium within the body. Generally speaking, endocrine diseases can be classified either as diseases of underproduction or overproduction, or as conditions involving the development of mass lesions—which themselves may be associated with underproduction or overproduction of hormones. Therefore, study the endocrine system first by learning the glands, their hormones, and their regulation, and then by integrating disease manifestations with diagnosis and management. Take time to learn the multisystem connections.

▶ ENDOCRINE—EMBRYOLOGY

Thyroid development

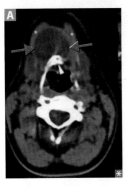

Thyroid diverticulum arises from floor of primitive pharynx and descends into neck. Connected to tongue by thyroglossal duct, which normally disappears but may persist as cysts or the pyramidal lobe of thyroid. Foramen cecum is normal remnant of thyroglossal duct.

Most common ectopic thyroid tissue site is the tongue (lingual thyroid). Removal may result in hypothyroidism if it is the only thyroid tissue present.

Thyroglossal duct cyst A presents as an anterior midline neck mass that moves with swallowing or protrusion of the tongue (vs persistent cervical sinus leading to branchial cleft cyst in lateral neck).

Thyroid follicular cells are derived from endoderm; parafollicular cells (aka, **C** cells, produce **C**alcitonin) are derived from neural crest.

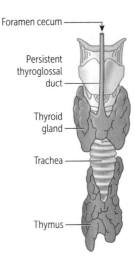

▶ ENDOCRINE—ANATOMY

Adrenal cortex and medulla

Adrenal cortex (derived from mesoderm) and medulla (derived from neural crest).

ANATOMY	HISTOLOGY			1° REGULATION BY	HORMONE CLASS	1° HORMONE PRODUCED
	Zona **G**lomerulosa			Angiotensin II	Mineralocorticoids	Aldosterone
CORTEX	Zona **F**asciculata			ACTH, CRH	Glucocorticoids	Cortisol
	Zona **R**eticularis			ACTH, CRH	Androgens	DHEA
MEDULLA	Chromaffin cells			Preganglionic sympathetic fibers	Catecholamines	Epi, NE

GFR corresponds with **S**alt (mineralocorticoids), **S**ugar (glucocorticoids), and **S**ex (androgens). "The deeper you go, **the sweeter it gets**."

Pituitary gland

Anterior pituitary (adenohypophysis)	Secretes FSH, LH, ACTH, TSH, prolactin, GH, and β-endorphin. Melanotropin (MSH) secreted from intermediate lobe of pituitary. Derived from oral ectoderm (Rathke pouch). ▪ α subunit—hormone subunit common to TSH, LH, FSH, and hCG. ▪ β subunit—determines hormone specificity.	ACTH, MSH, and β-endorphin are derivatives of proopiomelanocortin. **FLAT PiG**: FSH, LH, ACTH, TSH, PRL, GH. **B-FLAT**: Basophils—FSH, LH, ACTH, TSH. Acidophils: GH, PRL.
Posterior pituitary (neurohypophysis)	Stores and releases vasopressin (antidiuretic hormone, or ADH) and oxytocin, both made in the hypothalamus (supraoptic and paraventricular nuclei) and transported to posterior pituitary via neurophysins (carrier proteins). Derived from neuroectoderm.	

Endocrine pancreas cell types	Islets of Langerhans are collections of α, β, and δ endocrine cells. Islets arise from pancreatic buds. ▪ α = glucagon (peripheral) ▪ β = insulin (central) ▪ δ = somatostatin (interspersed)	Insulin (β cells) inside.

Insulin

SYNTHESIS	Preproinsulin (synthesized in RER) → cleavage of "presignal" → proinsulin (stored in secretory granules) → cleavage of proinsulin → exocytosis of insulin and C-peptide equally. Insulin and C-peptide are ↑ in insulinoma and sulfonylurea use, whereas exogenous insulin lacks C-peptide.

Proinsulin — C peptide — S–S — α-chain — β-chain

FUNCTION	Released from pancreatic β cells. Binds insulin receptors (tyrosine kinase activity ❶), inducing glucose uptake (carrier-mediated transport) into insulin-dependent tissue ❷ and gene transcription.

Anabolic effects of insulin:
- ↑ glucose transport in skeletal muscle and adipose tissue
- ↑ glycogen synthesis and storage
- ↑ triglyceride synthesis
- ↑ Na^+ retention (kidneys)
- ↑ protein synthesis (muscles)
- ↑ cellular uptake of K^+ and amino acids
- ↓ glucagon release
- ↓ lipolysis in adipose tissue

Unlike glucose, insulin does not cross placenta.

Insulin-dependent glucose transporters:
- GLUT4: adipose tissue, striated muscle (exercise can also ↑ GLUT4 expression)

Insulin-independent transporters:
- GLUT1: RBCs, brain, cornea, placenta
- GLUT2 (**bidirectional**): β islet cells, liver, kidney, small intestine (think 2-way street)
- GLUT3: brain, placenta
- GLUT5 (**Fructose**): spermatocytes, GI tract
- SGLT1/SGLT2 (Na^+-glucose cotransporters): kidney, small intestine

Brain utilizes glucose for metabolism but ketone bodies during starvation. RBCs utilize glucose, as they lack mitochondria for aerobic metabolism.

BRICK LIPS (insulin-independent glucose uptake): **B**rain, **R**BCs, **I**ntestine, **C**ornea, **K**idney, **L**iver, **I**slet (β) cells, **P**lacenta, **S**permatocytes

REGULATION	Glucose is the major regulator of insulin release. ↑ insulin response with oral vs IV glucose due to incretins (eg, glucagon-like peptide 1 [GLP-1], glucose-dependent insulinotropic polypeptide [GIP]), which are released after meals and ↑ β cell sensitivity to glucose. Release ↓ by α_2, ↑ by β_2 (2 = regulates insulin)

Glucose enters β cells ❸ → ↑ ATP generated from glucose metabolism ❹ closes K^+ channels (target of sulfonylureas) ❺ and depolarizes β cell membrane ❻. Voltage-gated Ca^{2+} channels open → Ca^{2+} influx ❼ and stimulation of insulin exocytosis ❽.

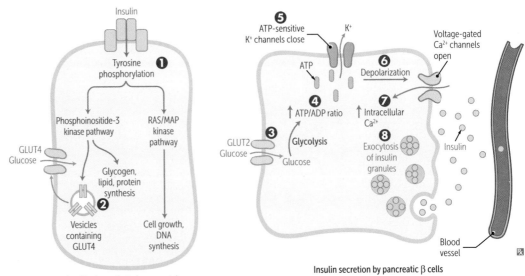

Insulin-dependent glucose uptake

Insulin secretion by pancreatic β cells

Glucagon

SOURCE	Made by α cells of pancreas.
FUNCTION	Promotes glycogenolysis, gluconeogenesis, lipolysis, and ketone production. Elevates blood sugar levels to maintain homeostasis when concentration of bloodstream glucose falls too low (ie, fasting state).
REGULATION	Secreted in response to hypoglycemia. Inhibited by insulin, hyperglycemia, and somatostatin.

Hypothalamic-pituitary hormones

HORMONE	FUNCTION	CLINICAL NOTES
ADH	↑ water permeability of distal convoluted tubule and collecting duct cells in kidney to ↑ water reabsorption	Stimulus for secretion is ↑ plasma osmolality, except in cases of SIADH, where ADH is inappropriately elevated despite ↓ plasma osmolality.
CRH	↑ ACTH, MSH, β-endorphin	↓ in chronic exogenous steroid use.
Dopamine	↓ prolactin, TSH	Dopamine antagonists (eg, antipsychotics) can cause galactorrhea due to hyperprolactinemia.
GHRH	↑ GH	Analog (tesamorelin) used to treat HIV-associated lipodystrophy.
GnRH	↑ FSH, LH	Suppressed by hyperprolactinemia. Tonic GnRH suppresses HPG axis. Pulsatile GnRH leads to puberty, fertility.
MSH	↑ melanogenesis by melanocytes	Causes hyperpigmentation in Cushing disease, as MSH and ACTH share the same precursor molecule, proopiomelanocortin.
Oxytocin	Causes uterine contractions during labor. Responsible for milk letdown reflex in response to suckling.	
Prolactin	↓ GnRH	Pituitary prolactinoma → amenorrhea, osteoporosis, hypogonadism, galactorrhea.
Somatostatin	↓ GH, TSH	Analogs used to treat acromegaly.
TRH	↑ TSH, prolactin	↑ TRH (eg, in 1°/2° hypothyroidism) may increase prolactin secretion → galactorrhea.

Prolactin

SOURCE	Secreted mainly by anterior pituitary.	Structurally homologous to growth hormone.
FUNCTION	Stimulates milk production in breast; inhibits ovulation in females and spermatogenesis in males by inhibiting GnRH synthesis and release.	Excessive amounts of prolactin associated with ↓ libido.
REGULATION	Prolactin secretion from anterior pituitary is tonically inhibited by dopamine from tuberoinfundibular pathway of hypothalamus. Prolactin in turn inhibits its own secretion by ↑ dopamine synthesis and secretion from hypothalamus. TRH ↑ prolactin secretion (eg, in 1° or 2° hypothyroidism).	Dopamine agonists (eg, bromocriptine) inhibit prolactin secretion and can be used in treatment of prolactinoma. Dopamine antagonists (eg, most antipsychotics) and estrogens (eg, OCPs, pregnancy) stimulate prolactin secretion.

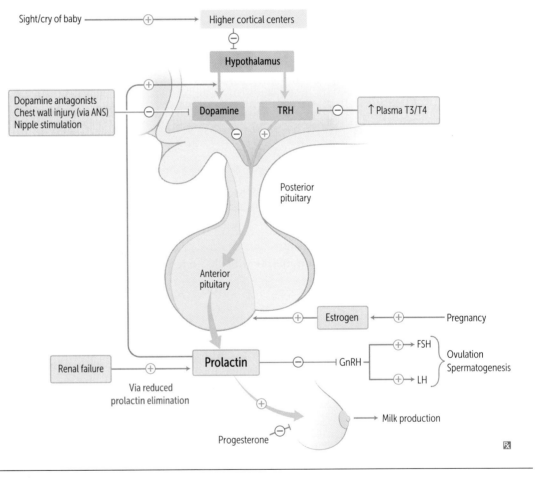

Growth hormone (somatotropin)

SOURCE	Secreted by anterior pituitary.	
FUNCTION	Stimulates linear growth and muscle mass through IGF-1 (somatomedin C) secretion by liver. ↑ insulin resistance (diabetogenic).	Somatostatin keeps your growth static. Somatomedin mediates your growth.
REGULATION	Released in pulses in response to growth hormone–releasing hormone (GHRH). Secretion ↑ during exercise, deep sleep, puberty, hypoglycemia. Secretion inhibited by glucose and somatostatin release via negative feedback by somatomedin.	Excess secretion of GH (eg, pituitary adenoma) may cause acromegaly (adults) or gigantism (children). Treat with somatostatin analogs (eg, octreotide) or surgery.

Appetite regulation

Ghrelin	Stimulates hunger (orexigenic effect) and GH release (via GH secretagogue receptor). Produced by stomach. Sleep deprivation or Prader-Willi syndrome → ↑ ghrelin production.	Ghrelin makes you hun**ghre** and **ghre**ow (grow). Acts via lateral area of hypothalamus to ↑ appetite (hunger center).
Leptin	Satiety hormone. Produced by adipose tissue. Mutation of leptin gene → congenital obesity. Sleep deprivation or starvation → ↓ leptin production.	Leptin keeps you t**hin**. Acts via ventromedial area of hypothalamus to ↓ appetite (satiety center).
Endocannabinoids	Act at cannabinoid receptors in hypothalamus and nucleus accumbens, two key brain areas for the homeostatic and hedonic control of food intake → ↑ appetite.	Exogenous cannabinoids cause "the munchies."

Antidiuretic hormone (vasopressin)

SOURCE	Synthesized in hypothalamus (supraoptic and paraventricular nuclei), stored and secreted by posterior pituitary.	
FUNCTION	Regulates serum osmolality (V_2-receptors) and blood pressure (V_1-receptors). Primary function is serum osmolality regulation (ADH ↓ serum osmolality, ↑ urine osmolality) via regulation of aquaporin channel insertion in principal cells of renal collecting duct.	ADH level is ↓ in central diabetes insipidus (DI), normal or ↑ in nephrogenic DI. Nephrogenic DI can be caused by mutation in V_2-receptor. Desmopressin (ADH analog) is a treatment for central DI and nocturnal enuresis.
REGULATION	Osmoreceptors in hypothalamus (1°); hypovolemia.	

Adrenal steroids and congenital adrenal hyperplasias

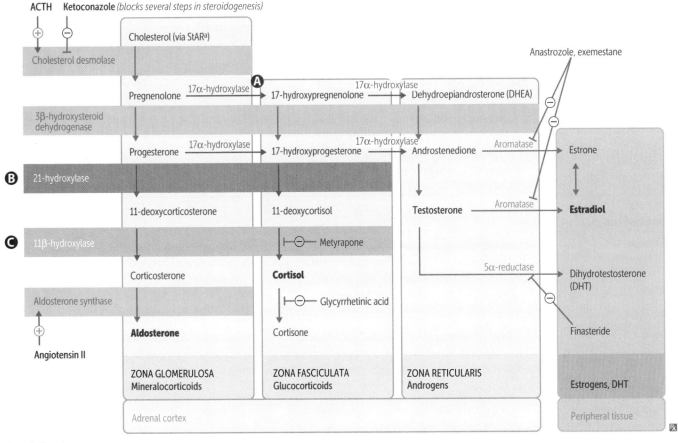

[a] Rate-limiting step.

ENZYME DEFICIENCY	MINERALOCORTICOIDS	CORTISOL	SEX HORMONES	BP	[K⁺]	LABS	PRESENTATION
Ⓐ 17α-hydroxylase[a]	↑	↓	↓	↑	↓	↓ androstenedione	XY: ambiguous genitalia, undescended testes XX: lacks 2° sexual development
Ⓑ 21-hydroxylase[a]	↓	↓	↑	↓	↑	↑ renin activity ↑ 17-hydroxy-progesterone	Most common Presents in infancy (salt wasting) or childhood (precocious puberty) XX: virilization
Ⓒ 11β-hydroxylase[a]	↓ aldosterone ↑ 11-deoxycorti-costerone (results in ↑ BP)	↓	↑	↑	↓	↓ renin activity	XX: virilization

[a] All congenital adrenal enzyme deficiencies are characterized by skin hyperpigmentation (due to ↑ MSH production, which is coproduced and secreted with ACTH) and bilateral adrenal gland enlargement (due to ↑ ACTH stimulation).
If deficient enzyme starts with 1, it causes hypertension; if deficient enzyme ends with 1, it causes virilization in females.

Cortisol

SOURCE	Adrenal zona fasciculata.	Bound to corticosteroid-binding globulin.

FUNCTION	↑ Appetite
	↑ Blood pressure:
	  ▪ Upregulates α_1-receptors on arterioles → ↑ sensitivity to norepinephrine and epinephrine (permissive action)
	  ▪ At high concentrations, can bind to mineralocorticoid (aldosterone) receptors
	↑ Insulin resistance (diabetogenic)
	↑ Gluconeogenesis, lipolysis, and proteolysis (↓ glucose utilization)
	↓ Fibroblast activity (poor wound healing, ↓ collagen synthesis, ↑ striae)
	↓ Inflammatory and Immune responses:
	  ▪ Inhibits production of leukotrienes and prostaglandins
	  ▪ Inhibits WBC adhesion → neutrophilia
	  ▪ Blocks histamine release from mast cells
	  ▪ Eosinopenia, lymphopenia
	  ▪ Blocks IL-2 production
	↓ Bone formation (↓ osteoblast activity)
		Cortisol is a **A BIG FIB**.
		Exogenous corticosteroids can cause reactivation of TB and candidiasis (blocks IL-2 production).

REGULATION	CRH (hypothalamus) stimulates ACTH release (pituitary) → cortisol production in adrenal zona fasciculata. Excess cortisol ↓ CRH, ACTH, and cortisol secretion.	Chronic stress induces prolonged secretion.

Calcium homeostasis	Plasma Ca^{2+} exists in three forms:
	  ▪ Ionized/free (~ 45%, active form)
	  ▪ Bound to albumin (~ 40%)
	  ▪ Bound to anions (~ 15%)
		↑ in pH → ↑ affinity of albumin (↑ negative charge) to bind Ca^{2+} → hypocalcemia (eg, cramps, pain, paresthesias, carpopedal spasm).
		Ionized/free Ca^{2+} is 1° regulator of PTH; changes in pH alter PTH secretion, whereas changes in albumin do not.

Parathyroid hormone

SOURCE	Chief cells of parathyroid.
FUNCTION	↑ bone resorption of Ca^{2+} and PO_4^{3-}. ↑ kidney reabsorption of Ca^{2+} in distal convoluted tubule. ↓ reabsorption of PO_4^{3-} in proximal convoluted tubule. ↑ 1,25-$(OH)_2 D_3$ (calcitriol) production by stimulating kidney 1α-hydroxylase in proximal convoluted tubule.	PTH ↑ serum Ca^{2+}, ↓ serum (PO_4^{3-}), ↑ urine (PO_4^{3-}), ↑ urine cAMP. ↑ RANK-L (receptor activator of NF-κB ligand) secreted by osteoblasts and osteocytes. Binds RANK (receptor) on osteoclasts and their precursors to stimulate osteoclasts and ↑ Ca^{2+} → bone resorption. Intermittent PTH release can also stimulate bone formation. PTH = Phosphate-Trashing Hormone. PTH-related peptide (PTHrP) functions like PTH and is commonly increased in malignancies (eg, squamous cell carcinoma of the lung, renal cell carcinoma).
REGULATION	↓ serum Ca^{2+} → ↑ PTH secretion. ↑ serum PO_4^{3-} → ↑ PTH secretion. ↓ serum Mg^{2+} → ↑ PTH secretion. ↓↓ serum Mg^{2+} → ↓ PTH secretion. Common causes of ↓ Mg^{2+} include diarrhea, aminoglycosides, diuretics, alcohol abuse.	

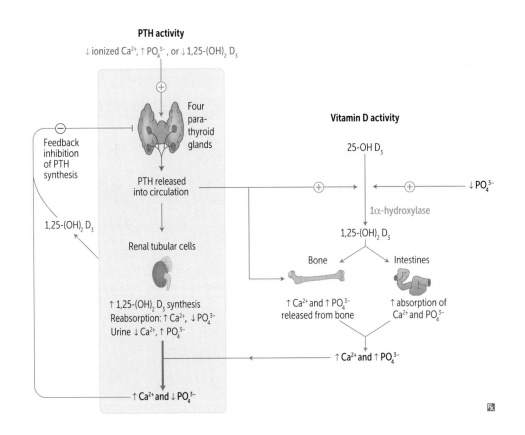

Calcitonin

SOURCE	Parafollicular cells (C cells) of thyroid.	Calcitonin opposes actions of PTH. Not important in normal Ca^{2+} homeostasis. Calcitonin tones down serum Ca^{2+} levels and keeps it in bones.
FUNCTION	↓ bone resorption of Ca^{2+}.	
REGULATION	↑ serum Ca^{2+} → calcitonin secretion.	

Thyroid hormones (T_3/T_4)

Iodine-containing hormones that control the body's metabolic rate.

SOURCE	Follicles of thyroid. 5'-deiodinase converts T_4 (the major thyroid product) to T_3 in peripheral tissue (5, 4, 3). Peripheral conversion is inhibited by glucocorticoids, β-blockers and propylthiouracil (PTU). Functions of thyroid peroxidase include oxidation, organification of iodide and coupling of monoiodotyrosine (MIT) and diiodotyrosine (DIT). Inhibited by PTU and methimazole. DIT + DIT = T_4. DIT + MIT = T_3. Wolff-Chaikoff effect—excess iodine temporarily ⊖ thyroid peroxidase → ↓ T_3/T_4 production.
FUNCTION	Only free hormone is active. T_3 binds nuclear receptor with greater affinity than T_4. T_3 functions —6 B's:
	▪ **Brain** maturation
	▪ **Bone** growth (synergism with GH)
	▪ **β-adrenergic** effects. ↑ β_1 receptors in heart → ↑ CO, HR, SV, contractility; β-blockers alleviate adrenergic symptoms in thyrotoxicosis
	▪ **Basal** metabolic rate ↑ (via Na^+/K^+-ATPase activity → ↑ O_2 consumption, RR, body temperature)
	▪ **Blood** sugar (↑ glycogenolysis, gluconeogenesis)
	▪ **Break** down lipids (↑ lipolysis)
REGULATION	TRH ⊕ TSH release → ⊕ follicular cells. Thyroid-stimulating immunoglobulin (TSI) may ⊕ follicular cells in Graves disease.
	Negative feedback primarily by free T_3/T_4:
	▪ Anterior pituitary → ↓ sensitivity to TRH
	▪ Hypothalamus → ↓ TRH secretion
	Thyroxine-binding globulin (TBG) binds most T_3/T_4 in blood. Bound T_3/T_4 = inactive.
	▪ ↑ TBG in pregnancy, OCP use (estrogen → ↑ TBG) → ↑ total T_3/T_4
	▪ ↓ TBG in hepatic failure, steroids, nephrotic syndrome

Signaling pathways of endocrine hormones

cAMP	FSH, LH, ACTH, TSH, CRH, hCG, ADH (V_2-receptor), MSH, PTH, calcitonin, GHRH, glucagon, histamine (H_2-receptor)	FLAT ChAMP
cGMP	BNP, ANP, EDRF (NO)	BAD GraMPa Think vasodilators
IP$_3$	GnRH, Oxytocin, ADH (V_1-receptor), TRH, Histamine (H_1-receptor), Angiotensin II, Gastrin	GOAT HAG
Intracellular receptor	Progesterone, Estrogen, Testosterone, Cortisol, Aldosterone, T_3/T_4, Vitamin D	PET CAT on TV
Receptor tyrosine kinase	Insulin, IGF-1, FGF, PDGF, EGF	MAP kinase pathway Think Growth Factors
Nonreceptor tyrosine kinase	Prolactin, Immunomodulators (eg, cytokines IL-2, IL-6, IFN), GH, G-CSF, Erythropoietin, Thrombopoietin	JAK/STAT pathway Think acidophils and cytokines PIGGLET

Signaling pathways of steroid hormones

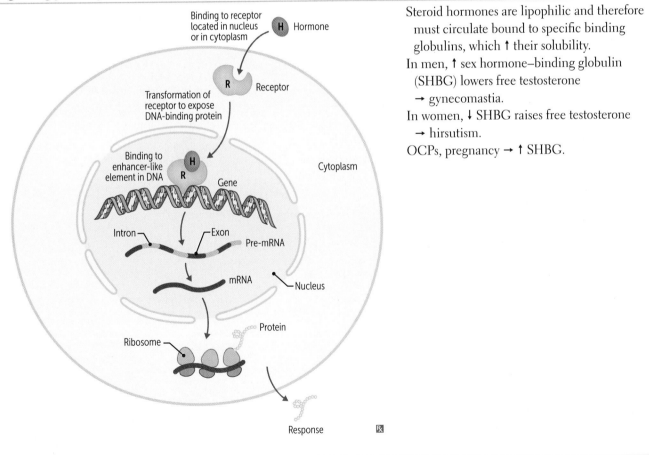

Steroid hormones are lipophilic and therefore must circulate bound to specific binding globulins, which ↑ their solubility.

In men, ↑ sex hormone–binding globulin (SHBG) lowers free testosterone → gynecomastia.

In women, ↓ SHBG raises free testosterone → hirsutism.

OCPs, pregnancy → ↑ SHBG.

▶ ENDOCRINE—PATHOLOGY

Cushing syndrome

ETIOLOGY	↑ cortisol due to a variety of causes: ▪ Exogenous corticosteroids—result in ↓ ACTH, bilateral adrenal atrophy. Most common cause. ▪ Primary adrenal adenoma, hyperplasia, or carcinoma—result in ↓ ACTH, atrophy of uninvolved adrenal gland. ▪ ACTH-secreting pituitary adenoma (Cushing disease); paraneoplastic ACTH secretion (eg, small cell lung cancer, bronchial carcinoids)—result in ↑ ACTH, bilateral adrenal hyperplasia. Cushing disease is responsible for the majority of endogenous cases of Cushing syndrome.
FINDINGS	Hypertension, weight gain, moon facies 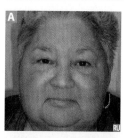, abdominal striae 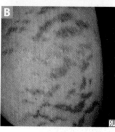 and truncal obesity, buffalo hump, skin changes (eg, thinning, striae), hirsutism, osteoporosis, hyperglycemia (insulin resistance), amenorrhea, immunosuppression. Can also present with pseudohyperaldosteronism.
DIAGNOSIS	Screening tests include: ↑ free cortisol on 24-hr urinalysis, ↑ midnight salivary cortisol, and no suppression with overnight low-dose dexamethasone test. Measure serum ACTH. If ↓, suspect adrenal tumor or exogenous glucocorticoids. If ↑, distinguish between Cushing disease and ectopic ACTH secretion (eg, from small cell lung cancer).

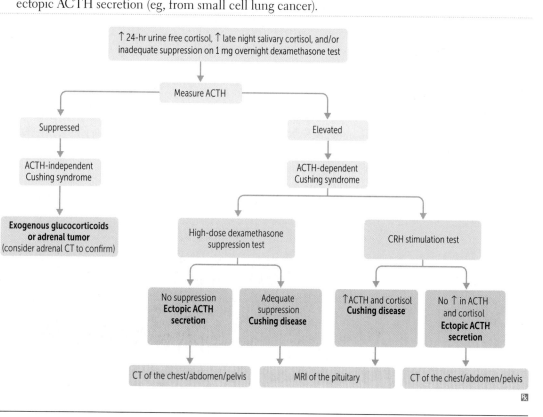

Adrenal insufficiency	Inability of adrenal glands to generate enough glucocorticoids +/– mineralocorticoids for the body's needs. Symptoms include weakness, fatigue, orthostatic hypotension, muscle aches, weight loss, GI disturbances, sugar and/or salt cravings. Treatment: glucocorticoid/mineralocorticoid replacement.	Diagnosis involves measurement of serum electrolytes, morning/random serum cortisol and ACTH (low cortisol, high ACTH in 1° adrenal insufficiency; low cortisol, low ACTH in 2°/3° adrenal insufficiency due to pituitary/hypothalamic disease), and response to ACTH stimulation test. Alternatively, can use metyrapone stimulation test: metyrapone blocks last step of cortisol synthesis (11-deoxycortisol → cortisol). Normal response is ↓ cortisol and compensatory ↑ ACTH and 11-deoxycortisol. In 1° adrenal insufficiency, ACTH is ↑ but 11-deoxycortisol remains ↓ after test. In 2°/3° adrenal insufficiency, both ACTH and 11-deoxycortisol remain ↓ after test.
Primary adrenal insufficiency 	Deficiency of aldosterone and cortisol production due to loss of gland function → hypotension (hyponatremic volume contraction), hyperkalemia, metabolic acidosis, skin and mucosal hyperpigmentation A (due to ↑ MSH, a byproduct of ACTH production from proopiomelanocortin). ▪ **Acute**—sudden onset (eg, due to massive hemorrhage). May present with shock in acute adrenal crisis. ▪ **Chronic**—**Addison disease**. Due to adrenal atrophy or destruction by disease (autoimmune destruction most common in the Western world; TB most common in the developing world).	Primary Pigments the skin/mucosa. Associated with autoimmune polyglandular syndromes. **Waterhouse-Friderichsen syndrome**—acute 1° adrenal insufficiency due to adrenal hemorrhage associated with septicemia (usually *Neisseria meningitidis*), DIC, endotoxic shock.
Secondary adrenal insufficiency	Seen with ↓ pituitary ACTH production. No skin/mucosal hyperpigmentation, no hyperkalemia (aldosterone synthesis preserved due to intact renin-angiotensin-aldosterone axis).	Secondary Spares the skin/mucosa.
Tertiary adrenal insufficiency	Seen in patients with chronic exogenous steroid use, precipitated by abrupt withdrawal. Aldosterone synthesis unaffected.	Tertiary from Treatment.
Hyperaldosteronism	Increased secretion of aldosterone from adrenal gland. Clinical features include hypertension, ↓ or normal K+, metabolic alkalosis. 1° hyperaldosteronism does not directly cause edema due to aldosterone escape mechanism. However, certain 2° causes of hyperaldosteronism (eg, heart failure) impair the aldosterone escape mechanism, leading to worsening of edema.	
Primary hyperaldosteronism	Seen with adrenal adenoma (Conn syndrome) or bilateral adrenal hyperplasia. ↑ aldosterone, ↓ renin. Causes resistant hypertension.	
Secondary hyperaldosteronism	Seen in patients with renovascular hypertension, juxtaglomerular cell tumors (renin-producing), and edema (eg, cirrhosis, heart failure, nephrotic syndrome).	

Neuroendocrine tumors

Heterogeneous group of neoplasms that begin in specialized cells called neuroendocrine cells (have traits similar to nerve cells and hormone-producing cells). Characteristics vary considerably depending on anatomical site, neuroendocrine cell(s) of origin (eg, enterochromaffin cells, enterochromaffin-like cells, insulin-producing β cells), and secretory products. Cells contain amine precursor uptake decarboxylase (APUD) and secrete different hormones (eg, serotonin, histamine, calcitonin, neuron-specific enolase [NSE], chromogranin A).

Most tumors arise in the GI system (eg, carcinoid, gastrinoma), pancreas (eg, insulinoma, glucagonoma), and lungs (eg, small cell carcinoma). Other organs include thyroid (eg, medullary carcinoma) and adrenals (eg, pheochromocytoma).

Neuroblastoma

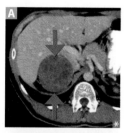

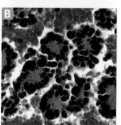

Most common tumor of the adrenal medulla in **children,** usually < 4 years old. Originates from Neural crest cells. Occurs anywhere along the sympathetic chain.

Most common presentation is abdominal distension and a firm, irregular mass that can cross the midline (vs Wilms tumor, which is smooth and unilateral). Less likely to develop hypertension than with pheochromocytoma (Neuroblastoma is Normotensive). Can also present with opsoclonus-myoclonus syndrome ("dancing eyes-dancing feet").

↑ HVA and VMA (catecholamine metabolites) in urine. Homer-Wright rosettes characteristic of neuroblastoma and medulloblastoma. Bombesin and NSE ⊕. Associated with overexpression of N-*myc* oncogene. Classified as an APUD tumor.

Pheochromocytoma

ETIOLOGY	Most common tumor of the adrenal medulla in **adults** . Derived from chromaffin cells (arise from neural crest). May be associated with germline mutations (eg, *NF-1, VHL, RET* [MEN 2A, 2B]).	**Rule of 10's:** 10% malignant 10% bilateral 10% extra-adrenal (eg, bladder wall, organ of Zuckerkandl) 10% calcify 10% kids
SYMPTOMS	Most tumors secrete epinephrine, norepinephrine, and dopamine, which can cause episodic hypertension. May also secrete EPO → polycythemia. Symptoms occur in "spells"—relapse and remit.	Episodic hyperadrenergic symptoms (5 P's): Pressure (↑ BP) Pain (headache) Perspiration Palpitations (tachycardia) Pallor
FINDINGS	↑ catecholamines and catecholamine metabolites (eg, metanephrines) in urine and plasma.	
TREATMENT	Irreversible α-antagonists (eg, phenoxybenzamine) followed by β-blockers prior to tumor resection. α-blockade must be achieved before giving β-blockers to avoid a hypertensive crisis. **A** before **B**.	**Phenoxybenzamine** (16 letters) is given for **pheochromocytoma** (also 16 letters).

VIPoma	Rare neuroendocrine tumor that secretes vasoactive intestinal peptide (VIP). Most commonly arises in pancreas. Associated with MEN-1. Primary symptom is secretory diarrhea. Associated with **WDHA** (**W**atery **D**iarrhea, **H**ypokalemia, **A**chlorhydria) syndrome.

Hypothyroidism vs hyperthyroidism

	Hypothyroidism	Hyperthyroidism
METABOLIC FINDINGS	Cold intolerance, ↓ sweating, weight gain (↓ basal metabolic rate → ↓ calorigenesis), hyponatremia (↓ free water clearance)	Heat intolerance, ↑ sweating, weight loss (↑ synthesis of Na^+-K^+ ATPase → ↑ basal metabolic rate → ↑ calorigenesis)
SKIN/HAIR FINDINGS	Dry, cool skin (due to ↓ blood flow); coarse, brittle hair; diffuse alopecia; brittle nails; puffy facies and generalized nonpitting edema (myxedema) due to ↑ GAGs in interstitial spaces → ↑ osmotic pressure → water retention	Warm, moist skin (due to vasodilation); fine hair; onycholysis (A); pretibial myxedema in Graves disease
OCULAR FINDINGS	Periorbital edema	Ophthalmopathy in Graves disease (including periorbital edema, exophthalmos), lid lag/retraction (↑ sympathetic stimulation of levator palpebrae superioris)
GASTROINTESTINAL FINDINGS	Constipation (↓ GI motility), ↓ appetite	Hyperdefecation/diarrhea (↑ GI motility), ↑ appetite
MUSCULOSKELETAL FINDINGS	Hypothyroid myopathy (proximal weakness, ↑ CK), carpal tunnel syndrome, myoedema (small lump rising on the surface of a muscle when struck with a hammer)	Thyrotoxic myopathy (proximal weakness, normal CK), osteoporosis/↑ fracture rate (T_3 directly stimulates bone resorption)
REPRODUCTIVE FINDINGS	Menorrhagia and/or oligomenorrhea; ↓ libido, infertility	Oligomenorrhea or amenorrhea, gynecomastia, ↓ libido, infertility
NEUROPSYCHIATRIC FINDINGS	Hypoactivity, lethargy, fatigue, weakness, depressed mood, ↓ reflexes (delayed/slow relaxing)	Hyperactivity, restlessness, anxiety, insomnia, fine tremors (due to ↑ β-adrenergic activity), ↑ reflexes (brisk)
CARDIOVASCULAR FINDINGS	Bradycardia, dyspnea on exertion (↓ cardiac output)	Tachycardia, palpitations, dyspnea, arrhythmias (eg, atrial fibrillation), chest pain and systolic HTN due to ↑ number and sensitivity of β-adrenergic receptors, ↑ expression of cardiac sarcolemmal ATPase and ↓ expression of phospholamban
LAB FINDINGS	↑ TSH (if 1°) ↓ free T_3 and T_4 Hypercholesterolemia (due to ↓ LDL receptor expression)	↓ TSH (if 1°) ↑ free T_3 and T_4 ↓ LDL, HDL, and total cholesterol

Hypothyroidism

Hashimoto thyroiditis	Most common cause of hypothyroidism in iodine-sufficient regions; an autoimmune disorder with antithyroid peroxidase (antimicrosomal) and antithyroglobulin antibodies. Associated with HLA-DR3, ↑ risk of non-Hodgkin lymphoma (typically of B-cell origin). May be hyperthyroid early in course due to thyrotoxicosis during follicular rupture. Histology: Hürthle cells, lymphoid aggregates with germinal centers 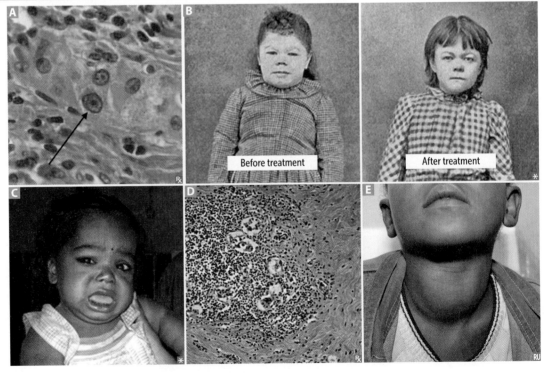. Findings: moderately enlarged, **nontender** thyroid.
Postpartum thyroiditis	Self-limited thyroiditis arising up to 1 year after delivery. Presents as transient hyperthyroidism, hypothyroidism, or hyperthyroidism followed by hypothyroidism. Majority of women are euthyroid following resolution. Thyroid usually painless and normal in size. Histology: lymphocytic infiltrate with occasional germinal center formation.
Congenital hypothyroidism (cretinism)	Severe fetal hypothyroidism due to antibody-mediated maternal hypothyroidism, thyroid agenesis, thyroid dysgenesis (most common cause in US), iodine deficiency, dyshormonogenetic goiter. Findings: Pot-bellied, Pale, Puffy-faced child with Protruding umbilicus, Protuberant tongue, and Poor brain development: the 6 P's B C.
Subacute granulomatous thyroiditis (de Quervain)	Self-limited disease often following a flu-like illness (eg, viral infection). May be hyperthyroid early in course, followed by hypothyroidism (permanent in ~15% of cases). Histology: granulomatous inflammation. Findings: ↑ ESR, jaw pain, very **tender** thyroid. (de Quervain is associated with **pain**.)
Riedel thyroiditis	Thyroid replaced by fibrous tissue with inflammatory infiltrate D. Fibrosis may extend to local structures (eg, trachea, esophagus), mimicking anaplastic carcinoma. ⅓ are hypothyroid. Considered a manifestation of IgG$_4$-related systemic disease (eg, autoimmune pancreatitis, retroperitoneal fibrosis, noninfectious aortitis). Findings: fixed, hard (rock-like), **painless** goiter.
Other causes	Iodine deficiency E, goitrogens (eg, amiodarone, lithium), Wolff-Chaikoff effect (thyroid gland downregulation in response to ↑ iodide).

Before treatment   After treatment

Hyperthyroidism

Graves disease	Most common cause of hyperthyroidism. Thyroid-stimulating immunoglobulin (IgG; type II hypersensitivity) stimulates TSH receptors on thyroid (hyperthyroidism, diffuse goiter) and dermal fibroblasts (pretibial myxedema). Infiltration of retroorbital space by activated T-cells → ↑ cytokines (eg, TNF-α, IFN-γ) → ↑ fibroblast secretion of hydrophilic GAGs → ↑ osmotic muscle swelling, muscle inflammation, and adipocyte count → exophthalmos . Often presents during stress (eg, pregnancy). Associated with HLA-DR3 and HLA-B8. Histology: tall, crowded follicular epithelial cells; scalloped colloid .
Toxic multinodular goiter	Focal patches of hyperfunctioning follicular cells distended with colloid working independently of TSH (due to TSH receptor mutations in 60% of cases). ↑ release of T_3 and T_4. Hot nodules are rarely malignant.
Thyroid storm	Uncommon but serious complication that occurs when hyperthyroidism is incompletely treated/untreated and then significantly worsens in the setting of acute stress such as infection, trauma, surgery. Presents with agitation, delirium, fever, diarrhea, coma, and tachyarrhythmia (cause of death). May see ↑ LFTs. Treat with the 4 P's: β-blockers (eg, Propranolol), Propylthiouracil, corticosteroids (eg, Prednisolone), Potassium iodide (Lugol iodine).
Jod-Basedow phenomenon	Thyrotoxicosis if a patient with iodine deficiency and partially autonomous thyroid tissue (eg, autonomous nodule) is made iodine replete. Can happen after iodine IV contrast. Opposite to Wolff-Chaikoff effect.

Causes of goiter

Smooth/diffuse	Nodular
Graves disease	Toxic multinodular goiter
Hashimoto thyroiditis	Thyroid adenoma
Iodine deficiency	Thyroid cancer
TSH-secreting pituitary adenoma	Thyroid cyst

Thyroid adenoma

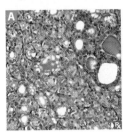

Benign solitary growth of the thyroid. Most are nonfunctional ("cold"), can rarely cause hyperthyroidism via autonomous thyroid hormone production ("hot" or "toxic"). Most common histology is follicular **A**; absence of capsular or vascular invasion (unlike follicular carcinoma).

Thyroid cancer

Typically diagnosed with fine needle aspiration; treated with thyroidectomy. Complications of surgery include hoarseness (due to recurrent laryngeal nerve damage), hypocalcemia (due to removal of parathyroid glands), and transection of recurrent and superior laryngeal nerves (during ligation of inferior thyroid artery and superior laryngeal artery, leading to dysphagia, dysphonia).

Papillary carcinoma

Most common, excellent prognosis. Empty-appearing nuclei with central clearing ("Orphan Annie" eyes) **A**, psam**M**oma bodies, nuclear grooves (**Papi** and **Moma** adopted **Orphan Annie**). ↑ risk with *RET/PTC* rearrangements and *BRAF* mutations, childhood irradiation.

Follicular carcinoma

Good prognosis. Invades thyroid capsule and vasculature (unlike follicular adenoma), uniform follicles; hematogenous spread is common. Associated with *RAS* mutation and *PAX8-PPAR-γ* translocations.

Medullary carcinoma

From parafollicular "C cells"; produces calcitonin, sheets of cells in an amyloid stroma (stains with Congo red **B**). Associated with MEN 2A and 2B (*RET* mutations).

Undifferentiated/ anaplastic carcinoma

Older patients; invades local structures, very poor prognosis.

Lymphoma

Associated with Hashimoto thyroiditis.

Diagnosing parathyroid disease

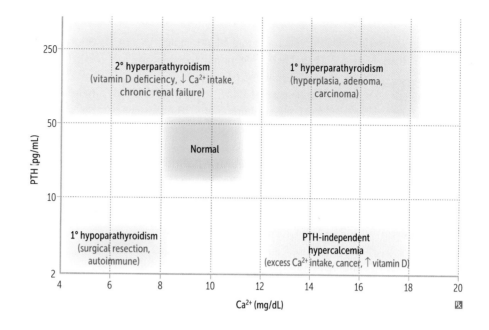

2° hyperparathyroidism (vitamin D deficiency, ↓ Ca²⁺ intake, chronic renal failure)

1° hyperparathyroidism (hyperplasia, adenoma, carcinoma)

Normal

1° hypoparathyroidism (surgical resection, autoimmune)

PTH-independent hypercalcemia (excess Ca²⁺ intake, cancer, ↑ vitamin D)

PTH (pg/mL): 250, 50, 10, 2

Ca²⁺ (mg/dL): 4, 6, 8, 10, 12, 14, 16, 18, 20

Hypoparathyroidism

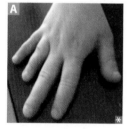

Due to accidental surgical excision of parathyroid glands, autoimmune destruction, or DiGeorge syndrome. Findings: tetany, hypocalcemia, hyperphosphatemia.

Chvostek sign—tapping of facial nerve (tap the Cheek) → contraction of facial muscles.

Trousseau sign—occlusion of brachial artery with BP cuff (cuff the Triceps) → carpal spasm.

Pseudohypoparathyroidism type 1A—unresponsiveness of kidney to PTH → hypocalcemia despite ↑ PTH levels. Presents as a constellation of physical findings known as Albright hereditary osteodystrophy: shortened 4th/5th digits 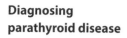, short stature, obesity, developmental delay. Autosomal dominant. Due to defective G$_s$ protein α-subunit causing end-organ resistance to PTH. Defect must be inherited from mother due to imprinting.

Pseudopseudohypoparathyroidism—physical exam features of Albright hereditary osteodystrophy but without end-organ PTH resistance (PTH level normal). Occurs when defective G$_s$ protein α-subunit is inherited from father.

Hyperparathyroidism

Primary hyperparathyroidism 	Usually due to parathyroid adenoma or hyperplasia. **Hypercalcemia**, hypercalciuria (renal **stones**), polyuria (**thrones**), hypophosphatemia, ↑ PTH, ↑ ALP, ↑ cAMP in urine. Most often asymptomatic. May present with weakness and constipation ("**groans**"), abdominal/flank pain (kidney stones, acute pancreatitis), neuropsychiatric disturbances ("**psychiatric overtones**").	**Osteitis fibrosa cystica**—cystic bone spaces filled with brown fibrous tissue **A** ("brown tumor" consisting of osteoclasts and deposited hemosiderin from hemorrhages; causes bone pain). Due to ↑ PTH, classically associated with 1° (but also seen with 2°) hyperparathyroidism. "Stones, thrones, bones, groans, and psychiatric overtones."
Secondary hyperparathyroidism	2° hyperplasia due to ↓ Ca^{2+} absorption and/or ↑ PO_4^{3-}, most often in chronic renal disease (causes hypovitaminosis D and hyperphosphatemia → ↓ Ca^{2+}). **Hypocalcemia**, hyperphosphatemia in chronic renal failure (vs hypophosphatemia with most other causes), ↑ ALP, ↑ PTH.	**Renal osteodystrophy**—renal disease → 2° and 3° hyperparathyroidism → bone lesions.
Tertiary hyperparathyroidism	Refractory (autonomous) hyperparathyroidism resulting from chronic renal disease. ↑↑ PTH, ↑ Ca^{2+}.	

Familial hypocalciuric hypercalcemia	Defective G-coupled Ca^{2+}-sensing receptors in multiple tissues (eg, parathyroids, kidneys). Higher than normal Ca^{2+} levels required to suppress PTH. Excessive renal Ca^{2+} reuptake → mild hypercalcemia and hypocalciuria with normal to ↑ PTH levels.

Nelson syndrome	Enlargement of existing ACTH-secreting pituitary adenoma after bilateral adrenalectomy for refractory Cushing disease (due to removal of cortisol feedback mechanism). Presents with hyperpigmentation, headaches and bitemporal hemianopia. Treatment: pituitary irradiation or surgical resection.

Acromegaly	Excess GH in adults. Typically caused by pituitary adenoma.	
FINDINGS	Large tongue with deep furrows, deep voice, large hands and feet, coarsening of facial features with aging **A**, frontal bossing, diaphoresis (excessive sweating), impaired glucose tolerance (insulin resistance), hypertension. ↑ risk of colorectal polyps and cancer.	↑ GH in children → gigantism (↑ linear bone growth). HF most common cause of death. Baseline
DIAGNOSIS	↑ serum IGF-1; failure to suppress serum GH following oral glucose tolerance test; pituitary mass seen on brain MRI.	
TREATMENT	Pituitary adenoma resection. If not cured, treat with octreotide (somatostatin analog) or pegvisomant (growth hormone receptor antagonist), dopamine agonists (eg, cabergoline).	

Laron syndrome (dwarfism)	Defective growth hormone receptors → ↓ linear growth. ↑ GH, ↓ IGF-1. Clinical features: short height, small head circumference, characteristic facies with saddle nose and prominent forehead, delayed skeletal maturation, small genitalia.

Diabetes insipidus	Characterized by intense thirst and polyuria with inability to concentrate urine due to lack of ADH (central) or failure of response to circulating ADH (nephrogenic).	
	Central DI	**Nephrogenic DI**
ETIOLOGY	Pituitary tumor, autoimmune, trauma, surgery, ischemic encephalopathy, idiopathic	Hereditary (ADH receptor mutation), 2° to hypercalcemia, hypokalemia, lithium, demeclocycline (ADH antagonist)
FINDINGS	↓ ADH	Normal or ↑ ADH levels
	Urine specific gravity < 1.006 Serum osmolality > 290 mOsm/kg Hyperosmotic volume contraction	
WATER DEPRIVATION TEST[a]	> 50% ↑ in urine osmolality only after administration of ADH analog	Minimal change in urine osmolality, even after administration of ADH analog
TREATMENT	Desmopressin Hydration	HCTZ, indomethacin, amiloride Hydration, dietary salt restriction, avoidance of offending agent

[a]No water intake for 2–3 hr followed by hourly measurements of urine volume and osmolality and plasma Na^+ concentration and osmolality. ADH analog (desmopressin) is administered if serum osmolality > 295–300 mOsm/kg, plasma Na^+ ≥ 145 mEq/L, or urine osmolality does not rise despite a rising plasma osmolality.

| **Syndrome of inappropriate antidiuretic hormone secretion** | Characterized by:
■ Excessive free water retention
■ Euvolemic hyponatremia with continued urinary Na^+ excretion
■ Urine osmolality > serum osmolality
Body responds to water retention with ↓ aldosterone and ↑ ANP and BNP → ↑ urinary Na^+ secretion → normalization of extracellular fluid volume → euvolemic hyponatremia. Very low serum Na^+ levels can lead to cerebral edema, seizures. Correct slowly to prevent osmotic demyelination syndrome (formerly known as central pontine myelinolysis). | SIADH causes include:
■ Ectopic ADH (eg, small cell lung cancer)
■ CNS disorders/head trauma
■ Pulmonary disease
■ Drugs (eg, cyclophosphamide)
Treatment: fluid restriction (first line), salt tablets, IV hypertonic saline, diuretics, conivaptan, tolvaptan, demeclocycline.
Increased urine osmolality during water deprivation test indicates psychogenic polydipsia. |

Hypopituitarism

Undersecretion of pituitary hormones due to:

- Nonsecreting pituitary adenoma, craniopharyngioma
- Sheehan syndrome—ischemic infarct of pituitary following postpartum bleeding; pregnancy-induced pituitary growth → ↑ susceptibility to hypoperfusion. Usually presents with failure to lactate, absent menstruation, cold intolerance
- Empty sella syndrome—atrophy or compression of pituitary (which lies in the sella turcica), often idiopathic, common in obese women; associated with idiopathic intracranial hypertension
- Pituitary apoplexy—sudden hemorrhage of pituitary gland, often in the presence of an existing pituitary adenoma. Usually presents with sudden onset severe headache, visual impairment (eg, bitemporal hemianopia, diplopia due to CN III palsy), and features of hypopituitarism.
- Brain injury
- Radiation

Treatment: hormone replacement therapy (corticosteroids, thyroxine, sex steroids, human growth hormone).

Diabetes mellitus

ACUTE MANIFESTATIONS	Polydipsia, polyuria, polyphagia, weight loss, DKA (type 1), hyperosmolar hyperglycemic state (type 2). Rarely, can be caused by unopposed secretion of GH and epinephrine. Also seen in patients on glucocorticoid therapy (steroid diabetes).
CHRONIC COMPLICATIONS	Nonenzymatic glycation: ▪ Small vessel disease (diffuse thickening of basement membrane) → retinopathy (hemorrhage, exudates, microaneurysms, vessel proliferation), glaucoma, neuropathy, nephropathy (nodular glomerulosclerosis, aka Kimmelstiel-Wilson nodules → progressive proteinuria [initially microalbuminuria; ACE inhibitors are renoprotective] and arteriolosclerosis → hypertension; both lead to chronic renal failure). ▪ Large vessel atherosclerosis, CAD, peripheral vascular occlusive disease, gangrene → limb loss, cerebrovascular disease. MI most common cause of death. Osmotic damage (sorbitol accumulation in organs with aldose reductase and ↓ or absent sorbitol dehydrogenase): ▪ Neuropathy (motor, sensory [glove and stocking distribution], and autonomic degeneration) ▪ Cataracts

DIAGNOSIS	TEST	DIAGNOSTIC CUTOFF	NOTES
	HbA_{1c}	≥ 6.5%	Reflects average blood glucose over prior 3 months
	Fasting plasma glucose	≥ 126 mg/dL	Fasting for > 8 hours
	2-hour oral glucose tolerance test	≥ 200 mg/dL	2 hours after consumption of 75 g of glucose in water

Insulin deficiency or severe insulin insensitivity

Type 1 vs type 2 diabetes mellitus

	Type 1	Type 2
1° DEFECT	Autoimmune destruction of β cells (eg, due to glutamic acid decarboxylase antibodies)	↑ resistance to insulin, progressive pancreatic β-cell failure
INSULIN NECESSARY IN TREATMENT	Always	Sometimes
AGE (EXCEPTIONS COMMONLY OCCUR)	< 30 yr	> 40 yr
ASSOCIATION WITH OBESITY	No	Yes
GENETIC PREDISPOSITION	Relatively weak (50% concordance in identical twins), polygenic	Relatively strong (90% concordance in identical twins), polygenic
ASSOCIATION WITH HLA SYSTEM	Yes, HLA-DR4 and -DR3 (4 – 3 = type 1)	No
GLUCOSE INTOLERANCE	Severe	Mild to moderate
INSULIN SENSITIVITY	High	Low
KETOACIDOSIS	Common	Rare
β-CELL NUMBERS IN THE ISLETS	↓	Variable (with amyloid deposits)
SERUM INSULIN LEVEL	↓	Variable
CLASSIC SYMPTOMS OF POLYURIA, POLYDIPSIA, POLYPHAGIA, WEIGHT LOSS	Common	Sometimes
HISTOLOGY	Islet leukocytic infiltrate	Islet amyloid polypeptide (IAPP) deposits

Diabetic ketoacidosis

One of the most feared complications of diabetes. Usually due to insulin noncompliance or ↑ insulin requirements from ↑ stress (eg, infection). Excess fat breakdown and ↑ ketogenesis from ↑ free fatty acids, which are then made into ketone bodies (β-hydroxybutyrate > acetoacetate). Usually occurs in type 1 diabetes, as endogenous insulin in type 2 diabetes usually prevents lipolysis.

SIGNS/SYMPTOMS	**DKA** is **D**eadly: **D**elirium/psychosis, **K**ussmaul respirations (rapid, deep breathing), **A**bdominal pain/nausea/vomiting, **D**ehydration. Fruity breath odor (due to exhaled acetone).
LABS	Hyperglycemia, ↑ H^+, ↓ HCO_3^- (↑ anion gap metabolic acidosis), ↑ blood ketone levels, leukocytosis. Hyperkalemia, but depleted intracellular K^+ due to transcellular shift from ↓ insulin and acidosis. Osmotic diuresis → ↑ K^+ loss in urine → total body K^+ depletion.
COMPLICATIONS	Life-threatening mucormycosis (usually caused by *Rhizopus* infection), cerebral edema, cardiac arrhythmias, heart failure.
TREATMENT	IV fluids, IV insulin, and K^+ (to replete intracellular stores); glucose if necessary to prevent hypoglycemia.

Hyperosmolar hyperglycemic state

State of profound hyperglycemia-induced dehydration and ↑ serum osmolality, classically seen in elderly type 2 diabetics with limited ability to drink. Hyperglycemia → excessive osmotic diuresis → dehydration → eventual onset of HHS. Symptoms: thirst, polyuria, lethargy, focal neurological deficits (eg, seizures), can progress to coma and death if left untreated. Labs: hyperglycemia (often > 600 mg/dL), ↑ serum osmolality (> 320 mOsm/kg), no acidosis (pH > 7.35, ketone production inhibited by presence of insulin). Treatment: aggressive IV fluids, insulin therapy.

Glucagonoma

Tumor of pancreatic α cells → overproduction of glucagon. Presents with dermatitis (necrolytic migratory erythema), diabetes (hyperglycemia), DVT, declining weight, depression. Treatment: octreotide, surgery.

Insulinoma

Tumor of pancreatic β cells → overproduction of insulin → hypoglycemia. May see Whipple triad: low blood glucose, symptoms of hypoglycemia (eg, lethargy, syncope, diplopia), and resolution of symptoms after normalization of glucose levels. Symptomatic patients have ↓ blood glucose and ↑ C-peptide levels (vs exogenous insulin use). ~ 10% of cases associated with MEN 1 syndrome. Treatment: surgical resection.

Somatostatinoma

Tumor of pancreatic δ cells → overproduction of somatostatin → ↓ secretion of secretin, cholecystokinin, glucagon, insulin, gastrin, gastric inhibitory peptide (GIP). May present with diabetes/glucose intolerance, steatorrhea, gallstones, achlorhydria. Treatment: surgical resection; somatostatin analogs (eg, octreotide) for symptom control.

Carcinoid syndrome

Rare syndrome caused by carcinoid tumors (neuroendocrine cells **A**; note prominent rosettes [arrow]), especially metastatic small bowel tumors, which secrete high levels of serotonin (5-HT). Not seen if tumor is limited to GI tract (5-HT undergoes first-pass metabolism in liver).

Results in recurrent diarrhea, cutaneous flushing, asthmatic wheezing, right-sided valvular heart disease (tricuspid regurgitation, pulmonic stenosis) due to lung MAO-A enzymatic breakdown of 5-HT before left heart return. ↑ 5-hydroxyindoleacetic acid (5-HIAA) in urine, niacin deficiency (pellagra). Associated with neuroendocrine tumor markers chromogranin A and synaptophysin.

Treatment: surgical resection, somatostatin analog (eg, octreotide).

Rule of 1/3s:
  1/3 metastasize
  1/3 present with 2nd malignancy
  1/3 are multiple
Most common malignancy in the small intestine.

Zollinger-Ellison syndrome	Gastrin-secreting tumor (gastrinoma) of pancreas or duodenum. Acid hypersecretion causes recurrent ulcers in duodenum and jejunum. Presents with abdominal pain (peptic ulcer disease, distal ulcers), diarrhea (malabsorption). Positive secretin stimulation test: gastrin levels remain elevated after administration of secretin, which normally inhibits gastrin release. May be associated with MEN 1.

Multiple endocrine neoplasias

All **MEN** syndromes have autosomal dominant inheritance.
"All **MEN** are dominant" (or so they think).

SUBTYPE	CHARACTERISTICS	COMMENTS
MEN 1	Pituitary tumors (prolactin or GH) Pancreatic endocrine tumors—Zollinger-Ellison syndrome, insulinomas, VIPomas, glucagonomas (rare) Parathyroid adenomas Associated with mutation of *MEN1* (menin, a tumor suppressor, chromosome 11), angiofibromas, collagenomas, meningiomas	
MEN 2A	Parathyroid hyperplasia Medullary thyroid carcinoma—neoplasm of parafollicular or C cells; secretes calcitonin; prophylactic thyroidectomy required Pheochromocytoma (secretes catecholamines) Associated with mutation in *RET* (codes for receptor tyrosine kinase) in cells of neural crest origin	
MEN 2B	Medullary thyroid carcinoma Pheochromocytoma Mucosal neuromas A (oral/intestinal ganglioneuromatosis) Associated with marfanoid habitus; mutation in *RET* gene	

MEN 1 = 3 P's: Pituitary, Parathyroid, and Pancreas
MEN 2A = 2 P's: Parathyroid and Pheochromocytoma
MEN 2B = 1 P: Pheochromocytoma

▶ ENDOCRINE—PHARMACOLOGY

Diabetes mellitus management	All patients with diabetes mellitus should receive education on diet, exercise, blood glucose monitoring, and complication management. Treatment differs based on the type of diabetes:

- Type 1 DM—insulin replacement
- Type 2 DM—oral agents (metformin is first line), non-insulin injectables, insulin replacement; weight loss particularly helpful in lowering blood glucose
- Gestational DM—insulin replacement if nutrition therapy and exercise alone fail

Regular (short-acting) insulin is preferred for DKA (IV), hyperkalemia (+ glucose), stress hyperglycemia.

DRUG CLASS	MECHANISM	ADVERSE EFFECTS
Injectables		
Insulin preparations Rapid acting (1-hr peak): Lispro, Aspart, Glulisine (no LAG) Short acting (2–3 hr peak): regular Intermediate acting (4–10 hr peak): NPH Long acting (no real peak): detemir, glargine	Bind insulin receptor (tyrosine kinase activity). Liver: ↑ glucose stored as glycogen. Muscle: ↑ glycogen, protein synthesis. Fat: ↑ TG storage. Cell membrane: ↑ K^+ uptake.	Hypoglycemia, lipodystrophy, rare hypersensitivity reactions.
Amylin analogs Pramlintide	↓ glucagon release, ↓ gastric emptying, ↑ satiety.	Hypoglycemia (in setting of mistimed prandial insulin), nausea.
GLP-1 analogs Exenatide, liraglutide	↓ glucagon release, ↓ gastric emptying, ↑ glucose-dependent insulin release, ↑ satiety.	Nausea, vomiting, pancreatitis. Promote weight loss (often desired).
Oral drugs		
Biguanides Metformin	Inhibit hepatic gluconeogenesis and the action of glucagon, by inhibiting mGPD. ↑ glycolysis, peripheral glucose uptake (↑ insulin sensitivity).	GI upset, lactic acidosis (use with caution in renal insufficiency), B_{12} deficiency. Promote weight loss (often desired).
Sulfonylureas 1st generation: chlorpropamide, tolbutamide 2nd generation: glimepiride, glipizide, glyburide	Close K^+ channel in pancreatic β cell membrane → cell depolarizes → insulin release via ↑ Ca^{2+} influx.	Hypoglycemia (↑ risk with renal failure), weight gain. 1st generation: disulfiram-like effects. 2nd generation: hypoglycemia.
Meglitinides Nateglinide, repaglinide	Close K^+ channel in pancreatic β cell membrane → cell depolarizes → insulin release via ↑ Ca^{2+} influx (binding site differs from sulfonylureas).	Hypoglycemia (↑ risk with renal failure), weight gain.

Diabetes mellitus management (continued)

DRUG CLASS	MECHANISM	ADVERSE EFFECTS
Oral drugs (continued)		
DPP-4 inhibitors Linagliptin, saxagliptin, sitagliptin	Inhibit DPP-4 enzyme that deactivates GLP-1. ↓ glucagon release, gastric emptying. ↑ glucose-dependent insulin release, satiety.	Mild urinary or respiratory infections, weight neutral.
Glitazones/ thiazolidinediones Pioglitazone, rosiglitazone	Binds to PPAR-γ nuclear transcription regulator → ↑ insulin sensitivity and levels of adiponectin → regulation of glucose metabolism and fatty acid storage.	Weight gain, edema, HF, ↑ risk of fractures. Delayed onset of action (several weeks).
Sodium-glucose co-transporter 2 (SGLT2) inhibitors Canagliflozin, dapagliflozin, empagliflozin	Block reabsorption of glucose in proximal convoluted tubule.	Glucosuria, UTIs, vaginal yeast infections, hyperkalemia, dehydration (orthostatic hypotension), weight loss.
α-glucosidase inhibitors Acarbose, miglitol	Inhibit intestinal brush-border α-glucosidases → delayed carbohydrate hydrolysis and glucose absorption → ↓ postprandial hyperglycemia.	GI upset. Not recommended if kidney function is impaired.

Thioamides

Propylthiouracil, methimazole.

MECHANISM	Block thyroid peroxidase, inhibiting the oxidation of iodide and the organification and coupling of iodine → inhibition of thyroid hormone synthesis. PTU also blocks 5'-deiodinase → ↓ peripheral conversion of T_4 to T_3.
CLINICAL USE	Hyperthyroidism. PTU blocks **P**eripheral conversion. PTU used in first trimester of pregnancy (due to methimazole teratogenicity); methimazole used in second and third trimesters of pregnancy (due to risk of PTU-induced hepatotoxicity). Not used to treat Graves ophthalmopathy (treated with corticosteroids).
ADVERSE EFFECTS	Skin rash, agranulocytosis (rare), aplastic anemia, hepatotoxicity. Methimazole is a possible teratogen (can cause aplasia cutis).

Levothyroxine (T_4), liothyronine (T_3)

MECHANISM	Thyroid hormone replacement.
CLINICAL USE	Hypothyroidism, myxedema. May be abused for weight loss.
ADVERSE EFFECTS	Tachycardia, heat intolerance, tremors, arrhythmias.

Hypothalamic/pituitary drugs

DRUG	CLINICAL USE
ADH antagonists (conivaptan, tolvaptan)	SIADH, block action of ADH at V_2-receptor.
Desmopressin	Central (not nephrogenic) DI, von Willebrand disease, sleep enuresis, hemophilia A.
GH	GH deficiency, Turner syndrome.
Oxytocin	Labor induction (stimulates uterine contractions), milk letdown; controls uterine hemorrhage.
Somatostatin (octreotide)	Acromegaly, carcinoid syndrome, gastrinoma, glucagonoma, esophageal varices.

Demeclocycline

MECHANISM	ADH antagonist (member of tetracycline family).
CLINICAL USE	SIADH.
ADVERSE EFFECTS	Nephrogenic DI, photosensitivity, abnormalities of bone and teeth.

Fludrocortisone

MECHANISM	Synthetic analog of aldosterone with little glucocorticoid effects.
CLINICAL USE	Mineralocorticoid replacement in 1° adrenal insufficiency.
ADVERSE EFFECTS	Similar to glucocorticoids; also edema, exacerbation of heart failure, hyperpigmentation.

Cinacalcet

MECHANISM	Sensitizes Ca^{2+}-sensing receptor (CaSR) in parathyroid gland to circulating Ca^{2+} → ↓ PTH.
CLINICAL USE	Refractory hypercalcemia in 1° hyperparathyroidism, 2° hyperparathyroidism, or parathyroid carcinoma.
ADVERSE EFFECTS	Hypocalcemia.

Sevelamer

MECHANISM	Nonabsorbable phosphate binder that prevents phosphate absorption from the GI tract.
CLINICAL USE	Hyperphosphatemia in CKD.
ADVERSE EFFECTS	Hypophosphatemia, GI upset.

Gastrointestinal

"A good set of bowels is worth more to a man than any quantity of brains."
—Josh Billings

"Man should strive to have his intestines relaxed all the days of his life."
—Moses Maimonides

"Is life worth living? It all depends on the liver."

—William James

When studying the gastrointestinal system, be sure to understand the normal embryology, anatomy, and physiology and how it is affected in the various pathologic diseases. Study not only what a disease entails, but also its specific findings, so that you can differentiate between two similar diseases. For example, what specifically makes ulcerative colitis different than Crohn disease? Also, it is important to understand bile metabolism and which lab values increase or decrease depending on the disease process. Be comfortable reading abdominal X-rays, CT scans, and endoscopy exams.

▶ GASTROINTESTINAL—EMBRYOLOGY

Normal gastrointestinal embryology	Foregut—esophagus to upper duodenum. Midgut—lower duodenum to proximal $^2/_3$ of transverse colon. Hindgut—distal $^1/_3$ of transverse colon to anal canal above pectinate line. Midgut development: ▪ 6th week—physiologic midgut herniates through umbilical ring ▪ 10th week—returns to abdominal cavity + rotates around superior mesenteric artery (SMA), total 270° counterclockwise

Ventral wall defects	Developmental defects due to failure of rostral fold closure (eg, sternal defects [ectopia cordis]), lateral fold closure (eg, omphalocele, gastroschisis), or caudal fold closure (eg, bladder exstrophy).

	Gastroschisis	Omphalocele
ETIOLOGY	Extrusion of abdominal contents through abdominal folds (typically right of umbilicus)	Failure of lateral walls to migrate at umbilical ring → persistent midline herniation of abdominal contents into umbilical cord
COVERAGE	Not covered by peritoneum or amnion; "the abdominal contents are coming out of the **G**"	Surrounded by peritoneum (light gray shiny sac); "abdominal contents are sealed in the **Θ**"
ASSOCIATIONS	Not associated with chromosome abnormalities	Associated with congenital anomalies (eg, trisomies 13 and 18, Beckwith-Wiedemann syndrome) and other structural abnormalities (eg, cardiac, GU, neural tube)
	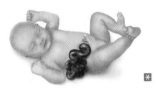	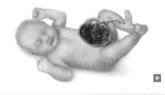

Congenital umbilical hernia	Failure of umbilical ring to close after physiologic herniation of the intestines. Small defects usually close spontaneously.

Tracheoesophageal anomalies	Esophageal atresia (EA) with distal tracheoesophageal fistula (TEF) is the most common (85%) and often presents as polyhydramnios in utero (due to inability of fetus to swallow amniotic fluid). Neonates drool, choke, and vomit with first feeding. TEFs allow air to enter stomach (visible on CXR). Cyanosis is 2° to laryngospasm (to avoid reflux-related aspiration). Clinical test: failure to pass nasogastric tube into stomach. In **H**-type, the fistula resembles the letter **H**. In pure EA, CXR shows gasless abdomen.

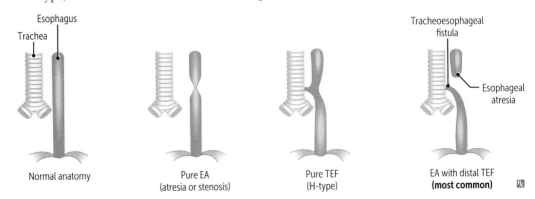

Normal anatomy | Pure EA (atresia or stenosis) | Pure TEF (H-type) | EA with distal TEF **(most common)**

Intestinal atresia

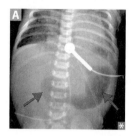

Presents with bilious vomiting and abdominal distension within first 1–2 days of life.
Duodenal atresia—failure to recanalize. Associated with "double bubble" (dilated stomach, proximal duodenum) on x-ray). Associated with Down syndrome.
Jejunal and ileal atresia—disruption of mesenteric vessels → ischemic necrosis → segmental resorption (bowel discontinuity or "apple peel").

Hypertrophic pyloric stenosis

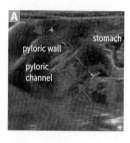

Most common cause of gastric outlet obstruction in infants (1:600). Palpable olive-shaped mass in epigastric region, visible peristaltic waves, and nonbilious projectile vomiting at ~ 2–6 weeks old. More common in firstborn males; associated with exposure to macrolides. Results in hypokalemic hypochloremic metabolic alkalosis (2° to vomiting of gastric acid and subsequent volume contraction). Ultrasound shows thickened and lengthened pylorus A. Treatment is surgical incision (pyloromyotomy).

Pancreas and spleen embryology

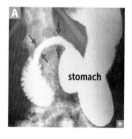

Pancreas—derived from foregut. Ventral pancreatic buds contribute to uncinate process and main pancreatic duct. The dorsal pancreatic bud alone becomes the body, tail, isthmus, and accessory pancreatic duct. Both the ventral and dorsal buds contribute to pancreatic head.
Annular pancreas—abnormal rotation of ventral pancreatic bud forms a ring of pancreatic tissue → encircles 2nd part of duodenum; may cause duodenal narrowing (arrows in A) and vomiting.
Pancreas divisum—ventral and dorsal parts fail to fuse at 8 weeks. Common anomaly; mostly asymptomatic, but may cause chronic abdominal pain and/or pancreatitis.
Spleen—arises in mesentery of stomach (hence is mesodermal) but has foregut supply (celiac trunk → splenic artery).

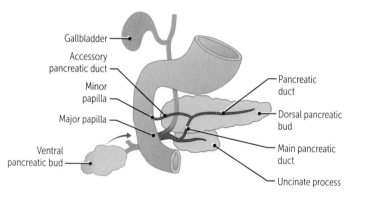

- Gallbladder
- Accessory pancreatic duct
- Minor papilla
- Major papilla
- Ventral pancreatic bud
- Pancreatic duct
- Dorsal pancreatic bud
- Main pancreatic duct
- Uncinate process
- stomach

▶ GASTROINTESTINAL—ANATOMY

Retroperitoneal structures

Retroperitoneal structures 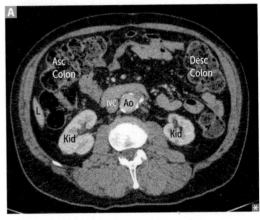 include GI structures that lack a mesentery and non-GI structures. Injuries to retroperitoneal structures can cause blood or gas accumulation in retroperitoneal space.

SAD PUCKER:
Suprarenal (adrenal) glands [not shown]
Aorta and IVC
Duodenum (2nd through 4th parts)
Pancreas (except tail)
Ureters [not shown]
Colon (descending and ascending)
Kidneys
Esophagus (thoracic portion) [not shown]
Rectum (partially) [not shown]

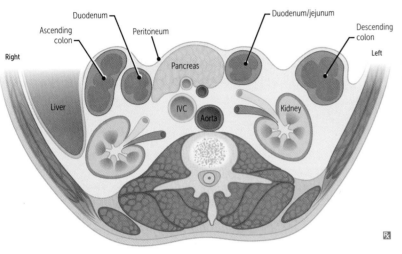

Important gastrointestinal ligaments

LIGAMENT	CONNECTS	STRUCTURES CONTAINED	NOTES
Falciform ligament	Liver to anterior abdominal wall	Ligamentum teres hepatis (derivative of fetal umbilical vein), patent paraumbilical veins	Derivative of ventral mesentery
Hepatoduodenal ligament	Liver to duodenum	Portal triad: proper hepatic artery, portal vein, common bile duct	Pringle maneuver—ligament may be compressed between thumb and index finger placed in omental foramen to control bleeding Borders the omental foramen, which connects the greater and lesser sacs Part of lesser omentum
Gastrohepatic ligament	Liver to lesser curvature of stomach	Gastric vessels	Separates greater and lesser sacs on the right May be cut during surgery to access lesser sac Part of lesser omentum
Gastrocolic ligament (not shown)	Greater curvature and transverse colon	Gastroepiploic arteries	Part of greater omentum
Gastrosplenic ligament	Greater curvature and spleen	Short gastrics, left gastroepiploic vessels	Separates greater and lesser sacs on the left Part of greater omentum
Splenorenal ligament	Spleen to posterior abdominal wall	Splenic artery and vein, tail of pancreas	

Digestive tract anatomy

Layers of gut wall (inside to outside—**MSMS**):

- Mucosa—epithelium, lamina propria, muscularis mucosa
- Submucosa—includes Submucosal nerve plexus (Meissner), Secretes fluid
- Muscularis externa—includes Myenteric nerve plexus (Auerbach), Motility
- Serosa (when intraperitoneal), adventitia (when retroperitoneal)

Ulcers can extend into submucosa, inner or outer muscular layer. Erosions are in the mucosa only.

Frequencies of basal electric rhythm (slow waves):

- Stomach—3 waves/min
- Duodenum—12 waves/min
- Ileum—8–9 waves/min

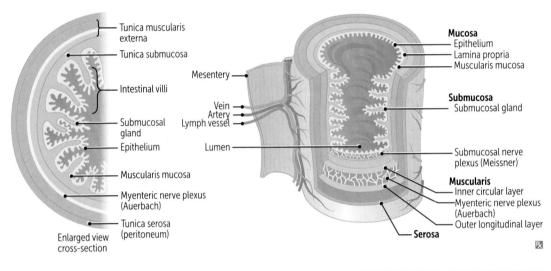

Digestive tract histology

Esophagus	Nonkeratinized stratified squamous epithelium.
Stomach	Gastric glands.
Duodenum	Villi and microvilli ↑ absorptive surface. Brunner glands (HCO_3^--secreting cells of submucosa) and crypts of Lieberkühn (contain stem cells that replace enterocytes/goblet cells and Paneth cells that secrete defensins, lysozyme, and TNF).
Jejunum	Plicae circulares (also present in distal duodenum) and crypts of Lieberkühn.
Ileum	Peyer patches (lymphoid aggregates in lamina propria, submucosa), plicae circulares (proximal ileum), and crypts of Lieberkühn. Largest number of goblet cells in the small intestine.
Colon	Crypts of Lieberkühn but no villi; abundant goblet cells.

Abdominal aorta and branches

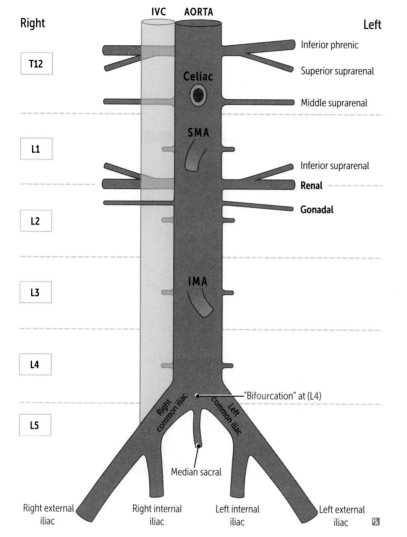

Right | IVC | AORTA | Left

T12

Inferior phrenic

Celiac

Superior suprarenal

Middle suprarenal

SMA

L1

Inferior suprarenal

Renal

Gonadal

L2

IMA

L3

L4

"Bifourcation" at (L4)

Right common iliac | Left common iliac

L5

Median sacral

Right external iliac | Right internal iliac | Left internal iliac | Left external iliac ℞

Arteries supplying GI structures are single and branch anteriorly.

Arteries supplying non-GI structures are paired and branch laterally and posteriorly.

Superior mesenteric artery syndrome— characterized by intermittent intestinal obstruction symptoms (primarily postprandial pain) when SMA and aorta compress transverse (third) portion of duodenum. Typically occurs in conditions associated with diminished mesenteric fat (eg, low body weight/malnutrition).

Two areas of the colon have dual blood supply from distal arterial branches ("watershed regions") → susceptible in colonic ischemia:
- Splenic flexure—SMA and IMA
- Rectosigmoid junction—the last sigmoid arterial branch from the IMA and superior rectal artery

Gastrointestinal blood supply and innervation

EMBRYONIC GUT REGION	ARTERY	PARASYMPATHETIC INNERVATION	VERTEBRAL LEVEL	STRUCTURES SUPPLIED
Foregut	Celiac	Vagus	T12/L1	Pharynx (vagus nerve only) and lower esophagus (celiac artery only) to proximal duodenum; liver, gallbladder, pancreas, spleen (mesoderm)
Midgut	SMA	Vagus	L1	Distal duodenum to proximal $^2/_3$ of transverse colon
Hindgut	IMA	Pelvic	L3	Distal $^1/_3$ of transverse colon to upper portion of rectum

Celiac trunk

Branches of celiac trunk: common hepatic, splenic, and left gastric. These constitute the main blood supply of the stomach.

Strong anastomoses exist between:

- Left and right gastroepiploics
- Left and right gastrics

Posterior duodenal ulcers penetrate gastroduodenal artery causing hemorrhage.

Anterior duodenal ulcers perforate into the anterior abdominal cavity, potentially leading to pneumoperitoneum.

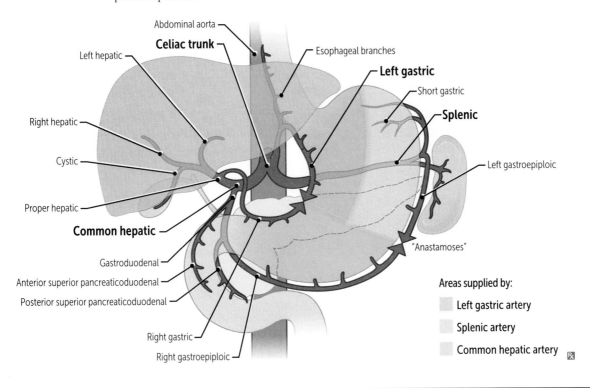

Areas supplied by:

Left gastric artery

Splenic artery

Common hepatic artery

Portosystemic anastomoses

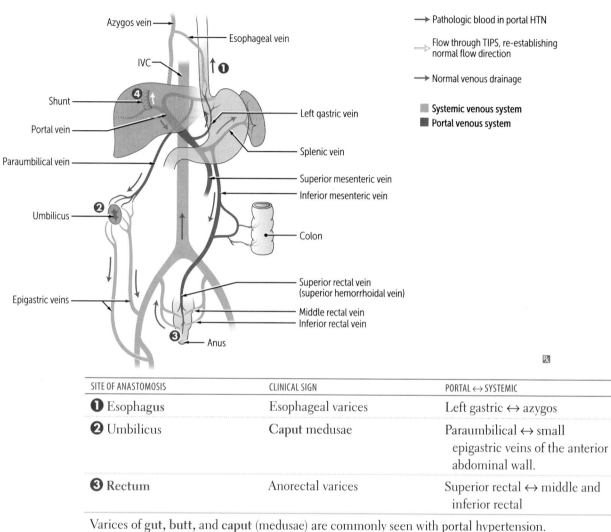

SITE OF ANASTOMOSIS	CLINICAL SIGN	PORTAL ↔ SYSTEMIC
❶ Esophagus	Esophageal varices	Left gastric ↔ azygos
❷ Umbilicus	Caput medusae	Paraumbilical ↔ small epigastric veins of the anterior abdominal wall.
❸ Rectum	Anorectal varices	Superior rectal ↔ middle and inferior rectal

Varices of **gut**, **butt**, and **caput** (medusae) are commonly seen with portal hypertension.

❹ Treatment with a transjugular intrahepatic portosystemic shunt (**TIPS**) between the portal vein and hepatic vein relieves portal hypertension by shunting blood to the systemic circulation, bypassing the liver. Can precipitate hepatic encephalopathy.

Pectinate (dentate) line

Formed where endoderm (hindgut) meets ectoderm.

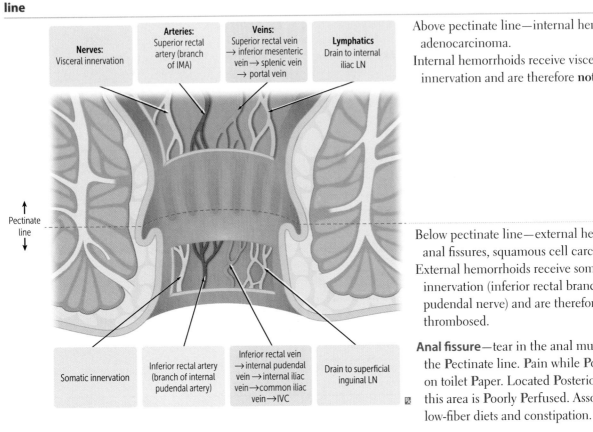

Nerves:
Visceral innervation

Arteries:
Superior rectal artery (branch of IMA)

Veins:
Superior rectal vein → inferior mesenteric vein → splenic vein → portal vein

Lymphatics
Drain to internal iliac LN

Pectinate line

Somatic innervation

Inferior rectal artery (branch of internal pudendal artery)

Inferior rectal vein → internal pudendal vein → internal iliac vein → common iliac vein → IVC

Drain to superficial inguinal LN

Above pectinate line—internal hemorrhoids, adenocarcinoma.

Internal hemorrhoids receive visceral innervation and are therefore **not painful**.

Below pectinate line—external hemorrhoids, anal fissures, squamous cell carcinoma.

External hemorrhoids receive somatic innervation (inferior rectal branch of pudendal nerve) and are therefore **painful** if thrombosed.

Anal fissure—tear in the anal mucosa below the Pectinate line. Pain while Pooping; blood on toilet Paper. Located Posteriorly because this area is Poorly Perfused. Associated with low-fiber diets and constipation.

Liver tissue architecture

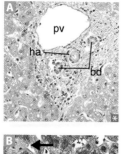

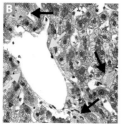

The functional unit of the liver is made up of hexagonally arranged lobules surrounding the central vein with portal triads on the edges (consisting of a portal vein, hepatic artery, bile ducts, as well lymphatics) .

Apical surface of hepatocytes faces bile canaliculi. Basolateral surface faces sinusoids.

Kupffer cells, which are specialized macrophages, are located in the sinusoids (black arrows in **B**; 2 yellow arrows show hepatic venule).

Hepatic stellate (Ito) cells in space of Disse store vitamin A (when quiescent) and produce extracellular matrix (when activated). Responsible for hepatic fibrosis.

Zone I—periportal zone:
- Affected 1st by viral hepatitis
- Ingested toxins (eg, cocaine)

Zone II—intermediate zone:
- Yellow fever

Zone III—pericentral vein (centrilobular) zone:
- Affected 1st by ischemia
- High concentration of cytochrome P-450
- Most sensitive to metabolic toxins (eg, ethanol, CCl_4, halothane, rifampin)
- Site of alcoholic hepatitis

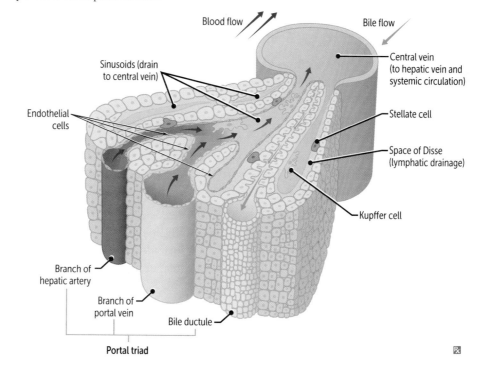

Biliary structures

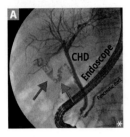

Gallstones that reach the confluence of the common bile and pancreatic ducts at the ampulla of Vater can block both the common bile and pancreatic ducts (double duct sign), causing both cholangitis and pancreatitis, respectively.

Tumors that arise in head of pancreas (usually ductal adenocarcinoma) can cause obstruction of common bile duct → enlarged gallbladder with painless jaundice (Courvoisier sign).

Cholangiography shows filling defects in gallbladder (blue arrow) and cystic duct (red arrow) **A**.

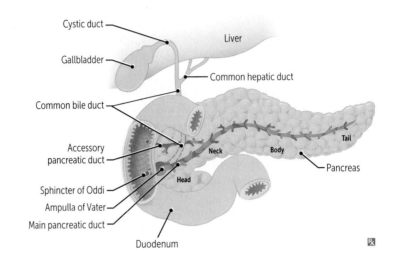

Femoral region

ORGANIZATION	Lateral to medial: Nerve-Artery-Vein-Lymphatics.	You go from lateral to medial to find your NAVeL.
Femoral triangle	Contains femoral nerve, artery, vein.	Venous near the penis.
Femoral sheath	Fascial tube 3–4 cm below inguinal ligament. Contains femoral vein, artery, and canal (deep inguinal lymph nodes) but not femoral nerve.	

Inguinal canal

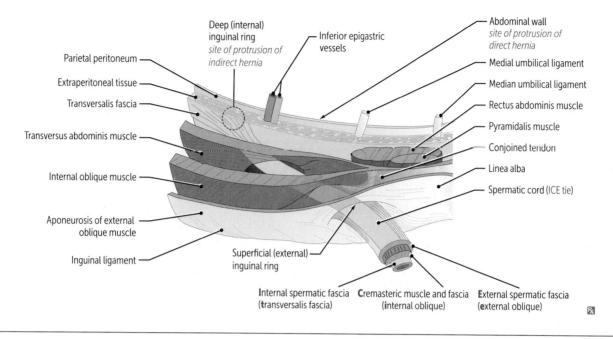

Deep (internal) inguinal ring
site of protrusion of indirect hernia

Inferior epigastric vessels

Abdominal wall
site of protrusion of direct hernia

Parietal peritoneum

Extraperitoneal tissue

Transversalis fascia

Transversus abdominis muscle

Internal oblique muscle

Aponeurosis of external oblique muscle

Inguinal ligament

Medial umbilical ligament

Median umbilical ligament

Rectus abdominis muscle

Pyramidalis muscle

Conjoined tendon

Linea alba

Spermatic cord (ICE tie)

Superficial (external) inguinal ring

Internal spermatic fascia (transversalis fascia)

Cremasteric muscle and fascia (internal oblique)

External spermatic fascia (external oblique)

Hernias	Protrusion of peritoneum through an opening, usually at a site of weakness. Contents may be at risk for incarceration (not reducible back into abdomen/pelvis) and strangulation (ischemia and necrosis). Complicated hernias can present with tenderness, erythema, fever.

Diaphragmatic hernia

Abdominal structures enter the thorax **A**; may occur due to congenital defect of pleuroperitoneal membrane or from trauma. Commonly occurs on left side due to relative protection of right hemidiaphragm by liver.

Most commonly a hiatal hernia, in which stomach herniates upward through the esophageal hiatus of the diaphragm.

Sliding hiatal hernia—gastroesophageal junction is displaced upward as gastric cardia slides into hiatus; "hourglass stomach." Most common type.

Paraesophageal hiatal hernia—gastroesophageal junction is usually normal but gastric fundus protrudes into the thorax.

Herniated gastric cardia — Sliding hiatal hernia
Herniated gastric fundus — Paraesophageal hiatal hernia

Indirect inguinal hernia

Goes through the internal (deep) inguinal ring, external (superficial) inguinal ring, and into the scrotum. Enters internal inguinal ring lateral to inferior epigastric vessels. Caused by failure of processus vaginalis to close (can form hydrocele). May be noticed in infants or discovered in adulthood. Much more common in males **B**.

An indirect inguinal hernia follows the path of descent of the testes. Covered by all 3 layers of spermatic fascia.

Direct inguinal hernia

Protrudes through the inguinal (Hesselbach) triangle. Bulges directly through parietal peritoneum medial to the inferior epigastric vessels but lateral to the rectus abdominis. Goes through the external (superficial) inguinal ring only. Covered by external spermatic fascia. Usually occurs in older men due to an acquired weakness in the transversalis fascia.

MDs don't LIe:
Medial to inferior epigastric vessels = Direct hernia.
Lateral to inferior epigastric vessels = Indirect hernia.

Femoral hernia

Protrudes below inguinal ligament through femoral canal below and lateral to pubic tubercle. More common in females, but overall inguinal hernias are the most common.

More likely to present with incarceration or strangulation than inguinal hernias.

Inguinal ligament "inferior border"
Indirect inguinal hernia
Femoral vessels
Inferior epigastric vessels "superolateral border"
Rectus abdominis muscle "medial border"
Inguinal (Hesselbach) triangle *Direct inguinal hernia*
Femoral hernia

Inguinal (Hesselbach) triangle:
- Inferior epigastric vessels
- Lateral border of rectus abdominis
- Inguinal ligament

▶ GASTROINTESTINAL—PHYSIOLOGY

Gastrointestinal regulatory substances

REGULATORY SUBSTANCE	SOURCE	ACTION	REGULATION	NOTES
Gastrin	G cells (antrum of stomach, duodenum)	↑ gastric H⁺ secretion ↑ growth of gastric mucosa ↑ gastric motility	↑ by stomach distention/alkalinization, amino acids, peptides, vagal stimulation via gastrin-releasing peptide (GRP) ↓ by pH < 1.5	↑ by chronic PPI use. ↑ in chronic atrophic gastritis (eg, *H pylori*). ↑↑ in Zollinger-Ellison syndrome (gastrinoma).
Somatostatin	D cells (pancreatic islets, GI mucosa)	↓ gastric acid and pepsinogen secretion ↓ pancreatic and small intestine fluid secretion ↓ gallbladder contraction ↓ insulin and glucagon release	↑ by acid ↓ by vagal stimulation	Inhibits secretion of various hormones (encourages **somato-stasis**). Octreotide is an analog used to treat acromegaly, carcinoid syndrome, and variceal bleeding.
Cholecystokinin	I cells (duodenum, jejunum)	↑ pancreatic secretion ↑ gallbladder contraction ↓ gastric emptying ↑ sphincter of Oddi relaxation	↑ by fatty acids, amino acids	Acts on neural muscarinic pathways to cause pancreatic secretion.
Secretin	S cells (duodenum)	↑ pancreatic HCO₃⁻ secretion ↓ gastric acid secretion ↑ bile secretion	↑ by acid, fatty acids in lumen of duodenum	↑ HCO₃⁻ neutralizes gastric acid in duodenum, allowing pancreatic enzymes to function.
Glucose-dependent insulinotropic peptide	K cells (duodenum, jejunum)	Exocrine: ↓ gastric H⁺ secretion Endocrine: ↑ insulin release	↑ by fatty acids, amino acids, oral glucose	Also known as gastric inhibitory peptide (GIP). Oral glucose load leads to ↑ insulin compared to IV equivalent due to GIP secretion.
Motilin	Small intestine	Produces migrating motor complexes (MMCs)	↑ in fasting state	Motilin receptor agonists (eg, erythromycin) are used to stimulate intestinal peristalsis.
Vasoactive intestinal polypeptide	Parasympathetic ganglia in sphincters, gallbladder, small intestine	↑ intestinal water and electrolyte secretion ↑ relaxation of intestinal smooth muscle and sphincters	↑ by distention and vagal stimulation ↓ by adrenergic input	VIPoma—non-α, non-β islet cell pancreatic tumor that secretes VIP. Watery Diarrhea, Hypokalemia, and Achlorhydria (**WDHA** syndrome).
Nitric oxide		↑ smooth muscle relaxation, including lower esophageal sphincter (LES)		Loss of NO secretion is implicated in ↑ LES tone of achalasia.
Ghrelin	Stomach	↑ appetite	↑ in fasting state ↓ by food	↑ in Prader-Willi syndrome. ↓ after gastric bypass surgery.

Gastrointestinal secretory products

PRODUCT	SOURCE	ACTION	REGULATION	NOTES
Intrinsic factor	Parietal cells (stomach)	Vitamin B_{12}–binding protein (required for B_{12} uptake in terminal ileum)		Autoimmune destruction of parietal cells → chronic gastritis and pernicious anemia.
Gastric acid	Parietal cells (stomach)	↓ stomach pH	↑ by histamine, vagal stimulation (ACh), gastrin ↓ by somatostatin, GIP, prostaglandin, secretin	
Pepsin	Chief cells (stomach)	Protein digestion	↑ by vagal stimulation (ACh), local acid	Pepsinogen (inactive) is converted to pepsin (active) in the presence of H^+.
Bicarbonate	Mucosal cells (stomach, duodenum, salivary glands, pancreas) and Brunner glands (duodenum)	Neutralizes acid	↑ by pancreatic and biliary secretion with secretin	Trapped in mucus that covers the gastric epithelium.

Locations of gastrointestinal secretory cells

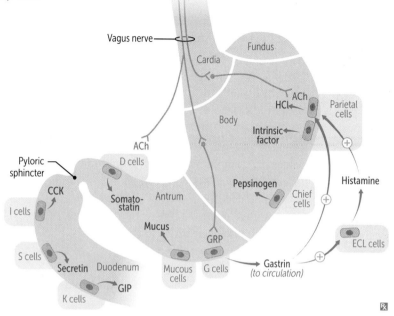

Gastrin ↑ acid secretion primarily through its effects on enterochromaffin-like (ECL) cells (leading to histamine release) rather than through its direct effect on parietal cells.

Pancreatic secretions	Isotonic fluid; low flow → high Cl^-, high flow → high HCO_3^-.	

ENZYME	ROLE	NOTES
α-amylase	Starch digestion	Secreted in active form
Lipases	Fat digestion	
Proteases	Protein digestion	Includes trypsin, chymotrypsin, elastase, carboxypeptidases Secreted as proenzymes also known as zymogens
Trypsinogen	Converted to active enzyme trypsin → activation of other proenzymes and cleaving of additional trypsinogen molecules into active trypsin (positive feedback loop)	Converted to trypsin by enterokinase/enteropeptidase, a brush-border enzyme on duodenal and jejunal mucosa

Carbohydrate absorption	Only monosaccharides (glucose, galactose, fructose) are absorbed by enterocytes. Glucose and galactose are taken up by SGLT1 (Na^+ dependent). Fructose is taken up via Facilitated diffusion by GLUT5. All are transported to blood by GLUT2. D-xylose absorption test: distinguishes GI mucosal damage from other causes of malabsorption.

Vitamin/mineral absorption

Iron	Absorbed as Fe^{2+} in duodenum.	Iron Fist, Bro
Folate	Absorbed in small bowel.	Clinically relevant in patients with small bowel disease or after resection.
B_{12}	Absorbed in terminal ileum along with bile salts, requires intrinsic factor.	

Peyer patches	Unencapsulated lymphoid tissue found in lamina propria and submucosa of ileum. Contain specialized **M** cells that sample and present antigens to i**M**mune cells. B cells stimulated in germinal centers of Peyer patches differentiate into IgA-secreting plasma cells, which ultimately reside in lamina propria. IgA receives protective secretory component and is then transported across the epithelium to the gut to deal with intraluminal antigen.	Think of **IgA**, the **I**ntra-gut **A**ntibody. And always say "secretory IgA."

Bile	Composed of bile salts (bile acids conjugated to glycine or taurine, making them water soluble), phospholipids, cholesterol, bilirubin, water, and ions. Cholesterol 7α-hydroxylase catalyzes rate-limiting step of bile acid synthesis. Functions: <ul><li>Digestion and absorption of lipids and fat-soluble vitamins</li><li>Cholesterol excretion (body's 1° means of eliminating cholesterol)</li><li>Antimicrobial activity (via membrane disruption)</li></ul>	↓ absorption of enteric bile salts at distal ileum (as in short bowel syndrome, Crohn disease) prevents normal fat absorption. Calcium, which normally binds oxalate, binds fat instead, so free oxalate is absorbed by gut → ↑ frequency of calcium oxalate kidney stones.

Bilirubin

Heme is metabolized by heme oxygenase to biliverdin, which is subsequently reduced to bilirubin. Unconjugated bilirubin is removed from blood by liver, conjugated with glucuronate, and excreted in bile.

Direct bilirubin—conjugated with glucuronic acid; water soluble.

Indirect bilirubin—unconjugated; water insoluble.

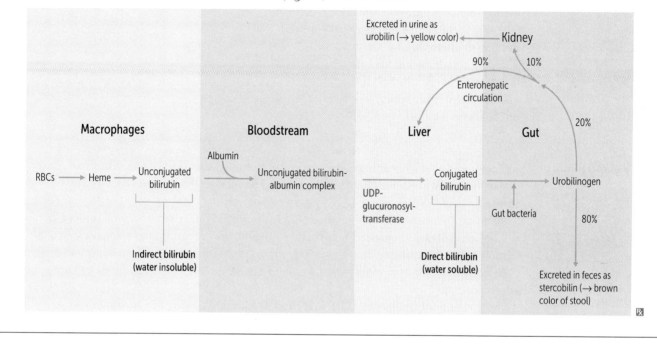

▶ GASTROINTESTINAL—PATHOLOGY

Sialolithiasis

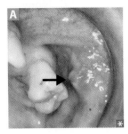

Stone(s) in salivary gland duct 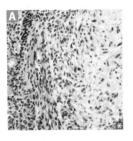. Can occur in 3 major salivary glands (parotid, submandibular, sublingual). Single stone more common in submandibular gland (Wharton duct).

Presents as recurrent pre-/periprandial pain and swelling in affected gland.

Caused by dehydration or trauma.

Treat conservatively with NSAIDs, gland massage, warm compresses, sour candies (to promote salivary flow).

Sialadenitis—inflammation of salivary gland due to obstruction, infection, or immune-mediated mechanisms.

Salivary gland tumors

Most commonly benign and in parotid gland. Tumors in smaller glands more likely malignant. Typically present as painless mass/swelling. Facial pain or paralysis suggests malignant involvement of CN VII.

- Pleomorphic adenoma (benign mixed tumor)—most common salivary gland tumor . Composed of chondromyxoid stroma and epithelium and recurs if incompletely excised or ruptured intraoperatively. May undergo malignant transformation.
- Mucoepidermoid carcinoma—most common malignant tumor, has mucinous and squamous components.
- Warthin tumor (papillary cystadenoma lymphomatosum)—benign cystic tumor with germinal centers. Typically found in **smokers**. Bilateral in 10%; multifocal in 10%. "**Warriors from Germany love smoking.**"

Achalasia

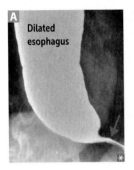
Dilated esophagus

Failure of LES to relax due to loss of myenteric (Auerbach) plexus due to loss of postganglionic inhibitory neurons (which contain NO and VIP).

Manometry findings include uncoordinated or absent peristalsis with high LES resting pressure → progressive dysphagia to solids and liquids (vs obstruction—solids only). Barium swallow shows dilated esophagus with an area of distal stenosis ("bird's beak").

Associated with ↑ risk of esophageal cancer.

A-*chalasia* = absence of relaxation.
2° achalasia (pseudoachalasia) may arise from Chagas disease (*T cruzi* infection) or extraesophageal malignancies (mass effect or paraneoplastic).

Esophageal pathologies

Boerhaave syndrome	Transmural, usually distal esophageal rupture with pneumomediastinum (arrows in **A**) due to violent retching. Subcutaneous emphysema may be due to dissecting air (crepitus may be felt in the neck region or chest wall). Surgical emergency.
Eosinophilic esophagitis	Infiltration of eosinophils in the esophagus often in atopic patients. Food allergens → dysphagia, food impaction. Esophageal rings and linear furrows often seen on endoscopy. Typically unresponsive to GERD therapy.
Esophageal strictures	Associated with caustic ingestion and acid reflux.
Esophageal varices	Dilated submucosal veins (red arrows in **B** **C**) in lower ⅓ of esophagus **A** 2° to portal hypertension. Common in cirrhotics, may be source of life-threatening hematemesis.
Esophagitis	Associated with reflux, infection in immunocompromised (*Candida*: white pseudomembrane; HSV-1: punched-out ulcers; CMV: linear ulcers), caustic ingestion, or pill esophagitis (eg, bisphosphonates, tetracycline, NSAIDs, iron, and potassium chloride).
Gastroesophageal reflux disease	Commonly presents as heartburn, regurgitation, dysphagia. May also present as chronic cough, hoarseness (laryngopharyngeal reflux). Associated with asthma. Transient decreases in LES tone.
Mallory-Weiss syndrome	Partial-thickness mucosal lacerations at gastroesophageal junction due to severe vomiting. Often presents with hematemesis. Usually found in alcoholics and bulimics.
Plummer-Vinson syndrome	Triad of Dysphagia, Iron deficiency anemia, and Esophageal webs. May be associated with glossitis. Increased risk of esophageal squamous cell carcinoma ("Plumbers DIE").
Sclerodermal esophageal dysmotility	Esophageal smooth muscle atrophy → ↓ LES pressure and dysmotility → acid reflux and dysphagia → stricture, Barrett esophagus, and aspiration. Part of CREST syndrome.

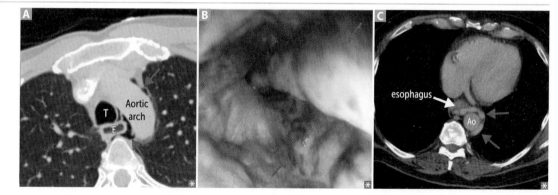

Barrett esophagus

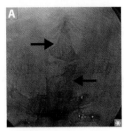

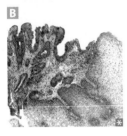

Specialized intestinal metaplasia 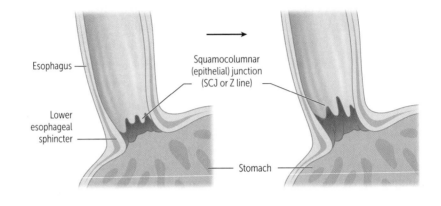—replacement of nonkeratinized stratified squamous epithelium with intestinal epithelium (nonciliated columnar with goblet cells [stained blue in **B**]) in distal esophagus. Due to chronic gastroesophageal reflux disease (GERD). Associated with ↑ risk of esophageal adenocarcinoma.

Esophageal cancer

Typically presents with progressive dysphagia (first solids, then liquids) and weight loss; poor prognosis.

CANCER	PART OF ESOPHAGUS AFFECTED	RISK FACTORS	PREVALENCE
Squamous cell carcinoma	Upper 2/3	Alcohol, hot liquids, caustic strictures, smoking, achalasia	More common worldwide
Adenocarcinoma	Lower 1/3	Chronic GERD, Barrett esophagus, obesity, smoking, achalasia	More common in America

Gastritis

Acute gastritis	Erosions can be caused by: ▪ NSAIDs—↓ PGE_2 → ↓ gastric mucosa protection ▪ Burns (Curling ulcer)—hypovolemia → mucosal ischemia ▪ Brain injury (Cushing ulcer)—↑ vagal stimulation → ↑ ACh → ↑ H^+ production	Especially common among alcoholics and patients taking daily NSAIDs (eg, patients with rheumatoid arthritis). Burned by the Curling iron. Always Cushion the brain.
Chronic gastritis	Mucosal inflammation, often leading to atrophy (hypochlorhydria → hypergastrinemia) and intestinal metaplasia (↑ risk of gastric cancers).	
H pylori	Most common. ↑ risk of peptic ulcer disease, MALT lymphoma.	Affects antrum first and spreads to body of stomach.
Autoimmune	Autoantibodies to parietal cells and intrinsic factor. ↑ risk of pernicious anemia.	Affects body/fundus of stomach.

Ménétrier disease 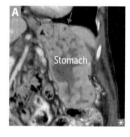	Hyperplasia of gastric mucosa → hypertrophied rugae (look like brain gyri 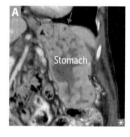). Causes excess mucus production with resultant protein loss and parietal cell atrophy with ↓ acid production. Precancerous. Presents with epigastric pain, anorexia, weight loss, vomiting, edema (due to protein loss).

Gastric cancer 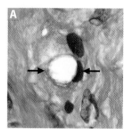	Most commonly gastric adenocarcinoma; lymphoma, GI stromal tumor, carcinoid (rare). Early aggressive local spread with node/liver metastases. Often presents late, with weight loss, abdominal pain, early satiety, and in some cases acanthosis nigricans or Leser-Trélat sign. Associated with blood type A. ▪ Intestinal—associated with *H pylori*, dietary nitrosamines (smoked foods), tobacco smoking, achlorhydria, chronic gastritis. Commonly on lesser curvature; looks like ulcer with raised margins. ▪ Diffuse—not associated with *H pylori*; signet ring cells (mucin-filled cells with peripheral nuclei) 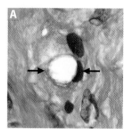; stomach wall grossly thickened and leathery (linitis plastica).	Virchow node—involvement of left supraclavicular node by metastasis from stomach. Krukenberg tumor—bilateral metastases to ovaries. Abundant mucin-secreting, signet ring cells. Sister Mary Joseph nodule—subcutaneous periumbilical metastasis.

Peptic ulcer disease

	Gastric ulcer	Duodenal ulcer
PAIN	Can be Greater with meals—weight loss	Decreases with meals—weight gain
H PYLORI INFECTION	~ 70%	~ 90%
MECHANISM	↓ mucosal protection against gastric acid	↓ mucosal protection or ↑ gastric acid secretion
OTHER CAUSES	NSAIDs	Zollinger-Ellison syndrome
RISK OF CARCINOMA	↑	Generally benign
OTHER	Biopsy margins to rule out malignancy	Hypertrophy of Brunner glands

Ulcer complications

Hemorrhage	Gastric, duodenal (posterior > anterior). Most common complication. Ruptured gastric ulcer on the lesser curvature of stomach → bleeding from left gastric artery. An ulcer on the posterior wall of duodenum → bleeding from gastroduodenal artery.
Obstruction	Pyloric channel, duodenal.
Perforation	Duodenal (anterior > posterior). May see free air under diaphragm A with referred pain to the shoulder via irritation of phrenic nerve.

Malabsorption syndromes	Can cause diarrhea, steatorrhea, weight loss, weakness, vitamin and mineral deficiencies. Screen for fecal fat (eg, Sudan stain).	
Celiac disease	Gluten-sensitive enteropathy, celiac sprue. Autoimmune-mediated intolerance of gliadin (gluten protein found in wheat) → malabsorption and steatorrhea. Associated with HLA-DQ2, HLA-DQ8, northern European descent, dermatitis herpetiformis, ↓ bone density. Findings: IgA anti-tissue transglutaminase (IgA tTG), anti-endomysial, anti-deamidated gliadin peptide antibodies; villous atrophy (arrow in A shows blunting), crypt hyperplasia (double arrows in A), and intraepithelial lymphocytosis. Moderately ↑ risk of malignancy (eg, T-cell lymphoma).	↓ mucosal absorption primarily affects distal duodenum and/or proximal jejunum. D-xylose test: passively absorbed in proximal small intestine; blood and urine levels ↓ with mucosa defects or bacterial overgrowth, normal in pancreatic insufficiency. Treatment: gluten-free diet.
Lactose intolerance	Lactase deficiency. Normal-appearing villi, except when 2° to injury at tips of villi (eg, viral enteritis). Osmotic diarrhea with ↓ stool pH (colonic bacteria ferment lactose).	Lactose hydrogen breath test: ⊕ for lactose malabsorption if post-lactose breath hydrogen value rises > 20 ppm compared with baseline.
Pancreatic insufficiency	Due to chronic pancreatitis, cystic fibrosis, obstructing cancer. Causes malabsorption of fat and fat-soluble vitamins (A, D, E, K) as well as vitamin B_{12}.	↓ duodenal pH (bicarbonate) and fecal elastase.
Tropical sprue	Similar findings as celiac sprue (affects small bowel), but responds to antibiotics. Cause is unknown, but seen in residents of or recent visitors to tropics.	↓ mucosal absorption affecting duodenum and jejunum but can involve ileum with time. Associated with megaloblastic anemia due to folate deficiency and, later, B_{12} deficiency.
Whipple disease	Infection with *Tropheryma whipplei* (intracellular gram ⊕); PAS ⊕ **foamy** macrophages in intestinal lamina propria B, **mesenteric** nodes. **Cardiac** symptoms, **Arthralgias**, and **Neurologic** symptoms are common. Diarrhea/steatorrhea occur later in disease course. Most common in older men.	Foamy Whipped cream in a CAN.

Inflammatory bowel disease

	Crohn disease	Ulcerative colitis
LOCATION	Any portion of the GI tract, usually the terminal ileum and colon. Skip lesions, rectal sparing.	Colitis = colon inflammation. Continuous colonic lesions, always with rectal involvement.
GROSS MORPHOLOGY	Transmural inflammation → fistulas. Cobblestone mucosa, creeping fat, bowel wall thickening ("string sign" on barium swallow x-ray A), linear ulcers, fissures.	Mucosal and submucosal inflammation only. Friable mucosa with superficial and/or deep ulcerations (compare normal B with diseased C). Loss of haustra → "lead pipe" appearance on imaging.
MICROSCOPIC MORPHOLOGY	Noncaseating granulomas and lymphoid aggregates. Th1 mediated.	Crypt abscesses and ulcers, bleeding, no granulomas. Th2 mediated.
COMPLICATIONS	Malabsorption/malnutrition, colorectal cancer (↑ risk with pancolitis).	
	Fistulas (eg, enterovesical fistulae, which can cause recurrent UTI and pneumaturia), phlegmon/abscess, strictures (causing obstruction), perianal disease.	Fulminant colitis, toxic megacolon, perforation.
INTESTINAL MANIFESTATION	Diarrhea that may or may not be bloody.	Bloody diarrhea.
EXTRAINTESTINAL MANIFESTATIONS	Rash (pyoderma gangrenosum, erythema nodosum), eye inflammation (episcleritis, uveitis), oral ulcerations (aphthous stomatitis), arthritis (peripheral, spondylitis).	
	Kidney stones (usually calcium oxalate), gallstones. May be ⊕ for anti-*Saccharomyces cerevisiae* antibodies (ASCA).	1° sclerosing cholangitis. Associated with p-ANCA.
TREATMENT	Corticosteroids, azathioprine, antibiotics (eg, ciprofloxacin, metronidazole), infliximab, adalimumab.	5-aminosalicylic preparations (eg, mesalamine), 6-mercaptopurine, infliximab, colectomy.
	For Crohn, think of a fat granny and an old crone skipping down a cobblestone road away from the wreck (rectal sparing).	Ulcerative colitis causes ULCCCERS: Ulcers Large intestine Continuous, Colorectal carcinoma, Crypt abscesses Extends proximally Red diarrhea Sclerosing cholangitis

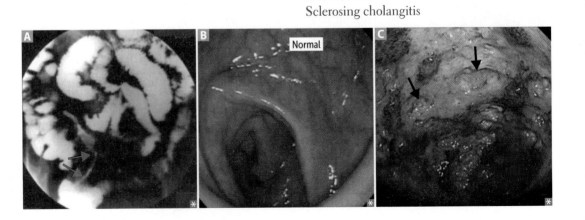

Irritable bowel syndrome

Recurrent abdominal pain associated with ≥ 2 of the following:
- Related to defecation
- Change in stool frequency
- Change in form (consistency) of stool

No structural abnormalities. Most common in middle-aged women. Chronic symptoms may be diarrhea-predominant, constipation-predominant, or mixed. Pathophysiology is multifaceted. First-line treatment is lifestyle modification and dietary changes.

Appendicitis

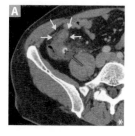

Acute inflammation of the appendix (yellow arrows in Ⓐ), can be due to obstruction by fecalith (red arrow in Ⓐ) (in adults) or lymphoid hyperplasia (in children).

Initial diffuse periumbilical pain migrates to McBurney point (⅓ the distance from right anterior superior iliac spine to umbilicus). Nausea, fever; may perforate → peritonitis; may elicit psoas, obturator, and Rovsing signs, guarding and rebound tenderness on exam.

Differential: diverticulitis (elderly), ectopic pregnancy (use β-hCG to rule out), pseudoappendicitis. Treatment: appendectomy.

Diverticula of the GI tract

Diverticulum	Blind pouch Ⓐ protruding from the alimentary tract that communicates with the lumen of the gut. Most diverticula (esophagus, stomach, duodenum, colon) are acquired and are termed "false diverticula."	"True" diverticulum—all gut wall layers outpouch (eg, Meckel). "False" diverticulum or pseudodiverticulum— only mucosa and submucosa outpouch. Occur especially where vasa recta perforate muscularis externa.
Diverticulosis	Many false diverticula of the colon Ⓑ, commonly sigmoid. Common (in ~ 50% of people > 60 years). Caused by ↑ intraluminal pressure and focal weakness in colonic wall. Associated with obesity and diets low in fiber, high in total fat/red meat.	Often asymptomatic or associated with vague discomfort. Complications include diverticular bleeding (painless hematochezia), diverticulitis.
Diverticulitis	Inflammation of diverticula with wall thickening Ⓒ classically causing LLQ pain, fever, leukocytosis. Treat with antibiotics.	Complications: abscess, fistula (colovesical fistula → pneumaturia), obstruction (inflammatory stenosis), perforation (→ peritonitis).

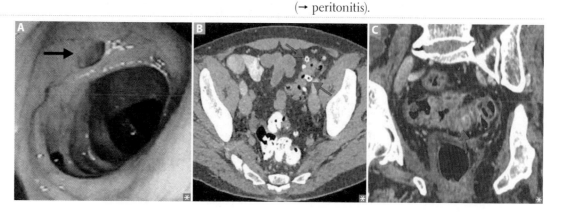

Zenker diverticulum

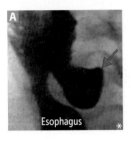

A

Esophagus

Pharyngoesophageal **false** diverticulum **A**. Esophageal dysmotility causes herniation of mucosal tissue at Killian triangle between the thyropharyngeal and cricopharyngeal parts of the inferior pharyngeal constrictor. Presenting symptoms: dysphagia, obstruction, gurgling, aspiration, foul breath, neck mass. Most common in elderly males.

Elder MIKE has bad breath.
  Elderly
  Males
  Inferior pharyngeal constrictor
  Killian triangle
  Esophageal dysmotility
  Halitosis

Meckel diverticulum

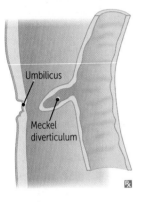

Umbilicus

Meckel
diverticulum

True diverticulum. Persistence of the vitelline (omphalomesenteric) duct. May contain ectopic acid–secreting gastric mucosa and/or pancreatic tissue. Most common congenital anomaly of GI tract. Can cause hematochezia/melena (less commonly), RLQ pain, intussusception, volvulus, or obstruction near terminal ileum.
Contrast with omphalomesenteric cyst = cystic dilation of vitelline duct.
Diagnosis: pertechnetate study for uptake by heterotopic gastric mucosa.

The rule of 2's:
  2 times as likely in males.
  2 inches long.
  2 feet from the ileocecal valve.
  2% of population.
  Commonly presents in first 2 years of life.
  May have 2 types of epithelia (gastric/pancreatic).

Hirschsprung disease

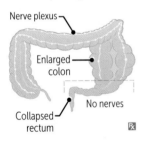

Nerve plexus

Enlarged
colon

No nerves

Collapsed
rectum

Congenital megacolon characterized by lack of ganglion cells/enteric nervous plexuses (Auerbach and Meissner plexuses) in distal segment of colon. Due to failure of neural crest cell migration. Associated with mutations in *RET*.
Presents with bilious emesis, abdominal distention, and failure to pass meconium within 48 hours → chronic constipation. Normal portion of the colon proximal to the aganglionic segment is dilated, resulting in a "transition zone."

Risk ↑ with Down syndrome.
Explosive expulsion of feces (squirt sign)
  → empty rectum on digital exam.
Diagnosed by absence of ganglionic cells on rectal suction biopsy.
Treatment: resection.
RET mutation in the REcTum.

Malrotation

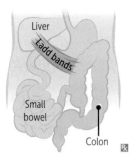

Anomaly of midgut rotation during fetal development → improper positioning of bowel (small bowel clumped on the right side) 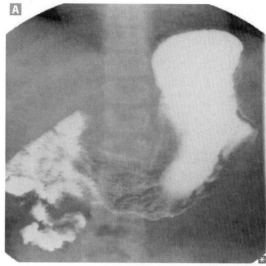, formation of fibrous bands (Ladd bands). Can lead to volvulus, duodenal obstruction.

Volvulus

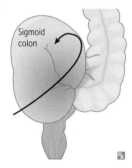

Twisting of portion of bowel around its mesentery; can lead to obstruction and infarction. Can occur throughout the GI tract. Midgut volvulus more common in infants and children. Sigmoid volvulus (coffee bean sign on x-ray 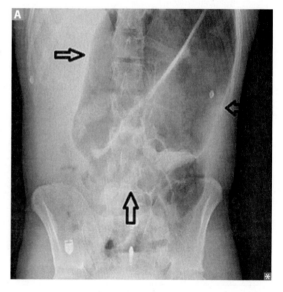) more common in elderly.

Intussusception

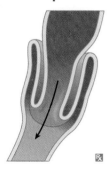

Telescoping 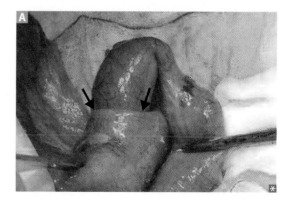 of proximal bowel segment into a distal segment, commonly at ileocecal junction. Compromised blood supply → intermittent abdominal pain often with "currant jelly" stools. Patient may draw legs to chest to ease pain. Exam may reveal sausage-shaped mass. Ultrasound shows "target sign." Often due to a lead point, but can be idiopathic. Most common pathologic lead point is a Meckel diverticulum (children) or intraluminal mass/tumor (adults). Majority of cases occur in children; unusual in adults. May be associated with rotavirus vaccine, Henoch-Schönlein purpura, and recent viral infection (eg, adenovirus; Peyer patch hypertrophy creates lead point).

Other intestinal disorders

Acute mesenteric ischemia	Critical blockage of intestinal blood flow (often embolic occlusion of SMA) → small bowel necrosis 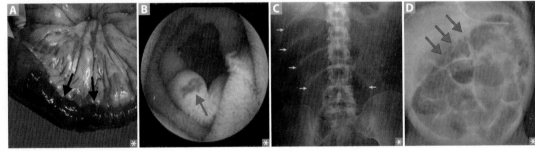 → abdominal pain out of proportion to physical findings. May see red "currant jelly" stools.
Chronic mesenteric ischemia	"Intestinal angina": atherosclerosis of celiac artery, SMA, or IMA → intestinal hypoperfusion → postprandial epigastric pain → food aversion and weight loss.
Colonic ischemia	Reduction in intestinal blood flow causes ischemia. Crampy abdominal pain followed by hematochezia. Commonly occurs at watershed areas (splenic flexure, distal colon). Typically affects elderly. Thumbprint sign on imaging due to mucosal edema/hemorrhage.
Angiodysplasia	Tortuous dilation of vessels B → hematochezia. Most often found in the right-sided colon. More common in older patients. Confirmed by angiography. Associated with aortic stenosis and von Willebrand disease.
Adhesion	Fibrous band of scar tissue; commonly forms after surgery. Most common cause of small bowel obstruction, demonstrated by multiple dilated small bowel loops on x-ray (arrows in C).
Ileus	Intestinal hypomotility without obstruction → constipation and ↓ flatus; distended/tympanic abdomen with ↓ bowel sounds. Associated with abdominal surgeries, opiates, hypokalemia, sepsis. Treatment: bowel rest, electrolyte correction, cholinergic drugs (stimulate intestinal motility).
Meconium ileus	In cystic fibrosis, meconium plug obstructs intestine, preventing stool passage at birth.
Necrotizing enterocolitis	Seen in premature, formula-fed infants with immature immune system. Necrosis of intestinal mucosa (primarily colonic) with possible perforation, which can lead to pneumatosis intestinalis D, free air in abdomen, portal venous gas.

Colonic polyps	Growths of tissue within the colon 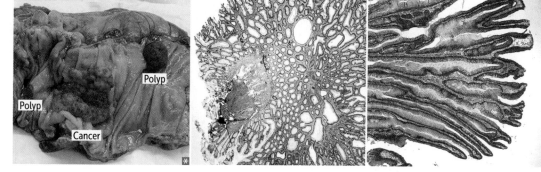. May be neoplastic or non-neoplastic. Grossly characterized as flat, sessile, or pedunculated (on a stalk) on the basis of protrusion into colonic lumen. Generally classified by histologic type.

HISTOLOGIC TYPE	CHARACTERISTICS
Generally non-neoplastic	
Hamartomatous polyps	Solitary lesions do not have significant risk of transformation. Growths of normal colonic tissue with distorted architecture. Associated with Peutz-Jeghers syndrome and juvenile polyposis.
Mucosal polyps	Small, usually < 5 mm. Look similar to normal mucosa. Clinically insignificant.
Inflammatory pseudopolyps	Due to mucosal erosion in inflammatory bowel disease.
Submucosal polyps	May include lipomas, leiomyomas, fibromas, and other lesions.
Hyperplastic polyps	Most common; generally smaller and predominantly located in rectosigmoid region. Occasionally evolves into serrated polyps and more advanced lesions.
Malignant potential	
Adenomatous polyps	Neoplastic, via chromosomal instability pathway with mutations in *APC* and *KRAS*. Tubular B histology has less malignant potential than villous C ("**villous** histology is **villainous**"); tubulovillous has intermediate malignant potential. Usually asymptomatic; may present with occult bleeding.
Serrated polyps	Premalignant. Characterized by CpG island methylator phenotype (CIMP; cytosine base followed by guanine, linked by a phosphodiester bond). Defect may silence *MMR* gene (DNA mismatch repair) expression. Mutations lead to microsatellite instability and mutations in *BRAF*. "Sawtooth" pattern of crypts on biopsy. Up to 20% of cases of sporadic CRC.

Polyposis syndromes

Familial adenomatous polyposis	Autosomal dominant mutation of *APC* tumor suppressor gene on chromosome 5q21. 2-hit hypothesis. Thousands of polyps arise starting after puberty; pancolonic; always involves rectum. Prophylactic colectomy or else 100% progress to CRC.
Gardner syndrome	FAP + osseous and soft tissue tumors, congenital hypertrophy of retinal pigment epithelium, impacted/supernumerary teeth.
Turcot syndrome	FAP/Lynch syndrome + malignant CNS tumor (eg, medulloblastoma, glioma). **Turcot** = **Turban**.
Peutz-Jeghers syndrome	Autosomal dominant syndrome featuring numerous hamartomas throughout GI tract, along with hyperpigmented mouth, lips, hands, genitalia. Associated with ↑ risk of breast and GI cancers (eg, colorectal, stomach, small bowel, pancreatic).
Juvenile polyposis syndrome	Autosomal dominant syndrome in children (typically < 5 years old) featuring numerous hamartomatous polyps in the colon, stomach, small bowel. Associated with ↑ risk of CRC.

Lynch syndrome	Previously known as hereditary nonpolyposis colorectal cancer (HNPCC). Autosomal dominant mutation of DNA mismatch repair genes with subsequent microsatellite instability. ~ 80% progress to CRC. Proximal colon is always involved. Associated with endometrial, ovarian, and skin cancers.

Colorectal cancer

EPIDEMIOLOGY	Most patients are > 50 years old. ~ 25% have a family history.	
RISK FACTORS	Adenomatous and serrated polyps, familial cancer syndromes, IBD, tobacco use, diet of processed meat with low fiber.	
PRESENTATION	Rectosigmoid > ascending > descending. Ascending—exophytic mass, iron deficiency anemia, weight loss. Descending—infiltrating mass, partial obstruction, colicky pain, hematochezia. Rarely, presents with S bovis (gallolyticus) bacteremia.	Right side bleeds; left side obstructs (narrower lumen).
DIAGNOSIS	Iron deficiency anemia in males (especially > 50 years old) and postmenopausal females raises suspicion. Screen low-risk patients starting at age 50 with colonoscopy A; alternatives include flexible sigmoidoscopy, fecal occult blood testing (FOBT), fecal immunochemical testing (FIT), and CT colonography. Patients with a first-degree relative who has colon cancer should be screened via colonoscopy at age 40, or starting 10 years prior to their relative's presentation. Patients with IBD have a distinct screening protocol. "Apple core" lesion seen on barium enema x-ray B. CEA tumor marker: good for monitoring recurrence, should not be used for screening.	

Molecular pathogenesis of colorectal cancer	Chromosomal instability pathway: mutations in *APC* cause FAP and most sporadic CRC (via adenoma-carcinoma sequence; (**firing** order of events is **AK-53**). Microsatellite instability pathway: mutations or methylation of mismatch repair genes (eg, *MLH1*) cause Lynch syndrome and some sporadic CRC (via serrated polyp pathway). Overexpression of COX-2 has been linked to colorectal cancer, NSAIDs may be chemopreventive.

Chromosomal instability pathway

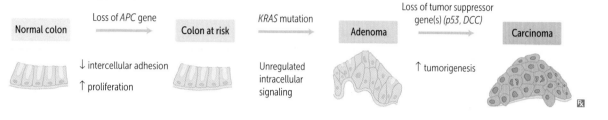

Normal colon — Loss of *APC* gene → Colon at risk — *KRAS* mutation → Adenoma — Loss of tumor suppressor gene(s) *(p53, DCC)* → Carcinoma

↓ intercellular adhesion
↑ proliferation

Unregulated intracellular signaling

↑ tumorigenesis

Cirrhosis and portal hypertension

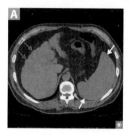

Cirrhosis—diffuse bridging fibrosis (via stellate cells) and regenerative nodules (red arrows in A; white arrows show splenomegaly) disrupt normal architecture of liver; ↑ risk for hepatocellular carcinoma (HCC). Etiologies include alcohol, nonalcoholic steatohepatitis, chronic viral hepatitis, autoimmune hepatitis, biliary disease, genetic/metabolic disorders.

Portal hypertension—↑ pressure in portal venous system. Etiologies include cirrhosis (most common cause in Western countries), vascular obstruction (eg, portal vein thrombosis, Budd-Chiari syndrome), schistosomiasis.

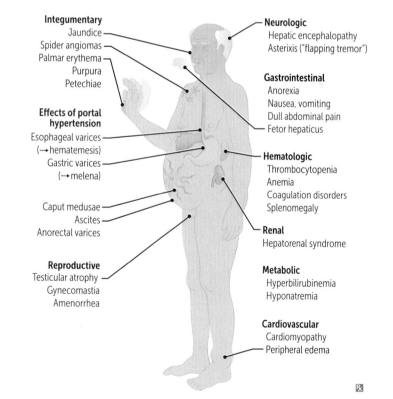

Integumentary
Jaundice
Spider angiomas
Palmar erythema
Purpura
Petechiae

Effects of portal hypertension
Esophageal varices
(→hematemesis)
Gastric varices
(→melena)

Caput medusae
Ascites
Anorectal varices

Reproductive
Testicular atrophy
Gynecomastia
Amenorrhea

Neurologic
Hepatic encephalopathy
Asterixis ("flapping tremor")

Gastrointestinal
Anorexia
Nausea, vomiting
Dull abdominal pain
Fetor hepaticus

Hematologic
Thrombocytopenia
Anemia
Coagulation disorders
Splenomegaly

Renal
Hepatorenal syndrome

Metabolic
Hyperbilirubinemia
Hyponatremia

Cardiovascular
Cardiomyopathy
Peripheral edema

Spontaneous bacterial peritonitis

Also known as 1° bacterial peritonitis. Common and potentially fatal bacterial infection in patients with cirrhosis and ascites. Often asymptomatic, but can cause fevers, chills, abdominal pain, ileus, or worsening encephalopathy. Commonly caused by aerobic gram ⊖ organisms (eg, *E coli*, *Klebsiella*) or less commonly gram ⊕ *Streptococcus*.

Diagnosis: paracentesis with ascitic fluid absolute neutrophil count (ANC) > 250 cells/mm³.

Empiric first-line treatment is 3rd generation cephalosporin (eg, cefotaxime).

Serum markers of liver pathology

ENZYMES RELEASED IN LIVER DAMAGE	
Aspartate aminotransferase and alanine aminotransferase	↑ in most liver disease: ALT > AST ↑ in alcoholic liver disease: AST > ALT AST > ALT in nonalcoholic liver disease suggests progression to advanced fibrosis or cirrhosis
Alkaline phosphatase	↑ in cholestasis (eg, biliary obstruction), infiltrative disorders, bone disease
γ-glutamyl transpeptidase	↑ in various liver and biliary diseases (just as ALP can), but not in bone disease; associated with alcohol use
FUNCTIONAL LIVER MARKERS	
Bilirubin	↑ in various liver diseases (eg, biliary obstruction, alcoholic or viral hepatitis, cirrhosis), hemolysis
Albumin	↓ in advanced liver disease (marker of liver's biosynthetic function)
Prothrombin time	↑ in advanced liver disease (↓ production of clotting factors, thereby measuring the liver's biosynthetic function)
Platelets	↓ in advanced liver disease (↓ thrombopoietin, liver sequestration) and portal hypertension (splenomegaly/splenic sequestration)

Reye syndrome

Rare, often fatal childhood hepatic encephalopathy. Findings: mitochondrial abnormalities, fatty liver (microvesicular fatty change), hypoglycemia, vomiting, hepatomegaly, coma. Associated with viral infection (especially VZV and influenza) that has been treated with aspirin. Mechanism: aspirin metabolites ↓ β-oxidation by reversible inhibition of mitochondrial enzymes. Avoid aspirin in children, except in those with Kawasaki disease.

Reye of sunSHINE:
Steatosis of liver/hepatocytes
Hypoglycemia/Hepatomegaly
Infection (VZV, influenza)
Not awake (coma)
Encephalopathy

Alcoholic liver disease

Hepatic steatosis	Macrovesicular fatty change A that may be reversible with alcohol cessation.	
Alcoholic hepatitis	Requires sustained, long-term consumption. Swollen and necrotic hepatocytes with neutrophilic infiltration. Mallory bodies B (intracytoplasmic eosinophilic inclusions of damaged keratin filaments).	Make a toAST with alcohol: AST > ALT (ratio usually > 2:1).
Alcoholic cirrhosis	Final and usually irreversible form. Sclerosis around central vein (arrows in C) may be seen in early disease. Regenerative nodules surrounded by fibrous bands in response to chronic liver injury → portal hypertension and end-stage liver disease.	

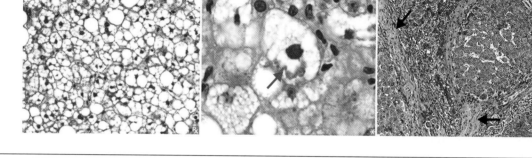

Nonalcoholic fatty liver disease	Metabolic syndrome (insulin resistance); obesity → fatty infiltration of hepatocytes A → cellular "ballooning" and eventual necrosis. May cause cirrhosis and HCC. Independent of alcohol use.	ALT > AST (Lipids)

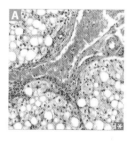

Hepatic encephalopathy	Cirrhosis → portosystemic shunts → ↓ NH_3 metabolism → neuropsychiatric dysfunction. Reversible neuropsychiatric dysfunction ranging from disorientation/asterixis (mild) to difficult arousal or coma (severe). Triggers: ▪ ↑ NH_3 production and absorption (due to dietary protein, GI bleed, constipation, infection). ▪ ↓ NH_3 removal (due to renal failure, diuretics, bypassed hepatic blood flow post-TIPS). Treatment: lactulose (↑ NH_4^+ generation) and rifaximin or neomycin (↓ NH_3 producing gut bacteria).

Hepatocellular carcinoma/hepatoma	Most common 1° malignant tumor of liver in adults 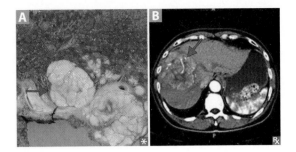. Associated with HBV (+/– cirrhosis) and all other causes of cirrhosis (including HCV, alcoholic and nonalcoholic fatty liver disease, autoimmune disease, hemochromatosis, α_1-antitrypsin deficiency) and specific carcinogens (eg, aflatoxin from *Aspergillus*). May lead to Budd-Chiari syndrome. Findings: jaundice, tender hepatomegaly, ascites, polycythemia, anorexia. Spreads hematogenously. Diagnosis: ↑ α-fetoprotein; ultrasound or contrast CT/MRI **B**, biopsy.

Other liver tumors

Cavernous hemangioma	Most common benign liver tumor **A**; typically occurs at age 30–50 years. Biopsy contraindicated because of risk of hemorrhage.
Hepatic adenoma	Rare, benign liver tumor, often related to oral contraceptive or anabolic steroid use; may regress spontaneously or rupture (abdominal pain and shock).
Angiosarcoma	Malignant tumor of endothelial origin; associated with exposure to arsenic, vinyl chloride.
Metastases	GI malignancies, breast and lung cancer. Most common overall; metastases are rarely solitary.

Budd-Chiari syndrome	Thrombosis or compression of hepatic veins with centrilobular congestion and necrosis → congestive liver disease (hepatomegaly, ascites, varices, abdominal pain, liver failure). Absence of JVD. Associated with hypercoagulable states, polycythemia vera, postpartum state, HCC. May cause nutmeg liver (mottled appearance).

α_1-antitrypsin deficiency	Misfolded gene product protein aggregates in hepatocellular ER → cirrhosis with PAS ⊕ globules **A** in liver. Codominant trait. Often presents in young patients with liver damage and dyspnea without a history of smoking.	In lungs, ↓ α_1-antitrypsin → uninhibited elastase in alveoli → ↓ elastic tissue → panacinar emphysema.

Jaundice	Abnormal yellowing of the skin and/or sclera A due to bilirubin deposition. Hyperbilirubinemia 2° to ↑ production or ↓ disposition (impaired hepatic uptake, conjugation, excretion).	**HOT Liver**—common causes of ↑ bilirubin level: **H**emolysis **O**bstruction **T**umor **Liver** disease

Unconjugated (indirect) hyperbilirubinemia	Hemolytic, physiologic (newborns), Crigler-Najjar, Gilbert syndrome.

Conjugated (direct) hyperbilirubinemia	Biliary tract obstruction: gallstones, cholangiocarcinoma, pancreatic or liver cancer, liver fluke.
	Biliary tract disease:
	  ▪ 1° sclerosing cholangitis
	  ▪ 1° biliary cholangitis
	Excretion defect: Dubin-Johnson syndrome, Rotor syndrome.

Mixed (direct and indirect) hyperbilirubinemia	Hepatitis, cirrhosis.

Physiologic neonatal jaundice	At birth, immature UDP-glucuronosyltransferase → unconjugated hyperbilirubinemia → jaundice/kernicterus (deposition of unconjugated, lipid-soluble bilirubin in the brain, particularly basal ganglia). Occurs after first 24 hours of life and usually resolves without treatment in 1–2 weeks. Treatment: phototherapy (non-UV) isomerizes unconjugated bilirubin to water-soluble form.

Hereditary hyperbilirubinemias	All autosomal recessive.	
❶ Gilbert syndrome	Mildly ↓ UDP-glucuronosyltransferase conjugation and impaired bilirubin uptake. Asymptomatic or mild jaundice usually with stress, illness, or fasting. ↑ unconjugated bilirubin without overt hemolysis.	Relatively common, benign condition. Go! (asymptomatic/benign)
❷ Crigler-Najjar syndrome, type I	Absent UDP-glucuronosyltransferase. Presents early in life; patients die within a few years. Findings: jaundice, kernicterus (bilirubin deposition in brain), ↑ unconjugated bilirubin. Treatment: plasmapheresis and phototherapy. Liver transplant is curative.	Type II is less severe and responds to phenobarbital, which ↑ liver enzyme synthesis. No-go! (symptomatic)
❸ Dubin-Johnson syndrome	Conjugated hyperbilirubinemia due to defective liver excretion. Grossly black (Dark) liver. Benign.	❹ Rotor syndrome is similar, but milder in presentation without black (Regular) liver. Due to impaired hepatic uptake and excretion.

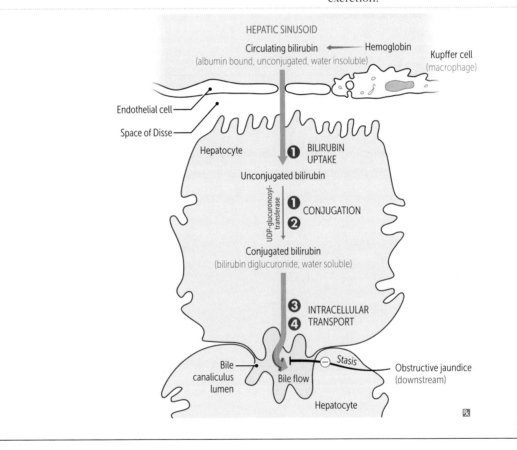

Wilson disease (hepatolenticular degeneration) 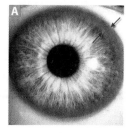	Autosomal recessive mutations in hepatocyte copper-transporting ATPase (*ATP7B* gene; chromosome 13) → ↓ copper incorporation into apoceruloplasmin and excretion into bile → ↓ serum ceruloplasmin. Copper accumulates, especially in liver, brain, cornea, kidneys; ↑ urine copper. Presents before age 40 with liver disease (eg, hepatitis, acute liver failure, cirrhosis), neurologic disease (eg, dysarthria, dystonia, tremor, parkinsonism), psychiatric disease, Kayser-Fleischer rings (deposits in Descemet membrane of cornea) **A**, hemolytic anemia, renal disease (eg, Fanconi syndrome). Treatment: chelation with penicillamine or trientine, oral zinc.
Hemochromatosis 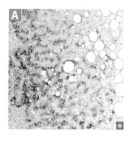	Autosomal recessive. C282Y mutation > H63D mutation on *HFE* gene, located on chromosome 6; associated with HLA-A3. Leads to abnormal **iron** sensing and ↑ intestinal absorption (↑ ferritin, ↑ iron, ↓ TIBC → ↑ transferrin saturation). Iron overload can also be 2° to chronic transfusion therapy (eg, β-thalassemia major). Iron accumulates, especially in liver, pancreas, skin, heart, pituitary, joints. Hemosiderin (iron) can be identified on liver MRI or biopsy with Prussian blue stain **A**. Presents after age 40 when total body iron > 20 g; iron loss through menstruation slows progression in women. Classic triad of cirrhosis, diabetes mellitus, skin pigmentation ("bronze diabetes"). Also causes restrictive cardiomyopathy (classic) or dilated cardiomyopathy (reversible), hypogonadism, arthropathy (calcium pyrophosphate deposition; especially metacarpophalangeal joints). HCC is common cause of death. Treatment: repeated phlebotomy, chelation with deferasirox, deferoxamine, oral deferiprone.
Biliary tract disease	May present with pruritus, jaundice, dark urine, light-colored stool, hepatosplenomegaly. Typically with cholestatic pattern of LFTs (↑ conjugated bilirubin, ↑ cholesterol, ↑ ALP).

	PATHOLOGY	EPIDEMIOLOGY	ADDITIONAL FEATURES
Primary sclerosing cholangitis	Unknown cause of concentric "onion skin" bile duct fibrosis → alternating strictures and dilation with "beading" of intra- and extrahepatic bile ducts on ERCP, magnetic resonance cholangiopancreatography (MRCP).	Classically in middle-aged men with IBD.	Associated with ulcerative colitis. p-ANCA ⊕. ↑ IgM. Can lead to 2° biliary cholangitis. ↑ risk of cholangiocarcinoma and gallbladder cancer.
Primary biliary cholangitis	Autoimmune reaction → lymphocytic infiltrate + granulomas → destruction of lobular bile ducts.	Classically in middle-aged women.	Anti-mitochondrial antibody ⊕, ↑ IgM. Associated with other autoimmune conditions (eg, Sjögren syndrome, Hashimoto thyroiditis, CREST, rheumatoid arthritis, celiac disease).
Secondary biliary cholangitis	Extrahepatic biliary obstruction → ↑ pressure in intrahepatic ducts → injury/fibrosis and bile stasis.	Patients with known obstructive lesions (gallstones, biliary strictures, pancreatic carcinoma).	May be complicated by ascending cholangitis.

Gallstones (cholelithiasis)

↑ cholesterol and/or bilirubin, ↓ bile salts, and gallbladder stasis all cause stones.

2 types of stones:
- Cholesterol stones (radiolucent with 10–20% opaque due to calcifications)—80% of stones. Associated with obesity, Crohn disease, advanced age, estrogen therapy, multiparity, rapid weight loss, Native American origin.
- Pigment stones A (black = radiopaque, Ca^{2+} bilirubinate, hemolysis; brown = radiolucent, infection). Associated with Crohn disease, chronic hemolysis, alcoholic cirrhosis, advanced age, biliary infections, total parenteral nutrition (TPN).

Risk factors (**4 F's**):
1. Female
2. Fat
3. Fertile (multiparity)
4. Forty

Most common complication is cholecystitis; can also cause acute pancreatitis, ascending cholangitis.

Diagnose with ultrasound. Treat with elective cholecystectomy if symptomatic.

RELATED PATHOLOGIES	CHARACTERISTICS
Biliary colic	Associated with nausea/vomiting and dull RUQ pain. Neurohormonal activation (eg, by CCK after a fatty meal) triggers contraction of gallbladder, forcing stone into cystic duct. Labs are normal, ultrasound shows cholelithiasis.
Choledocholithiasis	Presence of gallstone(s) in common bile duct, often leading to elevated ALP, GGT, direct bilirubin, and/or AST/ALT.
Cholecystitis	Acute or chronic inflammation of gallbladder. Calculous cholecystitis—most common type; due to gallstone impaction in the cystic duct resulting in inflammation and gallbladder wall thickening (arrows in B); can produce 2° infection. Acalculous cholecystitis—due to gallbladder stasis, hypoperfusion, or infection (CMV); seen in critically ill patients. Murphy sign: inspiratory arrest on RUQ palpation due to pain. Pain may radiate to right shoulder (due to irritation of phrenic nerve). ↑ ALP if bile duct becomes involved (eg, ascending cholangitis). Diagnose with ultrasound or cholescintigraphy (HIDA scan). Failure to visualize gallbladder on HIDA scan suggests obstruction. Gallstone ileus—fistula between gallbladder and GI tract → stone enters GI lumen → obstructs at ileocecal valve (narrowest point); can see air in biliary tree (pneumobilia).
Porcelain gallbladder	Calcified gallbladder due to chronic cholecystitis; usually found incidentally on imaging C. Treatment: prophylactic cholecystectomy due to high rates of gallbladder cancer (mostly adenocarcinoma).
Ascending cholangitis	Infection of biliary tree usually due to obstruction that leads to stasis/bacterial overgrowth. Charcot triad of cholangitis includes jaundice, fever, RUQ pain. Reynolds pentad is Charcot triad plus altered mental status and shock (hypotension).

Acute pancreatitis

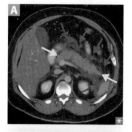
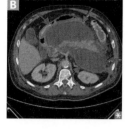

Autodigestion of pancreas by pancreatic enzymes (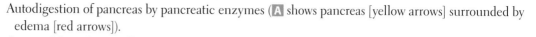 **A** shows pancreas [yellow arrows] surrounded by edema [red arrows]).

Causes: Idiopathic, Gallstones, Ethanol, Trauma, Steroids, Mumps, Autoimmune disease, Scorpion sting, Hypercalcemia/Hypertriglyceridemia (> 1000 mg/dL), ERCP, Drugs (eg, sulfa drugs, NRTIs, protease inhibitors). **I GET SMASHED.**

Diagnosis by 2 of 3 criteria: acute epigastric pain often radiating to the back, ↑ serum amylase or lipase (more specific) to 3× upper limit of normal, or characteristic imaging findings.

Complications: pseudocyst **B** (lined by granulation tissue, not epithelium), abscess, necrosis, hemorrhage, infection, organ failure (ARDS, shock, renal failure), hypocalcemia (precipitation of Ca^{2+} soaps).

Chronic pancreatitis

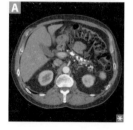

Chronic inflammation, atrophy, calcification of the pancreas **A**. Major causes include alcohol abuse and genetic predisposition (ie, cystic fibrosis); can be idiopathic. Complications include pancreatic insufficiency and pseudocysts.

Pancreatic insufficiency (typically when <10% pancreatic function) may manifest with steatorrhea, fat-soluble vitamin deficiency, diabetes mellitus.

Amylase and lipase may or may not be elevated (almost always elevated in acute pancreatitis).

Pancreatic adenocarcinoma

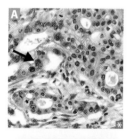
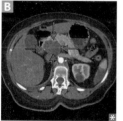

Very aggressive tumor arising from pancreatic ducts (disorganized glandular structure with cellular infiltration **A**); often metastatic at presentation, with average survival ~ 1 year after diagnosis. Tumors more common in pancreatic head **B** (→ obstructive jaundice). Associated with CA 19-9 tumor marker (also CEA, less specific).

Risk factors:
- Tobacco use
- Chronic pancreatitis (especially > 20 years)
- Diabetes
- Age > 50 years
- Jewish and African-American males

Often presents with:
- Abdominal pain radiating to back
- Weight loss (due to malabsorption and anorexia)
- Migratory thrombophlebitis—redness and tenderness on palpation of extremities (Trousseau syndrome)
- Obstructive jaundice with palpable, nontender gallbladder (Courvoisier sign)

Treatment: Whipple procedure, chemotherapy, radiation therapy.

▶ **GASTROINTESTINAL—PHARMACOLOGY**

Acid suppression therapy

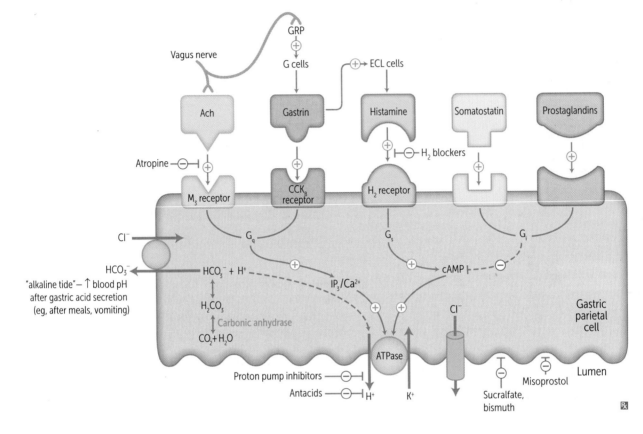

Histamine-2 blockers	Cimetidine, ranitidine, famotidine, nizatidine.	Take H_2 blockers before you **dine**. Think "table for 2" to remember H_2.
MECHANISM	Reversible block of histamine H_2-receptors → ↓ H^+ secretion by parietal cells.	
CLINICAL USE	Peptic ulcer, gastritis, mild esophageal reflux.	
ADVERSE EFFECTS	Cimetidine is a potent inhibitor of cytochrome P-450 (multiple drug interactions); it also has antiandrogenic effects (prolactin release, gynecomastia, impotence, ↓ libido in males); can cross blood-brain barrier (confusion, dizziness, headaches) and placenta. Both cimetidine and ranitidine ↓ renal excretion of creatinine. Other H_2 blockers are relatively free of these effects.	

Proton pump inhibitors	Omeprazole, lansoprazole, esomeprazole, pantoprazole, dexlansoprazole.
MECHANISM	Irreversibly inhibit H^+/K^+ ATPase in stomach parietal cells.
CLINICAL USE	Peptic ulcer, gastritis, esophageal reflux, Zollinger-Ellison syndrome, component of therapy for *H pylori*, stress ulcer prophylaxis.
ADVERSE EFFECTS	↑ risk of *C difficile* infection, pneumonia, acute interstitial nephritis. ↓ serum Mg^{2+} with long-term use; ↓ serum Mg^{2+} and ↓ Ca^{2+} absorption (potentially leading to increased fracture risk in elderly).

Antacids	Can affect absorption, bioavailability, or urinary excretion of other drugs by altering gastric and urinary pH or by delaying gastric emptying. All can cause hypokalemia. Overuse can also cause the following problems.	
Aluminum hydroxide	Constipation and hypophosphatemia; proximal muscle weakness, osteodystrophy, seizures	**Alumin**imum amount of feces.
Calcium carbonate	Hypercalcemia (milk-alkali syndrome), rebound acid ↑	Can chelate and ↓ effectiveness of other drugs (eg, tetracycline).
Magnesium hydroxide	Diarrhea, hyporeflexia, hypotension, cardiac arrest	Mg^{2+} = Must go to the bathroom.

Bismuth, sucralfate

MECHANISM	Bind to ulcer base, providing physical protection and allowing HCO_3^- secretion to reestablish pH gradient in the mucous layer. Require acidic environment; usually not given with PPIs/H_2 blockers.
CLINICAL USE	↑ ulcer healing, travelers' diarrhea (bismuth).

Misoprostol

MECHANISM	PGE_1 analog. ↑ production and secretion of gastric mucous barrier, ↓ acid production.
CLINICAL USE	Prevention of NSAID-induced peptic ulcers (NSAIDs block PGE_1 production). Also used off-label for induction of labor (ripens cervix).
ADVERSE EFFECTS	Diarrhea. Contraindicated in women of childbearing potential (abortifacient).

Octreotide

MECHANISM	Long-acting somatostatin analog; inhibits secretion of various splanchnic vasodilatory hormones.
CLINICAL USE	Acute variceal bleeds, acromegaly, VIPoma, carcinoid tumors.
ADVERSE EFFECTS	Nausea, cramps, steatorrhea. ↑ risk of cholelithiasis due to CCK inhibition.

Sulfasalazine

MECHANISM	A combination of sulfapyridine (antibacterial) and 5-aminosalicylic acid (anti-inflammatory). Activated by colonic bacteria.
CLINICAL USE	Ulcerative colitis, Crohn disease (colitis component).
ADVERSE EFFECTS	Malaise, nausea, sulfonamide toxicity, reversible oligospermia.

Loperamide

MECHANISM	Agonist at μ-opioid receptors; slows gut motility. Poor CNS penetration (low addictive potential).
CLINICAL USE	Diarrhea.
ADVERSE EFFECTS	Constipation, nausea.

Ondansetron

MECHANISM	5-HT$_3$ antagonist; ↓ vagal stimulation. Powerful central-acting antiemetic.
CLINICAL USE	Control vomiting postoperatively and in patients undergoing cancer chemotherapy.
ADVERSE EFFECTS	Headache, constipation, QT interval prolongation, serotonin syndrome.

Metoclopramide

MECHANISM	D$_2$ receptor antagonist. ↑ resting tone, contractility, LES tone, motility, promotes gastric emptying. Does not influence colon transport time.
CLINICAL USE	Diabetic and postsurgery gastroparesis, antiemetic, persistent GERD.
ADVERSE EFFECTS	↑ parkinsonian effects, tardive dyskinesia. Restlessness, drowsiness, fatigue, depression, diarrhea. Drug interaction with digoxin and diabetic agents. Contraindicated in patients with small bowel obstruction or Parkinson disease (due to D$_2$-receptor blockade).

Orlistat

MECHANISM	Inhibits gastric and pancreatic lipase → ↓ breakdown and absorption of dietary fats.
CLINICAL USE	Weight loss.
ADVERSE EFFECTS	Abdominal pain, flatulence, bowel urgency/frequent bowel movements; ↓ absorption of fat-soluble vitamins.

Laxatives

Indicated for constipation or patients on opiates requiring a bowel regimen.

	EXAMPLES	MECHANISM	ADVERSE EFFECTS
Bulk-forming laxatives	Psyllium, methylcellulose	Soluble fibers draw water into gut lumen, forming a viscous liquid that promotes peristalsis	Bloating
Osmotic laxatives	Magnesium hydroxide, magnesium citrate, polyethylene glycol, lactulose	Provides osmotic load to draw water into GI lumen. Lactulose also treats hepatic encephalopathy: gut flora degrade lactulose into metabolites (lactic acid, acetic acid) that promote nitrogen excretion as NH$_4^+$	Diarrhea, dehydration; may be abused by bulimics
Stimulants	Senna	Enteric nerve stimulation → colonic contraction	Diarrhea, melanosis coli
Emollients	Docusate	Promotes incorporation of water and fat into stool	Diarrhea

Aprepitant

MECHANISM	Substance P antagonist. Blocks NK$_1$ (neurokinin-1) receptors in brain.
CLINICAL USE	Antiemetic for chemotherapy-induced nausea and vomiting.

Hematology and Oncology

"Of all that is written, I love only what a person has written with his own blood."

— Friedrich Nietzsche

"All the soarings of my mind begin in my blood."

— Rainer Maria Rilke

"The best blood will at some time get into a fool or a mosquito."

— Austin O'Malley

When studying hematology, pay close attention to the many cross connections to immunology. Make sure you master the different types of anemias. Be comfortable interpreting blood smears. Please note that solid tumors are covered in the other organ systems. When reviewing oncologic drugs, focus on mechanisms and adverse effects rather than details of clinical uses, which may be lower yield.

▶ HEMATOLOGY AND ONCOLOGY—ANATOMY

Erythrocytes

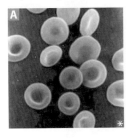

Carry O_2 to tissues and CO_2 to lungs. Anucleate and lack organelles; biconcave , with large surface area-to-volume ratio for rapid gas exchange. Life span of 120 days. Source of energy is glucose (90% used in glycolysis, 10% used in HMP shunt). Membranes contain Cl^-/HCO_3^- antiporter, which allow RBCs to export HCO_3^- and transport CO_2 from the periphery to the lungs for elimination.

Eryth = red; *cyte* = cell.

Erythrocytosis = polycythemia = ↑ Hct.
Anisocytosis = varying sizes.
Poikilocytosis = varying shapes.

Reticulocyte = immature RBC; reflects erythroid proliferation.
Bluish color (polychromasia) on Wright-Giemsa stain of reticulocytes represents residual ribosomal RNA.

Thrombocytes (platelets)

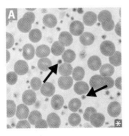

Involved in 1° hemostasis. Small cytoplasmic fragments derived from megakaryocytes. Life span of 8–10 days. When activated by endothelial injury, aggregate with other platelets and interact with fibrinogen to form platelet plug. Contain dense granules (ADP, Ca^{2+}) and α granules (vWF, fibrinogen, fibronectin). Approximately ⅓ of platelet pool is stored in the spleen.

Thrombocytopenia or ↓ platelet function results in petechiae.
vWF receptor: GpIb.
Fibrinogen receptor: GpIIb/IIIa.
Thrombopoietin stimulates megakaryocyte proliferation.
Alfa granules contain vwF, fibrinogen, fibronectin.

Leukocytes

Divided into granulocytes (neutrophils, eosinophils, basophils, mast cells) and mononuclear cells (monocytes, lymphocytes). WBC differential count from highest to lowest (normal ranges per USMLE):
    Neutrophils (~ 60%)
    Lymphocytes (~ 30%)
    Monocytes (~ 6%)
    Eosinophils (~ 3%)
    Basophils (~ 1%)

Leuk = white; *cyte* = cell.

Neutrophils Like Making Everything Better.

Neutrophils

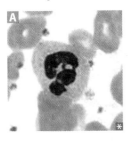

Acute inflammatory response cells. Numbers ↑ in bacterial infections. Phagocytic. Multilobed nucleus . Specific granules contain leukocyte alkaline phosphatase (LAP), collagenase, lysozyme, and lactoferrin. Azurophilic granules (lysosomes) contain proteinases, acid phosphatase, myeloperoxidase, and β-glucuronidase.

Hypersegmented neutrophils (nucleus has 6+ lobes) are seen in vitamin B_{12}/ folate deficiency.
↑ band cells (immature neutrophils) reflect states of ↑ myeloid proliferation (bacterial infections, CML).
Important neutrophil chemotactic agents: C5a, IL-8, LTB_4, kallikrein, platelet-activating factor.

Monocytes

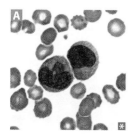

Found in blood, differentiate into macrophages in tissues.

Large, kidney-shaped nucleus A. Extensive "frosted glass" cytoplasm.

Mono = one (nucleus); *cyte* = cell.

Macrophages

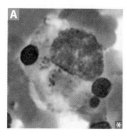

Phagocytose bacteria, cellular debris, and senescent RBCs. Long life in tissues. Differentiate from circulating blood monocytes A. Activated by γ-interferon. Can function as antigen-presenting cell via MHC II.

Macro = large; *phage* = eater.

Name differs in each tissue type (eg, Kupffer cells in liver, histiocytes in connective tissue, Langerhans cells in skin, osteoclasts in bone, microglial cells in brain).

Important component of granuloma formation (eg, TB, sarcoidosis).

Lipid A from bacterial LPS binds CD14 on macrophages to initiate septic shock.

Eosinophils

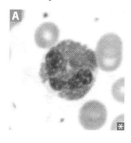

Defend against helminthic infections (major basic protein). Bilobate nucleus. Packed with large eosinophilic granules of uniform size A. Highly phagocytic for antigen-antibody complexes.

Produce histaminase, major basic protein (MBP, a helminthotoxin), eosinophil peroxidase, eosinophil cationic protein, and eosinophil-derived neurotoxin.

Eosin = pink dye; *philic* = loving.

Causes of eosinophilia = **PACCMAN**:

Parasites

Asthma

Churg-Strauss syndrome

Chronic adrenal insufficiency

Myeloproliferative disorders

Allergic processes

Neoplasia (eg, Hodgkin lymphoma)

Basophils

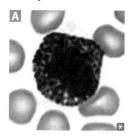

Mediate allergic reaction. Densely basophilic granules A contain heparin (anticoagulant) and histamine (vasodilator). Leukotrienes synthesized and released on demand.

Basophilic—stains readily with **basic** stains.

Basophilia is uncommon, but can be a sign of myeloproliferative disease, particularly CML.

Mast cells

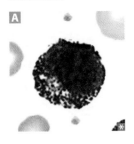

Mediate allergic reaction in local tissues. Contain basophilic granules and originate from the same precursor as basophils but are not the same cell type. Can bind the Fc portion of IgE to membrane. Activated by tissue trauma, C3a and C5a, surface IgE crosslinking by antigen (IgE receptor aggregation) → degranulation → release of histamine, heparin, tryptase, and eosinophil chemotactic factors.

Involved in type I hypersensitivity reactions. Cromolyn sodium prevents mast cell degranulation (used for asthma prophylaxis).

Dendritic cells

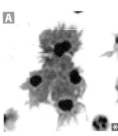

Highly phagocytic antigen-presenting cells (APCs) A. Function as link between innate and adaptive immune systems. Express MHC class II and Fc receptors on surface. Called Langerhans cell in the skin.

Lymphocytes

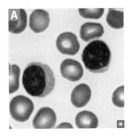

Refer to B cells, T cells, and NK cells. B cells and T cells mediate adaptive immunity. NK cells are part of the innate immune response. Round, densely staining nucleus with small amount of pale cytoplasm A.

B cells

Part of humoral immune response. Originate from stem cells in bone marrow and matures in marrow. Migrate to peripheral lymphoid tissue (follicles of lymph nodes, white pulp of spleen, unencapsulated lymphoid tissue). When antigen is encountered, B cells differentiate into plasma cells (which produce antibodies) and memory cells. Can function as an APC.

B = Bone marrow.

T cells

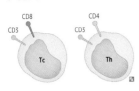

Mediate cellular immune response. Originate from stem cells in the bone marrow, but mature in the thymus. Differentiate into cytotoxic T cells (express CD8, recognize MHC I), helper T cells (express CD4, recognize MHC II), and regulatory T cells. CD28 (costimulatory signal) necessary for T-cell activation. Most circulating lymphocytes are T cells (80%).

T is for Thymus.
CD4+ helper T cells are the primary target of HIV.

Rule of 8: MHC II × CD4 = 8; MHC I × CD8 = 8.

Plasma cells

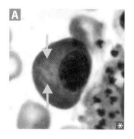

Produce large amounts of antibody specific to a particular antigen. "Clock-face" chromatin distribution and eccentric nucleus, abundant RER, and well-developed Golgi apparatus (arrows in **A**). Found in bone marrow and normally do not circulate in peripheral blood.

Multiple myeloma is a plasma cell cancer.

▶ HEMATOLOGY AND ONCOLOGY—PHYSIOLOGY

Fetal erythropoiesis	Fetal erythropoiesis occurs in: • Yolk sac (3–8 weeks) • Liver (6 weeks–birth) • Spleen (10–28 weeks) • Bone marrow (18 weeks to adult)	Young Liver Synthesizes Blood.
Hemoglobin development	Embryonic globins: ζ and ε. Fetal hemoglobin (HbF) = $\alpha_2\gamma_2$. Adult hemoglobin (HbA$_1$) = $\alpha_2\beta_2$. HbF has higher affinity for O_2 due to less avid binding of 2,3-BPG, allowing HbF to extract O_2 from maternal hemoglobin (HbA$_1$ and HbA$_2$) across the placenta. HbA$_2$ ($\alpha_2\delta_2$) is a form of adult hemoglobin present in small amounts.	From fetal to adult hemoglobin: Alpha Always; Gamma Goes, Becomes Beta.

BIRTH

Site of erythropoiesis

Yolk sac · Liver · Spleen · Bone marrow

% of total globin synthesis

50
40 — α — Fetal (HbF) — Adult (HbA₁)
30 — γ
20 — β
10 — ε · ζ · Embryonic globins

Weeks: 6 12 18 24 30 36   6 12 18 24 30 36 42 >>
FETUS (weeks)   POSTNATAL (months)   ADULT >>

Blood groups

	ABO classification				Rh classification	
	A	**B**	**AB**	**O**	**Rh⊕**	**Rh⊖**
RBC type						
Group antigens on RBC surface	A △	B ●	A & B △ ●	NONE	Rh (D) ⬠	NONE
Antibodies in plasma	Anti-B IgM	Anti-A IgM	NONE	Anti-A Anti-B IgM, IgG	NONE	Anti-D IgG
Clinical relevance	Receive B or AB → hemolytic reaction	Receive A or AB → hemolytic reaction	Universal recipient of RBCs; universal donor of plasma	Receive any non-O → hemolytic reaction Universal donor of RBCs; universal recipient of plasma	Can receive either Rh⊕ or Rh⊖ blood	Treat mother with anti-D Ig during and after each pregnancy to prevent anti-D IgG formation

Hemolytic disease of the newborn	Also known as erythroblastosis fetalis.	
	Rh hemolytic disease of the newborn	**ABO hemolytic disease of the newborn**
INTERACTION	Rh ⊖ mothers; Rh ⊕ fetus.	Type O mothers; type A or B fetus.
MECHANISM	First pregnancy: mother exposed to fetal blood (often during delivery) → formation of maternal anti-D IgG. Subsequent pregnancies: anti-D IgG crosses the placenta → HDN in the fetus.	Pre-existing maternal anti-A and/or anti-B IgG antibodies cross placenta → HDN in the fetus.
PRESENTATION	Jaundice shortly after birth, kernicterus, hydrops fetalis.	Mild jaundice in the neonate within 24 hours of birth. Usually less severe than Rh HDN.
TREATMENT/PREVENTION	Prevent by administration of anti-D IgG to Rh ⊖ pregnant women during third trimester and early postpartum period (if fetus tests ⊕ for Rh). Prevents maternal anti-D IgG production.	Treat newborn with phototherapy or exchange transfusion.

Hemoglobin electrophoresis

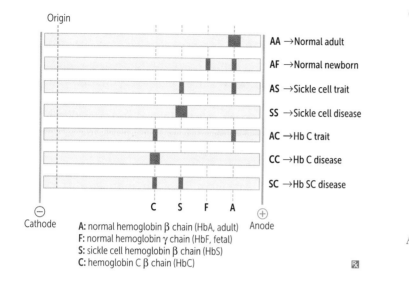

Origin

AA	→	Normal adult
AF	→	Normal newborn
AS	→	Sickle cell trait
SS	→	Sickle cell disease
AC	→	Hb C trait
CC	→	Hb C disease
SC	→	Hb SC disease

C   S   F   A

⊖ Cathode   ⊕ Anode

A: normal hemoglobin β chain (HbA, adult)
F: normal hemoglobin γ chain (HbF, fetal)
S: sickle cell hemoglobin β chain (HbS)
C: hemoglobin C β chain (HbC)

On a gel, hemoglobin migrates from the negatively charged cathode to the positively charged anode. HbA migrates the farthest, followed by HbF, HbS, and HbC. This is because the missense mutations in HbS and HbC replace glutamic acid ⊖ with valine (neutral) and lysine ⊕, respectively, impacting the net protein charge.

A Fat Santa Claus

Coagulation and kinin pathways

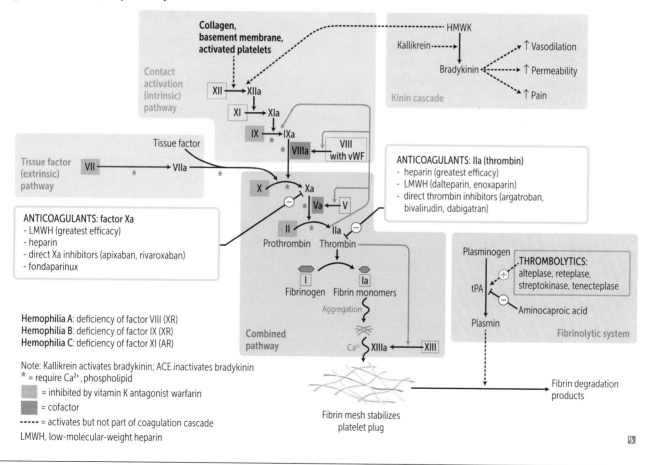

Collagen, basement membrane, activated platelets

HMWK

Kallikrein ----→

Bradykinin ◀---- ↑ Vasodilation
                 ↑ Permeability
                 ↑ Pain

Kinin cascade

Contact activation (intrinsic) pathway

XII → XIIa
XI → XIa
IX → IXa *
VIIIa
VIII with vWF

Tissue factor (extrinsic) pathway

VII → VIIa *
Tissue factor

X → Xa *
V → Va *
II → IIa *
Prothrombin   Thrombin

ANTICOAGULANTS: IIa (thrombin)
- heparin (greatest efficacy)
- LMWH (dalteparin, enoxaparin)
- direct thrombin inhibitors (argatroban, bivalirudin, dabigatran)

ANTICOAGULANTS: factor Xa
- LMWH (greatest efficacy)
- heparin
- direct Xa inhibitors (apixaban, rivaroxaban)
- fondaparinux

I → Ia
Fibrinogen   Fibrin monomers
Aggregation

Combined pathway

Ca^{2+} XIIIa ← XIII

Plasminogen

tPA ⊕ **THROMBOLYTICS:** alteplase, reteplase, streptokinase, tenecteplase
⊖ Aminocaproic acid

Plasmin

Fibrinolytic system

Fibrin degradation products

Hemophilia A: deficiency of factor VIII (XR)
Hemophilia B: deficiency of factor IX (XR)
Hemophilia C: deficiency of factor XI (AR)

Note: Kallikrein activates bradykinin; ACE inactivates bradykinin
* = require Ca^{2+}, phospholipid
▨ = inhibited by vitamin K antagonist warfarin
▨ = cofactor
---- = activates but not part of coagulation cascade
LMWH, low-molecular-weight heparin

Fibrin mesh stabilizes platelet plug

Coagulation cascade components

Procoagulation

Oxidized vitamin K →(epoxide reductase)→ reduced vitamin K →(acts as cofactor)→ γ-glutamyl carboxylase

- inactive II, VII, IX, X, C, S
- mature (active) II, VII, IX, X, C, S

Warfarin ⊖ (inhibits epoxide reductase)

Vitamin K deficiency: ↓ synthesis of factors II, VII, IX, X, protein C, protein S.

Warfarin inhibits vitamin K epoxide reductase. Vitamin K administration can potentially reverse inhibitory effect of warfarin on clotting factor synthesis. FFP or PCC administration reverses action of warfarin immediately and can be given with vitamin K in cases of severe bleeding.

Neonates lack enteric bacteria, which produce vitamin K. Early administration of vitamin K overcomes neonatal deficiency/coagulopathy.

Factor VII—Shortest half life.

Factor II—Longest half life.

vWF carries/protects factor VIII; volksWagen Factories make gr8 cars.

Anticoagulation

Protein C →(thrombin-thrombomodulin complex (endothelial cells))→ activated protein C →(protein S)→ cleaves and inactivates Va, VIIIa

Plasminogen →(tPA)→ plasmin → fibrinolysis:
1. cleavage of fibrin mesh
2. destruction of coagulation factors

Antithrombin inhibits activated forms of factors II, VII, IX, X, XI, XII.

Heparin enhances the activity of antithrombin.

Principal targets of antithrombin: thrombin and factor Xa.

Factor V Leiden mutation produces a factor V resistant to inhibition by activated protein C.

tPA is used clinically as a thrombolytic.

Platelet plug formation (primary hemostasis)

① INJURY
Endothelial damage → transient vasoconstriction via neural stimulation reflex and endothelin (released from damaged cell)

② EXPOSURE
vWF binds to exposed collagen
vWF is from Weibel-Palade bodies of endothelial cells and α-granules of platelets

③ ADHESION
Platelets bind vWF via GpIb receptor at the site of injury only (specific) → platelets undergo conformational change

Platelets release ADP and Ca^{2+} (necessary for coagulation cascade), TXA_2

ADP helps platelets adhere to endothelium

④A ACTIVATION
ADP binding to $P2Y_{12}$ receptor induces GpIIb/IIIa expression at platelet surface

④B AGGREGATION
Fibrinogen binds GpIIb/IIIa receptors and links platelets

Balance between

Pro-aggregation factors:
TXA_2 (released by platelets)
↓ blood flow
↑ platelet aggregation

Anti-aggregation factors:
PGI_2 and NO (released by endothelial cells)
↑ blood flow
↓ platelet aggregation

Temporary plug stops bleeding; unstable, easily dislodged

2° hemostasis
Coagulation cascade

Thrombogenesis

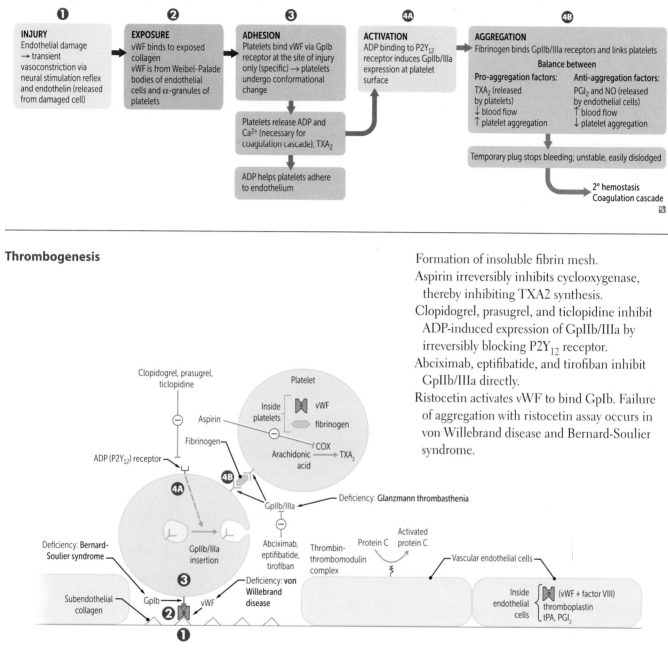

Formation of insoluble fibrin mesh.

Aspirin irreversibly inhibits cyclooxygenase, thereby inhibiting TXA2 synthesis.

Clopidogrel, prasugrel, and ticlopidine inhibit ADP-induced expression of GpIIb/IIIa by irreversibly blocking $P2Y_{12}$ receptor.

Abciximab, eptifibatide, and tirofiban inhibit GpIIb/IIIa directly.

Ristocetin activates vWF to bind GpIb. Failure of aggregation with ristocetin assay occurs in von Willebrand disease and Bernard-Soulier syndrome.

▸ HEMATOLOGY AND ONCOLOGY—PATHOLOGY

Pathologic RBC forms

TYPE	EXAMPLE	ASSOCIATED PATHOLOGY	NOTES
Acanthocytes ("spur cells") A		Liver disease, abetalipoproteinemia (states of cholesterol dysregulation).	*Acantho* = spiny.
Basophilic stippling B		Sideroblastic anemias (eg, lead poisoning, myelodysplastic syndromes), thalassemias.	Seen primarily in peripheral smear, vs ringed sideroblasts seen in bone marrow. Aggregation of residual ribosomes.
Dacrocytes ("teardrop cells") C		Bone marrow infiltration (eg, myelofibrosis), thalassemias.	RBC "sheds a **tear**" because it's mechanically squeezed out of its home in the bone marrow.
Degmacytes ("bite cells") D		G6PD deficiency.	
Echinocytes ("burr cells") E		End-stage renal disease, liver disease, pyruvate kinase deficiency.	Different from acanthocyte; its projections are more uniform and smaller.
Elliptocytes F		Hereditary elliptocytosis, usually asymptomatic; caused by mutation in genes encoding RBC membrane proteins (eg, spectrin).	
Macro-ovalocytes G		Megaloblastic anemia (also hypersegmented PMNs).	

Pathologic RBC forms (continued)

TYPE	EXAMPLE	ASSOCIATED PATHOLOGY	NOTES
Ringed sideroblasts H		Sideroblastic anemia. Excess iron in mitochondria.	Seen in bone marrow with special staining (Prussian blue), vs basophilic stippling in peripheral smear.
Schistocytes I		Microangiopathic hemolytic anemias, including DIC, TTP/HUS, HELLP syndrome, mechanical hemolysis (eg, heart valve prosthesis).	Fragmented RBCs (eg, helmet cells).
Sickle cells J		Sickle cell anemia.	Sickling occurs with dehydration, deoxygenation, and at high altitude.
Spherocytes K		Hereditary spherocytosis, drug- and infection-induced hemolytic anemia.	Small, spherical cells without central pallor.
Target cells L		HbC disease, Asplenia, Liver disease, Thalassemia.	"HALT," said the hunter to his target.

Other RBC abnormalities

TYPE	EXAMPLE	ASSOCIATED PATHOLOGY	NOTES
Heinz bodies A		Seen in G6PD deficiency.	Oxidation of Hb -SH groups to -S—S- → Hb precipitation (Heinz bodies), with subsequent phagocytic damage to RBC membrane → bite cells.
Howell-Jolly bodies B		Seen in patients with functional hyposplenia or asplenia.	Basophilic nuclear remnants found in RBCs. Howell-Jolly bodies are normally removed from RBCs by splenic macrophages.

Anemias

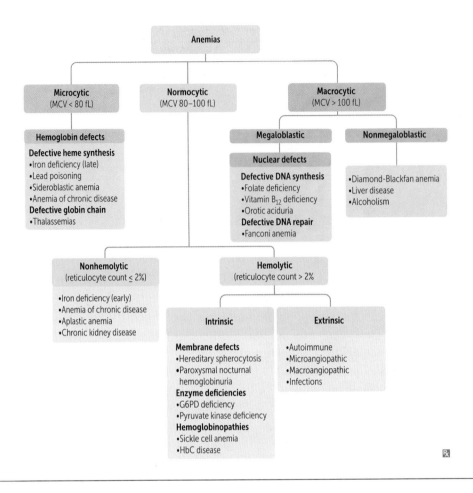

Microcytic, hypochromic anemia	MCV < 80 fL.
Iron deficiency	↓ iron due to chronic bleeding (eg, GI loss, menorrhagia), malnutrition, absorption disorders, GI surgery (eg, gastrectomy), or ↑ demand (eg, pregnancy) → ↓ final step in heme synthesis. Labs: ↓ iron, ↑ TIBC, ↓ ferritin, ↑ free erythrocyte protoporphyrin, ↑ RDW. Microcytosis and hypochromasia (↑ central pallor) **A**. Symptoms: fatigue, conjunctival pallor **B**, pica (consumption of nonfood substances), spoon nails (koilonychia). May manifest as glossitis, cheilosis, Plummer-Vinson syndrome (triad of iron deficiency anemia, esophageal webs, and dysphagia).
α-thalassemia	α-globin gene deletions → ↓ α-globin synthesis. *cis* deletion (deletions occur on same chromosome) prevalent in Asian populations; *trans* deletion (deletions occur on separate chromosomes) prevalent in African populations. Normal is αα/αα.

NUMBER OF α-GLOBIN GENES DELETED	DISEASE	CLINICAL OUTCOME
1 (α α/α −)	α-thalassemia minima	No anemia (silent carrier)
2 (α −/α −; *trans*) or (α α/− −; *cis*)	α-thalassemia minor	Mild microcytic, hypochromic anemia; *cis* deletion may worsen outcome for the carrier's offspring
3 (− −/− α)	Hemoglobin H disease (HbH); excess β-globin forms β_4	Moderate to severe microcytic hypochromic anemia
4 (− −/− −)	Hemoglobin Barts disease (Hb Barts); no α-globin, excess γ-globin forms γ_4	Hydrops fetalis; incompatible with life

Microcytic, hypochromic anemia *(continued)*

β-thalassemia	Point mutations in splice sites and promoter sequences → ↓ β-globin synthesis. Prevalent in Mediterranean populations.
	β-thalassemia minor (heterozygote): β chain is underproduced. Usually asymptomatic. Diagnosis confirmed by ↑ HbA$_2$ (> 3.5%) on electrophoresis.
	β-thalassemia major (homozygote): β chain is absent → severe microcytic, hypochromic anemia with target cells and increased anisopoikilocytosis requiring blood transfusion (2° hemochromatosis). Marrow expansion ("crew cut" on skull x-ray) → skeletal deformities. "Chipmunk" facies. Extramedullary hematopoiesis → hepatosplenomegaly. ↑ risk of parvovirus B19–induced aplastic crisis. ↑ HbF ($\alpha_2\gamma_2$), HbA$_2$ ($\alpha_2\delta_2$). HbF is protective in the infant and disease becomes symptomatic only after 6 months, when fetal hemoglobin declines.
	HbS/β-thalassemia heterozygote: mild to moderate sickle cell disease depending on amount of β-globin production.
Lead poisoning	Lead inhibits ferrochelatase and ALA dehydratase → ↓ heme synthesis and ↑ RBC protoporphyrin. Also inhibits rRNA degradation → RBCs retain aggregates of rRNA (basophilic stippling).
	Symptoms of **LEAD** poisoning:
	▪ **L**ead **L**ines on gingivae (Burton lines) and on metaphyses of long bones **D** on x-ray.
	▪ **E**ncephalopathy and **E**rythrocyte basophilic stippling.
	▪ **A**bdominal colic and sideroblastic **A**nemia.
	▪ **D**rops—wrist and foot drop. Dimercaprol and EDTA are 1st line of treatment.
	Succimer used for chelation for kids (It "**suc**ks" to be a kid who eats lead).
	Exposure risk ↑ in old houses with chipped paint.
Sideroblastic anemia	Causes: genetic (eg, X-linked defect in ALA synthase gene), acquired (myelodysplastic syndromes), and reversible (alcohol is most common; also lead, vitamin B$_6$ deficiency, copper deficiency, isoniazid, chloramphenicol).
	Lab findings: ↑ iron, normal/↓ TIBC, ↑ ferritin. Ringed sideroblasts (with iron-laden, Prussian blue–stained mitochondria) seen in bone marrow **E**. Peripheral blood smear: basophilic stippling of RBCs.
	Treatment: pyridoxine (B$_6$, cofactor for ALA synthase).

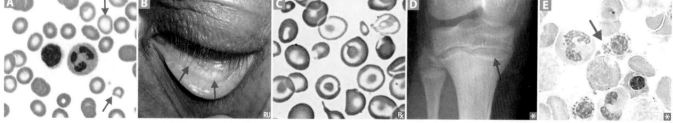

Macrocytic anemia   MCV > 100 fL.

	DESCRIPTION	FINDINGS
Megaloblastic anemia A 	Impaired DNA synthesis → maturation of nucleus of precursor cells in bone marrow delayed relative to maturation of cytoplasm.	RBC macrocytosis, hypersegmented neutrophils A, glossitis.
Folate deficiency	Causes: malnutrition (eg, alcoholics), malabsorption, drugs (eg, methotrexate, trimethoprim, phenytoin), ↑ requirement (eg, hemolytic anemia, pregnancy).	↑ homocysteine, normal methylmalonic acid. **No neurologic symptoms** (vs B_{12} deficiency).
Vitamin B_{12} (cobalamin) deficiency	Causes: pernicious anemia, malabsorption (eg, Crohn disease), gastrectomy, insufficient intake (eg, veganism), *Diphyllobothrium latum* (fish tapeworm).	↑ homocysteine, ↑ methylmalonic acid. **Neurologic symptoms:** reversible dementia, subacute combined degeneration (due to involvement of B_{12} in fatty acid pathways and myelin synthesis): spinocerebellar tract, lateral corticospinal tract, dorsal column dysfunction. Historically diagnosed with the Schilling test, a 4-stage test that determines if the cause is dietary insufficiency vs malabsorption. Anemia 2° to insufficient intake may take several years to develop due to liver's ability to store B_{12} (as opposed to folate deficiency).
Orotic aciduria	Inability to convert orotic acid to UMP (de novo pyrimidine synthesis pathway) because of defect in UMP synthase. Autosomal recessive. Presents in children as failure to thrive, developmental delay, and megaloblastic anemia refractory to folate and B_{12}. No hyperammonemia (vs ornithine transcarbamylase deficiency—↑ orotic acid with hyperammonemia).	Orotic acid in urine. Treatment: uridine monophosphate or uridine triacetate to bypass mutated enzyme.
Nonmegaloblastic anemia	Macrocytic anemia in which DNA synthesis is unimpaired. Causes: alcoholism, liver disease.	RBC macrocytosis without hypersegmented neutrophils.
Diamond-Blackfan anemia	Rapid-onset anemia within 1st year of life due to intrinsic defect in erythroid progenitor cells.	↑ % HbF (but ↓ total Hb). Short stature, craniofacial abnormalities, and upper extremity malformations (triphalangeal thumbs) in up to 50% of cases.

Normocytic, normochromic anemia	Normocytic, normochromic anemias are classified as nonhemolytic or hemolytic. The hemolytic anemias are further classified according to the cause of the hemolysis (intrinsic vs extrinsic to the RBC) and by the location of the hemolysis (intravascular vs extravascular). Hemolysis can lead to increases in LDH, reticulocytes, unconjugated bilirubin, urobilinogen in urine.
Intravascular hemolysis	Findings: ↓ haptoglobin, ↑ schistocytes on blood smear. Characteristic hemoglobinuria, hemosiderinuria, and urobilinogen in urine. May also see ↑ unconjugated bilirubin. Notable causes are mechanical hemolysis (eg, prosthetic valve), paroxysmal nocturnal hemoglobinuria, microangiopathic hemolytic anemias.
Extravascular hemolysis	Findings: macrophages in spleen clear RBCs. Spherocytes in peripheral smear (most commonly hereditary spherocytosis and autoimmune hemolytic anemia), no hemoglobinuria/hemosiderinuria. Can present with urobilinogen in urine.

Nonhemolytic, normocytic anemia

	DESCRIPTION	FINDINGS
Anemia of chronic disease	Inflammation → ↑ hepcidin (released by liver, binds ferroportin on intestinal mucosal cells and macrophages, thus inhibiting iron transport) → ↓ release of iron from macrophages and ↓ iron absorption from gut. Associated with conditions such as rheumatoid arthritis, SLE, neoplastic disorders, and chronic kidney disease.	↓ iron, ↓ TIBC, ↑ ferritin. Normocytic, but can become microcytic. Treatment: address underlying cause of inflammation, judicious use of blood transfusion, consider erythropoiesis-stimulating agents such as EPO (eg, in chronic kidney disease).
Aplastic anemia	Caused by failure or destruction of myeloid stem cells due to: ▪ Radiation and drugs (eg, benzene, chloramphenicol, alkylating agents, antimetabolites) ▪ Viral agents (EBV, HIV, hepatitis viruses) ▪ Fanconi anemia (DNA repair defect causing bone marrow failure; macrocytosis may be seen on CBC); also short stature, ↑ incidence of tumors/leukemia, café-au-lait spots, thumb/radial defects ▪ Idiopathic (immune mediated, 1° stem cell defect); may follow acute hepatitis	↓ reticulocyte count, ↑ EPO. Pancytopenia characterized by anemia, leukopenia, and thrombocytopenia. Normal cell morphology, but hypocellular bone marrow with fatty infiltration A (dry bone marrow tap). Symptoms: fatigue, malaise, pallor, purpura, mucosal bleeding, petechiae, infection. Treatment: withdrawal of offending agent, immunosuppressive regimens (eg, antithymocyte globulin, cyclosporine), bone marrow allograft, RBC/platelet transfusion, bone marrow stimulation (eg, GM-CSF).

Intrinsic hemolytic anemia

	DESCRIPTION	FINDINGS
Hereditary spherocytosis	Extravascular hemolysis due to defect in proteins interacting with RBC membrane skeleton and plasma membrane (eg, ankyrin, band 3, protein 4.2, spectrin). Mostly autosomal dominant inheritance. Results in small, round RBCs with less surface area and no central pallor (↑ MCHC) → premature removal by spleen.	Splenomegaly, aplastic crisis (parvovirus B19 infection). Labs: ↑ fragility in osmotic fragility test. Normal to ↓ MCV with abundance of cells. Treatment: splenectomy.
G6PD deficiency	Most common enzymatic disorder of RBCs. Causes extravascular and intravascular hemolysis. X-linked recessive. Defect in G6PD → ↓ reduced glutathione → ↑ RBC susceptibility to oxidant stress. Hemolytic anemia following oxidant stress (eg, sulfa drugs, antimalarials, infections, fava beans).	Back pain, hemoglobinuria a few days after oxidant stress. Labs: blood smear shows RBCs with Heinz bodies and bite cells. "Stress makes me eat bites of fava beans with Heinz ketchup."
Pyruvate kinase deficiency	Autosomal recessive pyruvate kinase defect → ↓ ATP → rigid RBCs → extravascular hemolysis. Increases levels of 2,3-BPG → ↓ hemoglobin affinity for O_2.	Hemolytic anemia in a newborn.
Paroxysmal nocturnal hemoglobinuria	↑ complement-mediated intravascular RBC lysis (acquired mutation in *PIGA* gene → impaired synthesis of GPI anchor for decay-accelerating factor [DAF/CD55] and membrane inhibitor of reactive lysis [MIRL/CD59] that protects RBC membrane from complement). Acquired mutation in a hematopoietic stem cell. ↑ incidence of acute leukemias.	Associated with aplastic anemia. Triad: Coombs ⊖ hemolytic anemia, pancytopenia, venous thrombosis. Patients may report red or pink urine (from hemoglobinuria). Labs: CD55/59 ⊖ RBCs on flow cytometry. Treatment: eculizumab (inhibits terminal complement formation).
Sickle cell anemia 	HbS point mutation causes a single amino acid replacement in β chain (substitution of glutamic acid with valine). Causes extravascular and intravascular hemolysis. Pathogenesis: low O_2, high altitude, or acidosis precipitates sickling (deoxygenated HbS polymerizes) → anemia, vaso-occlusive disease. Newborns are initially asymptomatic because of ↑ HbF and ↓ HbS. Heterozygotes (sickle cell trait) also have resistance to malaria. 8% of African Americans carry an HbS allele. Sickle cells are crescent-shaped RBCs **A**. "Crew cut" on skull x-ray due to marrow expansion from ↑ erythropoiesis (also seen in thalassemias).	Complications in sickle cell disease: <ul><li>Aplastic crisis (due to parvovirus B19).</li><li>Autosplenectomy (Howell-Jolly bodies) → ↑ risk of infection by encapsulated organisms (eg, *S pneumoniae*).</li><li>Splenic infarct/sequestration crisis.</li><li>*Salmonella* osteomyelitis.</li><li>Painful crises (vaso-occlusive): dactylitis **B** (painful swelling of hands/feet), priapism, acute chest syndrome, avascular necrosis, stroke.</li><li>Sickling in renal medulla (↓ P_{O_2}) → renal papillary necrosis → microhematuria.</li></ul> Diagnosis: hemoglobin electrophoresis. Treatment: hydroxyurea (↑ HbF), hydration.
HbC disease	Glutamic acid–to-lyCine (lysine) mutation in β-globin. Causes extravascular hemolysis.	Patients with HbSC (1 of each mutant gene) have milder disease than HbSS patients. Blood smear in homozygotes: hemoglobin Crystals inside RBCs, target cells.

Extrinsic hemolytic anemia

	DESCRIPTION	FINDINGS
Autoimmune hemolytic anemia	Warm (IgG)—chronic anemia seen in SLE and CLL and with certain drugs (eg, α-methyldopa) ("**warm** weather is **G**reat"). Cold (IgM and complement)—acute anemia triggered by cold; seen in CLL, *Mycoplasma pneumoniae* infections, and infectious Mononucleosis ("**cold** weather is **MMM**iserable"). RBC agglutinates A may cause painful, blue fingers and toes with cold exposure. Many warm and cold AIHAs are idiopathic.	Autoimmune hemolytic anemias are usually Coombs ⊕. Direct Coombs test—anti-Ig antibody (Coombs reagent) added to patient's RBCs. RBCs agglutinate if RBCs are coated with Ig. Indirect Coombs test—normal RBCs added to patient's serum. If serum has anti-RBC surface Ig, RBCs agglutinate when Coombs reagent added.

	Patient component	Reagent(s)	⊕ Result (agglutination)	⊖ Result (no agglutination)
Direct Coombs	RBCs +/− anti-RBC Ab	Anti-human globulin (Coombs reagent)	⊕ Result Anti-RBC Ab present	⊖ Result Anti-RBC Ab absent
Indirect Coombs	Patient serum +/− anti-donor RBC Ab	Donor blood / Anti-human globulin (Coombs reagent)	⊕ Result Anti−donor RBC Ab present	⊖ Result Anti−donor RBC Ab absent

Microangiopathic anemia	Pathogenesis: RBCs are damaged when passing through obstructed or narrowed vessel lumina. Seen in DIC, TTP/HUS, SLE, HELLP syndrome, hypertensive emergency.	Schistocytes (eg, "helmet cells") are seen on peripheral blood smear due to mechanical destruction (*schisto* = to split) of RBCs.
Macroangiopathic anemia	Prosthetic heart valves and aortic stenosis may also cause hemolytic anemia 2° to mechanical destruction of RBCs.	Schistocytes on peripheral blood smear.
Infections	↑ destruction of RBCs (eg, malaria, *Babesia*).	

Interpretation of iron studies

	Iron deficiency	Chronic disease	Hemochromatosis	Pregnancy/ OCP use
Serum iron	↓	↓	↑	—
Transferrin or TIBC	↑	↓[a]	↓	↑
Ferritin	↓	↑	↑	—
% transferrin saturation (serum iron/TIBC)	↓↓	—	↑↑	↓

↑↓ = 1° disturbance.

Transferrin—**trans**ports iron in blood.

TIBC—indirectly measures transferrin.

Ferritin—1° iron storage protein of body.

[a]Evolutionary reasoning—pathogens use circulating iron to thrive. The body has adapted a system in which iron is stored within the cells of the body and prevents pathogens from acquiring circulating iron.

Leukopenias

CELL TYPE	CELL COUNT	CAUSES
Neutropenia	Absolute neutrophil count < 1500 cells/mm^3 Severe infections typical when < 500 cells/mm^3	Sepsis/postinfection, drugs (including chemotherapy), aplastic anemia, SLE, radiation
Lymphopenia	Absolute lymphocyte count < 1500 cells/mm^3 (< 3000 cells/mm^3 in children)	HIV, DiGeorge syndrome, SCID, SLE, corticosteroids[a], radiation, sepsis, postoperative
Eosinopenia	Absolute eosinophil count < 30 cells/mm^3	Cushing syndrome, corticosteroids[a]

[a]Corticosteroids cause neutrophilia, despite causing eosinopenia and lymphopenia. Corticosteroids ↓ activation of neutrophil adhesion molecules, impairing migration out of the vasculature to sites of inflammation. In contrast, corticosteroids sequester eosinophils in lymph nodes and cause apoptosis of lymphocytes.

Left shift	↑ neutrophil precursors, such as band cells and metamyelocytes, in peripheral blood. Usually seen with neutrophilia in the acute response to infection or inflammation. Called **leukoerythroblastic reaction** when left shift is seen with immature RBCs. Occurs with severe anemia (physiologic response) or marrow response (eg, fibrosis, tumor taking up space in marrow).	A left shift is a shift to a more immature cell in the maturation process.

Heme synthesis, porphyrias, and lead poisoning	The porphyrias are hereditary or acquired conditions of defective heme synthesis that lead to the accumulation of heme precursors. Lead inhibits specific enzymes needed in heme synthesis, leading to a similar condition.

CONDITION	AFFECTED ENZYME	ACCUMULATED SUBSTRATE	PRESENTING SYMPTOMS
Lead poisoning	Ferrochelatase and ALA dehydratase	Protoporphyrin, ALA (blood)	Microcytic anemia (basophilic stippling in peripheral smear A, ringed sideroblasts in bone marrow), GI and kidney disease. Children—exposure to lead paint → mental deterioration. Adults—environmental exposure (eg, batteries, ammunition) → headache, memory loss, demyelination.
Acute intermittent porphyria	Porphobilinogen deaminase, previously known as uroporphyrinogen I synthase (autosomal dominant mutation)	Porphobilinogen, ALA	Symptoms (5 P's): ▪ Painful abdomen ▪ Port wine–colored urine ▪ Polyneuropathy ▪ Psychological disturbances ▪ Precipitated by drugs (eg, cytochrome P-450 inducers), alcohol, starvation Treatment: hemin and glucose, which inhibit ALA synthase.
Porphyria cutanea tarda	Uroporphyrinogen decarboxylase (autosomal dominant mutation)	Uroporphyrin (tea-colored urine)	Blistering cutaneous photosensitivity and hyperpigmentation B. Most common porphyria. Exacerbated with alcohol consumption. Associated with hepatitis C.

Location	Intermediates	Enzymes	Diseases
Mitochondria	Glycine + succinyl-CoA B₆ ↓ ⊖ ← Glucose, hemin Aminolevulinic acid	Aminolevulinate synthase (rate-limiting step)	Sideroblastic anemia (X-linked)
Cytoplasm	↓ Porphobilinogen	Aminolevulinate dehydratase	Lead poisoning
	↓ Hydroxymethylbilane	Porphobilinogen deaminase	Acute intermittent porphyria
	↓ Uroporphyrinogen III ↓ Coproporphyrinogen III	Uroporphyrinogen decarboxylase	Porphyria cutanea tarda
Mitochondria	↓ Protoporphyrin Fe²⁺ ↓ Heme	Ferrochelatase	Lead poisoning

↓ heme → ↑ ALA synthase activity
↑ heme → ↓ ALA synthase activity

Iron poisoning	High mortality rate with accidental ingestion by children (adult iron tablets may look like candy).
MECHANISM	Cell death due to peroxidation of membrane lipids.
SYMPTOMS/SIGNS	Nausea, vomiting, gastric bleeding, lethargy, scarring leading to GI obstruction.
TREATMENT	Chelation (eg, IV deferoxamine, oral deferasirox) and dialysis.

Coagulation disorders

PT—tests function of common and extrinsic pathway (factors I, II, V, VII, and X). Defect → ↑ PT (**P**lay **T**ennis outside [extrinsic pathway]).

INR (international normalized ratio)—calculated from PT. 1 = normal, > 1 = prolonged. Most common test used to follow patients on warfarin.

PTT—tests function of common and **in**trinsic pathway (all factors except VII and XIII). Defect → ↑ PTT (**P**lay **T**able **T**ennis inside).

Coagulation disorders can be due to clotting factor deficiencies or acquired inhibitors. Diagnosed with a mixing study, in which normal plasma is added to patient's plasma. Clotting factor deficiencies should correct (the PT or PTT returns to within the appropriate normal range), whereas factor inhibitors will not correct.

DISORDER	PT	PTT	MECHANISM AND COMMENTS
Hemophilia A, B, or C	—	↑	Intrinsic pathway coagulation defect (↑ PTT). ▪ A: deficiency of factor VIII; X-linked recessive. ▪ B: deficiency of factor IX; X-linked recessive. ▪ C: deficiency of factor XI; autosomal recessive. Hemorrhage in hemophilia—hemarthroses (bleeding into joints, eg, knee Ⓐ), easy bruising, bleeding after trauma or surgery (eg, dental procedures). Treatment: desmopressin + factor VIII concentrate (A); factor IX concentrate (B); factor XI concentrate (C).
Vitamin K deficiency	↑	↑	General coagulation defect. Bleeding time normal. ↓ activity of factors II, VII, IX, X, protein C, protein S.

Platelet disorders

Defects in platelet plug formation → ↑ bleeding time (BT).

Platelet abnormalities → microhemorrhage: mucous membrane bleeding, epistaxis, petechiae, purpura, ↑ bleeding time, possibly decreased platelet count (PC).

DISORDER	PC	BT	MECHANISM AND COMMENTS
Bernard-Soulier syndrome	−/↓	↑	Defect in platelet plug formation. Large platelets. ↓ GpIb → defect in platelet-to-vWF adhesion. Abnormal ristocetin test that does not correct with mixing studies.
Glanzmann thrombasthenia	−	↑	Defect in platelet integrin $\alpha_{IIb}\beta_3$ (GpIIb/IIIa) → defect in platelet-to-platelet aggregation, and therefore platelet plug formation. Labs: blood smear shows no platelet clumping.
Hemolytic-uremic syndrome	↓	↑	Characterized by thrombocytopenia, microangiopathic hemolytic anemia, and acute renal failure. Typical HUS is seen in children, accompanied by diarrhea and commonly caused by Shiga-like toxin of enterohemorrhagic *E coli* (EHEC) (eg, O157:H7). HUS in adults does not present with diarrhea; EHEC infection not required. Same spectrum as TTP, with a similar clinical presentation and same initial treatment of plasmapheresis.
Immune thrombocytopenia	↓	↑	Anti-GpIIb/IIIa antibodies → splenic macrophage consumption of platelet-antibody complex. May be 1° (idiopathic) or 2° to autoimmune disorder, viral illness, malignancy, or drug reaction. Labs: ↑ megakaryocytes on bone marrow biopsy. Treatment: steroids, IVIG; rituximab or splenectomy for refractory ITP.
Thrombotic thrombocytopenic purpura	↓	↑	Inhibition or deficiency of ADAMTS 13 (vWF metalloprotease) → ↓ degradation of vWF multimers. Pathogenesis: ↑ large vWF multimers → ↑ platelet adhesion → ↑ platelet aggregation and thrombosis. Labs: schistocytes, ↑ LDH, normal coagulation parameters. Symptoms (**FAT RN**): pentad of Fever, microangiopathic hemolytic Anemia, Thrombocytopenia, Renal failure, Neurologic symptoms. Treatment: plasmapheresis, steroids.

Mixed platelet and coagulation disorders

DISORDER	PC	BT	PT	PTT	MECHANISM AND COMMENTS
von Willebrand disease	—	↑	—	—/↑	Intrinsic pathway coagulation defect: ↓ vWF → ↑ PTT (vWF acts to carry/protect factor VIII). Defect in platelet plug formation: ↓ vWF → defect in platelet-to-vWF adhesion. Autosomal dominant. Mild but most common inherited bleeding disorder. No platelet aggregation with ristocetin cofactor assay. Treatment: desmopressin, which releases vWF stored in endothelium.
Disseminated intravascular coagulation	↓	↑	↑	↑	Widespread activation of clotting → deficiency in clotting factors → bleeding state. Causes: Sepsis (gram ⊖), Trauma, Obstetric complications, acute Pancreatitis, Malignancy, Nephrotic syndrome, Transfusion (STOP Making New Thrombi). Labs: schistocytes, ↑ fibrin degradation products (D-dimers), ↓ fibrinogen, ↓ factors V and VIII.

Hereditary thrombosis syndromes leading to hypercoagulability

DISEASE	DESCRIPTION
Antithrombin deficiency	Inherited deficiency of antithrombin: has no direct effect on the PT, PTT, or thrombin time but diminishes the increase in PTT following heparin administration. Can also be acquired: renal failure/nephrotic syndrome → antithrombin loss in urine → ↓ inhibition of factors IIa and Xa.
Factor V Leiden	Production of mutant factor V (G → A DNA point mutation → Arg506Gln mutation near the cleavage site) that is resistant to degradation by activated protein C. Most common cause of inherited hypercoagulability in Caucasians. Complications include DVT, cerebral vein thromboses, recurrent pregnancy loss.
Protein C or S deficiency	↓ ability to inactivate factors Va and VIIIa. ↑ risk of thrombotic skin necrosis with hemorrhage after administration of warfarin. If this occurs, think protein C deficiency. Together, protein C Cancels, and protein S Stops, coagulation.
Prothrombin gene mutation	Mutation in 3′ untranslated region → ↑ production of prothrombin → ↑ plasma levels and venous clots.

Blood transfusion therapy

COMPONENT	DOSAGE EFFECT	CLINICAL USE
Packed RBCs	↑ Hb and O_2 carrying capacity	Acute blood loss, severe anemia
Platelets	↑ platelet count (↑ ~ 5000/mm³/unit)	Stop significant bleeding (thrombocytopenia, qualitative platelet defects)
Fresh frozen plasma/prothrombin complex concentrate	↑ coagulation factor levels; FFP contains all coagulation factors and plasma proteins; PCC generally contains factors II, VII, IX, and X, as well as protein C and S	DIC, cirrhosis, immediate anticoagulation reversal
Cryoprecipitate	Contains fibrinogen, factor VIII, factor XIII, vWF, and fibronectin	Coagulation factor deficiencies involving fibrinogen and factor VIII

Blood transfusion risks include infection transmission (low), transfusion reactions, iron overload (may lead to 2° hemochromatosis), hypocalcemia (citrate is a Ca^{2+} chelator), and hyperkalemia (RBCs may lyse in old blood units).

Leukemia vs lymphoma

Leukemia	Lymphoid or myeloid neoplasm with widespread involvement of bone marrow. Tumor cells are usually found in peripheral blood.
Lymphoma	Discrete tumor mass arising from lymph nodes. Presentations often blur definitions.

Hodgkin vs non-Hodgkin lymphoma

Hodgkin	Non-Hodgkin
Both may present with constitutional ("B") signs/symptoms: low-grade fever, night sweats, weight loss (patients are **B**othered by **B** symptoms).	
Localized, single group of nodes; contiguous spread (stage is strongest predictor of prognosis). Overall prognosis better than that of non-Hodgkin lymphoma.	Multiple lymph nodes involved; extranodal involvement common; noncontiguous spread.
Characterized by Reed-Sternberg cells.	Majority involve B cells; a few are of T-cell lineage.
Bimodal distribution–young adulthood and > 55 years; more common in men except for nodular sclerosing type.	Can occur in children and adults.
Associated with EBV.	May be associated with HIV and autoimmune diseases.

Hodgkin lymphoma

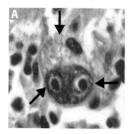

Contains Reed-Sternberg cells: distinctive tumor giant cells; binucleate or bilobed with the 2 halves as mirror images ("owl eyes" A). 2 owl eyes × 15 = 30. RS cells are CD15+ and CD30+ B-cell origin.

SUBTYPE	NOTES
Nodular sclerosis	Most common
Lymphocyte rich	Best prognosis
Mixed cellularity	Eosinophilia, seen in immunocompromised patients
Lymphocyte depleted	Seen in immunocompromised patients

Non-Hodgkin lymphoma

TYPE	OCCURS IN	GENETICS	COMMENTS
Neoplasms of mature B cells			
Burkitt lymphoma	Adolescents or young adults	t(8;14)—translocation of c-*myc* (8) and heavy-chain Ig (14)	"Starry sky" appearance, sheets of lymphocytes with interspersed "tingible body" macrophages (arrows in A). Associated with EBV. Jaw lesion B in endemic form in Africa; pelvis or abdomen in sporadic form.
Diffuse large B-cell lymphoma	Usually older adults, but 20% in children	Alterations in Bcl-2, Bcl-6	Most common type of non-Hodgkin lymphoma in adults.
Follicular lymphoma	Adults	t(14;18)—translocation of heavy-chain Ig (14) and *BCL*-2 (18)	Indolent course; Bcl-2 inhibits apoptosis. Presents with painless "waxing and waning" lymphadenopathy.
Mantle cell lymphoma	Adult males	t(11;14)—translocation of cyclin D1 (11) and heavy-chain Ig (14), CD 5+	Very aggressive, patients typically present with late-stage disease.
Marginal zone lymphoma	Adults	t(11;18)	Associated with chronic inflammation (eg, Sjögren syndrome, chronic gastritis [MALT lymphoma]).
Primary central nervous system lymphoma	Adults	Most commonly associated with HIV/AIDS; pathogenesis involves EBV infection	Considered an AIDS-defining illness. Variable presentation: confusion, memory loss, seizures. Mass lesion(s) (may be ring-enhancing in immunocompromised patient) on MRI C, needs to be distinguished from toxoplasmosis via CSF analysis or other lab tests.
Neoplasms of mature T cells			
Adult T-cell lymphoma	Adults	Caused by HTLV (associated with IV drug abuse)	Adults present with cutaneous lesions; common in Japan, West Africa, and the Caribbean. Lytic bone lesions, hypercalcemia.
Mycosis fungoides/ Sézary syndrome	Adults		Mycosis fungoides: skin patches D/plaques (cutaneous T-cell lymphoma), characterized by atypical CD4+ cells with "cerebriform" nuclei and intraepidermal neoplastic cell aggregates (Pautrier microabscess). May progress to Sézary syndrome (T-cell leukemia).

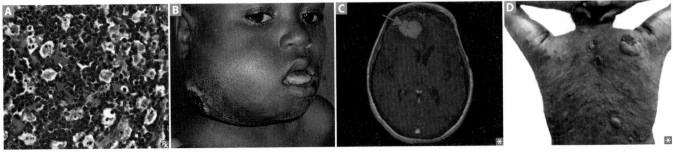

Multiple myeloma

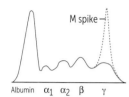

Monoclonal plasma cell ("fried egg" appearance) cancer that arises in the marrow and produces large amounts of IgG (55%) or IgA (25%). Bone marrow > 10% monoclonal plasma cells. Most common 1° tumor arising within bone in people > 40–50 years old. Associated with:

- ↑ susceptibility to infection
- Primary amyloidosis (AL)
- Punched-out lytic bone lesions on x-ray **A**
- M spike on serum protein electrophoresis
- Ig light chains in urine (Bence Jones protein)
- Rouleaux formation **B** (RBCs stacked like poker chips in blood smear)

Numerous plasma cells **C** with "clock-face" chromatin and intracytoplasmic inclusions containing immunoglobulin.

Monoclonal gammopathy of undetermined significance (MGUS)—monoclonal expansion of plasma cells (bone marrow < 10% monoclonal plasma cells), asymptomatic, may lead to multiple myeloma. No **CRAB** findings. Patients with MGUS develop multiple myeloma at a rate of 1–2% per year.

Think **CRAB**:
HyperCalcemia
Renal involvement
Anemia
Bone lytic lesions/Back pain
Multiple Myeloma: Monoclonal **M** protein spike
Distinguish from Waldenström macroglobulinemia → M spike = IgM → hyperviscosity syndrome (eg, blurred vision, Raynaud phenomenon); no **CRAB** findings.

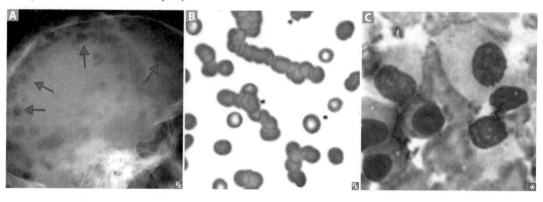

Myelodysplastic syndromes

Stem-cell disorders involving ineffective hematopoiesis → defects in cell maturation of nonlymphoid lineages. Caused by de novo mutations or environmental exposure (eg, radiation, benzene, chemotherapy). Risk of transformation to AML.

Pseudo–Pelger-Huet anomaly—neutrophils with bilobed ("**duet**") nuclei. Typically seen after chemotherapy.

Leukemias	Unregulated growth and differentiation of WBCs in bone marrow → marrow failure → anemia (↓ RBCs), infections (↓ mature WBCs), and hemorrhage (↓ platelets). Usually presents with ↑ circulating WBCs (malignant leukocytes in blood); rare cases present with normal/↓ WBCs. Leukemic cell infiltration of liver, spleen, lymph nodes, and skin (leukemia cutis) possible.

TYPE	NOTES
Lymphoid neoplasms	
Acute lymphoblastic leukemia/lymphoma	Most frequently occurs in children; less common in adults (worse prognosis). T-cell ALL can present as mediastinal mass (presenting as SVC-like syndrome). Associated with Down syndrome. Peripheral blood and bone marrow have ↑↑↑ lymphoblasts 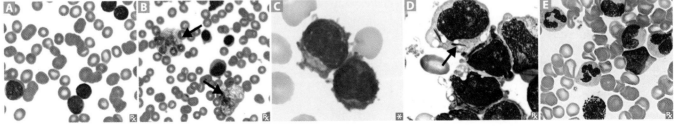. TdT+ (marker of pre-T and pre-B cells), CD10+ (marker of pre-B cells). Most responsive to therapy. May spread to CNS and testes. t(12;21) → better prognosis.
Chronic lymphocytic leukemia/small lymphocytic lymphoma	Age > 60 years. Most common adult leukemia. CD20+, CD23+, CD5+ B-cell neoplasm. Often asymptomatic, progresses slowly; smudge cells **B** in peripheral blood smear; autoimmune hemolytic anemia. CLL = Crushed Little Lymphocytes (smudge cells). Richter transformation—CLL/SLL transformation into an aggressive lymphoma, most commonly diffuse large B-cell lymphoma (DLBCL).
Hairy cell leukemia	Adult males. Mature B-cell tumor. Cells have filamentous, hair-like projections (fuzzy appearing on LM **C**). Peripheral lymphadenopathy is uncommon. Causes marrow fibrosis → dry tap on aspiration. Patients usually present with massive splenomegaly and pancytopenia. Stains TRAP (tartrate-resistant acid phosphatase) ⊕. TRAP stain largely replaced with flow cytometry. Treatment: cladribine, pentostatin.
Myeloid neoplasms	
Acute myelogenous leukemia	Median onset 65 years. Auer rods **D**; myeloperoxidase ⊕ cytoplasmic inclusions seen mostly in APL (formerly M3 AML); ↑↑↑ circulating myeloblasts on peripheral smear; adults. Risk factors: prior exposure to alkylating chemotherapy, radiation, myeloproliferative disorders, Down syndrome. APL: t(15;17), responds to all-*trans* retinoic acid (vitamin A), inducing differentiation of promyelocytes; DIC is a common presentation.
Chronic myelogenous leukemia	Occurs across the age spectrum with peak incidence 45–85 years, median age at diagnosis 64 years. Defined by the Philadelphia chromosome (t[9;22], *BCR-ABL*) and myeloid stem cell proliferation. Presents with dysregulated production of mature and maturing granulocytes (eg, neutrophils, metamyelocytes, myelocytes, basophils **E**) and splenomegaly. May accelerate and transform to AML or ALL ("blast crisis"). Very low LAP as a result of low activity in malignant neutrophils (vs benign neutrophilia [leukemoid reaction], in which LAP is ↑). Responds to *bcr-abl* tyrosine kinase inhibitors (eg, imatinib, dasatinib).

Chronic myeloproliferative disorders	The myeloproliferative disorders (polycythemia vera, essential thrombocythemia, myelofibrosis, and CML) are malignant hematopoietic neoplasms with varying impacts on WBCs and myeloid cell lines. Associated with V617F *JAK2* mutation.
Polycythemia vera	Primary polycythemia. Disorder of ↑ RBCs. May present as intense itching after hot shower. Rare but classic symptom is erythromelalgia (severe, burning pain and red-blue coloration) due to episodic blood clots in vessels of the extremities **A**. ↓ EPO (vs 2° polycythemia, which presents with endogenous or artificially ↑ EPO). Treatment: phlebotomy, hydroxyurea, ruxolitinib (JAK1/2 inhibitor).
Essential thrombocythemia	Characterized by massive proliferation of megakaryocytes and platelets. Symptoms include bleeding and thrombosis. Blood smear shows markedly increased number of platelets, which may be large or otherwise abnormally formed **B**. Erythromelalgia may occur.
Myelofibrosis	Obliteration of bone marrow with fibrosis **C** due to ↑ fibroblast activity. Often associated with massive splenomegaly and "**teardrop**" RBCs **D**. "Bone marrow is **crying** because it's fibrosed and is a dry tap."

	RBCs	WBCs	PLATELETS	PHILADELPHIA CHROMOSOME	*JAK2* MUTATIONS
Polycythemia vera	↑	↑	↑	⊖	⊕
Essential thrombocythemia	–	–	↑	⊖	⊕ (30–50%)
Myelofibrosis	↓	Variable	Variable	⊖	⊕ (30–50%)
CML	↓	↑	↑	⊕	⊖

Polycythemia

	PLASMA VOLUME	RBC MASS	O₂ SATURATION	EPO LEVELS	ASSOCIATIONS
Relative	↓	–	–	–	Dehydration, burns.
Appropriate absolute	–	↑	↓	↑	Lung disease, congenital heart disease, high altitude.
Inappropriate absolute	–	↑	–	↑	Malignancy (eg, renal cell carcinoma, hepatocellular carcinoma), hydronephrosis. Due to ectopic EPO secretion.
Polycythemia vera	↑	↑↑	–	↓	EPO ↓ in PCV due to negative feedback suppressing renal EPO production.

↑↓ = 1° disturbance

Chromosomal translocations

TRANSLOCATION	ASSOCIATED DISORDER	
t(8;14)	Burkitt (Burk-8) lymphoma (*c-myc* activation)	
t(9;22) (**Philadelphia chromosome**)	**CML** (*BCR-ABL* hybrid), ALL (less common, poor prognostic factor)	**Philadelphia CreaML cheese.** The Ig heavy chain genes on chromosome 14 are constitutively expressed. When other genes (eg, *c-myc* and *BCL-2*) are translocated next to this heavy chain gene region, they are overexpressed.
t(11;14)	Mantle cell lymphoma (cyclin D1 activation)	
t(14;18)	Follicular lymphoma (*BCL-2* activation)	
t(15;17)	APL (M3 type of AML)	Responds to all-*trans* retinoic acid.

Langerhans cell histiocytosis	Collective group of proliferative disorders of dendritic (Langerhans) cells. Presents in a child as lytic bone lesions A and skin rash or as recurrent otitis media with a mass involving the mastoid bone. Cells are functionally immature and do not effectively stimulate primary T cells via antigen presentation. Cells express S-100 (mesodermal origin) and CD1a. Birbeck granules ("tennis rackets" or rod shaped on EM) are characteristic B.	Birbeck granules

Tumor lysis syndrome	Oncologic emergency triggered by massive tumor cell lysis, most often in lymphomas/leukemias. Release of K^+ → hyperkalemia, release of PO_4^{3-} → hyperphosphatemia, hypocalcemia due to Ca^{2+} sequestration by PO_4^{3-}. ↑ nucleic acid breakdown → hyperuricemia → acute kidney injury. Prevention and treatment include aggressive hydration, allopurinol, rasburicase.

▶ HEMATOLOGY AND ONCOLOGY—PHARMACOLOGY

Heparin

MECHANISM	Activates antithrombin, which ↓ action of IIa (thrombin) and factor Xa. Short half-life.
CLINICAL USE	Immediate anticoagulation for pulmonary embolism (PE), acute coronary syndrome, MI, deep venous thrombosis (DVT). Used during pregnancy (does not cross placenta). Follow PTT.
ADVERSE EFFECTS	Bleeding, thrombocytopenia (HIT), osteoporosis, drug-drug interactions. For rapid reversal (antidote), use protamine sulfate (positively charged molecule that binds negatively charged heparin).
NOTES	Low-molecular-weight heparins (eg, enoxaparin, dalteparin) act predominantly on factor Xa. Fondaparinux acts only on factor Xa. Have better bioavailability and 2–4× longer half life than unfractionated heparin; can be administered subcutaneously and without laboratory monitoring. Not easily reversible.

Heparin-induced thrombocytopenia (HIT)—development of IgG antibodies against heparin-bound platelet factor 4 (PF4). Antibody-heparin-PF4 complex activates platelets → thrombosis and thrombocytopenia. |

Direct thrombin inhibitors	Bivalirudin (related to hirudin, the anticoagulant used by leeches), Argatroban, Dabigatran (only oral agent in class).
MECHANISM	Directly inhibits activity of free and clot-associated thrombin.
CLINICAL USE	Venous thromboembolism, atrial fibrillation. Can be used in HIT, when heparin is **BAD** for the patient. Does not require lab monitoring.
ADVERSE EFFECTS	Bleeding; can reverse dabigatran with idarucizumab. Consider PCC and/or antifibrinolytics (eg, tranexamic acid) if no reversal agent available.

Warfarin

MECHANISM	Interferes with γ-carboxylation of vitamin K–dependent clotting factors II, VII, IX, and X, and proteins C and S. Metabolism affected by polymorphisms in the gene for vitamin K epoxide reductase complex (*VKORC1*). In laboratory assay, has effect on EXtrinsic pathway and ↑ PT. Long half-life.	The EX-PresidenT went to war(farin).
CLINICAL USE	Chronic anticoagulation (eg, venous thromboembolism prophylaxis, and prevention of stroke in atrial fibrillation). Not used in pregnant women (because warfarin, unlike heparin, crosses placenta). Follow PT/INR.	
ADVERSE EFFECTS	Bleeding, teratogenic, skin/tissue necrosis A, drug-drug interactions. Initial risk of hypercoagulation: protein C has a shorter half-life than factors II and X. Existing protein C depletes before existing factors II and X deplete, and before warfarin can reduce factors II and X production → hypercoagulation. Skin/tissue necrosis within first few days of large doses believed to be due to small vessel microthrombosis.	For reversal of warfarin, give vitamin K. For rapid reversal, give fresh frozen plasma (FFP) or PCC. Heparin "bridging": heparin frequently used when starting warfarin. Heparin's activation of antithrombin enables anticoagulation during initial, transient hypercoagulable state caused by warfarin. Initial heparin therapy reduces risk of recurrent venous thromboembolism and skin/tissue necrosis. Cytochrome P-450 inhibitors increase warfarin effect.

Heparin vs warfarin

	Heparin	Warfarin
ROUTE OF ADMINISTRATION	Parenteral (IV, SC)	Oral
SITE OF ACTION	Blood	Liver
ONSET OF ACTION	Rapid (seconds)	Slow, limited by half-lives of normal clotting factors
MECHANISM OF ACTION	Activates antithrombin, which ↓ the action of IIa (thrombin) and factor Xa	Impairs synthesis of vitamin K–dependent clotting factors II, VII, IX, and X, and anti-clotting proteins C and S
DURATION OF ACTION	Hours	Days
AGENTS FOR REVERSAL	Protamine sulfate	Vitamin K, FFP, PCC
MONITORING	PTT (intrinsic pathway)	PT/INR (extrinsic pathway)
CROSSES PLACENTA	No	Yes (teratogenic)

Direct factor Xa inhibitors	ApiXaban, rivaroXaban.
MECHANISM	Bind to and directly inhibit factor **Xa**.
CLINICAL USE	Treatment and prophylaxis for DVT and PE; stroke prophylaxis in patients with atrial fibrillation. Oral agents do not usually require coagulation monitoring.
ADVERSE EFFECTS	Bleeding. Not easily reversible.

Thrombolytics	Alteplase (tPA), reteplase (rPA), streptokinase, tenecteplase (TNK-tPA).
MECHANISM	Directly or indirectly aid conversion of plasminogen to plasmin, which cleaves thrombin and fibrin clots. ↑ PT, ↑ PTT, no change in platelet count.
CLINICAL USE	Early MI, early ischemic stroke, direct thrombolysis of severe PE.
ADVERSE EFFECTS	Bleeding. Contraindicated in patients with active bleeding, history of intracranial bleeding, recent surgery, known bleeding diatheses, or severe hypertension. Nonspecific reversal with antifibrinolytics (eg, aminocaproic acid, tranexamic acid), platelet transfusions, and factor corrections (eg, cryoprecipitate, FFP, PCC).

ADP receptor inhibitors	Clopidogrel, prasugrel, ticagrelor (reversible), ticlopidine.
MECHANISM	Inhibit platelet aggregation by irreversibly blocking ADP (P2Y$_{12}$) receptor. Prevent expression of glycoproteins IIb/IIIa on platelet surface.
CLINICAL USE	Acute coronary syndrome; coronary stenting. ↓ incidence or recurrence of thrombotic stroke.
ADVERSE EFFECTS	Neutropenia (ticlopidine). TTP may be seen.

Cilostazol, dipyridamole	
MECHANISM	Phosphodiesterase inhibitors; ↑ cAMP in platelets, resulting in inhibition of platelet aggregation; vasodilators.
CLINICAL USE	Intermittent claudication, coronary vasodilation, prevention of stroke or TIAs (combined with aspirin).
ADVERSE EFFECTS	Nausea, headache, facial flushing, hypotension, abdominal pain.

Glycoprotein IIb/IIIa inhibitors	Abciximab, eptifibatide, tirofiban.
MECHANISM	Bind to the glycoprotein receptor IIb/IIIa on activated platelets, preventing aggregation. Abciximab is made from monoclonal antibody Fab fragments.
CLINICAL USE	Unstable angina, percutaneous coronary intervention.
ADVERSE EFFECTS	Bleeding, thrombocytopenia.

Cancer drugs—cell cycle

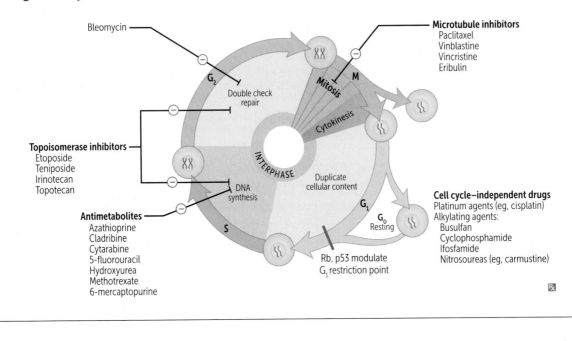

Cancer drugs—targets

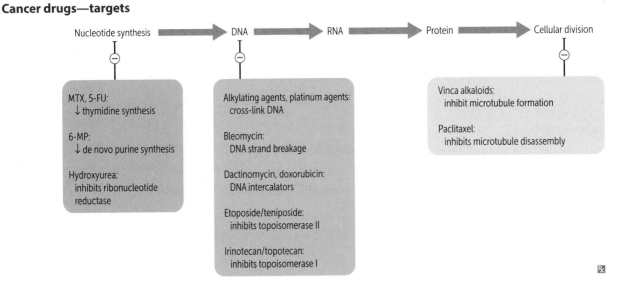

Antimetabolites

DRUG	MECHANISM[a]	CLINICAL USE	ADVERSE EFFECTS
Azathioprine, 6-mercaptopurine	Purine (thiol) analogs → ↓ de novo purine synthesis. Activated by HGPRT. Azathioprine is metabolized into 6-MP.	Preventing organ rejection, rheumatoid arthritis, IBD, SLE; used to wean patients off steroids in chronic disease and to treat steroid-refractory chronic disease.	Myelosuppression; GI, liver toxicity. Azathioprine and 6-MP are metabolized by xanthine oxidase; thus both have ↑ toxicity with allopurinol or febuxostat.
Cladribine	Purine analog → multiple mechanisms (eg, inhibition of DNA polymerase, DNA strand breaks).	Hairy cell leukemia.	Myelosuppression, nephrotoxicity, and neurotoxicity.
Cytarabine (arabinofuranosyl cytidine)	Pyrimidine analog → DNA chain termination. At higher concentrations, inhibits DNA polymerase.	Leukemias (AML), lymphomas.	Myelosuppression with megaloblastic anemia. CYTarabine causes panCYTopenia.
5-fluorouracil	Pyrimidine analog bioactivated to 5-FdUMP, which covalently complexes with thymidylate synthase and folic acid. Capecitabine is a prodrug with similar activity. This complex inhibits thymidylate synthase → ↓ dTMP → ↓ DNA synthesis.	Colon cancer, pancreatic cancer, actinic keratosis, basal cell carcinoma (topical). Effects enhanced with the addition of leucovorin.	Myelosuppression, palmar-plantar erythrodysesthesia (hand-foot syndrome).
Methotrexate	Folic acid analog that competitively inhibits dihydrofolate reductase → ↓ dTMP → ↓ DNA synthesis.	Cancers: leukemias (ALL), lymphomas, choriocarcinoma, sarcomas. Non-neoplastic: ectopic pregnancy, medical abortion (with misoprostol), rheumatoid arthritis, psoriasis, IBD, vasculitis.	Myelosuppression, which is reversible with leucovorin "rescue." Hepatotoxicity. Mucositis (eg, mouth ulcers). Pulmonary fibrosis. Folate deficiency, which may be teratogenic (neural tube defects) without supplementation. Nephrotoxicity (rare).

[a]All are S-phase specific.

Antitumor antibiotics

DRUG	MECHANISM	CLINICAL USE	ADVERSE EFFECTS
Bleomycin	Induces free radical formation → breaks in DNA strands.	Testicular cancer, Hodgkin lymphoma.	Pulmonary fibrosis, skin hyperpigmentation. Minimal myelosuppression.
Dactinomycin (actinomycin D)	Intercalates into DNA, preventing RNA synthesis.	Wilms tumor, Ewing sarcoma, rhabdomyosarcoma. Used for childhood tumors.	Myelosuppression.
Doxorubicin, daunorubicin	Generate free radicals. Intercalate in DNA → breaks in DNA → ↓ replication. Interferes with topoisomerase II enzyme.	Solid tumors, leukemias, lymphomas.	Cardiotoxicity (dilated cardiomyopathy), myelosuppression, alopecia. Dexrazoxane (iron chelating agent), used to prevent cardiotoxicity.

Alkylating agents

DRUG	MECHANISM	CLINICAL USE	ADVERSE EFFECTS
Busulfan	Cross-links DNA.	Used to ablate patient's bone marrow before bone marrow transplantation.	Severe myelosuppression (in almost all cases), pulmonary fibrosis, hyperpigmentation.
Cyclophosphamide, ifosfamide	Cross-link DNA at guanine. Require bioactivation by liver. A nitrogen mustard.	Solid tumors, leukemia, lymphomas.	Myelosuppression; SIADH; hemorrhagic cystitis, prevented with mesna (thiol group of mesna binds toxic metabolites) or adequate hydration.
Nitrosoureas	Require bioactivation. Cross blood-brain barrier → CNS. Cross-link DNA.	Brain tumors (including glioblastoma multiforme).	CNS toxicity (convulsions, dizziness, ataxia).
Procarbazine	Cell cycle phase–nonspecific alkylating agent, mechanism not yet defined.	Hodgkin lymphoma, brain tumors.	Bone marrow suppression, pulmonary toxicity, leukemia.

Microtubule inhibitors

DRUG	MECHANISM	CLINICAL USE	ADVERSE EFFECTS
Paclitaxel, other taxanes	Hyperstabilize polymerized microtubules in M phase so that mitotic spindle cannot break down (anaphase cannot occur).	Ovarian and breast carcinomas.	Myelosuppression, neuropathy, hypersensitivity. Taxes stabilize society.
Vincristine, vinblastine	Vinca alkaloids that bind β-tubulin and inhibit its polymerization into microtubules → prevent mitotic spindle formation (M-phase arrest).	Solid tumors, leukemias, Hodgkin (vinblastine) and non-Hodgkin (vincristine) lymphomas.	Vincristine: neurotoxicity (areflexia, peripheral neuritis), constipation (including paralytic ileus). Crisps the nerves. Vinblastine: bone marrow suppression. Blasts the bone marrow.

Cisplatin, carboplatin

MECHANISM	Cross-link DNA.
CLINICAL USE	Testicular, bladder, ovary, and lung carcinomas.
ADVERSE EFFECTS	Nephrotoxicity, peripheral neuropathy, ototoxicity. Prevent nephrotoxicity with amifostine (free radical scavenger) and chloride (saline) diuresis.

Etoposide, teniposide

MECHANISM	Inhibit topoisomerase II → ↑ DNA degradation.
CLINICAL USE	Solid tumors (particularly testicular and small cell lung cancer), leukemias, lymphomas.
ADVERSE EFFECTS	Myelosuppression, alopecia.

Irinotecan, topotecan

MECHANISM	Inhibit topoisomerase I and prevent DNA unwinding and replication.
CLINICAL USE	Colon cancer (irinotecan); ovarian and small cell lung cancers (topotecan).
ADVERSE EFFECTS	Severe myelosuppression, diarrhea.

Hydroxyurea

MECHANISM	Inhibits ribonucleotide reductase → ↓ DNA Synthesis (S-phase specific).
CLINICAL USE	Myeloproliferative disorders (eg, CML, polycythemia vera), sickle cell (↑ HbF).
ADVERSE EFFECTS	Severe myelosuppression.

Bevacizumab

MECHANISM	Monoclonal antibody against VEGF. Inhibits angiogenesis (BeVacizumab inhibits Blood Vessel formation).
CLINICAL USE	Solid tumors (colorectal cancer, renal cell carcinoma), wet age-related macular degeneration.
ADVERSE EFFECTS	Hemorrhage, blood clots, and impaired wound healing.

Erlotinib

MECHANISM	EGFR tyrosine kinase inhibitor.
CLINICAL USE	Non-small cell lung carcinoma.
ADVERSE EFFECTS	Rash.

Cetuximab

MECHANISM	Monoclonal antibody against EGFR.
CLINICAL USE	Stage IV colorectal cancer (wild-type *KRAS*), head and neck cancer.
ADVERSE EFFECTS	Rash, elevated LFTs, diarrhea.

Imatinib

MECHANISM	Tyrosine kinase inhibitor of *BCR-ABL* (Philadelphia chromosome fusion gene in CML) and c-*kit* (common in GI stromal tumors).
CLINICAL USE	CML, GI stromal tumors (GIST).
ADVERSE EFFECTS	Fluid retention.

Rituximab

MECHANISM	Monoclonal antibody against CD20, which is found on most B-cell neoplasms.
CLINICAL USE	Non-Hodgkin lymphoma, CLL, ITP, rheumatoid arthritis.
ADVERSE EFFECTS	↑ risk of progressive multifocal leukoencephalopathy.

Bortezomib, carfilzomib

MECHANISM	Proteasome inhibitors, induce arrest at G2-M phase and apoptosis.
CLINICAL USE	Multiple myeloma, mantle cell lymphoma.
ADVERSE EFFECTS	Peripheral neuropathy, herpes zoster reactivation.

Tamoxifen, raloxifene

MECHANISM	Selective estrogen receptor modulators (SERMs)—receptor antagonists in breast and agonists in bone. Block the binding of estrogen to ER ⊕ cells.
CLINICAL USE	Breast cancer treatment (tamoxifen only) and prevention. Raloxifene also useful to prevent osteoporosis.
ADVERSE EFFECTS	Tamoxifen—partial agonist in endometrium, which ↑ the risk of endometrial cancer; "hot flashes." **Raloxifene**—no ↑ in endometrial carcinoma (so you can **relax**!), because it is an estrogen receptor antagonist in endometrial tissue. Both ↑ risk of thromboembolic events (eg, DVT, PE).

Trastuzumab (Herceptin)

MECHANISM	Monoclonal antibody against HER-2 (*c-erbB2*), a tyrosine kinase receptor. Helps kill cancer cells that overexpress HER-2 through inhibition of HER-2 initiated cellular signaling and antibody-dependent cytotoxicity.
CLINICAL USE	HER-2 ⊕ breast cancer and gastric cancer (tras2zumab).
ADVERSE EFFECTS	Cardiotoxicity. "**Heart**ceptin" damages the **heart**.

Vemurafenib

MECHANISM	Small molecule inhibitor of *BRAF* oncogene ⊕ melanoma. **VEmuRAF-enib** is for V600E-mutated *BRAF* inhibition.
CLINICAL USE	Metastatic melanoma.

Rasburicase

MECHANISM	Recombinant uricase that catalyzes metabolism of uric acid to allantoin.
CLINICAL USE	Prevention and treatment of tumor lysis syndrome.

Common chemotoxicities

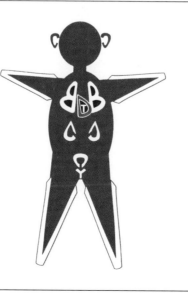

Cisplatin/Carboplatin → ototoxicity

Vincristine → peripheral neuropathy
Bleomycin, Busulfan → pulmonary fibrosis
Doxorubicin → cardiotoxicity
Trastuzumab (Herceptin) → cardiotoxicity
Cisplatin/Carboplatin → nephrotoxicity

CYclophosphamide → hemorrhagic cystitis

▶ NOTES

Musculoskeletal, Skin, and Connective Tissue

"Rigid, the skeleton of habit alone upholds the human frame."
—Virginia Woolf

"Beauty may be skin deep, but ugly goes clear to the bone."
—Redd Foxx

"The function of muscle is to pull and not to push, except in the case of the genitals and the tongue."
—Leonardo da Vinci

"To thrive in life you need three bones. A wishbone. A backbone. And a funny bone."
—Reba McEntire

This chapter provides information you will need to understand certain anatomical dysfunctions, rheumatic diseases, and dermatologic conditions. Be able to interpret 3D anatomy in the context of radiologic imaging. For the rheumatic diseases, create instructional cases or personas that includes the most likely presentation and symptoms: risk factors, gender, important markers (eg, autoantibodies), and other epidemiologic factors. Doing so will allow you to answer the higher order questions that are likely to be asked on the exam.

▶ MUSCULOSKELETAL, SKIN, AND CONNECTIVE TISSUE—ANATOMY AND PHYSIOLOGY

Arm abduction

DEGREE	MUSCLE	NERVE
0°–15°	Supraspinatus	Suprascapular
15°–100°	Deltoid	Axillary
> 90°	Trapezius	Accessory
> 100°	Serratus Anterior	Long Thoracic (SALT)

Rotator cuff muscles

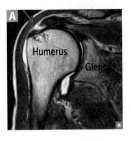

Shoulder muscles that form the rotator cuff:

- Supraspinatus (suprascapular nerve)—abducts arm initially (before the action of the deltoid); most common rotator cuff injury (trauma or degeneration and impingement → tendinopathy or tear [arrow in A]), assessed by "empty/full can" test.
- Infraspinatus (suprascapular nerve)—externally rotates arm; pitching injury.
- teres minor (axillary nerve)—adducts and externally rotates arm.
- Subscapularis (upper and lower subscapular nerves)—internally rotates and adducts arm.

Innervated primarily by C5-C6.

SItS (small t is for teres minor).

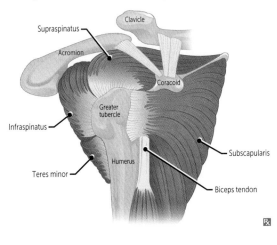

Overuse injuries of the elbow

Medial epicondylitis (golfer's elbow)	Repetitive flexion (forehand shots) or idiopathic → pain near medial epicondyle.
Lateral epicondylitis (tennis elbow)	Repetitive extension (backhand shots) or idiopathic → pain near lateral epicondyle.

Wrist region

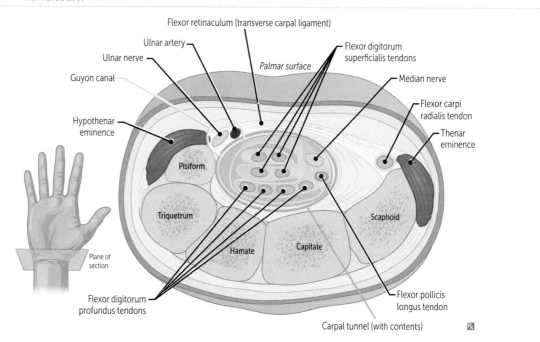

Scaphoid, Lunate, Triquetrum, Pisiform, Hamate, Capitate, Trapezoid, Trapezium **A**. (So Long To Pinky, Here Comes The Thumb).

Scaphoid (palpable in anatomic snuff box **B**) is the most commonly fractured carpal bone, typically due to a fall on an outstretched hand. Complications of proximal scaphoid fractures include avascular necrosis and nonunion due to retrograde blood supply. Fracture not always seen on initial x-ray.

Dislocation of lunate may cause acute carpal tunnel syndrome.

Metacarpal neck fracture

Also called boxer's fracture. Common fracture caused by direct blow with a closed fist (eg, from punching a wall or individual). Most commonly seen in 4th and 5th metacarpals.

Carpal tunnel syndrome

Entrapment of median nerve in carpal tunnel (between transverse carpal ligament and carpal bones); nerve compression → paresthesia, pain, and numbness in distribution of median nerve. Thenar eminence atrophies **C** but sensation spared, because palmar cutaneous branch enters hand external to carpal tunnel.

Suggested by ⊕ Tinel sign (percussion of wrist causes tingling) and Phalen maneuver (90° flexion of wrist causes tingling).

Associated with pregnancy (due to edema), rheumatoid arthritis, hypothyroidism, diabetes, acromegaly, dialysis-related amyloidosis; may be associated with repetitive use.

Guyon canal syndrome

Compression of ulnar nerve at wrist. Classically seen in cyclists due to pressure from handlebars.

1st MC

Trapezoid Capitate Hamate

Trapezium

Scaphoid

Triquetrum

Pisiform

Lunate

Radius Ulna

Flexor retinaculum (transverse carpal ligament)

Ulnar artery

Ulnar nerve

Guyon canal

Hypothenar eminence

Pisiform

Palmar surface

Flexor digitorum superficialis tendons

Median nerve

Flexor carpi radialis tendon

Thenar eminence

Triquetrum

Hamate

Capitate

Scaphoid

Plane of section

Flexor digitorum profundus tendons

Flexor pollicis longus tendon

Carpal tunnel (with contents)

Common pediatric fractures

Greenstick fracture	Incomplete fracture extending partway through width of bone **A** following bending stress; bone fails on tension side; compression side intact (compare to torus fracture). Bone is bent like a green twig.	
Torus (buckle) fracture	Axial force applied to immature bone → cortex buckles on compression side and fractures **B**. Tension side (other side of cortex) remains intact.	

Normal   Greenstick fracture   Torus fracture   Complete fracture

Hand muscles Thenar eminence Hypothenar eminence	Thenar (median)—Opponens pollicis, Abductor pollicis brevis, Flexor pollicis brevis, superficial head (deep head by ulnar nerve). Hypothenar (ulnar)—Opponens digiti minimi, Abductor digiti minimi, Flexor digiti minimi brevis. Dorsal interossei (ulnar)—abduct the fingers. Palmar interossei (ulnar)—adduct the fingers. Lumbricals (1st/2nd, median; 3rd/4th, ulnar)—flex at the MCP joint, extend PIP and DIP joints.	Both groups perform the same functions: Oppose, Abduct, and Flex (OAF). DAB = Dorsals ABduct. PAD = Palmars ADduct.

Upper extremity nerves

NERVE	CAUSES OF INJURY	PRESENTATION
Axillary (C5-C6)	Fractured surgical neck of humerus Anterior dislocation of humerus	Flattened deltoid Loss of arm abduction at shoulder (> 15°) Loss of sensation over deltoid muscle and lateral arm
Musculocutaneous (C5-C7)	Upper trunk compression	Loss of forearm flexion and supination Loss of sensation over lateral forearm
Radial (C5-T1)	Compression of axilla, eg, due to crutches or sleeping with arm over chair ("Saturday night palsy") Midshaft fracture of humerus Repetitive pronation/supination of forearm, eg, due to screwdriver use ("finger drop")	Wrist drop: loss of elbow, wrist, and finger extension ↓ grip strength (wrist extension necessary for maximal action of flexors) Loss of sensation over posterior arm/forearm and dorsal hand
Median (C5-T1)	Supracondylar fracture of humerus (proximal lesion) Carpal tunnel syndrome and wrist laceration (distal lesion)	"Ape hand" and "Pope's blessing" Loss of wrist flexion, flexion of lateral fingers, thumb opposition, lumbricals of 2nd and 3rd digits Loss of sensation over thenar eminence and dorsal and palmar aspects of lateral 3½ fingers with proximal lesion
Ulnar (C8-T1)	Fracture of medial epicondyle of humerus "funny bone" (proximal lesion) Fractured hook of hamate (distal lesion) from fall on outstretched hand	"Ulnar claw" on digit extension Radial deviation of wrist upon flexion (proximal lesion) Loss of wrist flexion, flexion of medial fingers, abduction and adduction of fingers (interossei), actions of medial 2 lumbrical muscles Loss of sensation over medial 1½ fingers including hypothenar eminence
Recurrent branch of median nerve (C5-T1)	Superficial laceration of palm	"Ape hand" Loss of thenar muscle group: opposition, abduction, and flexion of thumb No loss of sensation

Humerus fractures, proximally to distally, follow the **ARM** (**A**xillary → **R**adial → **M**edian)

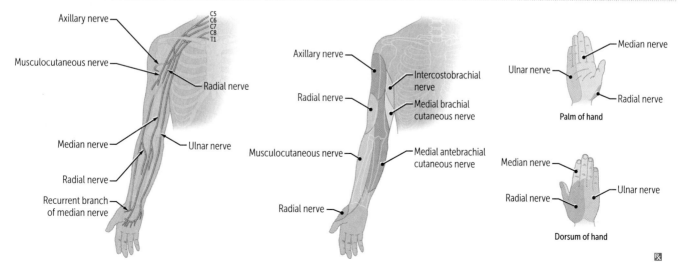

Brachial plexus lesions

❶ Erb palsy ("waiter's tip")
❷ Klumpke palsy (claw hand)
❸ Wrist drop
❹ Winged scapula
❺ Deltoid paralysis
❻ "Saturday night palsy" (wrist drop)
❼ Difficulty flexing elbow, variable sensory loss
❽ Decreased thumb function, "Pope's blessing"
❾ Intrinsic muscles of hand, claw hand

Randy
Travis
Drinks
Cold
Beer

CONDITION	INJURY	CAUSES	MUSCLE DEFICIT	FUNCTIONAL DEFICIT	PRESENTATION
Erb palsy ("waiter's tip")	Traction or tear of **upper** ("Erb-er") trunk: C5-C6 roots	Infants—lateral traction on neck during delivery Adults—trauma	Deltoid, supraspinatus	Abduction (arm hangs by side)	
			Infraspinatus	Lateral rotation (arm medially rotated)	
			Biceps brachii	Flexion, supination (arm extended and pronated)	
Klumpke palsy	Traction or tear of **lower** trunk: C8-T1 root	Infants—upward force on arm during delivery Adults—trauma (eg, grabbing a tree branch to break a fall)	Intrinsic hand muscles: lumbricals, interossei, thenar, hypothenar	Total claw hand: lumbricals normally flex MCP joints and extend DIP and PIP joints	
Thoracic outlet syndrome	Compression of **lower** trunk and subclavian vessels	Cervical rib (arrows in A), Pancoast tumor	Same as Klumpke palsy	Atrophy of intrinsic hand muscles; ischemia, pain, and edema due to vascular compression	
Winged scapula	Lesion of long thoracic nerve, roots C5-C7 ("wings of heaven")	Axillary node dissection after mastectomy, stab wounds	Serratus anterior	Inability to anchor scapula to thoracic cage → cannot abduct arm above horizontal position B	

Distortions of the hand At rest, a balance exists between the extrinsic flexors and extensors of the hand, as well as the intrinsic muscles of the hand—particularly the lumbrical muscles (flexion of MCP, extension of DIP and PIP joints).

"Clawing"—seen best with **distal** lesions of median or ulnar nerves. Remaining extrinsic flexors of the digits exaggerate the loss of the lumbricals → fingers extend at MCP, flex at DIP and PIP joints.

Deficits less pronounced in **proximal** lesions; deficits present during voluntary flexion of the digits.

PRESENTATION				
CONTEXT	Extending fingers/at rest	Making a fist	Extending fingers/at rest	Making a fist
LOCATION OF LESION	Distal ulnar nerve	Proximal median nerve	Distal median nerve	Proximal ulnar nerve
SIGN	"Ulnar claw"	"Pope's blessing"	"Median claw"	"OK gesture"

Note: Atrophy of the thenar eminence (unopposable thumb → "ape hand") can be seen in median nerve lesions, while atrophy of the hypothenar eminence can be seen in ulnar nerve lesions.

Knee exam

Lateral femoral condyle to anterior tibia: ACL.
Medial femoral condyle to posterior tibia: PCL.
LAMP.

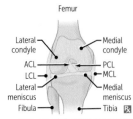

TEST	PROCEDURE		
Anterior drawer sign	Bending knee at 90° angle, ↑ anterior gliding of tibia (relative to femur) due to ACL injury. Lachman test also tests ACL, but is more sensitive (↑ anterior gliding of tibia [relative to femur] with knee bent at 30° angle).		ACL tear Anterior drawer sign
Posterior drawer sign	Bending knee at 90° angle, ↑ posterior gliding of tibia due to PCL injury.		PCL tear Posterior drawer sign
Abnormal passive abduction	Knee either extended or at ~ 30° angle, lateral (valgus) force → medial space widening of tibia → MCL injury.	Abduction (valgus) force	MCL tear
Abnormal passive adduction	Knee either extended or at ~ 30° angle, medial (varus) force → lateral space widening of tibia → LCL injury.	Adduction (varus) force	LCL tear
McMurray test	During flexion and extension of knee with rotation of tibia/foot: ▪ Pain, "popping" on external rotation → medial meniscal tear (external rotation stresses medial meniscus) ▪ Pain, "popping" on internal rotation → lateral meniscal tear (internal rotation stresses lateral meniscus)	External rotation Internal rotation	Medial tear Lateral tear

Common hip and knee conditions

Trochanteric bursitis	Inflammation of the gluteal tendon and bursa lateral to greater trochanter of femur. Treat pain with NSAIDs, heat, stretching.
"Unhappy triad"	Common injury in contact sports due to lateral force applied to a planted leg. Classically, consists of damage to the ACL **A**, MCL, and medial meniscus (attached to MCL); however, lateral meniscus injury is more common. Presents with acute knee pain and signs of joint injury/instability.
Prepatellar bursitis	Inflammation of the prepatellar bursa in front of the kneecap (red arrow in **B**). Can be caused by repeated trauma or pressure from excessive kneeling (also called "housemaid's knee").
Baker cyst	Popliteal fluid collection (red arrow in **C**) in gastrocnemius-semimembranosus bursa commonly communicating with synovial space and related to chronic joint disease (eg, osteoarthritis, rheumatoid arthritis).

Unhappy triad figure (Right knee): Lateral force, ACL, LCL, PCL, MCL, Medial meniscus

A: Fem, Pat, ACL, Tib
B: Fem, Ant meniscus, Tib, Post meniscus
C: Fem (lat cond), Fem (med cond), Pop a

Ankle sprains	Anterior TaloFibular ligament—most common ankle sprain overall, classified as a low ankle sprain. Due to overinversion/supination of foot. Always Tears First. Anterior inferior tibiofibular ligament—most common high ankle sprain.

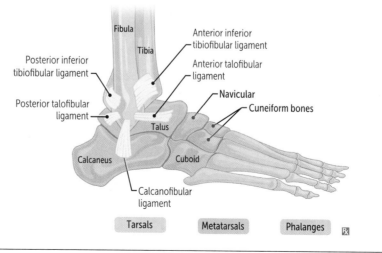

Fibula, Tibia, Anterior inferior tibiofibular ligament, Anterior talofibular ligament, Navicular, Cuneiform bones, Posterior inferior tibiofibular ligament, Posterior talofibular ligament, Talus, Calcaneus, Cuboid, Calcanofibular ligament, Tarsals, Metatarsals, Phalanges

Lower extremity nerves

NERVE	INNERVATION	CAUSE OF INJURY	PRESENTATION/COMMENTS
Iliohypogastric (T12-L1)	Sensory—suprapubic region Motor—transversus abdominis and internal oblique	Abdominal surgery	Burning or tingling pain in surgical incision site radiating to inguinal and suprapubic region
Genitofemoral nerve (L1-L2)	Sensory—scrotum/labia majora, medial thigh Motor—cremaster	Laparoscopic surgery	↓ anterior thigh sensation beneath inguinal ligament; absent cremasteric reflex
Lateral femoral cutaneous (L2-L3)	Sensory—anterior and lateral thigh	Tight clothing, obesity, pregnancy, pelvic procedures	↓ thigh sensation (anterior and lateral)
Obturator (L2-L4)	Sensory—medial thigh Motor—obturator externus, adductor longus, adductor brevis, gracilis, pectineus, adductor magnus	Pelvic surgery	↓ thigh sensation (medial) and adduction
Femoral (L2-L4)	Sensory—anterior thigh, medial leg Motor—quadriceps, iliacus, pectineus, sartorius	Pelvic fracture	↓ thigh flexion and leg extension
Sciatic (L4-S3)	Motor—semitendinosus, semimembranosus, biceps femoris, adductor magnus	Herniated disc, posterior hip dislocation	Splits into common peroneal and tibial nerves
Common peroneal (L4-S2)	Superficial peroneal nerve: ▪ Sensory—dorsum of foot (except webspace between hallux and 2nd digit) ▪ Motor—peroneus longus and brevis Deep peroneal nerve: ▪ Sensory—webspace between hallux and 2nd digit ▪ Motor—tibialis anterior	Trauma or compression of lateral aspect of leg, fibular neck fracture	**PED** = **P**eroneal **E**verts and **D**orsiflexes; if injured, foot drop**PED** Loss of sensation on dorsum of foot Foot drop—inverted and plantarflexed at rest, loss of eversion and dorsiflexion; "steppage gait"
Tibial (L4-S3)	Sensory—sole of foot Motor—biceps femoris (long head), triceps surae, plantaris, popliteus, flexor muscles of foot	Knee trauma, Baker cyst (proximal lesion); tarsal tunnel syndrome (distal lesion)	**TIP** = **T**ibial **I**nverts and **P**lantarflexes; if injured, can't stand on **TIP**toes Inability to curl toes and loss of sensation on sole; in proximal lesions, foot everted at rest with loss of inversion and plantarflexion

Lower extremity nerves *(continued)*

NERVE	INNERVATION	CAUSE OF INJURY	PRESENTATION/COMMENTS
Superior gluteal (L4-S1) 	Motor—gluteus medius, gluteus minimus, tensor fascia latae	Iatrogenic injury during intramuscular injection to superomedial gluteal region (prevent by choosing superolateral quadrant, preferably anterolateral region)	Trendelenburg sign/gait—pelvis tilts because weight-bearing leg cannot maintain alignment of pelvis through hip abduction Lesion is contralateral to the side of the hip that drops, ipsilateral to extremity on which the patient stands
Inferior gluteal (L5-S2)	Motor—gluteus maximus	Posterior hip dislocation	Difficulty climbing stairs, rising from seated position; loss of hip extension
Pudendal (S2-S4)	Sensory—perineum Motor—external urethral and anal sphincters	Stretch injury during childbirth	↓ sensation in perineum and genital area; can cause fecal or urinary incontinence Can be blocked with local anesthetic during childbirth using ischial spine as a landmark for injection

Actions of hip muscles

ACTION	MUSCLES
Abductors	Gluteus medius, gluteus minimus
Adductors	Adductor magnus, adductor longus, adductor brevis
Extensors	Gluteus maximus, semitendinosus, semimembranosus
Flexors	Iliopsoas, rectus femoris, tensor fascia lata, pectineus, sartorius
Internal rotation	Gluteus medius, gluteus minimus, tensor fascia latae
External rotation	Iliopsoas, gluteus maximus, piriformis, obturator

Common musculoskeletal conditions

Iliotibial band syndrome	Overuse injury of lateral knee that occurs primarily in runners. Pain develops 2° to friction of iliotibial band against lateral femoral epicondyle.
Medial tibial stress syndrome	Also called shin splints. Common cause of shin pain and diffuse tenderness in runners and military recruits. Caused by bone resorption that outpaces bone formation in tibial cortex.
Limb compartment syndrome	↑ pressure within a fascial compartment of a limb (defined by compartment pressure to diastolic blood pressure gradient of < 30 mm Hg) → venous outflow obstruction and arteriolar collapse → anoxia and necrosis. Causes include significant long bone fractures, reperfusion injury, animal venoms. Presents with severe pain and tense, swollen compartments with limb flexion. Motor deficits are late sign of irreversible muscle and nerve damage.
Plantar fasciitis	Inflammation of plantar aponeurosis characterized by heel pain (worse with first steps in the morning or after period of inactivity) and tenderness.
De Quervain tenosynovitis	Noninflammatory thickening of abductor pollicis longus and extensor pollicis brevis tendons characterized by pain or tenderness at radial styloid. ⊕ Finkelstein test (pain at radial styloid with active or passive stretch of thumb tendons).
Ganglion cyst	Fluid-filled swelling overlying joint or tendon sheath, most commonly at dorsal side of wrist. Arises from herniation of dense connective tissue.

Childhood musculoskeletal conditions

Developmental dysplasia of the hip	Abnormal acetabulum development in newborns. Results in hip instability/dislocation. Commonly tested with Ortolani and Barlow maneuvers (manipulation of newborn hip reveals a "clunk"). Confirmed via ultrasound (x-ray not used until ~4–6 months because cartilage is not ossified). Treatment: splint/harness.
Legg-Calvé-Perthes disease	Idiopathic avascular necrosis of femoral head. Commonly presents between 5–7 years with insidious onset of hip pain that may cause child to limp. More common in males (4:1 ratio). Initial x-ray often normal.
Slipped capital femoral epiphysis	Classically presents in an obese ~12-year-old child with hip/knee pain and altered gait. Increased axial force on femoral head → epiphysis displaces relative to femoral neck (like a scoop of ice cream slipping off a cone). Diagnosed via x-ray. Treatment: surgery.
Osgood-Schlatter disease (traction apophysitis)	Overuse injury caused by repetitive strain and chronic avulsion of the secondary ossification center of proximal tibial tubercle. Occurs in adolescents after growth spurt. Common in running and jumping athletes. Presents with progressive anterior knee pain.
Radial head subluxation (nursemaid's elbow)	Common elbow injury in children < 5 years. Caused by a sudden pull on the arm → immature annular ligament slips over head of radius. Injured arm held in flexed and pronated position.

Signs of lumbosacral radiculopathy

Paresthesia and weakness related to specific lumbosacral spinal nerves. Usually, the intervertebral disc herniates into central canal, affecting the inferior nerves (eg, herniation of L3/4 disc affects L4 spinal nerve, but not L3).

Intervertebral discs generally herniate posterolaterally, due to the thin posterior longitudinal ligament and thicker anterior longitudinal ligament along the midline of the vertebral bodies.

SPINAL LEVEL	FINDINGS
L3–L4	Weakness of knee extension, ↓ patellar reflex
L4–L5	Weakness of dorsiflexion, difficulty in heel-walking
L5-S1	Weakness of plantar flexion, difficulty in toe-walking, ↓ Achilles reflex

Neurovascular pairing

Nerves and arteries are frequently named together by the bones/regions with which they are associated. The following are exceptions to this naming convention.

LOCATION	NERVE	ARTERY
Axilla/lateral thorax	Long thoracic	Lateral thoracic
Surgical neck of humerus	Axillary	Posterior circumflex
Midshaft of humerus	Radial	Deep brachial
Distal humerus/ cubital fossa	Median	Brachial
Popliteal fossa	Tibial	Popliteal
Posterior to medial malleolus	Tibial	Posterior tibial

Motoneuron action potential to muscle contraction

T-tubules are extensions of plasma membrane in contact with the sarcoplasmic reticulum, allowing for coordinated contraction of striated muscles.

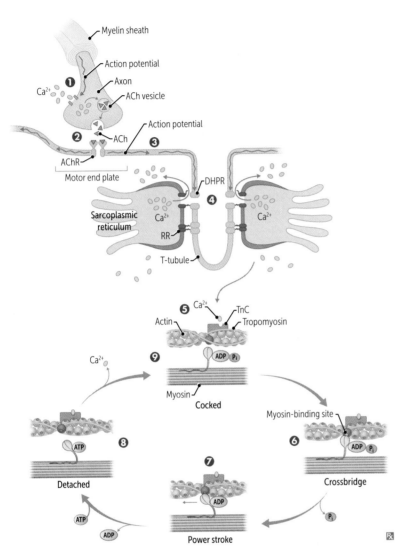

❶ Action potential opens presynaptic voltage-gated Ca^{2+} channels, inducing acetylcholine (ACh) release.

❷ Postsynaptic ACh binding leads to muscle cell depolarization at the motor end plate.

❸ Depolarization travels over the entire muscle cell and deep into the muscle via the T-tubules.

❹ Membrane depolarization induces conformational changes in the voltage-sensitive dihydropyridine receptor (DHPR) and its mechanically coupled ryanodine receptor (RR) → Ca^{2+} release from the sarcoplasmic reticulum into the cytoplasm.

❺ Tropomyosin is blocking myosin-binding sites on the actin filament. Released Ca^{2+} binds to troponin C (TnC), shifting tropomyosin to expose the myosin-binding sites.

❻ The myosin head binds strongly to actin, forming a crossbridge. P_i is then released, initiating the power stroke.

❼ During the power stroke, force is produced as myosin pulls on the thin filament. Muscle shortening occurs, with shortening of **H** and **I** bands and between **Z** lines (**HIZ** shrinkage). The A band remains the same length (**A** band is **A**lways the same length). ADP is released at the end of the power stroke.

❽ Binding of new ATP molecule causes detachment of myosin head from actin filament. Ca^{2+} is resequestered.

❾ ATP hydrolysis into ADP and P_i results in myosin head returning to high-energy position (cocked). The myosin head can bind to a new site on actin to form a crossbridge if Ca^{2+} remains available.

Types of muscle fibers

Type 1 muscle	Slow twitch; **red** fibers resulting from ↑ mitochondria and myoglobin concentration (↑ oxidative phosphorylation) → sustained contraction. Proportion ↑ after endurance training.	Think "**1** slow red ox."
Type 2 muscle	Fast twitch; white fibers resulting from ↓ mitochondria and myoglobin concentration (↑ anaerobic glycolysis). Proportion ↑ after weight/resistance training, sprinting.	

Smooth muscle contraction and relaxation

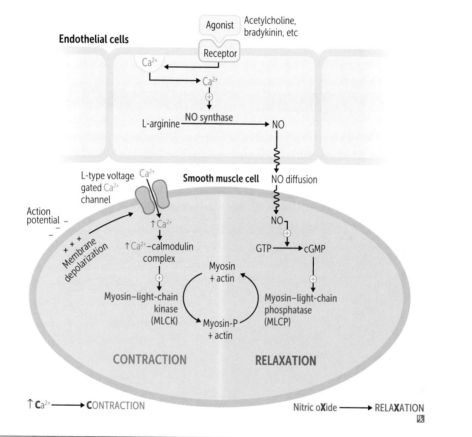

Bone formation

Endochondral ossification	Bones of axial skeleton, appendicular skeleton, and base of skull. Cartilaginous model of bone is first made by chondrocytes. Osteoclasts and osteoblasts later replace with woven bone and then remodel to lamellar bone. In adults, woven bone occurs after fractures and in Paget disease. Defective in achondroplasia.
Membranous ossification	Bones of calvarium, facial bones, and clavicle. Woven bone formed directly without cartilage. Later remodeled to lamellar bone.

Cell biology of bone

Osteoblast	Builds bone by secreting collagen and catalyzing mineralization in alkaline environment via ALP. Differentiates from mesenchymal stem cells in periosteum. Osteoblastic activity measured by bone ALP, osteocalcin, propeptides of type I procollagen.
Osteoclast	Dissolves ("crushes") bone by secreting H^+ and collagenases. Differentiates from a fusion of monocyte/macrophage lineage precursors. RANK receptors on osteoclasts are stimulated by RANKL (RANK ligand, secreted by osteoblasts). RANK receptors blocked by OPG (osteoprotegerin, a RANKL decoy receptor) → ↓ osteoclast activity.
Parathyroid hormone	At low, intermittent levels, exerts anabolic effects (building bone) on osteoblasts and osteoclasts (indirect). Chronically ↑ PTH levels (1° hyperparathyroidism) cause catabolic effects (osteitis fibrosa cystica).
Estrogen	Inhibits apoptosis in bone-forming osteoblasts and induces apoptosis in bone-resorbing osteoclasts. Causes closure of epiphyseal plate during puberty. Estrogen deficiency (surgical or postmenopausal) → ↑ cycles of remodeling and bone resorption → ↑ risk of osteoporosis.

▶ MUSCULOSKELETAL, SKIN, AND CONNECTIVE TISSUE—PATHOLOGY

Achondroplasia	Failure of longitudinal bone growth (endochondral ossification) → short limbs. Membranous ossification is affected → large head relative to limbs. Constitutive activation of fibroblast growth factor receptor (FGFR3) actually inhibits chondrocyte proliferation. > 85% of mutations occur sporadically; autosomal dominant with full penetrance (homozygosity is lethal). Associated with ↑ paternal age. Most common cause of dwarfism.

Osteoporosis

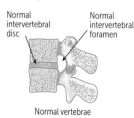

Normal intervertebral disc — Normal intervertebral foramen

Normal vertebrae

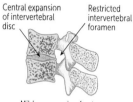

Central expansion of intervertebral disc — Restricted intervertebral foramen

Mild compression fracture

Trabecular (spongy) and cortical bone lose mass and interconnections despite normal bone mineralization and lab values (serum Ca^{2+} and PO_4^{3-}).

Most commonly due to ↑ bone resorption related to ↓ estrogen levels and old age. Can be 2° to drugs (eg, steroids, alcohol, anticonvulsants, anticoagulants, thyroid replacement therapy) or other medical conditions (eg, hyperparathyroidism, hyperthyroidism, multiple myeloma, malabsorption syndromes).

Diagnosed by bone mineral density measurement by DEXA (dual-energy X-ray absorptiometry) at the lumbar spine, total hip, and femoral neck, with a T-score of ≤ −2.5 or by a fragility fracture (eg, fall from standing height, minimal trauma) at hip or vertebra. One time screening recommended in women ≥ 65 years old.

Prophylaxis: regular weight-bearing exercise and adequate Ca^{2+} and vitamin D intake throughout adulthood.

Treatment: bisphosphonates, teriparatide, SERMs, rarely calcitonin; denosumab (monoclonal antibody against RANKL).

Can lead to vertebral compression fractures 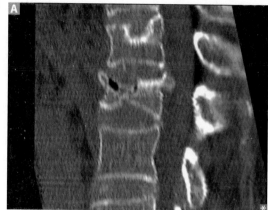—acute back pain, loss of height, kyphosis. Also can present with fractures of femoral neck, distal radius (Colles fracture).

Osteopetrosis

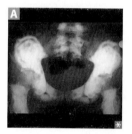

Failure of normal bone resorption due to defective osteoclasts → thickened, dense bones that are prone to fracture. Mutations (eg, carbonic anhydrase II) impair ability of osteoclast to generate acidic environment necessary for bone resorption. Overgrowth of cortical bone fills marrow space → pancytopenia, extramedulla ry hematopoiesis. Can result in cranial nerve impingement and palsies due to narrowed foramina.

X-rays show diffuse symmetric sclerosis (bone-in-bone, "stone bone"). Bone marrow transplant is potentially curative as osteoclasts are derived from monocytes.

Osteomalacia/rickets

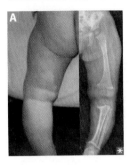

Defective mineralization of osteoid (osteomalacia) or cartilaginous growth plates (rickets, only in children). Most commonly due to vitamin D deficiency.

X-rays show osteopenia and "Looser zones" (pseudofractures) in osteomalacia, epiphyseal widening and metaphyseal cupping/fraying in rickets. Children with rickets have pathologic bow legs (genu varum A), bead-like costochondral junctions (rachitic rosary B), craniotabes (soft skull).

↓ vitamin D → ↓ serum Ca^{2+} → ↑ PTH secretion → ↓ serum PO_4^{3-}.

Hyperactivity of osteoblasts → ↑ ALP.

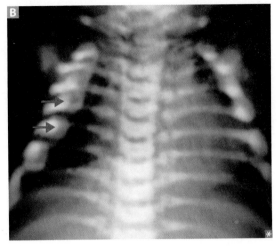

Paget disease of bone (osteitis deformans)

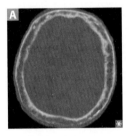

Common, localized disorder of bone remodeling caused by ↑ osteoclastic activity followed by ↑ osteoblastic activity that forms poor-quality bone. Serum Ca^{2+}, phosphorus, and PTH levels are normal. ↑ ALP. Mosaic pattern of woven and lamellar bone (osteocytes within lacunae in chaotic juxtapositions); long bone chalk-stick fractures. ↑ blood flow from ↑ arteriovenous shunts may cause high-output heart failure. ↑ risk of osteogenic sarcoma.

Hat size can be increased due to skull thickening A; hearing loss is common due to auditory foramen narrowing.

Stages of Paget disease:
- Lytic—osteoclasts
- Mixed—osteoclasts + osteoblasts
- Sclerotic—osteoblasts
- Quiescent—minimal osteoclast/osteoblast activity

Treatment: bisphosphonates.

Osteonecrosis (avascular necrosis)

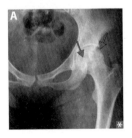

Infarction of bone and marrow, usually very painful. Most common site is femoral head (watershed zone) A (due to insufficiency of medial circumflex femoral artery). Causes include Corticosteroids, Alcoholism, Sickle cell disease, Trauma, "the Bends" (caisson/decompression disease), LEgg-Calvé-Perthes disease (idiopathic), Gaucher disease, Slipped capital femoral epiphysis—CAST Bent LEGS.

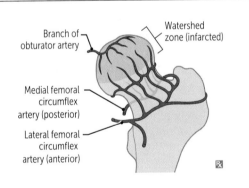

Lab values in bone disorders

DISORDER	SERUM Ca^{2+}	PO_4^{3-}	ALP	PTH	COMMENTS
Osteoporosis	—	—	—	—	↓ bone mass
Osteopetrosis	—/↓	—	—	—	Dense, brittle bones. Ca^{2+} ↓ in severe, malignant disease
Paget disease of bone	—	—	↑	—	Abnormal "mosaic" bone architecture
Osteitis fibrosa cystica					"Brown tumors" due to fibrous replacement of bone, subperiosteal thinning
Primary hyperparathyroidism	↑	↓	↑	↑	Idiopathic or parathyroid hyperplasia, adenoma, carcinoma
Secondary hyperparathyroidism	↓	↑	↑	↑	Often as compensation for CKD (↓ PO_4^{3-} excretion and production of activated vitamin D)
Osteomalacia/rickets	↓	↓	↑	↑	Soft bones; vitamin D deficiency also causes 2° hyperparathyroidism
Hypervitaminosis D	↑	↑	—	↓	Caused by oversupplementation or granulomatous disease (eg, sarcoidosis)

↑ ↓ = 1° change.

Primary bone tumors　Metastatic disease is more common than 1° bone tumors.

TUMOR TYPE	EPIDEMIOLOGY	LOCATION	CHARACTERISTICS
Benign tumors			
Osteochondroma	Most common benign bone tumor. Males < 25 years old.	Metaphysis of long bones.	Lateral bony projection of growth plate (continuous with marrow space) covered by cartilaginous cap **A**. Rarely transforms to chondrosarcoma.
Osteoma	Middle age.	Surface of facial bones.	Associated with Gardner syndrome.
Osteoid osteoma	Adults < 25 years old. Males > females.	Cortex of long bones.	Presents as bone pain (worse at night) that is relieved by NSAIDs. Bony mass (< 2 cm) with radiolucent osteoid core.
Osteoblastoma		Vertebrae.	Similar histology to osteoid osteoma. Larger size (> 2 cm), pain unresponsive to NSAIDs.
Chondroma		Medulla of small bones of hand and feet.	Benign tumor of cartilage.
Giant cell tumor	20–40 years old.	Epiphysis of long bones (often in knee region).	Locally aggressive benign tumor. Neoplastic mononuclear cells that express RANKL and reactive multinucleated giant (osteoclast-like) cells. "Osteoclastoma." "Soap bubble" appearance on x-ray **B**.
Malignant tumors			
Osteosarcoma (osteogenic sarcoma)	Accounts for 20% of 1° bone cancers. Peak incidence of 1° tumor in males < 20 years. Less common in elderly; usually 2° to predisposing factors, such as Paget disease of bone, bone infarcts, radiation, familial retinoblastoma, Li-Fraumeni syndrome.	Metaphysis of long bones (often in knee region) **C**.	Pleomorphic osteoid-producing cells (malignant osteoblasts). Presents as painful enlarging mass or pathologic fractures. Codman triangle (from elevation of periosteum) or sunburst pattern on x-ray. Think of an osteocod (bone fish) swimming in the sun. Aggressive. 1° usually responsive to treatment (surgery, chemotherapy), poor prognosis for 2°.
Chondrosarcoma		Medulla of pelvis and central skeleton.	Tumor of malignant chondrocytes.

Primary bone tumors *(continued)*

TUMOR TYPE	EPIDEMIOLOGY	LOCATION	CHARACTERISTICS
Ewing sarcoma	Most common in Caucasians. Generally boys < 15 years old.	Diaphysis of long bones (especially femur), pelvic flat bones.	Anaplastic small blue cells of neuroectodermal origin (resemble lymphocytes) **D**. Differentiate from conditions with similar morphology (eg, lymphoma, chronic osteomyelitis) by testing for t(11;22) (fusion protein EWS-FLI1). "Onion skin" periosteal reaction in bone. Aggressive with early metastases, but responsive to chemotherapy. 11 + 22 = **33** (Patrick **Ewing**'s jersey number).

Osteoarthritis and rheumatoid arthritis

	Osteoarthritis	Rheumatoid arthritis
PATHOGENESIS	Mechanical—wear and tear destroys articular cartilage (degenerative joint disorder) → inflammation with inadequate repair. Chondrocytes mediate degradation and inadequate repair.	Autoimmune—inflammation induces formation of pannus (proliferative granulation tissue **A**), which erodes articular cartilage and bone.
PREDISPOSING FACTORS	Age, female, obesity, joint trauma.	Female, HLA-DR4 (4-walled "**rheum**"), smoking. ⊕ rheumatoid factor (IgM antibody that targets IgG Fc region; in 80%), anti-cyclic citrullinated peptide antibody (more specific).
PRESENTATION	Pain in weight-bearing joints after use (eg, at the end of the day), improving with rest. Asymmetric joint involvement. Knee cartilage loss begins medially ("bowlegged"). No systemic symptoms.	Pain, swelling, and morning stiffness lasting > 1 hour, improving with use. Symmetric joint involvement. Systemic symptoms (fever, fatigue, weight loss). Extraarticular manifestations common.*
JOINT FINDINGS	Osteophytes (bone spurs), joint space narrowing, subchondral sclerosis and cysts. Synovial fluid noninflammatory (WBC < 2000/mm^3). Involves DIP (Heberden nodes **B**) and PIP (Bouchard nodes **C**), and 1st CMC; not MCP.	Erosions, juxta-articular osteopenia, soft tissue swelling, subchondral cysts, joint space narrowing. Deformities: cervical subluxation, ulnar finger deviation, swan neck **D**, boutonniere **E**. Involves MCP, PIP, wrist; not DIP or 1st CMC. Synovial fluid inflammatory.
TREATMENT	Acetaminophen, NSAIDs, intra-articular glucocorticoids.	NSAIDs, glucocorticoids, disease-modifying agents (methotrexate, sulfasalazine, hydroxychloroquine, leflunomide), biologic agents (eg, TNF-α inhibitors).

*Extraarticular manifestations include rheumatoid nodules (fibrinoid necrosis with palisading histiocytes) in subcutaneous tissue and lung (+ pneumoconiosis → Caplan syndrome), interstitial lung disease, pleuritis, pericarditis, anemia of chronic disease, neutropenia + splenomegaly (Felty syndrome), AA amyloidosis, Sjögren syndrome, scleritis, carpal tunnel syndrome.

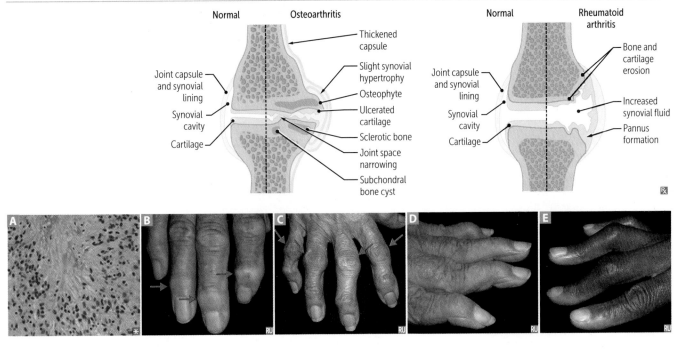

Gout

FINDINGS	Acute inflammatory monoarthritis caused by precipitation of monosodium urate crystals in joints A. Risk factors: male sex, hypertension, obesity, diabetes, dyslipidemia. Strongest risk factor is hyperuricemia, which can be caused by:
	▪ Underexcretion of uric acid (90% of patients)—largely idiopathic, potentiated by renal failure; can be exacerbated by certain medications (eg, thiazide diuretics).
	▪ Overproduction of uric acid (10% of patients)—Lesch-Nyhan syndrome, PRPP excess, ↑ cell turnover (eg, tumor lysis syndrome), von Gierke disease.
	Crystals are needle shaped and ⊖ birefringent under polarized light (yellow under parallel light, blue under perpendicular light B).
SYMPTOMS	Asymmetric joint distribution. Joint is swollen, red, and painful. Classic manifestation is painful MTP joint of big toe (podagra). Tophus formation C (often on external ear, olecranon bursa, or Achilles tendon). Acute attack tends to occur after a large meal with foods rich in purines (eg, red meat, seafood), trauma, surgery, dehydration, diuresis, or alcohol consumption (alcohol metabolites compete for same excretion sites in kidney as uric acid → ↓ uric acid secretion and subsequent buildup in blood).
TREATMENT	Acute: NSAIDs (eg, indomethacin), glucocorticoids, colchicine. Chronic (preventive): xanthine oxidase inhibitors (eg, allopurinol, febuxostat).

Calcium pyrophosphate deposition disease 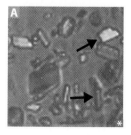	Previously called pseudogout. Deposition of calcium pyrophosphate crystals within the joint space. Occurs in patients > 50 years old; both sexes affected equally. Usually idiopathic, sometimes associated with hemochromatosis, hyperparathyroidism, joint trauma. Pain and swelling with acute inflammation (pseudogout) and/or chronic degeneration (pseudo-osteoarthritis). Knee most commonly affected joint. Chondrocalcinosis (cartilage calcification) on x-ray. Crystals are rhomboid and weakly ⊕ birefringent under polarized light (blue when parallel to light) A. Acute treatment: NSAIDs, colchicine, glucocorticoids. Prophylaxis: colchicine.	The blue P's—blue (when Parallel), Positive birefringent, calcium Pyrophosphate, Pseudogout

Systemic juvenile idiopathic arthritis

Childhood arthritis seen in < 12 year olds. Usually presents with daily spiking fevers, salmon-pink macular rash, uveitis, and arthritis (commonly 2+ joints). Frequently presents with leukocytosis, thrombocytosis, anemia, ↑ ESR, ↑ CRP. Treatment: NSAIDs, steroids, methotrexate, TNF inhibitors.

Sjögren syndrome

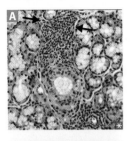
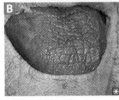

Autoimmune disorder characterized by destruction of exocrine glands (especially lacrimal and salivary) by lymphocytic infiltrates . Predominantly affects women 40–60 years old.

Findings:
- Inflammatory joint pain
- Keratoconjunctivitis sicca (↓ tear production and subsequent corneal damage)
- Xerostomia (↓ saliva production B)
- Presence of antinuclear antibodies, rheumatoid factor (can be in the absence of rheumatoid arthritis), antiribonucleoprotein antibodies: SS-A (anti-Ro) and/or SS-B (anti-La)
- Bilateral parotid enlargement

Anti-SSA and anti-SSB may also be seen in SLE. ⊕ Anti-SSA in pregnant women with SLE → ↑ risk of congenital heart block in the newborn.

A common 1° disorder or a 2° syndrome associated with other autoimmune disorders (eg, rheumatoid arthritis, SLE, systemic sclerosis).

Complications: dental caries; mucosa-associated lymphoid tissue (MALT) lymphoma (may present as parotid enlargement).

Focal lymphocytic sialadenitis on labial salivary gland biopsy can confirm diagnosis.

Septic arthritis

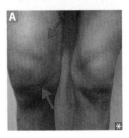

S aureus, Streptococcus, and *Neisseria gonorrhoeae* are common causes. Affected joint is swollen A, red, and painful. Synovial fluid purulent (WBC > 50,000/mm^3).

Gonococcal arthritis—STI that presents as either purulent arthritis (eg, knee) or triad of polyarthralgia, tenosynovitis (eg, hand), dermatitis (eg, pustules).

Seronegative spondyloarthritis	Arthritis without rheumatoid factor (no anti-IgG antibody). Strong association with HLA-B27 (MHC class I serotype). Subtypes (**PAIR**) share variable occurrence of inflammatory back pain (associated with morning stiffness, improves with exercise), peripheral arthritis, enthesitis (inflamed insertion sites of tendons, eg, Achilles), dactylitis ("sausage fingers"), uveitis.	
Psoriatic arthritis	Associated with skin psoriasis and nail lesions. Asymmetric and patchy involvement **A**. Dactylitis and "pencil-in-cup" deformity of DIP on x-ray **B**.	Seen in fewer than $\frac{1}{3}$ of patients with psoriasis.
Ankylosing spondylitis	Symmetric involvement of spine and sacroiliac joints → ankylosis (joint fusion), uveitis, aortic regurgitation.	Bamboo spine (vertebral fusion) **C**. Can cause restrictive lung disease due to limited chest wall expansion (costovertebral and costosternal ankylosis). More common in males.
Inflammatory bowel disease	Crohn disease and ulcerative colitis are often associated with spondyloarthritis.	
Reactive arthritis	Formerly known as Reiter syndrome. Classic triad: <ul><li>Conjunctivitis</li><li>Urethritis</li><li>Arthritis</li></ul>	"Can't see, can't pee, can't bend my knee." *Shigella, Yersinia, Chlamydia, Campylobacter, Salmonella* (ShY ChiCS).

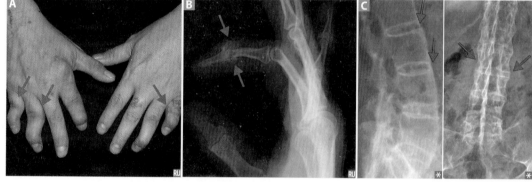

Systemic lupus erythematosus

Systemic, remitting, and relapsing autoimmune disease. Organ damage primarily due to a type III hypersensitivity reaction and, to a lesser degree, a type II hypersensitivity reaction. Associated with deficiency of early complement proteins (eg, C1q, C4, C2) → ↓ clearance of of immune complexes. Classic presentation: rash, joint pain, and fever in a female of reproductive age (especially of African-American or Hispanic descent).

Libman-Sacks Endocarditis—nonbacterial, verrucous thrombi usually on mitral or aortic valve and can be present on either surface of the valve (but usually on undersurface). LSE in SLE.

Lupus nephritis (glomerular deposition of DNA-anti-DNA immune complexes) can be nephritic or nephrotic (causing hematuria or proteinuria). Most common and severe type is diffuse proliferative.

Common causes of death in SLE: Renal disease (most common), Infections, Cardiovascular disease (accelerated CAD).

RASH OR PAIN:
Rash (malar A or discoid B)
Arthritis (nonerosive)
Serositis (eg, pleuritis, pericarditis)
Hematologic disorders (eg, cytopenias)
Oral/nasopharyngeal ulcers (usually painless)
Renal disease
Photosensitivity
Antinuclear antibodies
Immunologic disorder (anti-dsDNA, anti-Sm, antiphospholipid)
Neurologic disorders (eg, seizures, psychosis)

Lupus patients die with Redness In their Cheeks.

Antiphospholipid syndrome

1° or 2° autoimmune disorder (most commonly in SLE).

Diagnose based on clinical criteria including history of thrombosis (arterial or venous) or spontaneous abortion along with laboratory findings of lupus anticoagulant, anticardiolipin, anti-β₂ glycoprotein antibodies. Treat with systemic anticoagulation.

Anticardiolipin antibodies can cause false-positive VDRL/RPR, and lupus anticoagulant can cause prolonged PTT that is not corrected by the addition of normal platelet-free plasma.

Mixed connective tissue disease

Features of SLE, systemic sclerosis, and/or polymyositis. Associated with anti-U1 RNP antibodies (speckled ANA).

Polymyalgia rheumatica

SYMPTOMS	Pain and stiffness in proximal muscles (eg, shoulders, hips), often with fever, malaise, weight loss. Does not cause muscular weakness. More common in women > 50 years old; associated with giant cell (temporal) arteritis.
FINDINGS	↑ ESR, ↑ CRP, normal CK.
TREATMENT	Rapid response to low-dose corticosteroids.

Fibromyalgia

Most common in women 20–50 years old. Chronic, widespread musculoskeletal pain associated with "tender points," stiffness, paresthesias, poor sleep, fatigue, cognitive disturbance ("fibro fog"). Treatment: regular exercise, antidepressants (TCAs, SNRIs), neuropathic pain agents (eg, gabapentin).

Polymyositis/ dermatomyositis	↑ CK, ⊕ ANA (nonspecific), ⊕ anti-Jo-1 (histidyl-tRNA synthetase) (specific), ⊕ anti-SRP (specific), ⊕ anti-Mi-2 (specific) antibodies. Both disorders associated with interstitial lung disease. Treatment: steroids followed by long-term immunosuppressant therapy (eg, methotrexate).
Polymyositis	Progressive symmetric proximal muscle weakness, characterized by endomysial inflammation with CD8+ T cells. Most often involves shoulders.
Dermatomyositis	Clinically similar to polymyositis, but also involves malar rash (similar to that in SLE but involves nasolabial folds), Gottron papules A, heliotrope (violaceous periorbital) rash B, "shawl and face" rash C, darkening and thickening of fingertips and sides resulting in irregular, "dirty"-appearing marks. ↑ risk of occult malignancy. Perimysial inflammation and atrophy with CD4+ T cells.

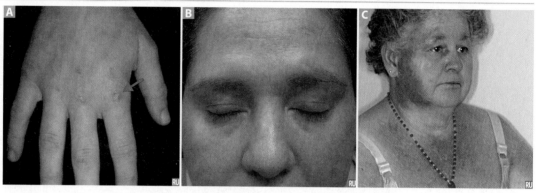

Neuromuscular junction diseases

	Myasthenia gravis	Lambert-Eaton myasthenic syndrome
FREQUENCY	Most common NMJ disorder	Uncommon
PATHOPHYSIOLOGY	Autoantibodies to postsynaptic ACh receptor	Autoantibodies to presynaptic Ca^{2+} channel → ↓ ACh release
CLINICAL	Ptosis, diplopia, weakness (respiratory muscle involvement can lead to dyspnea) Worsens with muscle use Improvement after edrophonium (tensilon) test	Proximal muscle weakness, autonomic symptoms (dry mouth, impotence) Improves with muscle use
ASSOCIATED WITH	Thymoma, thymic hyperplasia	Small cell lung cancer
AChE INHIBITOR ADMINISTRATION	Reverses symptoms (edrophonium to diagnose, pyridostigmine to treat)	Minimal effect

Raynaud phenomenon

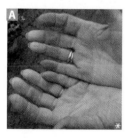

↓ blood flow to skin due to arteriolar (small vessel) vasospasm in response to cold or stress: color change from white (ischemia) to blue (hypoxia) to red (reperfusion). Most often in the fingers A and toes. Called Raynaud disease when 1° (idiopathic), Raynaud syndrome when 2° to a disease process such as mixed connective tissue disease, SLE, or CREST syndrome (limited form of systemic sclerosis). Digital ulceration (critical ischemia) seen in 2° Raynaud syndrome. Treat with Ca^{2+} channel blockers.

Scleroderma (systemic sclerosis)

Triad of autoimmunity, noninflammatory vasculopathy, and collagen deposition with fibrosis. Commonly sclerosis of skin, manifesting as puffy, taut skin 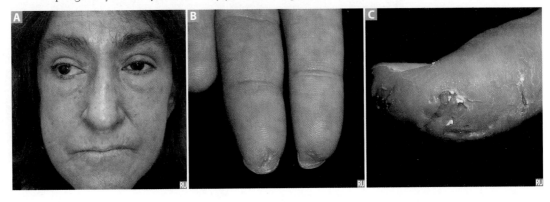 without wrinkles, fingertip pitting **B**. Can involve other systems, eg, renal (scleroderma renal crisis; treat with ACE inhibitors), pulmonary (interstitial fibrosis, pulmonary HTN), GI (esophageal dysmotility and reflux), cardiovascular. 75% female. 2 major types:

- **Diffuse scleroderma**—widespread skin involvement, rapid progression, early visceral involvement. Associated with anti-Scl-70 antibody (anti-DNA topoisomerase I antibody).

- **Limited scleroderma**—limited skin involvement confined to fingers and face. Also with CREST syndrome: Calcinosis cutis **C**, anti-Centromere antibody, Raynaud phenomenon, Esophageal dysmotility, Sclerodactyly, and Telangiectasia. More benign clinical course.

▶ MUSCULOSKELETAL, SKIN, AND CONNECTIVE TISSUE—DERMATOLOGY

Skin layers

Skin has 3 layers: epidermis, dermis, subcutaneous fat (hypodermis, subcutis).
Epidermis layers from surface to base 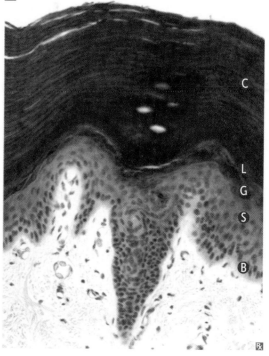:

- **Stratum Corneum** (keratin)
- **Stratum Lucidum** (most prominent in palms and soles)
- **Stratum Granulosum**
- **Stratum Spinosum** (desmosomes)
- **Stratum Basale** (stem cell site)

Californians Like Girls in String Bikinis.

Epithelial cell junctions

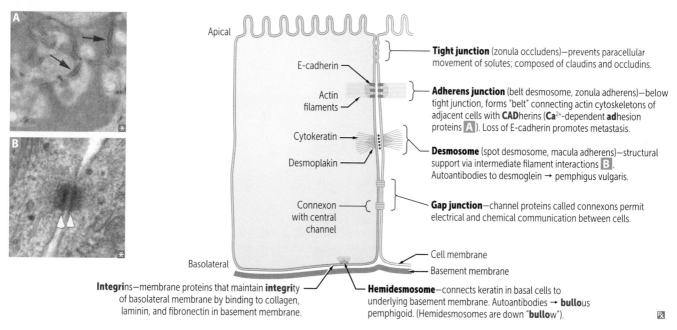

Tight junction (zonula occludens)—prevents paracellular movement of solutes; composed of claudins and occludins.

Adherens junction (belt desmosome, zonula adherens)—below tight junction, forms "belt" connecting actin cytoskeletons of adjacent cells with **CAD**herins (**Ca**²⁺-dependent **ad**hesion proteins A). Loss of E-cadherin promotes metastasis.

Desmosome (spot desmosome, macula adherens)—structural support via intermediate filament interactions B. Autoantibodies to desmoglein → pemphigus vulgaris.

Gap junction—channel proteins called connexons permit electrical and chemical communication between cells.

Apical

E-cadherin

Actin filaments

Cytokeratin

Desmoplakin

Connexon with central channel

Basolateral

Cell membrane

Basement membrane

Integrins—membrane proteins that maintain **integr**ity of basolateral membrane by binding to collagen, laminin, and fibronectin in basement membrane.

Hemidesmosome—connects keratin in basal cells to underlying basement membrane. Autoantibodies → **bull**ous pemphigoid. (Hemidesmosomes are down "**bull**ow").

Dermatologic macroscopic terms

LESION	CHARACTERISTICS	EXAMPLES
Macule	Flat lesion with well-circumscribed change in skin color < 1 cm	Freckle, labial macule 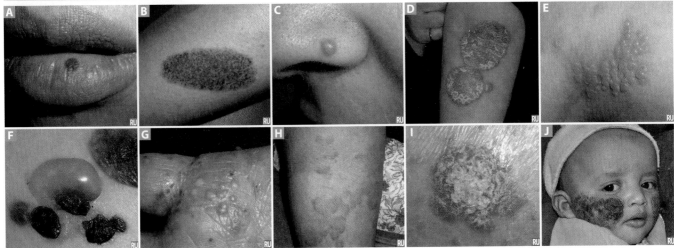 **A**
Patch	Macule > 1 cm	Large birthmark (congenital nevus) **B**
Papule	Elevated solid skin lesion < 1 cm	Mole (nevus) **C**, acne
Plaque	Papule > 1 cm	Psoriasis **D**
Vesicle	Small fluid-containing blister < 1 cm	Chickenpox (varicella), shingles (zoster) **E**
Bulla	Large fluid-containing blister > 1 cm	Bullous pemphigoid **F**
Pustule	Vesicle containing pus	Pustular psoriasis **G**
Wheal	Transient smooth papule or plaque	Hives (urticaria) **H**
Scale	Flaking off of stratum corneum	Eczema, psoriasis, SCC **I**
Crust	Dry exudate	Impetigo **J**

Dermatologic microscopic terms

LESION	CHARACTERISTICS	EXAMPLES
Hyperkeratosis	↑ thickness of stratum corneum	Psoriasis, calluses
Parakeratosis	Retention of nuclei in stratum corneum	Psoriasis
Hypergranulosis	↑ thickness of stratum granulosum	Lichen planus
Spongiosis	Epidermal accumulation of edematous fluid in intercellular spaces	Eczematous dermatitis
Acantholysis	Separation of epidermal cells	Pemphigus vulgaris
Acanthosis	Epidermal hyperplasia (↑ spinosum)	Acanthosis nigricans

Pigmented skin disorders

Albinism	Normal melanocyte number with ↓ melanin production 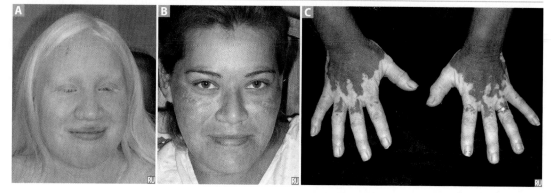 due to ↓ tyrosinase activity or defective tyrosine transport. ↑ risk of skin cancer.
Melasma (chloasma)	Hyperpigmentation associated with pregnancy ("mask of pregnancy" B) or OCP use.
Vitiligo	Irregular patches of complete depigmentation C. Caused by autoimmune destruction of melanocytes.

Seborrheic dermatitis

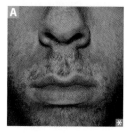

Erythematous, well-demarcated plaques with greasy yellow scales in areas rich in sebaceous glands, such as scalp, face, and periocular region. Common in both infants and adults, associated with Parkinson disease. Sebaceous glands are not inflamed, but play a role in disease development. Possibly associated with *Malassezia* spp. Treat with topical antifungals and corticosteroids.

Common skin disorders

Acne	Multifactorial etiology—↑ sebum/androgen production, abnormal keratinocyte desquamation, *Cutibacterium* (formerly *Propionibacterium*) *acnes* colonization of the pilosebaceous unit (comedones), and inflammation (papules/pustules **A**, nodules, cysts). Treatment includes retinoids, benzoyl peroxide, and antibiotics.
Atopic dermatitis (eczema)	Pruritic eruption, commonly on skin flexures. Associated with other atopic diseases (asthma, allergic rhinitis, food allergies); ↑ serum IgE. Mutations in filaggrin gene predispose (via skin barrier dysfunction). Often appears on face in infancy **B** and then in antecubital fossa **C** in children and adults.
Allergic contact dermatitis	Type IV hypersensitivity reaction that follows exposure to allergen. Lesions occur at site of contact (eg, nickel **D**, poison ivy, neomycin **E**).
Melanocytic nevus	Common mole. Benign, but melanoma can arise in congenital or atypical moles. Intradermal nevi are papular **F**. Junctional nevi are flat macules **G**.
Pseudofolliculitis barbae	Foreign body inflammatory facial skin disorder characterized by firm, hyperpigmented papules and pustules that are painful and pruritic. Located on cheeks, jawline, and neck. Commonly occurs as a result of shaving ("razor bumps"), primarily affects African-American males.
Psoriasis	Papules and plaques with silvery scaling **H**, especially on knees and elbows. Acanthosis with parakeratotic scaling (nuclei still in stratum corneum), Munro microabscesses. ↑ stratum spinosum, ↓ stratum granulosum. Auspitz sign (**I**)—pinpoint bleeding spots from exposure of dermal papillae when scales are scraped off. Associated with nail pitting and psoriatic arthritis.
Rosacea	Inflammatory facial skin disorder characterized by erythematous papules and pustules **J**, but no comedones. May be associated with facial flushing in response to external stimuli (eg, alcohol, heat). Phymatous rosacea can cause rhinophyma (bulbous deformation of nose).
Seborrheic keratosis	Flat, greasy, pigmented squamous epithelial proliferation with keratin-filled cysts (horn cysts) **K**. Looks "stuck on." Lesions occur on head, trunk, and extremities. Common benign neoplasm of older persons. Leser-Trélat sign **L**—sudden appearance of multiple seborrheic keratoses, indicating an underlying malignancy (eg, GI, lymphoid).
Verrucae	Warts; caused by low-risk HPV strains. Soft, tan-colored, cauliflower-like papules **M**. Epidermal hyperplasia, hyperkeratosis, koilocytosis. Condyloma acuminatum on anus or genitals **N**.
Urticaria	Hives. Pruritic wheals that form after mast cell degranulation **O**. Characterized by superficial dermal edema and lymphatic channel dilation.

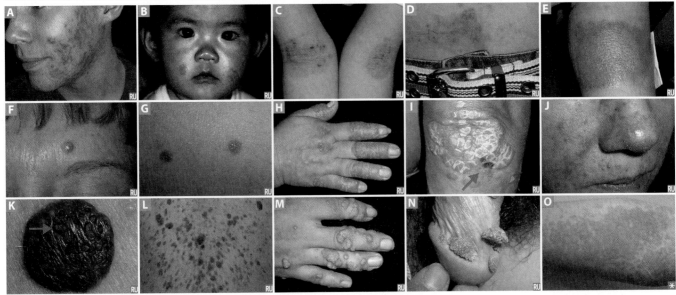

Vascular tumors of skin

Angiosarcoma	Rare blood vessel malignancy typically occurring in the head, neck, and breast areas. Usually in elderly, on sun-exposed areas. Associated with radiation therapy and chronic postmastectomy lymphedema. Hepatic angiosarcoma associated with vinyl chloride and arsenic exposures. Very aggressive and difficult to resect due to delay in diagnosis.
Bacillary angiomatosis	Benign capillary skin papules **A** found in AIDS patients. Caused by *Bartonella* infections. Frequently mistaken for Kaposi sarcoma, but has neutrophilic infiltrate.
Cherry hemangioma	Benign capillary hemangioma of the elderly **B**. Does not regress. Frequency ↑ with age.
Cystic hygroma	Cavernous lymphangioma of the neck **C**. Associated with Turner syndrome.
Glomus tumor	Benign, painful, red-blue tumor, commonly under fingernails **D**. Arises from modified smooth muscle cells of the thermoregulatory glomus body.
Kaposi sarcoma	Endothelial malignancy most commonly of the skin, but also mouth, GI tract, and respiratory tract. Associated with HHV-8 and HIV. Rarely mistaken for bacillary angiomatosis, but has lymphocytic infiltrate.
Pyogenic granuloma	Polypoid lobulated capillary hemangioma **E** that can ulcerate and bleed. Associated with trauma and pregnancy.
Strawberry hemangioma	Benign capillary hemangioma of infancy **F**. Appears in first few weeks of life (1/200 births); grows rapidly and regresses spontaneously by 5–8 years old.

Skin infections

Bacterial infections

Impetigo	Very superficial skin infection. Usually from *S aureus* or *S pyogenes*. Highly contagious. Honey-colored crusting **A**. Bullous impetigo **B** has bullae and is usually caused by *S aureus*.
Erysipelas	Infection involving upper dermis and superficial lymphatics, usually from *S pyogenes*. Presents with well-defined, raised demarcation between infected and normal skin **C**.
Cellulitis	Acute, painful, spreading infection of deeper dermis and subcutaneous tissues. Usually from *S pyogenes* or *S aureus*. Often starts with a break in skin from trauma or another infection **D**.
Abscess	Collection of pus from a walled-off infection within deeper layers of skin **E**. Offending organism is almost always *S aureus*.
Necrotizing fasciitis	Deeper tissue injury, usually from anaerobic bacteria or *S pyogenes*. Pain may be out of proportion to exam findings. Results in crepitus from methane and CO_2 production. "Flesh-eating bacteria." Causes bullae and a purple color to the skin **F**. Surgical emergency.
Staphylococcal scalded skin syndrome	Exotoxin destroys keratinocyte attachments in stratum granulosum only (vs toxic epidermal necrolysis, which destroys epidermal-dermal junction). Characterized by fever and generalized erythematous rash with sloughing of the upper layers of the epidermis **G** that heals completely. ⊕ Nikolsky sign (separation of epidermis upon manual stroking of skin). Seen in newborns and children, adults with renal insufficiency.

Viral infections

Herpes	Herpes virus infections (HSV1 and HSV2) of skin can occur anywhere from mucosal surfaces to normal skin. These include herpes labialis, herpes genitalis, herpetic whitlow **H** (finger).
Molluscum contagiosum	Umbilicated papules **I** caused by a poxvirus. While frequently seen in children, it may be sexually transmitted in adults.
Varicella zoster virus	Causes varicella (chickenpox) and zoster (shingles). Varicella presents with multiple crops of lesions in various stages from vesicles to crusts. Zoster is a reactivation of the virus in dermatomal distribution (unless it is disseminated).
Hairy leukoplakia	Irregular, white, painless plaques on lateral tongue that cannot be scraped off **J**. EBV mediated. Occurs in HIV-positive patients, organ transplant recipients. Contrast with thrush (scrapable) and leukoplakia (precancerous).

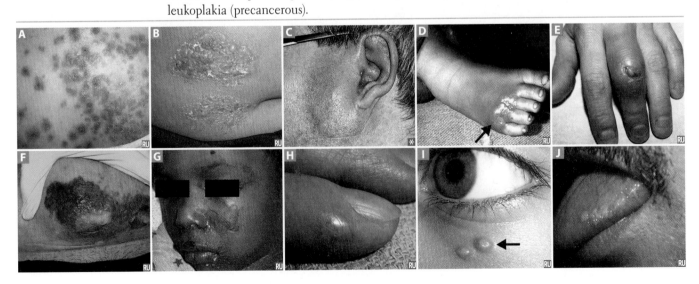

Blistering skin disorders

Pemphigus vulgaris	Potentially fatal autoimmune skin disorder with IgG antibody against desmoglein (component of desmosomes, which connect keratinocytes in the stratum spinosum). Flaccid intraepidermal bullae **A** caused by acantholysis (separation of keratinocytes, resembling a "row of tombstones"); oral mucosa is also involved. Type II hypersensitivity reaction. Immunofluorescence reveals antibodies around epidermal cells in a reticular (net-like) pattern **B**. Nikolsky sign ⊕.
Bullous pemphigoid	Less severe than pemphigus vulgaris. Type II hypersensitivity reaction: involves IgG antibody against hemidesmosomes (epidermal basement membrane; antibodies are "bullow" the epidermis). Tense blisters **C** containing eosinophils affect skin but spare oral mucosa. Immunofluorescence reveals linear pattern at epidermal-dermal junction **D**. Nikolsky sign ⊖.
Dermatitis herpetiformis	Pruritic papules, vesicles, and bullae (often found on elbows) **E**. Deposits of IgA at tips of dermal papillae. Associated with celiac disease. Treatment: dapsone, gluten-free diet.
Erythema multiforme	Associated with infections (eg, *Mycoplasma pneumoniae*, HSV), drugs (eg, sulfa drugs, β-lactams, phenytoin), cancers, autoimmune disease. Presents with multiple types of lesions—macules, papules, vesicles, target lesions (look like targets with multiple rings and dusky center showing epithelial disruption) **F**.
Stevens-Johnson syndrome	Characterized by fever, bullae formation and necrosis, sloughing of skin at dermal-epidermal junction, high mortality rate. Typically 2 mucous membranes are involved **G** **H**, and targetoid skin lesions may appear, as seen in erythema multiforme. Usually associated with adverse drug reaction. A more severe form of Stevens-Johnson syndrome (SJS) with > 30% of the body surface area involved is toxic epidermal necrolysis **I** **J** (TEN). 10–30% involvement denotes SJS-TEN.

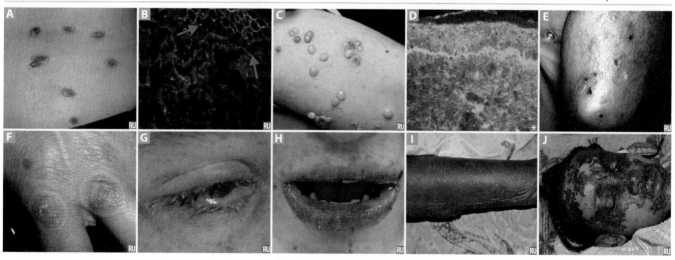

Miscellaneous skin disorders

Acanthosis nigricans	Epidermal hyperplasia causing symmetric, hyperpigmented thickening of skin, especially in axilla or on neck **A** **B**. Associated with insulin resistance (eg, diabetes, obesity, Cushing syndrome), visceral malignancy (eg, gastric adenocarcinoma).
Actinic keratosis	Premalignant lesions caused by sun exposure. Small, rough, erythematous or brownish papules or plaques **C** **D**. Risk of squamous cell carcinoma is proportional to degree of epithelial dysplasia.
Erythema nodosum	Painful, raised inflammatory lesions of subcutaneous fat (panniculitis), usually on anterior shins. Often idiopathic, but can be associated with sarcoidosis, coccidioidomycosis, histoplasmosis, TB, streptococcal infections **E**, leprosy **F**, inflammatory bowel disease.
Lichen Planus	Pruritic, Purple, Polygonal Planar Papules and Plaques are the 6 P's of lichen Planus **G** **H**. Mucosal involvement manifests as Wickham striae (reticular white lines) and hypergranulosis. Sawtooth infiltrate of lymphocytes at dermal-epidermal junction. Associated with hepatitis C.
Pityriasis rosea	"Herald patch" **I** followed days later by other scaly erythematous plaques, often in a "Christmas tree" distribution on trunk **J**. Multiple pink plaques with collarette scale. Self-resolving in 6–8 weeks.
Sunburn	Acute cutaneous inflammatory reaction due to excessive UV irradiation. Causes DNA mutations, inducing apoptosis of keratinocytes. UVB is dominant in sunBurn, UVA in tAnning and photoAging. Exposure to UVA and UVB ↑ risk of skin cancer. Can also lead to impetigo.

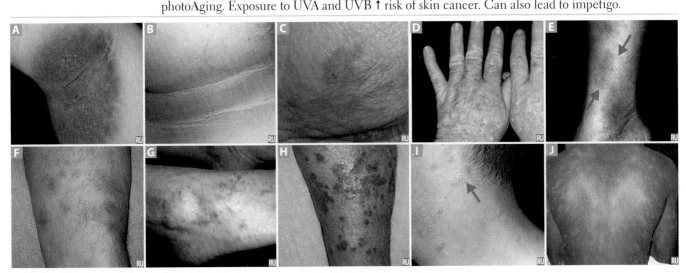

Burn classifications

First-degree burn	Superficial, through epidermis (eg, common sunburn).	Painful, erythematous, blanching
Second-degree burn	Partial-thickness burn through epidermis and dermis. Skin is blistered and usually heals **without scarring.**	Painful, erythematous, blanching
Third-degree burn	Full-thickness burn through epidermis, dermis, and hypodermis. **Skin scars** with wound healing.	Painless, waxy or leathery appearance, nonblanching

Skin cancer

| **Basal cell carcinoma** | Most common skin cancer. Found in sun-exposed areas of body (eg, face). Locally invasive, but rarely metastasizes. Waxy, pink, pearly nodules, commonly with telangiectasias, rolled borders, central crusting or ulceration **A**. BCCs also appear as nonhealing ulcers with infiltrating growth **B** or as a scaling plaque (superficial BCC) **C**. Basal cell tumors have "palisading" nuclei **D**. |

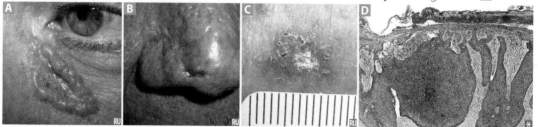

| **Squamous cell carcinoma** | Second most common skin cancer. Associated with excessive exposure to sunlight, immunosuppression, chronically draining sinuses, and occasionally arsenic exposure. Commonly appears on face **E**, lower lip **F**, ears, hands. Locally invasive, may spread to lymph nodes, and will rarely metastasize. Ulcerative red lesions with frequent scale. Histopathology: keratin "pearls" **G**.
Actinic keratosis, a scaly plaque, is a precursor to squamous cell carcinoma.
Keratoacanthoma is a variant that grows rapidly (4–6 weeks) and may regress spontaneously over months **H**. |

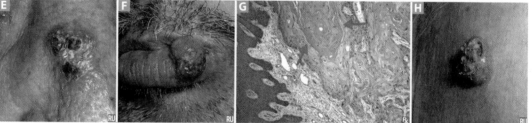

| **Melanoma** | Common tumor with significant risk of metastasis. S-100 tumor marker. Associated with sunlight exposure and dysplastic nevi; fair-skinned persons are at ↑ risk. Depth of tumor (Breslow thickness) correlates with risk of metastasis. Look for the **ABCDE**s: Asymmetry, Border irregularity, Color variation, Diameter > 6 mm, and Evolution over time. At least 4 different types of melanoma, including superficial spreading **I**, nodular **J**, lentigo maligna **K**, and acral lentiginous (highest prevalence in African-Americans and Asians) **L**. Often driven by activating mutation in BRAF kinase. Primary treatment is excision with appropriately wide margins. Metastatic or unresectable melanoma in patients with *BRAF* V600E mutation may benefit from vemurafenib, a BRAF kinase inhibitor. |

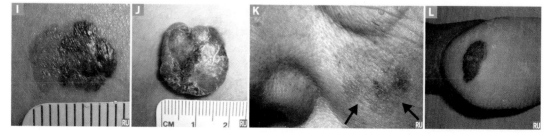

▶ MUSCULOSKELETAL, SKIN, AND CONNECTIVE TISSUE—PHARMACOLOGY

Arachidonic acid pathway

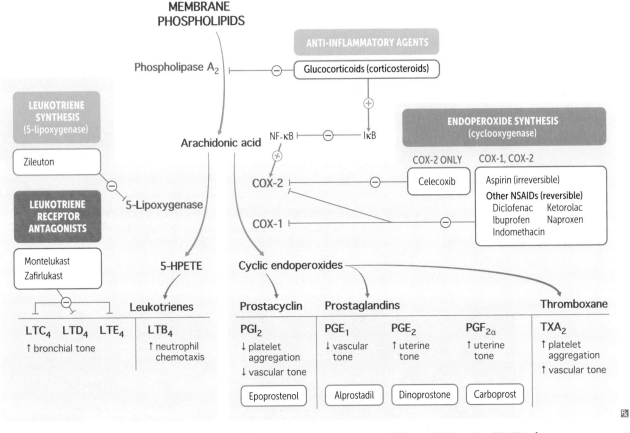

LTB$_4$ is a neutrophil chemotactic agent.   Neutrophils arrive "B4" others.
PGI$_2$ inhibits platelet aggregation and promotes   Platelet-Gathering Inhibitor.
   vasodilation.

Acetaminophen

MECHANISM	Reversibly inhibits cyclooxygenase, mostly in CNS. Inactivated peripherally.
CLINICAL USE	Antipyretic, analgesic, but not anti-inflammatory. Used instead of aspirin to avoid Reye syndrome in children with viral infection.
ADVERSE EFFECTS	Overdose produces hepatic necrosis; acetaminophen metabolite (NAPQI) depletes glutathione and forms toxic tissue byproducts in liver. N-acetylcysteine is antidote—regenerates glutathione.

Aspirin

MECHANISM	NSAID that irreversibly inhibits cyclooxygenase (both COX-1 and COX-2) by covalent acetylation → ↓ synthesis of TXA_2 and prostaglandins. ↑ bleeding time. No effect on PT, PTT. Effect lasts until new platelets are produced.
CLINICAL USE	Low dose (< 300 mg/day): ↓ platelet aggregation. Intermediate dose (300–2400 mg/day): antipyretic and analgesic. High dose (2400–4000 mg/day): anti-inflammatory.
ADVERSE EFFECTS	Gastric ulceration, tinnitus (CN VII), allergic reactions (especially in patients with asthma or nasal polyps). Chronic use can lead to acute renal failure, interstitial nephritis, GI bleeding. Risk of Reye syndrome in children treated with aspirin for viral infection. Toxic doses cause respiratory alkalosis early, but transitions to mixed metabolic acidosis-respiratory alkalosis.

Celecoxib

MECHANISM	Reversibly and selectively inhibits the cyclooxygenase (COX) isoform 2 ("Selecoxib"), which is found in inflammatory cells and vascular endothelium and mediates inflammation and pain; spares COX-1, which helps maintain gastric mucosa. Thus, does not have the corrosive effects of other NSAIDs on the GI lining. Spares platelet function as TXA_2 production is dependent on COX-1.
CLINICAL USE	Rheumatoid arthritis, osteoarthritis.
ADVERSE EFFECTS	↑ risk of thrombosis. Sulfa allergy.

Nonsteroidal anti-inflammatory drugs

Ibuprofen, naproxen, indomethacin, ketorolac, diclofenac, meloxicam, piroxicam.

MECHANISM	Reversibly inhibit cyclooxygenase (both COX-1 and COX-2). Block prostaglandin synthesis.
CLINICAL USE	Antipyretic, analgesic, anti-inflammatory. Indomethacin is used to close a PDA.
ADVERSE EFFECTS	Interstitial nephritis, gastric ulcer (prostaglandins protect gastric mucosa), renal ischemia (prostaglandins vasodilate afferent arteriole), aplastic anemia.

Leflunomide

MECHANISM	Reversibly inhibits dihydroorotate dehydrogenase, preventing pyrimidine synthesis. Suppresses T-cell proliferation.
CLINICAL USE	Rheumatoid arthritis, psoriatic arthritis.
ADVERSE EFFECTS	Diarrhea, hypertension, hepatotoxicity, teratogenicity.

Bisphosphonates

Alendronate, ibandronate, risedronate, zoledronate.

MECHANISM	Pyrophosphate analogs; bind hydroxyapatite in bone, inhibiting osteoclast activity.
CLINICAL USE	Osteoporosis, hypercalcemia, Paget disease of bone, metastatic bone disease, osteogenesis imperfecta.
ADVERSE EFFECTS	Esophagitis (if taken orally, patients are advised to take with water and remain upright for 30 minutes), osteonecrosis of jaw, atypical femoral stress fractures.

Teriparatide

MECHANISM	Recombinant PTH analog. ↑ osteoblastic activity when administered in pulsatile fashion.
CLINICAL USE	Osteoporosis. Causes ↑ bone growth compared to antiresorptive therapies (eg, bisphosphonates).
ADVERSE EFFECTS	↑ risk of osteosarcoma (avoid use in patients with Paget disease of the bone or unexplained elevation of alkaline phosphatase). Avoid in patients who have had prior cancers or radiation therapy. Transient hypercalcemia.

Gout drugs

Chronic gout drugs (preventive)

Probenecid	Inhibits reabsorption of uric acid in proximal convoluted tubule (also inhibits secretion of penicillin). Can precipitate uric acid calculi.	**Prevent A Painful Flare.**
Allopurinol	Competitive inhibitor of xanthine oxidase → ↓ conversion of hypoxanthine and xanthine to urate. Also used in lymphoma and leukemia to prevent tumor lysis–associated urate nephropathy. ↑ concentrations of azathioprine and 6-MP (both normally metabolized by xanthine oxidase).	
Pegloticase	Recombinant uricase catalyzing uric acid to allantoin (a more water-soluble product).	
Febuxostat	Inhibits xanthine oxidase.	

Acute gout drugs

NSAIDs	Any NSAID. Use salicylates with caution (may decrease uric acid excretion, particularly at low doses).
Glucocorticoids	Oral, intra-articular, or parenteral.
Colchicine	Binds and stabilizes tubulin to inhibit microtubule polymerization, impairing neutrophil chemotaxis and degranulation. Acute and prophylactic value. GI, neuromyopathic side effects.

TNF-α inhibitors

DRUG	MECHANISM	CLINICAL USE	ADVERSE EFFECTS
Etanercept	Fusion protein (decoy receptor for TNF-α + IgG$_1$ Fc), produced by recombinant DNA. Etanercept intercepts TNF.	Rheumatoid arthritis, psoriasis, ankylosing spondylitis	Predisposition to infection, including reactivation of latent TB, since TNF is important in granuloma formation and stabilization. Can also lead to drug-induced lupus.
Infliximab, adalimumab, certolizumab, golimumab	Anti-TNF-α monoclonal antibody.	Inflammatory bowel disease, rheumatoid arthritis, ankylosing spondylitis, psoriasis	

Neurology and Special Senses

> "We are all now connected by the Internet, like neurons in a giant brain."
> —Stephen Hawking

> "Anything's possible if you've got enough nerve."
> —J.K. Rowling, *Harry Potter and the Order of the Phoenix*

> "I like nonsense; it wakes up the brain cells."
> —Dr. Seuss

> "I believe in an open mind, but not so open that your brains fall out."
> —Arthur Hays Sulzberger

> "The chief function of the body is to carry the brain around."
> —Thomas Edison

> "Exactly how [the brain] operates remains one of the biggest unsolved mysteries, and it seems the more we probe its secrets, the more surprises we find."
>
> —Neil deGrasse Tyson

Know how to clinically interpret common patterns of neurologic symptoms and findings. Questions on the exam often correlate clinical scenarios with gross pathologic specimens or cross-sectional CT/MR imaging. With regard to neuropharmacology, antiparkinsonism, antiepileptic and opioid drugs tend to be highly testable.

▶ NEUROLOGY—EMBRYOLOGY

Neural development

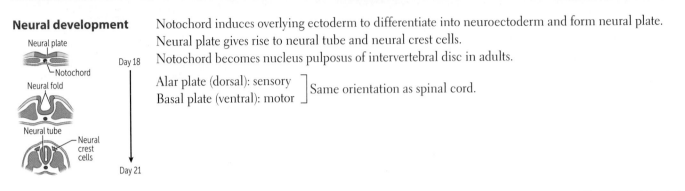

Notochord induces overlying ectoderm to differentiate into neuroectoderm and form neural plate.
Neural plate gives rise to neural tube and neural crest cells.
Notochord becomes nucleus pulposus of intervertebral disc in adults.

Alar plate (dorsal): sensory ⎤
Basal plate (ventral): motor ⎦ Same orientation as spinal cord.

Regional specification of developing brain

Telencephalon is the 1st part. Diencephalon is the 2nd part. The rest are arranged alphabetically: mesencephalon, metencephalon, myelencephalon.

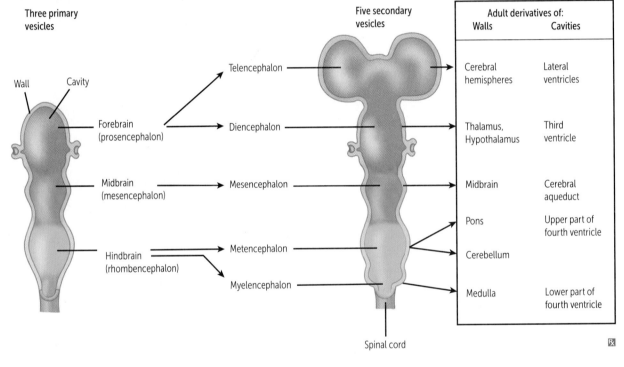

Central and peripheral nervous systems origins

Neuroepithelia in neural tube—CNS neurons, ependymal cells (inner lining of ventricles, make CSF), oligodendrocytes, astrocytes.
Neural crest—PNS neurons, Schwann cells.
Mesoderm—Microglia (like Macrophages).

Neural tube defects	Neuropores fail to fuse (4th week) → persistent connection between amniotic cavity and spinal canal. Associated with maternal diabetes as well as low folic acid intake before conception and during pregnancy. ↑ α-fetoprotein (AFP) in amniotic fluid and maternal serum (except spina bifida occulta = normal AFP). ↑ acetylcholinesterase (AChE) in amniotic fluid is a helpful confirmatory test.
Spina bifida occulta	Failure of caudal neuropore to close, but no herniation. Usually seen at lower vertebral levels. Dura is intact. Associated with tuft of hair or skin dimple at level of bony defect.
Meningocele	Meninges (but no neural tissue) herniate through bony defect. Associated with spina bifida cystica.
Meningomyelocele	Meninges and neural tissue (eg, cauda equina) herniate through bony defect.
Myeloschisis	Also known as rachischisis. Exposed unfused neural tissue without skin/meningeal covering.
Anencephaly	Failure of rostral neuropore to close → no forebrain, open calvarium. Clinical findings: polyhydramnios (no swallowing center in brain).

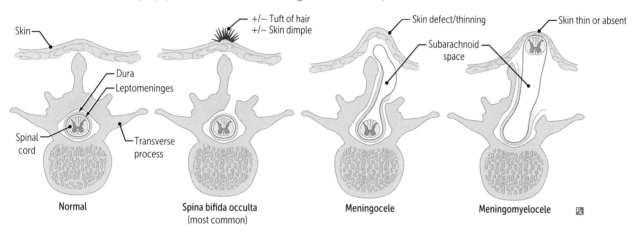

Holoprosencephaly	Failure of left and right hemispheres to separate; usually occurs during weeks 5–6. May be related to mutations in sonic hedgehog signaling pathway. Moderate form has cleft lip/palate, most severe form results in cyclopia. Seen in trisomy 13 and fetal alcohol syndrome. MRI 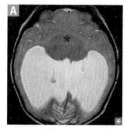 reveals monoventricle and fusion of basal ganglia (star in A).

Posterior fossa malformations

Chiari I malformation	Ectopia of cerebellar **tonsils** (1 structure) A. Congenital, usually asymptomatic in childhood, manifests in adulthood with headaches and cerebellar symptoms. Associated with spinal cavitations (eg, syringomyelia).
Chiari II malformation	Herniation of low-lying cerebellar **vermis** and **tonsils** (2 structures) through foramen magnum with aqueductal stenosis → hydrocephalus. Usually associated with lumbosacral meningomyelocele (may present as paralysis/sensory loss at and below the level of the lesion).
Dandy-Walker syndrome	Agenesis of cerebellar vermis leads to cystic enlargement of 4th ventricle (arrow in B) that fills the enlarged posterior fossa. Associated with noncommunicating hydrocephalus, spina bifida.

Syringomyelia	Cystic cavity (syrinx) within central canal of spinal cord (yellow arrows in A). Fibers crossing in anterior white commissure (spinothalamic tract) are typically damaged first. Results in a "cape-like," bilateral symmetrical loss of pain and temperature sensation in upper extremities (fine touch sensation is preserved). Associated with Chiari malformations (red arrow shows low-lying cerebellar tonsils in A) and other congenital malformations; acquired causes include trauma and tumors.	*Syrinx* = tube, as in syringe. Most common at C8–T1.

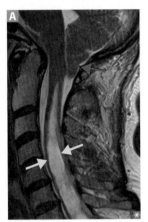

Tongue development

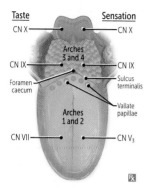

1st and 2nd branchial arches form anterior $^2/_3$ (thus sensation via CN V$_3$, taste via CN VII). 3rd and 4th branchial arches form posterior $^1/_3$ (thus sensation and taste mainly via CN IX, extreme posterior via CN X).

Motor innervation is via CN XII to hyoglossus (retracts and depresses tongue), genioglossus (**protrudes** tongue), and styloglossus (draws sides of tongue upward to create a trough for swallowing).

Motor innervation is via CN X to palatoglossus (elevates posterior tongue during swallowing).

Taste—CN VII, IX, X (solitary nucleus).
Pain—CN V$_3$, IX, X.
Motor—CN X, XII.

The **Genie sticks out** his tongue.

▶ NEUROLOGY—ANATOMY AND PHYSIOLOGY

Neurons	Signal-transmitting cells of the nervous system. Permanent cells—do not divide in adulthood. Signal-relaying cells with dendrites (receive input), cell bodies, and axons (send output). Cell bodies and dendrites can be seen on Nissl staining (stains RER). RER is not present in the axon. Injury to axon → Wallerian degeneration—degeneration of axon distal to site of injury and axonal retraction proximally; allows for potential regeneration of axon (if in PNS). Macrophages remove debris and myelin.

Astrocytes

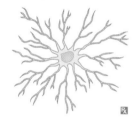

Most common glial cell type in CNS. Physical support, repair, extracellular K$^+$ buffer, removal of excess neurotransmitter, component of blood-brain barrier, glycogen fuel reserve buffer. Reactive gliosis in response to neural injury.

Derived from neuroectoderm. Astrocyte marker: GFAP.

Microglia

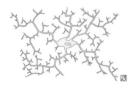

Phagocytic scavenger cells of CNS (mesodermal, mononuclear origin). Activated in response to tissue damage. Not readily discernible by Nissl stain.

HIV-infected microglia fuse to form multinucleated giant cells in CNS.

Ependymal cells

Glial cells with a ciliated simple columnar form that line the ventricles and central canal of spinal cord. Apical surfaces are covered in cilia (which circulate CSF) and microvilli (which help in CSF absorption).

Myelin

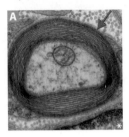

↑ conduction velocity of signals transmitted down axons → saltatory conduction of action potential at the nodes of Ranvier, where there are high concentrations of Na⁺ channels. Synthesis of myelin by oligodendrocytes in CNS (including CN I and II) and Schwann cells in PNS (including CN III-XII).

Wraps and insulates axons (arrow in A): ↑ space constant and ↑ conduction velocity.
COPS: CNS = Oligodendrocytes, PNS = Schwann cells.

Schwann cells

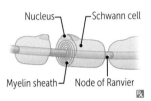

Each Schwann cell myelinates only 1 PNS axon. Also promote axonal regeneration. Derived from neural crest.

Injured in Guillain-Barré syndrome.

Oligodendrocytes

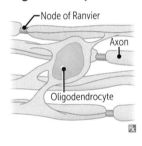

Myelinates axons of neurons in CNS. Each oligodendrocyte can myelinate many axons (~ 30). Predominant type of glial cell in white matter.

Derived from neuroectoderm.
"Fried egg" appearance histologically.
Injured in multiple sclerosis, progressive multifocal leukoencephalopathy (PML), leukodystrophies.

Sensory receptors

RECEPTOR TYPE	SENSORY NEURON FIBER TYPE	LOCATION	SENSES
Free nerve endings	C—slow, unmyelinated fibers Aδ—fAst, myelinated fibers	All skin, epidermis, some viscera	Pain, temperature
Meissner corpuscles	Large, myelinated fibers; adapt quickly	Glabrous (hairless) skin	Dynamic, fine/light touch, position sense
Pacinian corpuscles	Large, myelinated fibers; adapt quickly	Deep skin layers, ligaments, joints	Vibration, pressure
Merkel discs	Large, myelinated fibers; adapt slowly	Finger tips, superficial skin	Pressure, deep static touch (eg, shapes, edges), position sense
Ruffini corpuscles	Dendritic endings with capsule; adapt slowly	Finger tips, joints	Pressure, slippage of objects along surface of skin, joint angle change

Peripheral nerve

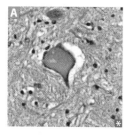

- Nerve trunk
- Epineurium
- Perineurium
- Endoneurium
- Nerve fiber

Endoneurium—invests single nerve fiber layers (inflammatory infiltrate in Guillain-Barré syndrome).

Perineurium (blood-nerve Permeability barrier)—surrounds a fascicle of nerve fibers. Must be rejoined in microsurgery for limb reattachment.

Epineurium—dense connective tissue that surrounds entire nerve (fascicles and blood vessels).

Endo = inner.
Peri = around.
Epi = outer.

Chromatolysis

Reaction of neuronal cell body to axonal injury. Changes reflect ↑ protein synthesis in effort to repair the damaged axon. Characterized by:
- Round cellular swelling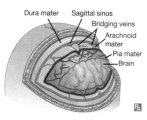
- Displacement of the nucleus to the periphery
- Dispersion of Nissl substance throughout cytoplasm

Concurrent with Wallerian degeneration.

Neurotransmitter changes with disease

	LOCATION OF SYNTHESIS	ANXIETY	DEPRESSION	SCHIZOPHRENIA	ALZHEIMER DISEASE	HUNTINGTON DISEASE	PARKINSON DISEASE
Acetylcholine	Basal nucleus of Meynert				↓	↓	↑
Dopamine	Ventral tegmentum, SNc		↓	↑		↑	↓
GABA	Nucleus accumbens	↓				↓	
Norepinephrine	Locus ceruleus	↑	↓				
Serotonin	Raphe nucleus	↓	↓				↓

Meninges

- Dura mater
- Sagittal sinus
- Bridging veins
- Arachnoid mater
- Pia mater
- Brain

Three membranes that surround and protect the brain and spinal cord:
- Dura mater—thick outer layer closest to skull. Derived from mesoderm.
- Arachnoid mater—middle layer, contains web-like connections. Derived from neural crest.
- Pia mater—thin, fibrous inner layer that firmly adheres to brain and spinal cord. Derived from neural crest.

CSF flows in the subarachnoid space, located between arachnoid and pia mater.

Epidural space—a potential space between the dura mater and skull containing fat and blood vessels.

Blood-brain barrier

Astrocyte foot processes

Capillary lumen

Tight junction

Basement membrane

Prevents circulating blood substances (eg, bacteria, drugs) from reaching the CSF/CNS. Formed by 3 structures:

- Tight junctions between nonfenestrated capillary endothelial cells
- Basement membrane
- Astrocyte foot processes

Glucose and amino acids cross slowly by carrier-mediated transport mechanisms.

Nonpolar/lipid-soluble substances cross rapidly via diffusion.

A few specialized brain regions with fenestrated capillaries and no blood-brain barrier allow molecules in blood to affect brain function (eg, area postrema—vomiting after chemo; OVLT [organum vasculosum lamina terminalis]—osmotic sensing) or neurosecretory products to enter circulation (eg, neurohypophysis—ADH release).

Infarction and/or neoplasm destroys endothelial cell tight junctions → vasogenic edema.

Other notable barriers include:

- Blood-testis barrier
- Maternal-fetal blood barrier of placenta

Hypothalamus	Maintains homeostasis by regulating Thirst and water balance, controlling Adenohypophysis (anterior pituitary) and Neurohypophysis (posterior pituitary) release of hormones produced in the hypothalamus, and regulating Hunger, Autonomic nervous system, Temperature, and Sexual urges (**TAN HATS**). Inputs (areas not protected by blood-brain barrier): OVLT (senses change in osmolarity), area postrema (found in medulla, responds to emetics).	
Lateral nucleus	Hunger. Destruction → anorexia, failure to thrive (infants). Stimulated by ghrelin, inhibited by leptin.	Lateral injury makes you Lean.
Ventromedial nucleus	Satiety. Destruction (eg, craniopharyngioma) → hyperphagia. Stimulated by leptin.	VentroMedial injury makes you Very Massive.
Anterior nucleus	Cooling, parasympathetic.	Anterior nucleus = cool off (cooling, pArasympathetic). A/C = anterior cooling.
Posterior nucleus	Heating, sympathetic.	Heating controlled by Posterior hypothalamus ("Hot Pot"). If you zap your posterior hypothalamus, you become a poikilotherm (cold-blooded, like a snake).
Suprachiasmatic nucleus	Circadian rhythm.	You need sleep to be charismatic (chiasmatic).
Supraoptic and paraventricular nuclei	Synthesize ADH and oxytocin.	ADH and oxytocin are carried by neurophysins down axons to posterior pituitary, where these hormones are stored and released.
Preoptic nucleus	Thermoregulation, sexual behavior. Releases GnRH. Failure of GnRH-producing neurons to migrate from olfactory pit → Kallmann syndrome.	

Vomiting center

Coordinated by nucleus tractus solitarius (NTS) in the medulla, which receives information from the chemoreceptor trigger zone (CTZ, located within area postrema in 4th ventricle), GI tract (via vagus nerve), vestibular system, and CNS.

CTZ and adjacent vomiting center nuclei receive input from 5 major receptors: muscarinic (M_1), dopamine (D_2), histamine (H_1), serotonin ($5\text{-}HT_3$), and neurokinin (NK-1) receptors.

- $5\text{-}HT_3$, D_2, and NK-1 antagonists used to treat chemotherapy-induced vomiting.
- M_1 and H_1 antagonists used to treat motion sickness and hyperemesis gravidarum.

Sleep physiology

Sleep cycle is regulated by the circadian rhythm, which is driven by suprachiasmatic nucleus (SCN) of hypothalamus. Circadian rhythm controls nocturnal release of ACTH, prolactin, melatonin, norepinephrine: SCN → norepinephrine release → pineal gland → melatonin. SCN is regulated by environment (eg, light).

Two stages: rapid-eye movement (REM) and non-REM.

Alcohol, benzodiazepines, and barbiturates are associated with ↓ REM sleep and delta wave sleep; norepinephrine also ↓ REM sleep.

Benzodiazepines are useful for night terrors and sleepwalking by ↓ N3 and REM sleep.

SLEEP STAGE (% OF TOTAL SLEEP TIME IN YOUNG ADULTS)	DESCRIPTION	EEG WAVEFORM
Awake (eyes open)	Alert, active mental concentration.	Beta (highest frequency, lowest amplitude)
Awake (eyes closed)		Alpha
Non-REM sleep		
Stage N1 (5%)	Light sleep.	Theta
Stage N2 (45%)	Deeper sleep; when bruxism (teeth grinding) occurs.	Sleep spindles and K complexes "Twoth" grinding
Stage N3 (25%)	Deepest non-REM sleep (slow-wave sleep); when sleepwalking, night terrors, and bedwetting occur.	Delta (lowest frequency, highest amplitude)
REM sleep (25%)	Loss of motor tone, ↑ brain O_2 use, ↑ and variable pulse and blood pressure ↑ ACh; when dreaming, nightmares, and penile/clitoral tumescence occur; may serve memory processing function. Depression increases total REM sleep but decreases REM latency. Extraocular movements due to activity of PPRF (paramedian pontine reticular formation/conjugate gaze center). Occurs every 90 minutes, and duration ↑ through the night.	Beta At night, **BATS** Drink Blood

Thalamus Major relay for all ascending sensory information except olfaction.

NUCLEI	INPUT	SENSES	DESTINATION	MNEMONIC
Ventral Postero-Lateral nucleus	Spinothalamic and dorsal columns/medial lemniscus	Vibration, Pain, Pressure, Proprioception, Light touch, temperature	1° somatosensory cortex	
Ventral postero-Medial nucleus	Trigeminal and gustatory pathway	Face sensation, taste	1° somatosensory cortex	Makeup goes on the face
Lateral geniculate nucleus	CN II, optic chiasm, optic tract	Vision	Calcarine sulcus	Lateral = Light
Medial geniculate nucleus	Superior olive and inferior colliculus of tectum	Hearing	Auditory cortex of temporal lobe	Medial = Music
Ventral lateral nucleus	Basal ganglia, cerebellum	Motor	Motor cortex	

Limbic system

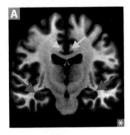

Collection of neural structures involved in emotion, long-term memory, olfaction, behavior modulation, ANS function.
Consists of hippocampus (red arrows in **A**), amygdalae, mammillary bodies, anterior thalamic nuclei, cingulate gyrus (yellow arrows in **A**), entorhinal cortex. Responsible for Feeding, Fleeing, Fighting, Feeling, and Sex.

The famous 5 F's.

Dopaminergic pathways Commonly altered by drugs (eg, antipsychotics) and movement disorders (eg, Parkinson disease).

PATHWAY	SYMPTOMS OF ALTERED ACTIVITY	NOTES
Mesocortical	↓ activity → "negative" symptoms (eg, anergia, apathy, lack of spontaneity).	Antipsychotic drugs have limited effect.
Mesolimbic	↑ activity → "positive" symptoms (eg, delusions, hallucinations).	1° therapeutic target of antipsychotic drugs → ↓ positive symptoms (eg, in schizophrenia).
Nigrostriatal	↓ activity → extrapyramidal symptoms (eg, dystonia, akathisia, parkinsonism, tardive dyskinesia).	Major dopaminergic pathway in brain. Significantly affected by movement disorders and antipsychotic drugs.
Tuberoinfundibular	↓ activity → ↑ prolactin → ↓ libido, sexual dysfunction, galactorrhea, gynecomastia (in men).	

Cerebellum

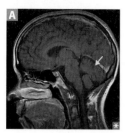

Modulates movement; aids in coordination and balance. Arrow in **A**.

Input:
- Contralateral cortex via middle cerebellar peduncle.
- Ipsilateral proprioceptive information via inferior cerebellar peduncle from spinal cord.

Output:
- The only output of cerebellar cortex = Purkinje cells (always inhibitory) → deep nuclei of cerebellum → contralateral cortex via superior cerebellar peduncle.
- Deep nuclei (lateral → medial)—Dentate, Emboliform, Globose, Fastigial.

Lateral lesions—affect voluntary movement of extremities (**lateral** structures); when injured, propensity to fall toward injured (ipsilateral) side.

Medial lesions (eg, vermis, fastigial nuclei, flocculonodular lobe)—truncal ataxia (wide-based cerebellar gait), nystagmus, head tilting. Generally result in bilateral motor deficits affecting axial and proximal limb musculature (**medial** structures).

Don't Eat Greasy Foods

Basal ganglia

Important in voluntary movements and making postural adjustments.

Receives cortical input, provides negative feedback to cortex to modulate movement.

Striatum = putamen (motor) + caudate (cognitive).

Lentiform = putamen + globus pallidus.

D_1-Receptor = D1Rect pathway.

Indirect (D_2) = Inhibitory.

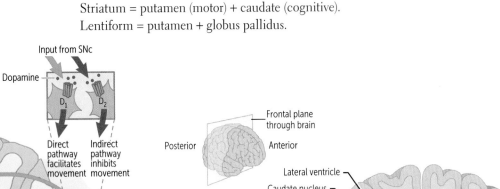

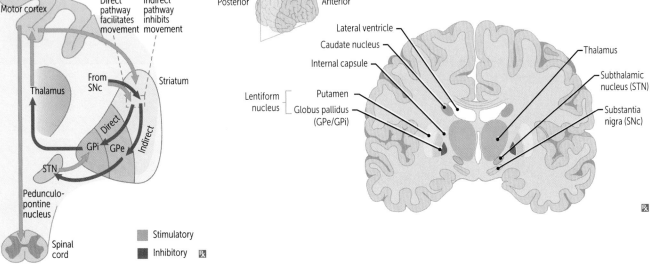

Direct (excitatory) pathway—SNc input stimulates the striatum, stimulating the release of GABA, which inhibits GABA release from the GPi, disinhibiting the thalamus via the GPi (↑ motion).

Indirect (inhibitory) pathway—SNc input stimulates the striatum, releasing GABA that disinhibits STN via GPe inhibition, and STN stimulates GPi to inhibit the thalamus (↓ motion).

Dopamine binds to D_1, stimulating the excitatory pathway, and to D_2, inhibiting the inhibitory pathway → ↑ motion.

Cerebral cortex regions

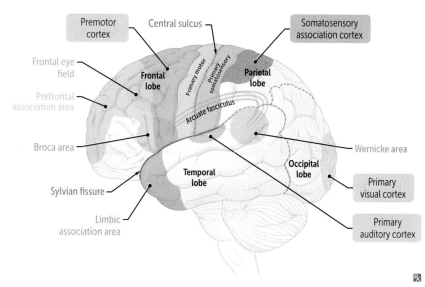

Homunculus

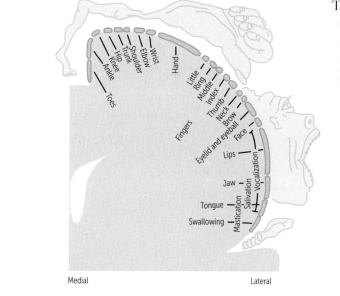

Topographic representation of motor (shown) and sensory areas in the cerebral cortex. Distorted appearance is due to certain body regions being more richly innervated and thus having ↑ cortical representation.

Cerebral perfusion

Brain perfusion relies on tight autoregulation. Cerebral perfusion is primarily driven by P_{CO_2} (P_{O_2} also modulates perfusion in severe hypoxia).

Cerebral perfusion relies on a pressure gradient between mean arterial pressure (MAP) and ICP. ↓ blood pressure or ↑ ICP → ↓ cerebral perfusion pressure (CPP).

Therapeutic hyperventilation → ↓ P_{CO_2} → vasoconstriction → ↓ cerebral blood flow → ↓ intracranial pressure (ICP). May be used to treat acute cerebral edema (eg, 2° to stroke) unresponsive to other interventions.

CPP = MAP − ICP. If CPP = 0, there is no cerebral perfusion → brain death.

Hypoxemia increases CPP only if P_{O_2} < 50 mm Hg.

CPP is directly proportional to P_{CO_2} until P_{CO_2} > 90 mm Hg.

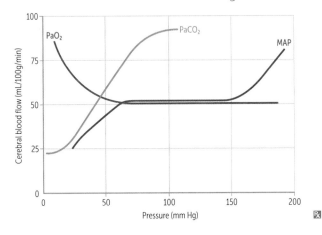

Cerebral arteries—cortical distribution

☐ Anterior cerebral artery (supplies anteromedial surface)

☐ Middle cerebral artery (supplies lateral surface)

☐ Posterior cerebral artery (supplies posterior and inferior surfaces)

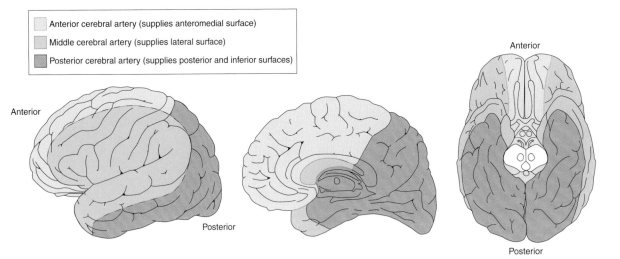

Watershed zones

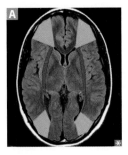

Between anterior cerebral/middle cerebral, posterior cerebral/middle cerebral arteries (cortical border zones) (blue areas in **A**); or may also occur between the superficial and deep vascular territories of the middle cerebral artery (internal border zones) (red areas in **A**).

Damage by severe hypotension → proximal upper and lower extremity weakness (if internal border zone stroke), higher order visual dysfunction (if posterior cerebral/middle cerebral cortical border zone stroke).

Circle of Willis   System of anastomoses between anterior and posterior blood supplies to brain.

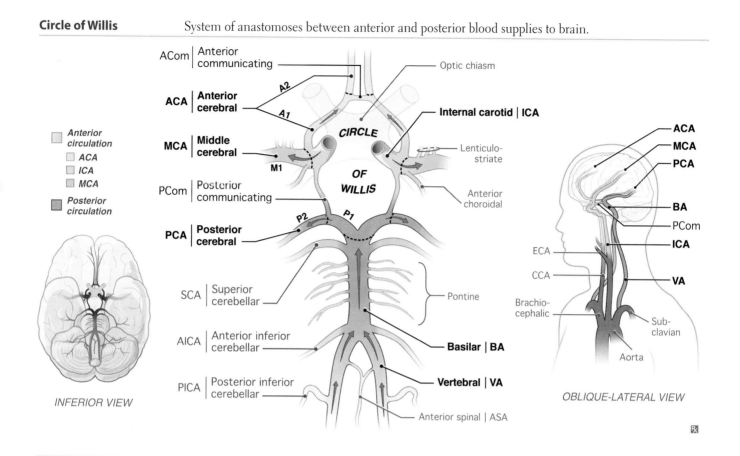

INFERIOR VIEW

OBLIQUE-LATERAL VIEW

Dural venous sinuses

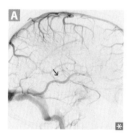

A

Large venous channels **A** that run through the periosteal and meningeal layers of the dura mater. Drain blood from cerebral veins (arrow) and receive CSF from arachnoid granulations. Empty into internal jugular vein.

Venous sinus thrombosis—presents with signs/symptoms of ↑ ICP (eg, headache, seizures, focal neurologic deficits). May lead to venous hemorrhage. Associated with hypercoagulable states (eg, pregnancy, OCP use, factor V Leiden).

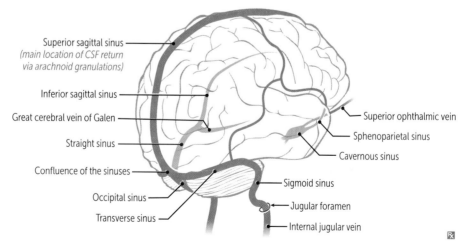

Ventricular system

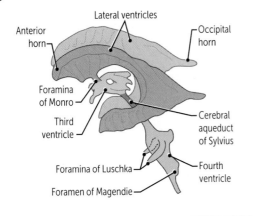

Lateral ventricles → 3rd ventricle via right and left interventricular foramina of Monro.

3rd ventricle → 4th ventricle via cerebral aqueduct of Sylvius.

4th ventricle → subarachnoid space via:
- Foramina of Luschka = Lateral.
- Foramen of Magendie = Medial.

CSF made by ependymal cells of choroid plexus. Travels to subarachnoid space via foramina of Luschka and Magendie, is reabsorbed by arachnoid granulations, and then drains into dural venous sinuses.

Brain stem—ventral view

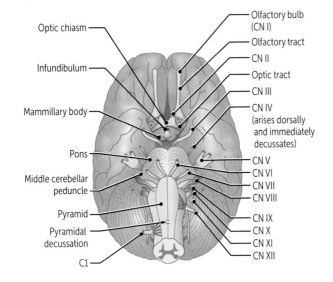

4 CN are above pons (I, II, III, IV).
4 CN exit the pons (V, VI, VII, VIII).
4 CN are in medulla (IX, X, XI, XII).
4 CN nuclei are medial (III, IV, VI, XII).
  "Factors of 12, except 1 and 2."

Brain stem—dorsal view (cerebellum removed)

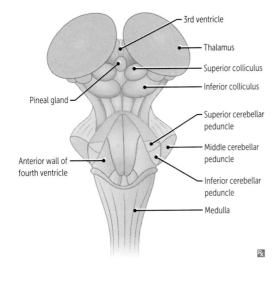

Pineal gland—melatonin secretion, circadian rhythms.

Superior colliculi—direct eye movements to stimuli (noise/movements) or objects of interest.

Inferior colliculi—auditory.

Your eyes are **above** your ears, and the superior colliculus (visual) is **above** the inferior colliculus (auditory).

Cranial nerve nuclei

Located in tegmentum portion of brain stem (between dorsal and ventral portions):
- Midbrain—nuclei of CN III, IV
- Pons—nuclei of CN V, VI, VII, VIII
- Medulla—nuclei of CN IX, X, XII
- Spinal cord—nucleus of CN XI

Lateral nuclei = sensory (aLar plate).
—Sulcus limitans—
Medial nuclei = Motor (basal plate).

Cranial nerve and vessel pathways

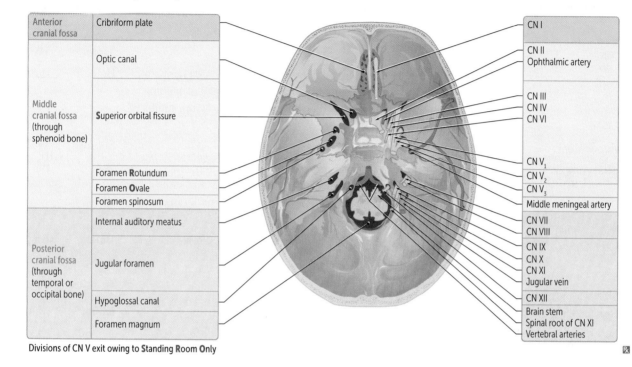

Anterior cranial fossa	Cribriform plate
Middle cranial fossa (through sphenoid bone)	Optic canal
	Superior orbital fissure
	Foramen **R**otundum
	Foramen **O**vale
	Foramen spinosum
Posterior cranial fossa (through temporal or occipital bone)	Internal auditory meatus
	Jugular foramen
	Hypoglossal canal
	Foramen magnum

CN I
CN II
Ophthalmic artery
CN III
CN IV
CN VI
CN V$_1$
CN V$_2$
CN V$_3$
Middle meningeal artery
CN VII
CN VIII
CN IX
CN X
CN XI
Jugular vein
CN XII
Brain stem
Spinal root of CN XI
Vertebral arteries

Divisions of CN V exit owing to **S**tanding **R**oom **O**nly

Cranial nerves

NERVE	CN	FUNCTION	TYPE	MNEMONIC
Olfactory	I	Smell (only CN without thalamic relay to cortex)	Sensory	Some
Optic	II	Sight	Sensory	Say
Oculomotor	III	Eye movement (SR, IR, MR, IO), pupillary constriction (sphincter pupillae: Edinger-Westphal nucleus, muscarinic receptors), accommodation, eyelid opening (levator palpebrae)	Motor	Marry
Trochlear	IV	Eye movement (SO)	Motor	Money
Trigeminal	V	Mastication, facial sensation (ophthalmic, maxillary, mandibular divisions), somatosensation from anterior $^2/_3$ of tongue	Both	But
Abducens	VI	Eye movement (LR)	Motor	My
Facial	VII	Facial movement, taste from anterior $^2/_3$ of tongue (chorda tympani), lacrimation, salivation (submandibular and sublingual glands are innervated by CN seven), eyelid closing (orbicularis oculi), auditory volume modulation (stapedius)	Both	Brother
Vestibulocochlear	VIII	Hearing, balance	Sensory	Says
Glossopharyngeal	IX	Taste and sensation from posterior $^1/_3$ of tongue, swallowing, salivation (parotid gland), monitoring carotid body and sinus chemo- and baroreceptors, and elevation of pharynx/larynx (stylopharyngeus)	Both	Big
Vagus	X	Taste from supraglottic region, swallowing, soft palate elevation, midline uvula, talking, cough reflex, parasympathetics to thoracoabdominal viscera, monitoring aortic arch chemo- and baroreceptors	Both	Brains
Accessory	XI	Head turning, shoulder shrugging (SCM, trapezius)	Motor	Matter
Hypoglossal	XII	Tongue movement	Motor	Most

Vagal nuclei

NUCLEUS	FUNCTION	CRANIAL NERVES
Nucleus Solitarius	Visceral Sensory information (eg, taste, baroreceptors, gut distention)	VII, IX, X
Nucleus aMbiguus	Motor innervation of pharynx, larynx, upper esophagus (eg, swallowing, palate elevation)	IX, X, XI (cranial portion)
Dorsal motor nucleus	Sends autonomic (parasympathetic) fibers to heart, lungs, upper GI	X

Cranial nerve reflexes

REFLEX	AFFERENT	EFFERENT
Corneal	V_1 ophthalmic (nasociliary branch)	Bilateral VII (temporal branch: orbicularis oculi)
Lacrimation	V_1 (loss of reflex does not preclude emotional tears)	VII
Jaw jerk	V_3 (sensory—muscle spindle from masseter)	V_3 (motor—masseter)
Pupillary	II	III
Gag	IX	X

Mastication muscles	3 muscles close jaw: Masseter, teMporalis, Medial pterygoid. 1 opens: Lateral pterygoid. All are innervated by trigeminal nerve (V_3).	M's Munch. Lateral Lowers (when speaking of pterygoids with respect to jaw motion). "It takes more muscle to keep your mouth shut."
Spinal nerves	There are 31 pairs of spinal nerves in total: 8 cervical, 12 thoracic, 5 lumbar, 5 sacral, 1 coccygeal. Nerves C1–C7 exit above the corresponding vertebra. C8 spinal nerve exits below C7 and above T1. All other nerves exit below (eg, C3 exits above the 3rd cervical vertebra; L2 exits below the 2nd lumbar vertebra). Vertebral disc herniation—nucleus pulposus (soft central disc) herniates through annulus fibrosus (outer ring); usually occurs posterolaterally at L4–L5 or L5–S1. Nerve usually affected is below the level of herniation (eg, L3–L4 disc spares L3 nerve and involves L4 nerve). Compression of S1 nerve root → absent ankle reflex.	
Spinal cord—lower extent	In adults, spinal cord ends at lower border of L1–L2 vertebrae. Subarachnoid space (which contains the CSF) extends to lower border of S2 vertebra. Lumbar puncture is usually performed between L3–L4 or L4–L5 (level of cauda equina).	Goal of lumbar puncture is to obtain sample of CSF without damaging spinal cord. To keep the cord **alive**, keep the spinal needle between **L3** and **L5**.

Spinal cord and associated tracts

Legs (Lumbosacral) are Lateral in Lateral corticospinal, spinothalamic tracts 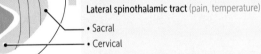.
Dorsal columns are organized as you are, with hands at sides. "Arms outside, legs inside."

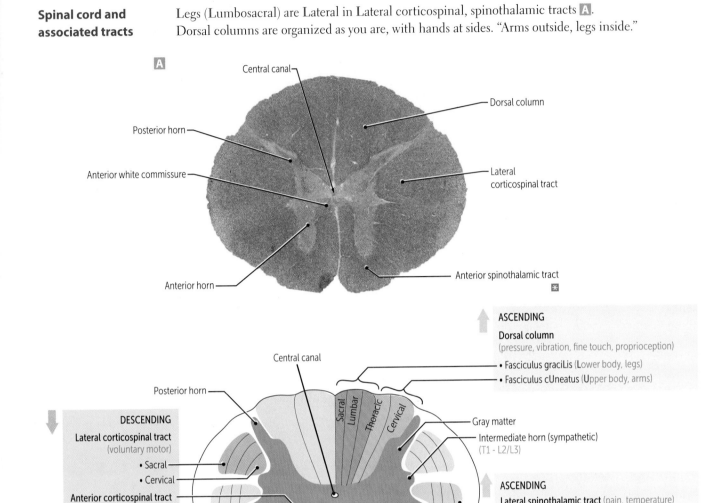

A

Central canal

Posterior horn

Anterior white commissure

Anterior horn

Dorsal column

Lateral corticospinal tract

Anterior spinothalamic tract

ASCENDING
↑

Dorsal column
(pressure, vibration, fine touch, proprioception)

• Fasciculus graciLis (Lower body, legs)
• Fasciculus cUneatus (Upper body, arms)

Central canal

Posterior horn

DESCENDING
↓

Lateral corticospinal tract
(voluntary motor)

• Sacral
• Cervical

Anterior corticospinal tract
(voluntary motor)

White matter

Anterior horn

Sacral
Lumbar
Thoracic
Cervical

Gray matter

Intermediate horn (sympathetic)
(T1 - L2/L3)

ASCENDING
↑

Lateral spinothalamic tract (pain, temperature)

• Sacral
• Cervical

Anterior spinothalamic tract (crude touch, pressure)

▶ NEUROLOGY—NEUROPATHOLOGY

Common brain lesions

AREA OF LESION	CONSEQUENCE	EXAMPLES/COMMENTS
Frontal lobe	Disinhibition and deficits in concentration, orientation, judgment; may have reemergence of primitive reflexes.	
Frontal eye fields	Eyes look toward (destructive) side of lesion. In seizures (irritative), eyes look away from side of the lesion.	
Paramedian pontine reticular formation	Eyes look away from side of lesion.	Ipsilateral gaze palsy (inability to look toward side of lesion).
Medial longitudinal fasciculus	Internuclear ophthalmoplegia (impaired adduction of ipsilateral eye; nystagmus of contralateral eye with abduction).	Multiple sclerosis.
Dominant parietal cortex	Agraphia, acalculia, finger agnosia, left-right disorientation.	Gerstmann syndrome.
Nondominant parietal cortex	Agnosia of the contralateral side of the world.	Hemispatial neglect syndrome.
Hippocampus (bilateral)	Anterograde amnesia—inability to make new memories.	
Basal ganglia	May result in tremor at rest, chorea, athetosis.	Parkinson disease, Huntington disease.
Subthalamic nucleus	Contralateral hemiballismus.	
Mammillary bodies (bilateral)	Wernicke-Korsakoff syndrome—Confusion, Ataxia, Nystagmus, Ophthalmoplegia, memory loss (anterograde and retrograde amnesia), confabulation, personality changes.	Wernicke problems come in a **CAN O'** beer.
Amygdala (bilateral)	Klüver-Bucy syndrome—disinhibited behavior (eg, hyperphagia, hypersexuality, hyperorality).	HSV-1 encephalitis.
Dorsal midbrain	Parinaud syndrome—vertical gaze palsy, pupillary light-near dissociation, lid retraction, convergence-retraction nystagmus.	Stroke, hydrocephalus, pinealoma.
Reticular activating system (midbrain)	Reduced levels of arousal and wakefulness (eg, coma).	
Cerebellar hemisphere	Intention tremor, limb ataxia, loss of balance; damage to cerebellum → ipsilateral deficits; fall toward side of lesion.	Cerebellar hemispheres are **laterally** located— affect **lateral** limbs.
Red nucleus	Decorticate (flexor) posturing—lesion above red nucleus, presents with flexion of upper extremities and extension of lower extremities. Decerebrate (extensor) posturing—lesion at or below red nucleus, presents with extension of upper and lower extremities.	Worse prognosis with decerebrate posturing.
Cerebellar vermis	Truncal ataxia (wide-based, "drunken sailor" gait), dysarthria.	Vermis is **centrally** located—affects **central** body. Degeneration associated with chronic alcohol use.

Ischemic brain disease/stroke

Irreversible damage begins after 5 minutes of hypoxia. Most vulnerable: hippocampus, neocortex, cerebellum (Purkinje cells), watershed areas. Irreversible neuronal injury. Hippocampus is most vulnerable to ischemic hypoxia ("**vulnerable hippos**").

Stroke imaging: noncontrast CT to exclude hemorrhage (before tPA can be given). CT detects ischemic changes in 6–24 hr. Diffusion-weighted MRI can detect ischemia within 3–30 min.

TIME SINCE ISCHEMIC EVENT	12–24 HOURS	24–72 HOURS	3–5 DAYS	1–2 WEEKS	> 2 WEEKS
Histologic features	Eosinophilic cytoplasm + pyknotic nuclei (red neurons)	Necrosis + neutrophils	Macrophages (microglia)	Reactive gliosis (astrocytes) + vascular proliferation	Glial scar

Ischemic stroke

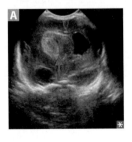

Acute blockage of vessels → disruption of blood flow and subsequent ischemia → liquefactive necrosis.

3 types:
- Thrombotic—due to a clot forming directly at site of infarction (commonly the MCA A), usually over an atherosclerotic plaque.
- Embolic—embolus from another part of the body obstructs vessel. Can affect multiple vascular territories. Examples: atrial fibrillation, carotid artery stenosis, DVT with patent foramen ovale.
- Hypoxic—due to hypoperfusion or hypoxemia. Common during cardiovascular surgeries, tends to affect watershed areas.

Treatment: tPA (if within 3–4.5 hr of onset and no hemorrhage/risk of hemorrhage). Reduce risk with medical therapy (eg, aspirin, clopidogrel); optimum control of blood pressure, blood sugars, lipids; and treat conditions that ↑ risk (eg, atrial fibrillation, carotid artery stenosis).

Transient ischemic attack

Brief, reversible episode of focal neurologic dysfunction without acute infarction (⊖ MRI), with the majority resolving in < 15 minutes; deficits due to focal ischemia.

Neonatal intraventricular hemorrhage

Bleeding into ventricles (arrow in A shows blood in right intraventricular blood, extending into periventricular white matter). Increased risk in premature and low-birth-weight infants. Originates in germinal matrix, a highly vascularized layer within the subventricular zone. Due to reduced glial fiber support and impaired autoregulation of BP in premature infants. Can present with altered level of consciousness, bulging fontanelle, hypotension, seizures, coma.

Intracranial hemorrhage

Epidural hematoma	Rupture of middle meningeal artery (branch of maxillary artery), often 2° to skull fracture (circle in **A**) involving the pterion (thinnest area of the lateral skull). Lucid interval. Scalp hematoma (arrows in **A**) and rapid intracranial expansion (arrows in **B**) under systemic arterial pressure → transtentorial herniation, CN III palsy. CT shows biconvex (lentiform), hyperdense blood collection **B** **not crossing suture lines.**

Subdural hematoma	Rupture of bridging veins. Can be acute (traumatic, high-energy impact → hyperdense on CT) or chronic (associated with mild trauma, cerebral atrophy, elderly, alcoholism → hypodense on CT). Also seen in shaken babies. Predisposing factors: brain atrophy, trauma. Crescent-shaped hemorrhage (red arrows in **C** and **D**) that crosses suture lines. Can cause midline shift (yellow arrow in **C**), findings of "acute on chronic" hemorrhage (blue arrows in **D**).

Subarachnoid hemorrhage	Bleeding **E** **F** due to trauma, or rupture of an aneurysm (such as a saccular aneurysm **E**) or arteriovenous malformation. Rapid time course. Patients complain of "worst headache of my life." Bloody or yellow (xanthochromic) spinal tap. Vasospasm can occur due to blood breakdown or rebleed 3–10 days after hemorrhage → ischemic infarct; nimodipine used to prevent/reduce vasospasm. ↑ risk of developing communicating and/or obstructive hydrocephalus.

Intraparenchymal hemorrhage	Most commonly caused by systemic hypertension. Also seen with amyloid angiopathy (recurrent lobar hemorrhagic stroke in elderly), vasculitis, neoplasm. May be 2° to reperfusion injury in ischemic stroke. Hypertensive hemorrhages (Charcot-Bouchard microaneurysm) most often occur in putamen of basal ganglia (lenticulostriate vessels **G**), followed by thalamus, pons, and cerebellum **H**.

Effects of strokes

ARTERY	AREA OF LESION	SYMPTOMS	NOTES
Anterior circulation			
Middle cerebral artery	Motor and sensory cortices A—upper limb and face. Temporal lobe (Wernicke area); frontal lobe (Broca area).	Contralateral paralysis and sensory loss—face and upper limb. Aphasia if in dominant (usually left) hemisphere. Hemineglect if lesion affects nondominant (usually right) side.	Wernicke aphasia is associated with right superior quadrant visual field defect due to temporal lobe involvement.
Anterior cerebral artery	Motor and sensory cortices—lower limb.	Contralateral paralysis and sensory loss—lower limb, urinary incontinence.	
Lenticulo-striate artery	Striatum, internal capsule.	Contralateral paralysis. Absence of cortical signs (eg, neglect, aphasia, visual field loss).	Common location of lacunar infarcts B, due to hyaline arteriosclerosis 2° to unmanaged hypertension.
Posterior circulation			
Anterior spinal artery	Lateral corticospinal tract. Medial lemniscus. Caudal medulla—hypoglossal nerve.	Contralateral paralysis—upper and lower limbs. ↓ contralateral proprioception. Ipsilateral hypoglossal dysfunction (tongue deviates ipsilaterally).	Medial medullary syndrome— caused by infarct of paramedian branches of ASA and/or vertebral arteries.
Posterior inferior cerebellar artery	Lateral medulla: Nucleus ambiguus (CN IX, X, XI) Vestibular nuclei Lateral spinothalamic tract, spinal trigeminal nucleus Sympathetic fibers Inferior cerebellar peduncle	**Dysphagia, hoarseness, ↓ gag reflex, hiccups** Vomiting, vertigo, nystagmus ↓ pain and temperature sensation from contralateral body, ipsilateral face Ipsilateral Horner syndrome Ipsilateral ataxia, dysmetria	Lateral medullary (Wallenberg) syndrome. Nucleus ambiguus effects are specific to PICA lesions C. "Don't pick a (PICA) horse (hoarseness) that **can't eat (dysphagia)**." Also supplies inferior cerebellar peduncle (part of cerebellum).
Anterior inferior cerebellar artery	Lateral pons: Facial nucleus Vestibular nuclei Spinothalamic tract, spinal trigeminal nucleus Sympathetic fibers Middle and inferior cerebellar peduncles Labyrinthine artery	**Paralysis of face (LMN lesion vs UMN lesion in cortical stroke),** ↓ lacrimation, ↓ salivation, ↓ taste from anterior 2/3 of tongue Vomiting, vertigo, nystagmus ↓ pain and temperature sensation from contralateral body, ipsilateral face Ipsilateral Horner syndrome Ataxia, dysmetria Ipsilateral sensorineural deafness, vertigo	Lateral pontine syndrome. Facial nucleus effects are specific to AICA lesions. "**Facial droop** means AICA's **pooped**." Also supplies middle and inferior cerebellar peduncles (part of cerebellum).

Effects of strokes *(continued)*

ARTERY	AREA OF LESION	SYMPTOMS	NOTES
Basilar artery	Pons, medulla, lower midbrain	RAS spared, therefore preserved consciousness	Locked-in syndrome (locked in the basement)
	Corticospinal and corticobulbar tracts	Quadriplegia; loss of voluntary facial, mouth, and tongue movements	
	Ocular cranial nerve nuclei, paramedian pontine reticular formation	Loss of horizontal, but not vertical, eye movements	
Posterior cerebral artery	Occipital lobe 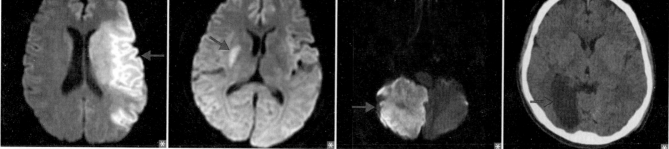.	Contralateral hemianopia with macular sparing; alexia without agraphia (dominant hemisphere).	

Central post-stroke pain syndrome	Neuropathic pain due to thalamic lesions. Initial paresthesias followed in weeks to months by allodynia (ordinarily painless stimuli cause pain) and dysesthesia on the contralateral side. Occurs in 10% of stroke patients.

Diffuse axonal injury	Caused by traumatic shearing forces during rapid acceleration and/or deceleration of the brain (eg, motor vehicle accident). Usually results in devastating neurologic injury, often causing coma or persistent vegetative state. A shows multiple lesions (punctate hemorrhages) involving the white matter tracts.

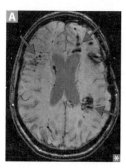

Aphasia	Aphasia—higher-order language deficit (inability to understand/produce/use language appropriately); caused by pathology in dominant cerebral hemisphere (usually left). Dysarthria—motor inability to speak (movement deficit).

TYPE	SPEECH FLUENCY	COMPREHENSION	COMMENTS
Repetition impaired			
Broca (expressive)	Nonfluent	Intact	Broca = Broken Boca (*boca* = mouth in Spanish). Broca area in inferior frontal gyrus of frontal lobe. Patient appears frustrated, insight intact.
Wernicke (receptive)	Fluent	Impaired	Wernicke is Wordy but makes no sense. Patients do not have insight. Wernicke area in superior temporal gyrus of temporal lobe.
Conduction	Fluent	Intact	Can be caused by damage to arCuate fasciculus.
Global	Nonfluent	Impaired	Arcuate fasciculus; Broca and Wernicke areas affected (all areas).
Repetition intact			
Transcortical motor	Nonfluent	Intact	Affects frontal lobe around Broca area, but Broca area is spared.
Transcortical sensory	Fluent	Impaired	Affects temporal lobe around Wernicke area, but Wernicke area is spared.
Transcortical, mixed	Nonfluent	Impaired	Broca and Wernicke areas and arcuate fasciculus remain intact; surrounding watershed areas affected.

Aneurysms	Abnormal dilation of an artery due to weakening of vessel wall.
Saccular aneurysm	Also known as berry aneurysm. Occurs at bifurcations in the circle of Willis. Most common site is junction of ACom and ACA. Associated with ADPKD, Ehlers-Danlos syndrome. Other risk factors: advanced age, hypertension, smoking, race (↑ risk in African-Americans). Usually clinically silent until rupture (most common complication) → subarachnoid hemorrhage ("worst headache of my life" or "thunderclap headache") → focal neurologic deficits. Can also cause symptoms via direct compression of surrounding structures by growing aneurysm. ■ ACom—compression → bitemporal hemianopia (compression of optic chiasm); visual acuity deficits; rupture → ischemia in ACA distribution → contralateral lower extremity hemiparesis, sensory deficits. ■ MCA—rupture → ischemia in MCA distribution → contralateral upper extremity and lower facial hemiparesis, sensory deficits. ■ PCom—compression → ipsilateral CN III palsy → mydriasis ("blown pupil"); may also see ptosis, "down and out" eye.
Charcot-Bouchard microaneurysm	Common, associated with chronic hypertension; affects small vessels (eg, lenticulostriate arteries in basal ganglia, thalamus) and can cause lacunar strokes. Not visible on angiography.

Seizures	Characterized by synchronized, high-frequency neuronal firing. Variety of forms.	
Partial (focal) seizures	Affect single area of the brain. Most commonly originate in medial temporal lobe. Types: ▪ Simple partial (consciousness intact)—motor, sensory, autonomic, psychic ▪ Complex partial (impaired consciousness, automatisms)	Epilepsy—a disorder of recurrent seizures (febrile seizures are not epilepsy). Status epilepticus—continuous (≥ 5 min) or recurring seizures that may result in brain injury. Causes of seizures by age: ▪ Children—genetic, infection (febrile), trauma, congenital, metabolic ▪ Adults—tumor, trauma, stroke, infection ▪ Elderly—stroke, tumor, trauma, metabolic, infection
Generalized seizures Tonic phase Clonic phase	Diffuse. Types: ▪ Absence (petit mal)—3 Hz spike-and-wave discharges, no postictal confusion, blank stare ▪ Myoclonic—quick, repetitive jerks ▪ Tonic-clonic (grand mal)—alternating stiffening and movement ▪ Tonic—stiffening ▪ Atonic—"drop" seizures (falls to floor); commonly mistaken for fainting	

Headaches		Pain due to irritation of structures such as the dura, cranial nerves, or extracranial structures. More common in females, except cluster headaches.		
CLASSIFICATION	LOCALIZATION	DURATION	DESCRIPTION	TREATMENT
Cluster[a]	Unilateral	15 min–3 hr; repetitive	Excruciating periorbital pain ("suicide headache") with lacrimation and rhinorrhea. May present with Horner syndrome. More common in males.	Acute: sumatriptan, 100% O_2 Prophylaxis: verapamil
Tension	Bilateral	> 30 min (typically 4–6 hr); constant	Steady, "band-like" pain. No photophobia or phonophobia. No aura.	Analgesics, NSAIDs, acetaminophen; amitriptyline for chronic pain
Migraine	Unilateral	4–72 hr	Pulsating pain with nausea, photophobia, or phonophobia. May have "aura." Due to irritation of CN V, meninges, or blood vessels (release of substance P, calcitonin gene-related peptide, vasoactive peptides).	Acute: NSAIDs, triptans, dihydroergotamine Prophylaxis: lifestyle changes (eg, sleep, exercise, diet), β-blockers, amitriptyline, topiramate, valproate. **POUND**–Pulsatile, One-day duration, Unilateral, Nausea, Disabling

Other causes of headache include subarachnoid hemorrhage ("worst headache of my life"), meningitis, hydrocephalus, neoplasia, giant cell (temporal) arteritis.

[a]Compare with **trigeminal neuralgia**, which produces repetitive, unilateral, shooting pain in the distribution of CN V. Triggered by chewing, talking, touching certain parts of the face. Lasts (typically) for seconds to minutes, but episodes often increase in intensity and frequency over time. First-line therapy: carbamazepine.

Movement disorders

DISORDER	PRESENTATION	CHARACTERISTIC LESION	NOTES
Akathisia	Restlessness and intense urge to move		Can be seen with neuroleptic use or as a side-effect of Parkinson treatment.
Asterixis	Extension of wrists causes "flapping" motion		Associated with hepatic encephalopathy, Wilson disease, and other metabolic derangements.
Athetosis	Slow, snake-like, writhing movements; especially seen in the fingers	Basal ganglia	
Chorea	Sudden, jerky, purposeless movements	Basal ganglia	*Chorea* = dancing. Seen in Huntington disease and in acute rheumatic fever (Sydenham chorea).
Dystonia	Sustained, involuntary muscle contractions		Writer's cramp, blepharospasm, torticollis.
Essential tremor	High-frequency tremor with sustained posture (eg, outstretched arms), worsened with movement or when anxious		Often familial. Patients often self-medicate with alcohol, which ↓ tremor amplitude. Treatment: nonselective β-blockers (eg, propranolol), primidone.
Hemiballismus	Sudden, wild flailing of 1 arm +/– ipsilateral leg	Contralateral subthalamic nucleus (eg, lacunar stroke)	Pronounce "**Half-of-body ballistic**." Contralateral lesion.
Intention tremor	Slow, zigzag motion when pointing/extending toward a target	Cerebellar dysfunction	
Myoclonus	Sudden, brief, uncontrolled muscle contraction		Jerks; hiccups; common in metabolic abnormalities such as renal and liver failure.
Resting tremor	Uncontrolled movement of distal appendages (most noticeable in hands); tremor alleviated by intentional movement	Substantia nigra (**Parkinson** disease)	Occurs at rest; "pill-rolling tremor" of Parkinson disease. When you **park** your car, it is at **rest**.
Restless legs syndrome	Worse at rest/nighttime. Relieved by movement		Associated with iron deficiency, CKD. Treat with dopamine agonists (pramipexole, ropinirole).

Neurodegenerative disorders	↓ in cognitive ability, memory, or function with intact consciousness. Must rule out depression as cause of dementia (known as pseudodementia).	
DISEASE	DESCRIPTION	HISTOLOGIC/GROSS FINDINGS

Parkinson disease	Parkinson **TRAPS** your body:
	  Tremor (pill-rolling tremor at rest)
	  Rigidity (cogwheel)
	  Akinesia (or bradykinesia)
	  Postural instability
	  Shuffling gait
	MPTP, a contaminant in illegal drugs, is metabolized to MPP+, which is toxic to substantia nigra.
		Loss of dopaminergic neurons (ie, depigmentation) of substantia nigra pars compacta.
		Lewy bodies: composed of α-synuclein (intracellular eosinophilic inclusions **A**).

Huntington disease	Autosomal dominant trinucleotide (CAG)$_n$ repeat expansion in the **huntingtin** (*HTT*) gene on chromosome 4 (**4 letters**). Symptoms manifest between ages 20 and 50: chorea, athetosis, aggression, depression, dementia (sometimes initially mistaken for substance abuse). Anticipation results from expansion of CAG repeats. Caudate loses ACh and GABA.	Atrophy of caudate and putamen with ex vacuo ventriculomegaly. ↑ dopamine, ↓ GABA, ↓ ACh in brain. Neuronal death via NMDA-R binding and glutamate excitotoxicity.

Alzheimer disease	Most common cause of dementia in elderly. Down syndrome patients have ↑ risk of developing Alzheimer disease, as APP is located on chromosome 21.
	↓ ACh.
	Associated with the following altered proteins:
	  ▪ ApoE-2: ↓ risk of sporadic form
	  ▪ ApoE-4: ↑ risk of sporadic form
	  ▪ APP, presenilin-1, presenilin-2: familial forms (10%) with earlier onset
		Widespread cortical atrophy (normal cortex **B**; cortex in Alzheimer disease **C**), especially hippocampus (arrows in **B** and **C**). Narrowing of gyri and widening of sulci.
		Senile plaques **D** in gray matter: extracellular β-amyloid core; may cause amyloid angiopathy → intracranial hemorrhage; Aβ (amyloid-β) synthesized by cleaving amyloid precursor protein (APP).
		Neurofibrillary tangles **E**: intracellular, hyperphosphorylated tau protein = insoluble cytoskeletal elements; number of tangles correlates with degree of dementia.

Frontotemporal dementia	Also known as Pick disease. Early changes in personality and behavior (behavioral variant), or aphasia (primary progressive aphasia). May have associated movement disorders (eg, parkinsonism).	Frontotemporal lobe degeneration **F**. Inclusions of hyperphosphorylated tau (round Pick bodies **G**) or ubiquitinated TDP-43.
Lewy body dementia	Visual hallucinations ("haLewycinations"), dementia with fluctuating cognition/alertness, REM sleep behavior disorder, and parkinsonism. Called Lewy body dementia if cognitive and motor symptom onset < 1 year apart, otherwise considered dementia 2° to Parkinson disease.	Intracellular Lewy bodies **A** primarily in cortex.

Neurodegenerative disorders *(continued)*

DISEASE	DESCRIPTION	HISTOLOGIC/GROSS FINDINGS
Vascular dementia	Result of multiple arterial infarcts and/or chronic ischemia. Step-wise decline in cognitive ability with late-onset memory impairment. 2nd most common cause of dementia in elderly.	MRI or CT shows multiple cortical and/or subcortical infarcts.
Creutzfeldt-Jakob disease	Rapidly progressive (weeks to months) dementia with myoclonus ("startle myoclonus") and ataxia. Commonly see periodic sharp waves on EEG and ↑ 14-3-3 protein in CSF.	Spongiform cortex. Prions (PrP^c → PrP^{sc} sheet [β-pleated sheet resistant to proteases]) **H**.

Idiopathic intracranial hypertension

Also known as pseudotumor cerebri. ↑ ICP with no apparent cause on imaging (eg, hydrocephalus, obstruction of CSF outflow). Risk factors include female gender, Tetracyclines, Obesity, vitamin A excess, Danazol (female TOAD).

Findings: headache, tinnitus, diplopia (usually from CN VI palsy), no change in mental status. Impaired optic nerve axoplasmic flow → papilledema. Visual field testing shows enlarged blind spot and peripheral constriction. Lumbar puncture reveals ↑ opening pressure and provides temporary headache relief.

Treatment: weight loss, acetazolamide, invasive procedures for refractory cases (eg, CSF shunt placement, optic nerve sheath fenestration surgery for visual loss).

Hydrocephalus	↑ CSF volume → ventricular dilation +/− ↑ ICP.
Communicating	
Communicating hydrocephalus	↓ CSF absorption by arachnoid granulations (eg, arachnoid scarring post-meningitis) → ↑ ICP, papilledema, herniation.
Normal pressure hydrocephalus	Affects the elderly; idiopathic; CSF pressure elevated only episodically; does not result in increased subarachnoid space volume. Expansion of ventricles A distorts the fibers of the corona radiata → triad of **urinary incontinence**, **gait apraxia** (magnetic gait), and **cognitive dysfunction** (sometimes reversible). "**Wet, wobbly, and wacky.**" Symptoms potentially reversible with CSF shunt placement.
Noncommunicating (obstructive)	
Noncommunicating hydrocephalus	Caused by structural blockage of CSF circulation within ventricular system (eg, stenosis of aqueduct of Sylvius; colloid cyst blocking foramen of Monro; tumor B).
Hydrocephalus mimics	
Ex vacuo ventriculomegaly	Appearance of ↑ CSF on imaging C, but is actually due to ↓ brain tissue and neuronal atrophy (eg, Alzheimer disease, advanced HIV, Pick disease, Huntington disease). ICP is normal; NPH triad is not seen.

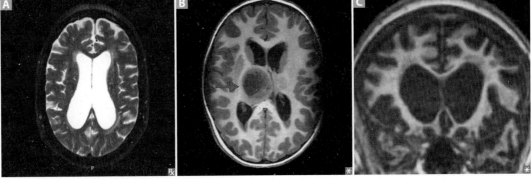

Multiple sclerosis

Autoimmune inflammation and demyelination of CNS (brain and spinal cord) with subsequent axonal damage. Can present with:

- Acute optic neuritis (painful unilateral visual loss associated with Marcus Gunn pupil)
- Brain stem/cerebellar syndromes (eg, diplopia, ataxia, scanning speech, intention tremor, nystagmus/INO (bilateral > unilateral)
- Pyramidal tract weakness
- Spinal cord syndromes (eg, electric shock-like sensation along spine on neck flexion [Lhermitte phenomenon], neurogenic bladder, paraparesis, sensory manifestations affecting the trunk or one or more extremity)

Symptoms may exacerbate with increased body temperature (eg, hot bath, exercise). Relapsing and remitting is most common clinical course. Most often affects women in their 20s and 30s; more common in Caucasians living farther from equator.

FINDINGS

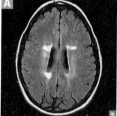

↑ IgG level and myelin basic protein in CSF. Oligoclonal bands are diagnostic. MRI is gold standard. Periventricular plaques (areas of oligodendrocyte loss and reactive gliosis). Multiple white matter lesions disseminated in space and time.

TREATMENT

Stop relapses and halt/slow progression with disease-modifying therapies (eg, β-interferon, glatiramer, natalizumab). Treat acute flares with IV steroids. Symptomatic treatment for neurogenic bladder (catheterization, muscarinic antagonists), spasticity (baclofen, GABA$_B$ receptor agonists), pain (TCAs, anticonvulsants).

Other demyelinating and dysmyelinating disorders

Osmotic demyelination syndrome	Also known as central pontine myelinolysis. Massive axonal demyelination in pontine white matter A 2° to rapid osmotic changes, most commonly iatrogenic correction of hyponatremia but also rapid shifts of other osmolytes (eg, glucose). Acute paralysis, dysarthria, dysphagia, diplopia, loss of consciousness. Can cause "locked-in syndrome." Correcting serum Na⁺ too fast: ▪ "From low to high, your pons will die" (osmotic demyelination syndrome). ▪ "From high to low, your brains will blow" (cerebral edema/herniation).
Acute inflammatory demyelinating polyradiculopathy	Most common subtype of **Guillain-Barré syndrome**. Autoimmune condition associated with infections (eg, *Campylobacter jejuni*, viruses [eg, Zika]) that destroys Schwann cells by inflammation and demyelination of peripheral nerves (including cranial nerves III-XII) and motor fibers likely due to molecular mimicry, inoculations, and stress, but no definitive link to pathogens. Results in symmetric ascending muscle weakness/paralysis and depressed/absent DTRs beginning in lower extremities. Facial paralysis (usually bilateral) and respiratory failure are common. May see autonomic dysregulation (eg, cardiac irregularities, hypertension, hypotension) or sensory abnormalities. Almost all patients survive; majority recover completely after weeks to months. ↑ CSF protein with normal cell count (albuminocytologic dissociation). Respiratory support is critical until recovery. Disease-modifying treatment: plasmapheresis, IV immunoglobulins. No role for steroids.
Acute disseminated (postinfectious) encephalomyelitis	Multifocal inflammation and demyelination after infection or vaccination. Presents with rapidly progressive multifocal neurologic symptoms, altered mental status.
Charcot-Marie-Tooth disease	Also known as hereditary motor and sensory neuropathy. Group of progressive hereditary nerve disorders related to the defective production of proteins involved in the structure and function of peripheral nerves or the myelin sheath. Typically autosomal dominant inheritance pattern and associated with foot deformities (eg, pes cavus, hammer toe), lower extremity weakness (eg, foot drop), and sensory deficits. Most common type, CMT1A, is caused by *PMP22* gene duplication.
Progressive multifocal leukoencephalopathy	Demyelination of CNS B due to destruction of oligodendrocytes (2° to reactivation of latent JC virus infection). Seen in 2–4% of patients with AIDS. Rapidly progressive, usually fatal. Predominantly involves parietal and occipital areas; visual symptoms are common. ↑ risk associated with natalizumab, rituximab.
Other disorders	Krabbe disease, metachromatic leukodystrophy, adrenoleukodystrophy.

Neurocutaneous disorders

Sturge-Weber syndrome	Also known as encephalotrigeminal angiomatosis. Congenital, noninherited (sporadic), developmental anomaly of neural crest derivatives due to somatic mosaicism for an activating mutation in one copy of the *GNAQ* gene. Affects small (capillary-sized) blood vessels → port-wine stain of the face **A** (nevus flammeus, a non-neoplastic "birthmark" in CN V_1/V_2 distribution); ipsilateral leptomeningeal angioma **B** → seizures/epilepsy; intellectual disability; and episcleral hemangioma → ↑ IOP → early-onset glaucoma. **STURGE**-Weber: **S**poradic, port-wine **S**tain; **T**ram track calcifications (opposing gyri); **U**nilateral; **R**etardation (intellectual disability); **G**laucoma, *GNAQ* gene; **E**pilepsy.
Tuberous sclerosis	*TSC1* mutation on chromosome 9 or *TSC2* mutation on chromosome 16. Tumor suppressor genes. Autosomal dominant, variable expression. **HAMARTOMAS**: **H**amartomas in CNS and skin; **A**ngiofibromas **C**; **M**itral regurgitation; **A**sh-leaf spots **D**; cardiac **R**habdomyoma; (**T**uberous sclerosis); autosomal d**O**minant; **M**ental retardation (intellectual disability); renal **A**ngiomyolipoma **E**; **S**eizures, **S**hagreen patches. ↑ incidence of subependymal giant cell astrocytomas and ungual fibromas.
Neurofibromatosis type I	Also known as von Recklinghausen disease. Mutation in *NF1* tumor suppressor gene on chromosome 17 (17 letters in "von Recklinghausen"), which normally codes for neurofibromin, a negative regulator of RAS. Autosomal dominant, 100% penetrance. Café-au-lait spots **F**, cutaneous neurofibromas **G**, optic gliomas, pheochromocytomas, Lisch nodules (pigmented iris hamartomas **H**).
Neurofibromatosis type II	Mutation in *NF2* tumor suppressor gene on chromosome 22. Autosomal dominant. Findings: bilateral acoustic schwannomas, juvenile cataracts, meningiomas, and ependymomas. NF2 affects 2 ears, 2 eyes, and 2 parts of the brain.
von Hippel-Lindau disease	Deletion of *VHL* gene on chromosome 3p (VHL = 3 letters). Autosomal dominant. pVHL ubiquitinates hypoxia-inducible factor 1a. Characterized by development of numerous tumors, both benign and malignant. **HARP**: **H**emangioblastomas (high vascularity with hyperchromatic nuclei **I**) in retina, brain stem, cerebellum, spine **J**; **A**ngiomatosis (eg, cavernous hemangiomas in skin, mucosa, organs); bilateral **R**enal cell carcinomas; **P**heochromocytomas.

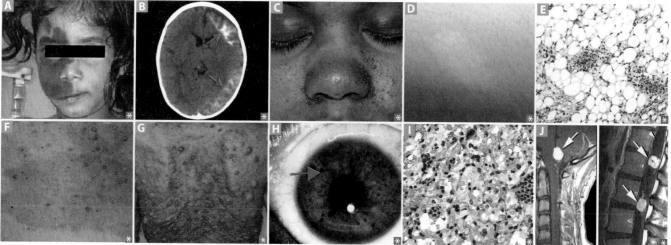

Adult primary brain tumors

TUMOR	DESCRIPTION	HISTOLOGY
Glioblastoma multiforme	Grade IV astrocytoma. Common, highly malignant 1° brain tumor with ~ 1-year median survival. Found in cerebral hemispheres A. Can cross corpus callosum ("butterfly glioma").	Astrocyte origin, GFAP ⊕. "Pseudopalisading" pleomorphic tumor cells B border central areas of necrosis, hemorrhage, and/or microvascular proliferation.
Oligodendroglioma	Relatively rare, slow growing. Most often in frontal lobes C. "Chicken-wire" capillary pattern.	Oligodendrocyte origin. "Fried egg" cells— round nuclei with clear cytoplasm D. Often calcified.
Meningioma	Common, typically benign. Females > males. Most often occurs near surfaces of brain and in parasagittal region. Extra-axial (external to brain parenchyma) and may have a dural attachment ("tail" E). Often asymptomatic; may present with seizures or focal neurologic signs. Resection and/or radiosurgery.	Arachnoid cell origin. Spindle cells concentrically arranged in a whorled pattern; psammoma bodies F (laminated calcifications).
Hemangioblastoma	Most often cerebellar G. Associated with von Hippel-Lindau syndrome when found with retinal angiomas. Can produce erythropoietin → 2° polycythemia.	Blood vessel origin. Closely arranged, thin-walled capillaries with minimal intervening parenchyma H.
Pituitary adenoma	Adenoma may be nonfunctioning (silent) or hyperfunctioning (hormone producing). Most commonly from lactotrophs (prolactinoma) I → hyperprolactinemia; less commonly adenoma of somatotrophs (GH) → acromegaly/ gigantism; corticotrophs (ACTH) → Cushing disease. Rarely, adenoma of thyrotrophs (TSH) and gonadotroph (FSH, LH). Nonfunctional tumors present with mass effect (bitemporal hemianopia, hypopituitarism, headache). Bitemporal hemianopia due to pressure on optic chiasm (J shows normal visual field above, patient's perspective below). Sequelae include hyper- or hypopituitarism, which may be caused by pituitary apoplexy.	Hyperplasia of only one type of endocrine cells found in pituitary (ie, lactotroph, gonadotroph, somatotroph, corticotroph). Prolactinoma in women classically presents as galactorrhea, amenorrhea, and ↓ bone density due to suppression of estrogen. Prolactinoma in men classically presents as low libido and infertility. Treatment: dopamine agonists (eg, bromocriptine, cabergoline), transsphenoidal resection.
Schwannoma	Classically at the cerebellopontine angle K involving both CNs VII and VIII, but can be along any peripheral nerve. Often localized to CN VIII in internal acoustic meatus → vestibular schwannoma. Bilateral vestibular schwannomas found in NF-2. Resection or stereotactic radiosurgery.	Schwann cell origin L, S-100 ⊕. Biphasic. Dense, hypercellular areas containing spindle cells alternating with hypocellular, myxoid areas.

Adult primary brain tumors *(continued)*

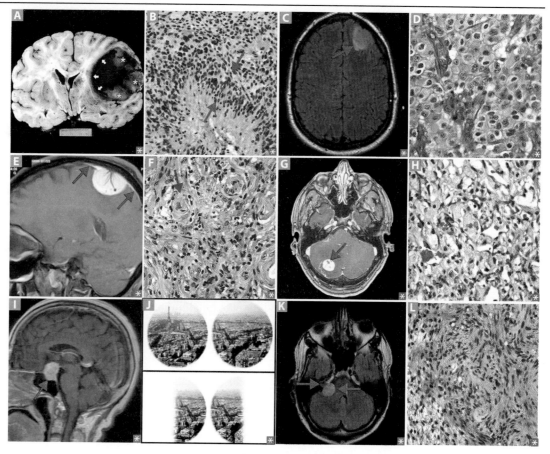

Childhood primary brain tumors

TUMOR	DESCRIPTION	HISTOLOGY
Pilocytic astrocytoma	Low-grade astrocytoma. Most common 1° brain tumor in childhood. Usually well circumscribed. In children, most often found in posterior fossa **A** (eg, cerebellum). May be supratentorial. Benign; good prognosis.	Glial cell origin, GFAP ⊕. Rosenthal fibers—eosinophilic, corkscrew fibers **B**. Cystic + solid (gross).
Medulloblastoma	Most common malignant brain tumor in childhood. Commonly involves cerebellum **C**. Can compress 4th ventricle, causing noncommunicating hydrocephalus → headaches, papilledema. Can send "drop metastases" to spinal cord.	Form of primitive neuroectodermal tumor (PNET). Homer-Wright rosettes, small blue cells **D**.
Ependymoma	Most commonly found in 4th ventricle **E**. Can cause hydrocephalus. Poor prognosis.	Ependymal cell origin. Characteristic perivascular pseudorosettes **F**. Rod-shaped blepharoplasts (basal ciliary bodies) found near the nucleus.
Craniopharyngioma	Most common childhood supratentorial tumor. May be confused with pituitary adenoma (both cause bitemporal hemianopia).	Derived from remnants of Rathke pouch (ectoderm). Calcification is common **G** **H**. Cholesterol crystals found in "motor oil"-like fluid within tumor.
Pinealoma	Tumor of pineal gland. Can cause Parinaud syndrome (compression of tectum → vertical gaze palsy); obstructive hydrocephalus (compression of cerebral aqueduct); precocious puberty in males (β-hCG production).	Similar to germ cell tumors (eg, testicular seminoma).

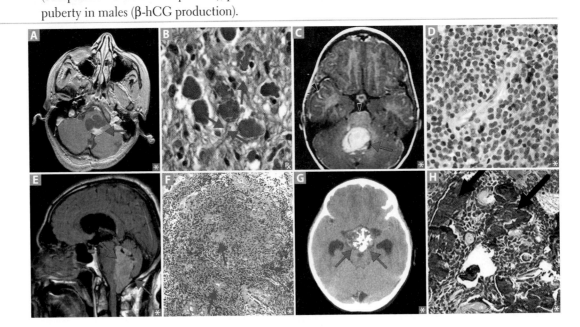

Herniation syndromes

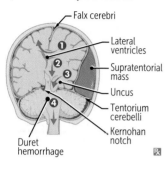

Falx cerebri
Lateral ventricles
❶
❷
❸
Supratentorial mass
Uncus
❹
Tentorium cerebelli
Kernohan notch
Duret hemorrhage

❶ Cingulate (subfalcine) herniation under falx cerebri	Can compress anterior cerebral artery.
❷ Transtentorial (central/downward) herniation	Caudal displacement of brain stem → rupture of paramedian basilar artery branches → Duret hemorrhages. Usually fatal.
❸ Uncal herniation	Uncus = medial temporal lobe. Herniation compresses ipsilateral CN III and contralateral crus cerebri against Kernohan notch (causes contralateral CN III palsy and/or ipsilateral hemiparesis, ie, a false localizing sign).
❹ Cerebellar tonsillar herniation into the foramen magnum	Coma and death result when these herniations compress the brain stem.

Motor neuron signs

SIGN	UMN LESION	LMN LESION	COMMENTS
Weakness	+	+	**Lower** motor neuron = everything **lowered** (less muscle mass, ↓ muscle tone, ↓ reflexes, downgoing toes).
Atrophy	–	+	
Fasciculations	–	+	
Reflexes	↑	↓	**Upper** motor neuron = everything **up** (tone, DTRs, toes).
Tone	↑	↓	
Babinski	+	–	Fasciculations = muscle twitching.
Spastic paresis	+	–	Positive Babinski is normal in infants.
Flaccid paralysis	–	+	
Clasp knife spasticity	+	–	

Spinal cord lesions

AREA AFFECTED	DISEASE	CHARACTERISTICS
	Spinal muscular atrophy	Congenital degeneration of anterior horns of spinal cord. LMN lesions only, symmetric weakness. "Floppy baby" with marked hypotonia (Flaccid paralysis) and tongue Fasciculations. Autosomal recessive inheritance of mutation in *SMN1*. SMA type 1 is called Werdnig-Hoffmann disease.
	Amyotrophic lateral sclerosis	Combined UMN (corticobulbar/corticospinal) and LMN (medullary and spinal cord) degeneration. No sensory or bowel/bladder deficits. Can be caused by defect in superoxide dismutase 1. LMN deficits due to anterior horn cell involvement (eg, dysarthria, dysphagia, asymmetric limb weakness, fasciculations, atrophy) and UMN deficits (pseudobulbar palsy, eg, dysarthria, dysphagia, emotional lability, spastic gait, clonus). Fatal. Commonly known as Lou Gehrig disease. Treatment: riluzole.
Posterior spinal arteries / Anterior spinal artery	Complete occlusion of anterior spinal artery	Spares dorsal columns and Lissauer tract; midthoracic ASA territory is watershed area, as artery of Adamkiewicz supplies ASA below T8. Can be caused by aortic aneurysm repair. Presents with UMN deficit below the lesion (corticospinal tract), LMN deficit at the level of the lesion (anterior horn), and loss of pain and temperature sensation below the lesion (spinothalamic tract).
	Tabes dorsalis	Caused by 3° syphilis. Results from degeneration (demyelination) of dorsal columns and roots → progressive sensory ataxia (impaired proprioception → poor coordination). ⊕ Romberg sign and absent DTRs. Associated with Charcot joints, shooting pain, Argyll Robertson pupils.
	Syringomyelia	Syrinx expands and damages anterior white commissure of spinothalamic tract (2nd-order neurons) → bilateral symmetrical loss of pain and temperature sensation in cape-like distribution. Seen with Chiari I malformation. Can affect other tracts.
	Vitamin B$_{12}$ deficiency	Subacute combined degeneration (SCD)—demyelination of Spinocerebellar tracts, lateral Corticospinal tracts, and Dorsal columns. Ataxic gait, paresthesia, impaired position/vibration sense.
	Cauda equina syndrome	Compression of spinal roots L2 and below, often due to intervertebral disc herniation or tumor. Unilateral radicular pain, absent knee and ankle reflex, loss of bladder and anal sphincter control, saddle anesthesia. Treatment: emergent surgery and steroids.

Poliomyelitis

Caused by poliovirus (fecal-oral transmission). Replicates in oropharynx and small intestine before spreading via bloodstream to CNS. Infection causes destruction of cells in anterior horn of spinal cord (LMN death).

Signs of LMN lesion: asymmetric weakness, hypotonia, flaccid paralysis, fasciculations, hyporeflexia, muscle atrophy. Respiratory muscle involvement leads to respiratory failure. Signs of infection: malaise, headache, fever, nausea, etc.

CSF shows ↑ WBCs (lymphocytic pleocytosis) and slight ↑ of protein (with no change in CSF glucose). Virus recovered from stool or throat.

Brown-Séquard syndrome

Hemisection of spinal cord. Findings:
❶ Ipsilateral loss of all sensation **at** level of lesion
❷ Ipsilateral LMN signs (eg, flaccid paralysis) **at** level of lesion
❸ Ipsilateral UMN signs **below** level of lesion (due to corticospinal tract damage)
❹ Ipsilateral loss of proprioception, vibration, light (2-point discrimination) touch, and tactile sense **below** level of lesion (due to dorsal column damage).
❺ Contralateral loss of pain, temperature, and crude (nonadiscriminative) touch **below** level of lesion (due to spinothalamic tract damage)

If lesion occurs above T1, patient may present with ipsilateral Horner syndrome due to damage of oculosympathetic pathway.

Level of lesion

❶ Loss of sensation
❷ LMN signs

❸ UMN signs
❹ Impaired proprioception, vibration, light touch, tactile sense

❺ Impaired pain, temperature, crude touch sensation

Friedreich ataxia

Autosomal recessive trinucleotide repeat disorder $(GAA)_n$ on chromosome 9 in gene that encodes frataxin (iron binding protein). Leads to impairment in mitochondrial functioning. Degeneration of lateral corticospinal tract (spastic paralysis), spinocerebellar tract (ataxia), dorsal columns (↓ vibratory sense, proprioception), and dorsal root ganglia (loss of DTRs). **Staggering** gait, frequent **falling**, nystagmus, dysarthria, pes cavus, hammer toes, **diabetes** mellitus, **hypertrophic cardiomyopathy** (cause of death). Presents in childhood with kyphoscoliosis A B.

Friedreich is Fratastic (**frataxin**): he's your favorite **frat** brother, always **staggering** and **falling** but has a **sweet**, **big heart**.

Ataxic **GAA**it.

A B

Common cranial nerve lesions

CN V motor lesion	Jaw deviates **toward** side of lesion due to unopposed force from the opposite pterygoid muscle.
CN X lesion	Uvula deviates **away** from side of lesion. Weak side collapses and uvula points away.
CN XI lesion	Weakness turning head to contralateral side of lesion (SCM). Shoulder droop on side of lesion (trapezius). The left SCM contracts to help turn the head to the right.
CN XII lesion	LMN lesion. Tongue deviates **toward** side of lesion ("lick your wounds") due to weakened tongue muscles on affected side.

Facial nerve lesions

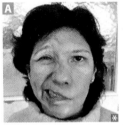

Bell palsy is the most common cause of peripheral facial palsy A. Usually develops after HSV reactivation. Treatment: corticosteroids ± acyclovir. Most patients gradually recover function, but aberrant regeneration can occur. Other causes of peripheral facial palsy include Lyme disease, herpes zoster (Ramsay Hunt syndrome), sarcoidosis, tumors (eg, parotid gland), diabetes mellitus.

	Upper motor neuron lesion	Lower motor neuron lesion
LESION LOCATION	Motor cortex, connection from motor cortex to facial nucleus in pons	Facial nucleus, anywhere along CN VII
AFFECTED SIDE	Contralateral	Ipsilateral
MUSCLES INVOLVED	Lower muscles of facial expression	Upper and lower muscles of facial expression
FOREHEAD INVOLVED?	Spared, due to bilateral UMN innervation	Affected
OTHER SYMPTOMS	None	Incomplete eye closure (dry eyes, corneal ulceration), hyperacusis, loss of taste sensation to anterior tongue

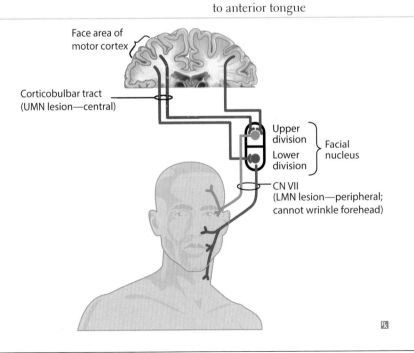

Face area of motor cortex

Corticobulbar tract (UMN lesion—central)

Upper division
Lower division
} Facial nucleus

CN VII (LMN lesion—peripheral; cannot wrinkle forehead)

▶ NEUROLOGY—OTOLOGY

Auditory physiology

Outer ear	Visible portion of ear (pinna), includes auditory canal and tympanic membrane. Transfers sound waves via vibration of tympanic membrane.
Middle ear	Air-filled space with three bones called the ossicles (malleus, incus, stapes). Ossicles conduct and amplify sound from tympanic membrane to inner ear.
Inner ear	Snail-shaped, fluid-filled cochlea. Contains basilar membrane that vibrates 2° to sound waves. Vibration transduced via specialized hair cells → auditory nerve signaling → brain stem. Each frequency leads to vibration at specific location on basilar membrane (tonotopy): ▪ Low frequency heard at apex near helicotrema (wide and flexible). ▪ High frequency heard best at base of cochlea (thin and rigid).

Diagnosing hearing loss

	WEBER TEST	RINNE TEST
Conductive hearing loss	Localizes to affected ear	Abnormal (bone > air)
Sensorineural hearing loss	Localizes to unaffected ear	Normal (air > bone)

Types of hearing loss

Noise-induced hearing loss	Damage to stereociliated cells in organ of Corti. Loss of high-frequency hearing first. Sudden extremely loud noises can produce hearing loss due to tympanic membrane rupture.
Presbycusis	Aging-related progressive bilateral/symmetric sensorineural hearing loss (often of higher frequencies) due to destruction of hair cells at the cochlear base (preserved low-frequency hearing at apex).

Cholesteatoma

Overgrowth of desquamated keratin debris within the middle ear space (**A**, arrows); may erode ossicles, mastoid air cells → conductive hearing loss. Often presents with painless otorrhea.

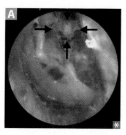

Vertigo	Sensation of spinning while actually stationary. Subtype of "dizziness," but distinct from "lightheadedness."
Peripheral vertigo	More common. Inner ear etiology (eg, semicircular canal debris, vestibular nerve infection, Ménière disease [triad: sensorineural hearing loss, vertigo, tinnitus], benign paroxysmal positional vertigo [BPPV]). Treatment: antihistamines, anticholinergics, antiemetics (symptomatic relief); low-salt diet ± diuretics (Ménière disease); Epley maneuver (BPPV).
Central vertigo	Brain stem or cerebellar lesion (eg, stroke affecting vestibular nuclei or posterior fossa tumor). Findings: directional or purely vertical nystagmus, skew deviation, diplopia, dysmetria. Focal neurologic findings.

▶ NEUROLOGY—OPHTHALMOLOGY

Normal eye

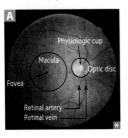

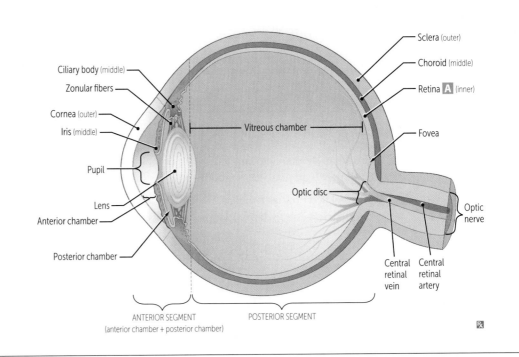

Conjunctivitis

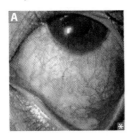

Inflammation of the conjunctiva → red eye A.
Allergic—itchy eyes, bilateral.
Bacterial—pus; treat with antibiotics.
Viral—most common, often adenovirus; sparse mucous discharge, swollen preauricular node; self-resolving.

Refractive errors	Common cause of impaired vision, correctable with glasses.
Hyperopia	Also known as "farsightedness." Eye too short for refractive power of cornea and lens → light focused behind retina. Correct with convex (converging) lenses.
Myopia	Also known as "nearsightedness." Eye too long for refractive power of cornea and lens → light focused in front of retina. Correct with concave (diverging) lens.
Astigmatism	Abnormal curvature of cornea → different refractive power at different axes. Correct with cylindrical lens.
Presbyopia	**Aging**-related impaired accommodation (focusing on near objects), primarily due to ↓ lens elasticity, changes in lens curvature, ↓ strength of the ciliary muscle. Patients often need "reading glasses" (magnifiers).

Cataract

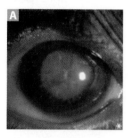

Painless, often bilateral, opacification of lens **A**, often resulting in glare and ↓ vision, especially at night. Acquired risk factors: ↑ age, smoking, excessive alcohol use, excessive sunlight, prolonged corticosteroid use, diabetes mellitus, trauma, infection. Congenital risk factors: classic galactosemia, galactokinase deficiency, trisomies (13, 18, 21), ToRCHeS infections (eg, rubella), Marfan syndrome, Alport syndrome, myotonic dystrophy, neurofibromatosis 2.

Aqueous humor pathway

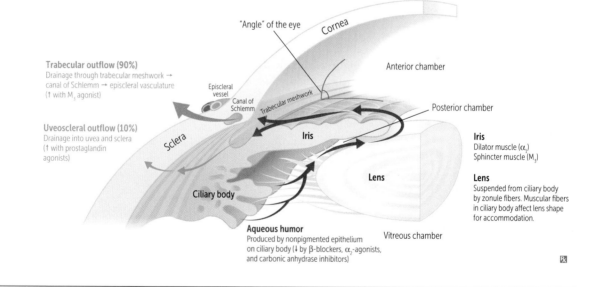

"Angle" of the eye

Cornea

Anterior chamber

Trabecular outflow (90%)
Drainage through trabecular meshwork → canal of Schlemm → episcleral vasculature
(↑ with M₃ agonist)

Episcleral vessel

Canal of Schlemm

Trabecular meshwork

Posterior chamber

Uveoscleral outflow (10%)
Drainage into uvea and sclera
(↑ with prostaglandin agonists)

Sclera

Iris

Iris
Dilator muscle (α₁)
Sphincter muscle (M₃)

Lens

Lens
Suspended from ciliary body by zonule fibers. Muscular fibers in ciliary body affect lens shape for accommodation.

Ciliary body

Aqueous humor
Produced by nonpigmented epithelium on ciliary body (↓ by β-blockers, α₂-agonists, and carbonic anhydrase inhibitors)

Vitreous chamber

Glaucoma	Optic disc atrophy with characteristic cupping (thinning of outer rim of optic nerve head **B** versus normal **A**), usually with elevated intraocular pressure (IOP) and progressive peripheral visual field loss if untreated. Treatment is through pharmacologic or surgical lowering of IOP.
Open-angle glaucoma	Associated with ↑ age, African-American race, family history. Painless, more common in US. Primary—cause unclear. Secondary—blocked trabecular meshwork from WBCs (eg, uveitis), RBCs (eg, vitreous hemorrhage), retinal elements (eg, retinal detachment).
Closed- or narrow-angle glaucoma	Primary—enlargement or anterior movement of lens against central iris (pupil margin) → obstruction of normal aqueous flow through pupil → fluid builds up behind iris, pushing peripheral iris against cornea **C** and impeding flow through trabecular meshwork. Secondary—hypoxia from retinal disease (eg, diabetes mellitus, vein occlusion) induces vasoproliferation in iris that contracts angle. Chronic closure—often asymptomatic with damage to optic nerve and peripheral vision. Acute closure—true ophthalmic emergency. ↑ IOP pushes iris forward → angle closes abruptly. Very painful, red eye **D**, sudden vision loss, halos around lights, frontal headache, fixed and mid-dilated pupil. Mydriatic agents contraindicated.

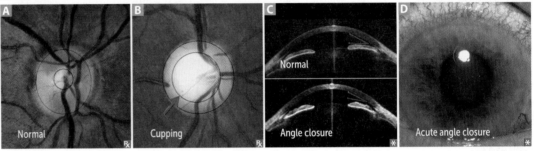

Uveitis	Inflammation of uvea; specific name based on location within affected eye. Anterior uveitis: iritis; posterior uveitis: choroiditis and/or retinitis. May have hypopyon (accumulation of pus in anterior chamber **A**) or conjunctival redness. Associated with systemic inflammatory disorders (eg, sarcoidosis, rheumatoid arthritis, juvenile idiopathic arthritis, HLA-B27–associated conditions).

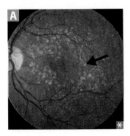

Age-related macular degeneration	Degeneration of macula (central area of retina). Causes distortion (metamorphopsia) and eventual loss of central vision (scotomas). ▪ Dry (nonexudative, > 80%)—Deposition of yellowish extracellular material in between Bruch membrane and retinal pigment epithelium ("Drusen") **A** with gradual ↓ in vision. Prevent progression with multivitamin and antioxidant supplements. ▪ Wet (exudative, 10–15%)—rapid loss of vision due to bleeding 2° to choroidal neovascularization. Treat with anti-VEGF (vascular endothelial growth factor) injections (eg, bevacizumab, ranibizumab).

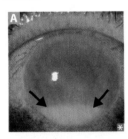

Diabetic retinopathy

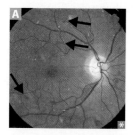

Retinal damage due to chronic hyperglycemia. Two types:
- Nonproliferative—damaged capillaries leak blood → lipids and fluid seep into retina → hemorrhages (arrows in) and macular edema. Treatment: blood sugar control.
- Proliferative—chronic hypoxia results in new blood vessel formation with resultant traction on retina. Treatment: peripheral retinal photocoagulation, surgery, anti-VEGF.

Hypertensive retinopathy

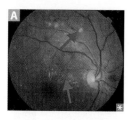

Retinal damage due to chronic uncontrolled HTN.

Flame-shaped retinal hemorrhages, arteriovenous nicking, microaneurysms, macular star (exudate, red arrow in A), cotton-wool spots (blue arrow in A). Presence of papilledema requires immediate lowering of BP.

Associated with ↑ risk of stroke, CAD, kidney disease.

Retinal vein occlusion

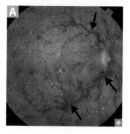

Blockage of central or branch retinal vein due to compression from nearby arterial atherosclerosis. Retinal hemorrhage and venous engorgement ("blood and thunder appearance"; arrows in A), edema in affected area.

Retinal detachment

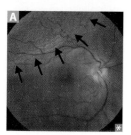

Separation of neurosensory layer of retina (photoreceptor layer with rods and cones) from outermost pigmented epithelium (normally shields excess light, supports retina) → degeneration of photoreceptors → vision loss. May be 2° to retinal breaks, diabetic traction, inflammatory effusions. Visualized on fundoscopy as crinkling of retinal tissue A and changes in vessel direction.

Breaks more common in patients with high myopia and/or history of head trauma. Often preceded by posterior vitreous detachment ("flashes" and "floaters") and eventual monocular loss of vision like a "curtain drawn down." Surgical emergency.

Central retinal artery occlusion

Acute, painless monocular vision loss. Retina cloudy with attenuated vessels and "cherry-red" spot at fovea (center of macula) 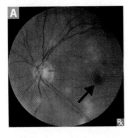. Evaluate for embolic source (eg, carotid artery atherosclerosis, cardiac vegetations, patent foramen ovale).

Retinitis pigmentosa

Inherited retinal degeneration. Painless, progressive vision loss beginning with night blindness (rods affected first). Bone spicule-shaped deposits around macula 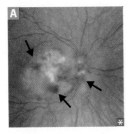.

Retinitis

Retinal edema and necrosis (arrows in 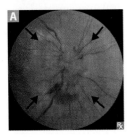) leading to scar. Often viral (CMV, HSV, VZV), but can be bacterial or parasitic. May be associated with immunosuppression.

Papilledema

Optic disc swelling (usually bilateral) due to ↑ ICP (eg, 2° to mass effect). Enlarged blind spot and elevated optic disc with blurred margins **A**.

Pupillary control

Miosis	Constriction, parasympathetic: ▪ 1st neuron: Edinger-Westphal nucleus to ciliary ganglion via CN III ▪ 2nd neuron: short ciliary nerves to sphincter pupillae muscles **Short** ciliary nerves **short**en the pupil diameter.
Pupillary light reflex	Light in either retina sends a signal via CN II to pretectal nuclei (dashed lines in image) in midbrain that activates bilateral Edinger-Westphal nuclei; pupils constrict bilaterally (direct and consensual reflex). Result: illumination of 1 eye results in bilateral pupillary constriction.
Mydriasis	Dilation, sympathetic: ▪ 1st neuron: hypothalamus to ciliospinal center of Budge (C8–T2) ▪ 2nd neuron: exit at T1 to superior cervical ganglion (travels along cervical sympathetic chain near lung apex, subclavian vessels) ▪ 3rd neuron: plexus along internal carotid, through cavernous sinus; enters orbit as long ciliary nerve to pupillary dilator muscles. Sympathetic fibers also innervate smooth muscle of eyelids (minor retractors) and sweat glands of forehead and face. **Long** ciliary nerves make the pupil diameter **long**er.
Marcus Gunn pupil	When the light shines into a normal eye, constriction of the ipsilateral (direct reflex) and contralateral eye (consensual reflex) is observed. When the light is then swung to the affected eye, both pupils dilate instead of constrict due to impaired conduction of light signal along the injured optic nerve.

Horner syndrome

Sympathetic denervation of face ➞:
- Ptosis (slight drooping of eyelid: superior tarsal muscle)
- Anhidrosis (absence of sweating) and flushing of affected side of face
- Miosis (pupil constriction)

Associated with lesions along the sympathetic chain:
- 1st neuron: pontine hemorrhage, lateral medullary syndrome, spinal cord lesion above T1 (eg, Brown-Séquard syndrome, late-stage syringomyelia)
- 2nd neuron (stellate ganglion): Pancoast tumor
- 3rd neuron: carotid dissection (painful)

PAM is horny (Horner).

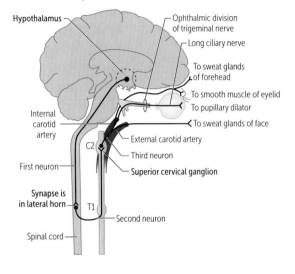

Ocular motility

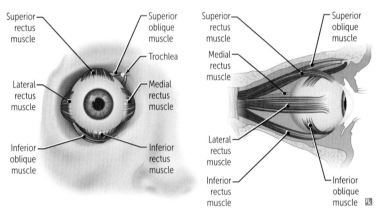

To test each muscle, ask patient to move his/her eye in the path diagrammed to the right, from neutral position toward the muscle being tested.

CN **VI** innervates the Lateral Rectus.
CN **IV** innervates the Superior Oblique.
CN **III** innervates the Rest.
The "chemical formula" $LR_6SO_4R_3$.
The strongest action of the superior oblique is depression when the eye is adducted. The further the eye is abducted, the more the superior oblique acts to intort the eye toward the nose.

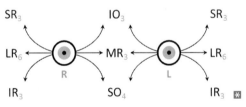

Obliques go Opposite (left SO and IO tested with patient looking right).
IOU: IO tested looking Up.

CN III, IV, VI palsies

CN III damage	CN III has both motor (central) and parasympathetic (peripheral) components. Common causes include:	

- Ischemia → pupil sparing
- Uncal herniation → coma
- PCA aneurysm → sudden-onset headache
- Cavernous sinus thrombosis → proptosis, involvement of CNs IV, V_1/V_2, VI
- Midbrain stroke → contralateral hemiplegia

CN III

Motor output to extraocular muscles—affected primarily by vascular disease (eg, diabetes mellitus: glucose → sorbitol) due to ↓ diffusion of oxygen and nutrients to the interior fibers from compromised vasculature that resides on outside of nerve. Signs: ptosis, "down and out" gaze.

Parasympathetic output—fibers on the periphery are first affected by compression (eg, PCom aneurysm, uncal herniation). Signs: diminished or absent pupillary light reflex, "blown pupil" often with "down-and-out" gaze A.

CN IV damage	Eye moves upward, particularly with contralateral gaze B (→ going down stairs, head may tilt in the opposite direction to compensate). Can't see the **floor** with CN **IV** damage.	

CN VI damage	Affected eye unable to abduct and is displaced medially in primary position of gaze C.	

Visual field defects

1. Right anopia
2. Bitemporal hemianopia
   (pituitary lesion, chiasm)
3. Left homonymous hemianopia
4. Left upper quadrantanopia
   (right temporal lesion, MCA)
5. Left lower quadrantanopia
   (right parietal lesion, MCA)
6. Left hemianopia with macular sparing
   (PCA infarct)
7. Central scotoma (eg, macular degeneration)

Meyer Loop—Lower retina; Loops around
   inferior horn of Lateral ventricle.
Dorsal optic radiation—superior retina; takes
   shortest path via internal capsule.

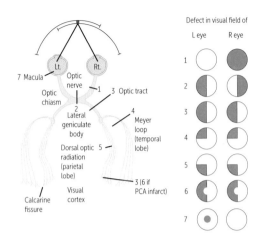

Note: When an image hits 1° visual cortex, it is upside
down and left-right reversed.

Cavernous sinus

Collection of venous sinuses on either side of pituitary. Blood from eye and superficial cortex
→ cavernous sinus → internal jugular vein.
CNs III, IV, V$_1$, VI, and V$_2$ plus postganglionic sympathetic pupillary fibers en route to orbit all
pass through cavernous sinus. Cavernous portion of internal carotid artery is also here.
Cavernous sinus syndrome—presents with variable ophthalmoplegia, ↓ corneal sensation, Horner
syndrome and occasional decreased maxillary sensation. 2° to pituitary tumor mass effect,
carotid-cavernous fistula, or cavernous sinus thrombosis related to infection. CN VI is most
susceptible to injury.

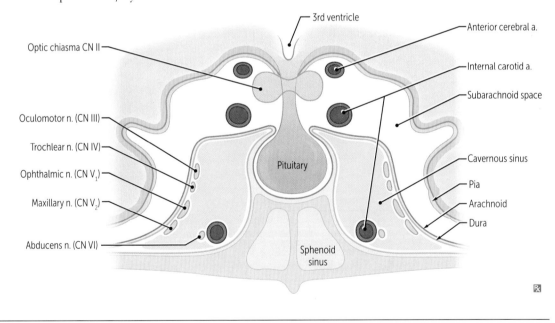

Internuclear ophthalmoplegia

Medial longitudinal fasciculus (MLF): pair of tracts that allows for crosstalk between CN VI and CN III nuclei. Coordinates both eyes to move in same horizontal direction. Highly myelinated (must communicate quickly so eyes move at same time). Lesions may be unilateral or bilateral (latter classically seen in multiple sclerosis).

Lesion in MLF = internuclear ophthalmoplegia (INO), a conjugate horizontal gaze palsy. Lack of communication such that when CN VI nucleus activates ipsilateral lateral rectus, contralateral CN III nucleus does not stimulate medial rectus to contract. Abducting eye gets nystagmus (CN VI overfires to stimulate CN III). Convergence normal.

MLF in MS.

When looking left, the left nucleus of CN VI fires, which contracts the left lateral rectus and stimulates the contralateral (right) nucleus of CN III via the right MLF to contract the right medial rectus.

Directional term (eg, right INO, left INO) refers to which eye is paralyzed.

INO = **I**psilateral adduction failure, **N**ystagmus **O**pposite.

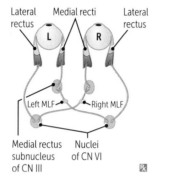

Lateral rectus — Medial recti — Lateral rectus
L   R
Left MLF — Right MLF
Medial rectus subnucleus of CN III   Nuclei of CN VI   Rx

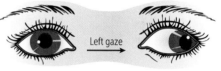

Right INO (right MLF lesion)

Left gaze

Impaired adduction (convergence normal)   Nystagmus

▶ NEUROLOGY—PHARMACOLOGY

Epilepsy drugs

	PARTIAL (FOCAL)	GENERALIZED			MECHANISM	SIDE EFFECTS	NOTES
		TONIC-CLONIC	ABSENCE	STATUS EPILEPTICUS			
Benzodiazepines				** ✓	↑ $GABA_A$ action	Sedation, tolerance, dependence, respiratory depression	Also for eclampsia seizures (1st line is $MgSO_4$)
Carbamazepine	* ✓	✓			Blocks Na^+ channels	Diplopia, ataxia, blood dyscrasias (agranulocytosis, aplastic anemia), liver toxicity, teratogenesis (cleft lip/palate, spina bifida), induction of cytochrome P-450, SIADH, Stevens-Johnson syndrome	1st line for trigeminal neuralgia
Ethosuximide			* ✓		Blocks thalamic T-type Ca^{2+} channels	**EFGHIJ**—Ethosuximide causes Fatigue, GI distress, Headache, Itching (and urticaria), and Stevens-Johnson syndrome	Sucks to have Silent (absence) Seizures
Gabapentin	✓				Primarily inhibits high-voltage-activated Ca^{2+} channels; designed as GABA analog	Sedation, ataxia	Also used for peripheral neuropathy, postherpetic neuralgia
Lamotrigine	✓	✓	✓		Blocks voltage-gated Na^+ channels, inhibits the release of glutamate	Stevens-Johnson syndrome (must be titrated slowly)	
Levetiracetam	✓	✓			Unknown; may modulate GABA and glutamate release	Neuropsychiatric symptoms (eg, personality change), fatigue, drowsiness, headache	
Phenobarbital	✓	✓		✓	↑ $GABA_A$ action	Sedation, tolerance, dependence, induction of cytochrome P-450, cardiorespiratory depression	1st line in **neonates** ("phenobabytal")
Phenytoin, fosphenytoin	✓	* ✓		*** ✓	Blocks Na^+ channels; zero-order kinetics	**PHENYTOIN**: P450 induction, Hirsutism, Enlarged gums, Nystagmus, Yellow-brown skin, Teratogenicity (fetal hydantoin syndrome), Osteopenia, Inhibited folate absorption, Neuropathy. Rare adverse reactions including Stevens-Johnson syndrome, DRESS syndrome, SLE-like syndrome. Toxicity leads to diplopia, ataxia, sedation.	
Tiagabine	✓				↑ GABA by inhibiting reuptake		
Topiramate	✓	✓			Blocks Na^+ channels, ↑ GABA action	Sedation, mental dulling, word-finding difficulty, kidney stones, weight loss, glaucoma	Also used for migraine prevention
Valproic acid	✓	* ✓	✓		↑ Na^+ channel inactivation, ↑ GABA concentration by inhibiting GABA transaminase	GI distress, rare but fatal hepatotoxicity (measure LFTs), pancreatitis, neural tube defects, tremor, weight gain, contraindicated in pregnancy	Also used for myoclonic seizures, bipolar disorder, migraine prophylaxis
Vigabatrin	✓				↑ GABA. Irreversible GABA transaminase inhibitor	Permanent visual loss (black box warning)	

* = Common use, ** = 1st line for acute, *** = 1st line for recurrent seizure prophylaxis.

Barbiturates	Phenobarbital, pentobarbital, thiopental, secobarbital.	
MECHANISM	Facilitate $GABA_A$ action by ↑ **duration** of Cl^- channel opening, thus ↓ neuron firing (barbi**dur**ates ↑ **dur**ation).	
CLINICAL USE	Sedative for anxiety, seizures, insomnia, induction of anesthesia (thiopental).	
ADVERSE EFFECTS	Respiratory and cardiovascular depression (can be fatal); CNS depression (can be exacerbated by alcohol use); dependence; drug interactions (induces cytochrome P-450). Overdose treatment is supportive (assist respiration and maintain BP). Contraindicated in porphyria.	

Benzodiazepines	Diazepam, lorazepam, triazolam, temazepam, oxazepam, midazolam, chlordiazepoxide, alprazolam.	
MECHANISM	Facilitate $GABA_A$ action by ↑ **frequency** of Cl^- channel opening. ↓ REM sleep. Most have long half-lives and active metabolites (exceptions [**ATOM**]: **A**lprazolam, **T**riazolam, **O**xazepam, and **M**idazolam are short acting → higher addictive potential).	"**Fren**zodiazepines" ↑ **fre**quency. Benzos, barbs, and alcohol all bind the $GABA_A$ receptor, which is a ligand-gated Cl^- channel. **O**xazepam, **T**emazepam, and **L**orazepam are **OK** for **T**errible **L**ivers: they can be used to treat alcohol withdrawal in patients with liver disease due to minimal first-pass metabolism.
CLINICAL USE	Anxiety, spasticity, status epilepticus (lorazepam, diazepam, midazolam), eclampsia, detoxification (especially alcohol withdrawal– DTs), night terrors, sleepwalking, general anesthetic (amnesia, muscle relaxation), hypnotic (insomnia).	
ADVERSE EFFECTS	Dependence, additive CNS depression effects with alcohol. Less risk of respiratory depression and coma than with barbiturates. Treat overdose with flumazenil (competitive antagonist at GABA benzodiazepine receptor). Can precipitate seizures by causing acute benzodiazepine withdrawal.	

Nonbenzodiazepine hypnotics	**Z**olpidem, **Z**aleplon, es**Z**opiclone. "These **ZZZ**s put you to sleep."	
MECHANISM	Act via the BZ_1 subtype of the GABA receptor. Effects reversed by flumazenil. Sleep cycle less affected as compared with benzodiazepine hypnotics.	
CLINICAL USE	Insomnia.	
ADVERSE EFFECTS	Ataxia, headaches, confusion. Short duration because of rapid metabolism by liver enzymes. Unlike older sedative-hypnotics, cause only modest day-after psychomotor depression and few amnestic effects. ↓ dependence risk than benzodiazepines.	

Suvorexant

MECHANISM	Orexin (hypocretin) receptor antagonist.
CLINICAL USE	Insomnia.
ADVERSE EFFECTS	CNS depression, headache, dizziness, abnormal dreams, upper respiratory tract infection. Contraindicated in patients with narcolepsy. Not recommended in patients with liver disease. No or low physical dependence. Contraindicated with strong CYP3A4 inhibitors.

Ramelteon

MECHANISM	Melatonin receptor agonist, binds MT1 and MT2 in suprachiasmatic nucleus.
CLINICAL USE	Insomnia.
ADVERSE EFFECTS	Dizziness, nausea, fatigue, headache. No dependence (not a controlled substance).

Triptans

Sumatriptan

MECHANISM	$5\text{-HT}_{1B/1D}$ agonists. Inhibit trigeminal nerve activation; prevent vasoactive peptide release; induce vasoconstriction.	A sumo wrestler **trips** and falls on your **head**.
CLINICAL USE	Acute migraine, cluster headache attacks.	
ADVERSE EFFECTS	Coronary vasospasm (contraindicated in patients with CAD or Prinzmetal angina), mild paresthesia, serotonin syndrome (in combination with other 5-HT agonists).	

Parkinson disease drugs	Parkinsonism is due to loss of dopaminergic neurons and excess cholinergic activity. Bromocriptine, Amantadine, Levodopa (with carbidopa), Selegiline (and COMT inhibitors), Antimuscarinics (**BALSA**).

STRATEGY	AGENTS
Dopamine agonists	Ergot—Bromocriptine. Non-ergot (preferred)—pramipexole, ropinirole; toxicity includes impulse control disorder (eg, gambling), postural hypotension, hallucinations/confusion.
↑ dopamine availability	Amantadine (↑ dopamine release and ↓ dopamine reuptake); toxicity = ataxia, livedo reticularis.
↑ L-DOPA availability	Agents prevent peripheral (pre-BBB) L-DOPA degradation → ↑ L-DOPA entering CNS → ↑ central L-DOPA available for conversion to dopamine. ▪ Levodopa (L-DOPA)/carbidopa—carbidopa blocks peripheral conversion of L-DOPA to dopamine by inhibiting DOPA decarboxylase. Also reduces side effects of peripheral L-DOPA conversion into dopamine (eg, nausea, vomiting). ▪ Entacapone prevents peripheral L-DOPA degradation to 3-O-methyldopa (3-OMD) by inhibiting COMT. Used in conjunction with levodopa.
Prevent dopamine breakdown	Agents act centrally (post-BBB) to inhibit breakdown of dopamine. ▪ Selegiline, rasagiline—block conversion of dopamine into DOPAC by selectively inhibiting MAO-B. ▪ Entacapone—blocks conversion of dopamine to 3-methoxytyramine (3-MT) by inhibiting central COMT.
Curb excess cholinergic activity	Benztropine, trihexyphenidyl (Antimuscarinic; improves tremor and rigidity but has little effect on bradykinesia in **Parkinson disease**). **Park** your **Mercedes-Benz**.

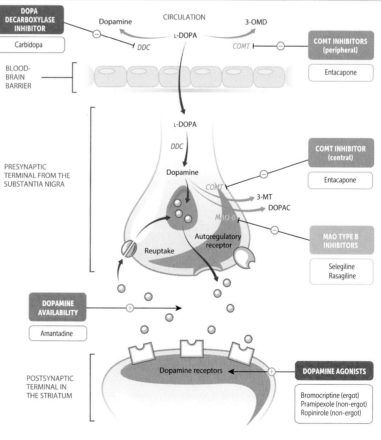

Levodopa/carbidopa

MECHANISM	↑ level of dopamine in brain. Unlike dopamine, L-DOPA can cross blood-brain barrier and is converted by dopa decarboxylase in the CNS to dopamine. Carbidopa, a peripheral DOPA decarboxylase inhibitor, is given with L-DOPA to ↑ the bioavailability of L-DOPA in the brain and to limit peripheral side effects.
CLINICAL USE	Parkinson disease.
ADVERSE EFFECTS	Nausea, hallucinations, postural hypotension from ↑ peripheral formation of catecholamines. Long-term use can lead to dyskinesia following administration ("on-off" phenomenon), akinesia between doses.

Selegiline, rasagiline

MECHANISM	Selectively inhibit MAO-B (metabolize dopamine) → ↑ dopamine availability.
CLINICAL USE	Adjunctive agent to L-DOPA in treatment of Parkinson disease.
ADVERSE EFFECTS	May enhance adverse effects of L-DOPA.

Tetrabenazine, reserpine

MECHANISM	Inhibit vesicular monoamine transporter (VMAT) dopamine → ↓ vesicle packaging and release.
CLINICAL USE	Huntington chorea, tardive dyskinesia

Riluzole

MECHANISM	↓ neuron glutamate excitotoxicity	For Lou Gehrig disease, give rilouzole.
CLINICAL USE	ALS, ↑ survival	

Alzheimer disease drugs

Memantine

MECHANISM	NMDA receptor antagonist; helps prevent excitotoxicity (mediated by Ca^{2+}).
ADVERSE EFFECTS	Dizziness, confusion, hallucinations.

Donepezil, rivastigmine, galantamine

MECHANISM	AChE inhibitors.	Dona Riva dances at the gala.
ADVERSE EFFECTS	Nausea, dizziness, insomnia.	

Anesthetics—general principles

CNS drugs must be lipid soluble (cross the blood-brain barrier) or be actively transported.
Drugs with ↓ solubility in blood = rapid induction and recovery times.

Drugs with ↑ solubility in lipids = ↑ potency = $\dfrac{1}{MAC}$

MAC = Minimal Alveolar Concentration (of inhaled anesthetic) required to prevent 50% of subjects from moving in response to noxious stimulus (eg, skin incision).

Examples: nitrous oxide (N_2O) has ↓ blood and lipid solubility, and thus fast induction and low potency. Halothane, propofol, and thiopental, in contrast, have ↑ lipid and blood solubility, and thus high potency and slow induction.

Inhaled anesthetics	Desflurane, halothane, enflurane, isoflurane, sevoflurane, methoxyflurane, N_2O.
MECHANISM	Mechanism unknown.
EFFECTS	Myocardial depression, respiratory depression, nausea/emesis, ↑ cerebral blood flow (↓ cerebral metabolic demand).
ADVERSE EFFECTS	Hepatotoxicity (halothane), **nephrotoxicity (methoxyflurane)**, proconvulsant (enflurane, epileptogenic), expansion of trapped gas in a body cavity (N_2O).
	Malignant hyperthermia—rare, life-threatening condition in which inhaled anesthetics or succinylcholine induce fever and severe muscle contractions. Susceptibility is often inherited as autosomal dominant with variable penetrance. Mutations in voltage-sensitive ryanodine receptor (*RYR1* gene) cause ↑ Ca^{2+} release from sarcoplasmic reticulum. Treatment: dantrolene (a ryanodine receptor antagonist).

Intravenous anesthetics

AGENT	MECHANISM	ANESTHESIA USE	NOTES
Thiopental	Facilitate $GABA_A$ (barbiturate).	Induction of anesthesia, short surgical procedures.	↓ cerebral blood flow. High lipid solubility. Effect terminated by rapid redistribution into tissue and fat.
Midazolam	Facilitate $GABA_A$ (benzodiazepine).	Procedural sedation (eg, endoscopy), anesthesia induction.	May cause severe postoperative respiratory depression, ↓ BP, anterograde amnesia.
Propofol	Potentiates $GABA_A$.	Rapid anesthesia induction, short procedures, ICU sedation.	
Ketamine	NMDA receptor antagonist.	Dissociative anesthesia. Sympathomimetic.	↑ cerebral blood flow. Emergence reaction possible with disorientation, hallucination, vivid dreams.

Local anesthetics	Esters—procaine, tetracaine, benzocaine, chloroprocaine. Amides—lIdocaIne, mepIvacaIne, bupIvacaIne, ropIvacaIne (amIdes have 2 I's in name).
MECHANISM	Block Na^+ channels by binding to specific receptors on inner portion of channel. Most effective in rapidly firing neurons. 3° amine local anesthetics penetrate membrane in uncharged form, then bind to ion channels as charged form.
	Can be given with vasoconstrictors (usually epinephrine) to enhance local action—↓ bleeding, ↑ anesthesia by ↓ systemic concentration.
	In infected (acidic) tissue, alkaline anesthetics are charged and cannot penetrate membrane effectively → need more anesthetic.
	Order of nerve blockade: small-diameter fibers > large diameter. Myelinated fibers > unmyelinated fibers. Overall, size factor predominates over myelination such that small myelinated fibers > small unmyelinated fibers > large myelinated fibers > large unmyelinated fibers.
	Order of loss: (1) pain, (2) temperature, (3) touch, (4) pressure.
CLINICAL USE	Minor surgical procedures, spinal anesthesia. If allergic to esters, give amides.
ADVERSE EFFECTS	CNS excitation, severe cardiovascular toxicity (bupivacaine), hypertension, hypotension, arrhythmias (cocaine), methemoglobinemia (benzocaine).

Neuromuscular blocking drugs	Muscle paralysis in surgery or mechanical ventilation. Selective for Nm nicotinic receptors at neuromuscular junction but not autonomic Nn receptors.
Depolarizing neuromuscular blocking drugs	Succinylcholine—strong ACh receptor agonist; produces sustained depolarization and prevents muscle contraction. Reversal of blockade: ▪ Phase I (prolonged depolarization)—no antidote. Block potentiated by cholinesterase inhibitors. ▪ Phase II (repolarized but blocked; ACh receptors are available, but desensitized)—may be reversed with cholinesterase inhibitors. Complications include hypercalcemia, hyperkalemia, malignant hyperthermia.
Nondepolarizing neuromuscular blocking drugs	Atracurium, cisatracurium, pancuronium, rocuronium, tubocurarine, vecuronium—competitive with ACh for receptors. Reversal of blockade—neostigmine (must be given with atropine or glycopyrrolate to prevent muscarinic effects such as bradycardia), edrophonium, and other cholinesterase inhibitors.

Dantrolene

MECHANISM	Prevents release of Ca^{2+} from the sarcoplasmic reticulum of skeletal muscle by binding to the ryanodine receptor.
CLINICAL USE	Malignant hyperthermia (a toxicity of inhaled anesthetics and succinylcholine) and neuroleptic malignant syndrome (a toxicity of antipsychotic drugs).

Baclofen

MECHANISM	Skeletal muscle relaxant. $GABA_B$ receptor agonist in spinal cord.
CLINICAL USE	Muscle spasticity, dystonia, multiple sclerosis.

Cyclobenzaprine

MECHANISM	Skeletal muscle relaxant. Acts within CNS.
CLINICAL USE	Muscle spasms.
ADVERSE EFFECTS	Anticholinergic side effects. Sedation.

Opioid analgesics

MECHANISM	Act as agonists at opioid receptors (μ = β-endorphin, δ = enkephalin, κ = dynorphin) to modulate synaptic transmission—close presynaptic Ca^{2+} channel, open postsynaptic K^+ channels → ↓ synaptic transmission. Inhibit release of ACh, norepinephrine, 5-HT, glutamate, substance P.
EFFICACY	Full agonist: morphine, heroin, meperidine, methadone, codeine. Partial agonist: buprenorphine. Mixed agonist/antagonist: nalbuphine, pentazocine. Antagonist: naloxone, naltrexone, methylnaltrexone.
CLINICAL USE	Moderate to severe or refractory pain, cough suppression (dextromethorphan), diarrhea (loperamide, diphenoxylate), acute pulmonary edema, maintenance programs for heroin addicts (methadone, buprenorphine + naloxone).
ADVERSE EFFECTS	Nausea, vomiting, pruritus, addiction, respiratory depression, constipation, sphincter of Oddi spasm, miosis (except meperidine → mydriasis), additive CNS depression with other drugs. Tolerance does not develop to miosis and constipation. Toxicity treated with naloxone (opioid receptor antagonist) and relapse prevention with naltrexone once detoxified.

Pentazocine

MECHANISM	κ-opioid receptor agonist and μ-opioid receptor weak antagonist or partial agonist.
CLINICAL USE	Analgesia for moderate to severe pain.
ADVERSE EFFECTS	Can cause opioid withdrawal symptoms if patient is also taking full opioid agonist (due to competition for opioid receptors).

Butorphanol

MECHANISM	κ-opioid receptor agonist and μ-opioid receptor partial agonist.
CLINICAL USE	Severe pain (eg, migraine, labor). Causes less respiratory depression than full opioid agonists.
ADVERSE EFFECTS	Use with full opioid agonist can precipitate withdrawal. Not easily reversed with naloxone.

Tramadol

MECHANISM	Very weak opioid agonist; also inhibits 5-HT receptors.
CLINICAL USE	Chronic pain.
ADVERSE EFFECTS	Similar to opioids. Decreases seizure threshold. Serotonin syndrome.

Glaucoma drugs

↓ IOP via ↓ amount of aqueous humor (inhibit synthesis/secretion or ↑ drainage).
BAD humor may not be **P**olitically **C**orrect.

DRUG CLASS	EXAMPLES	MECHANISM	ADVERSE EFFECTS
β-blockers	Timolol, betaxolol, carteolol	↓ aqueous humor synthesis	No pupillary or vision changes
α-agonists	Epinephrine (α_1), apraclonidine, brimonidine (α_2)	↓ aqueous humor synthesis via vasoconstriction (epinephrine) ↓ aqueous humor synthesis (apraclonidine, brimonidine)	Mydriasis (α_1); do not use in closed-angle glaucoma Blurry vision, ocular hyperemia, foreign body sensation, ocular allergic reactions, ocular pruritus
Diuretics	Acetazolamide	↓ aqueous humor synthesis via inhibition of carbonic anhydrase	No pupillary or vision changes
Prostaglandins	Bimatoprost, latanoprost ($PGF_{2\alpha}$)	↑ outflow of aqueous humor via ↓ resistance of flow through uveoscleral pathway	Darkens color of iris (browning), eyelash growth
Cholinomimetics (M_3)	Direct: pilocarpine, carbachol Indirect: physostigmine, echothiophate	↑ outflow of aqueous humor via contraction of ciliary muscle and opening of trabecular meshwork Use pilocarpine in acute angle closure glaucoma—very effective at opening meshwork into canal of Schlemm	Miosis (contraction of pupillary sphincter muscles) and cyclospasm (contraction of ciliary muscle)

▶ NOTES

Psychiatry

"Words of comfort, skillfully administered, are the oldest therapy known to man."

—Louis Nizer

"All men should strive to learn before they die what they are running from, and to, and why."

—James Thurber

"Man wishes to be happy even when he so lives as to make happiness impossible."

—St. Augustine

"It's no use going back to yesterday, because I was a different person then."
—Lewis Carroll, *Alice in Wonderland*

This chapter encompasses overlapping areas in psychiatry, psychology, sociology, and psychopharmacology. High-yield topics include schizophrenia, mood disorders, eating disorders, personality disorders, psychosomatic/somatoform disorders, and antipsychotic agents. Know the DSM-5 criteria for diagnosing common psychiatric disorders.

▸ PSYCHIATRY—PSYCHOLOGY

Classical conditioning	Learning in which a natural response (salivation) is elicited by a conditioned, or learned, stimulus (bell) that previously was presented in conjunction with an unconditioned stimulus (food).	Usually deals with **involuntary** responses. Pavlov's classical experiments with dogs— ringing the bell provoked salivation.

Operant conditioning	Learning in which a particular action is elicited because it produces a punishment or reward. Usually deals with **voluntary** responses.
Reinforcement	Target behavior (response) is followed by desired reward (positive reinforcement) or removal of aversive stimulus (negative reinforcement).
Extinction	Discontinuation of reinforcement (positive or negative) eventually eliminates behavior. Can occur in operant or classical conditioning.
Punishment	Repeated application of aversive stimulus (positive punishment) or removal of desired reward (negative punishment) to extinguish unwanted behavior (Skinner's operant conditioning quadrant).

	Increase behavior	Decrease behavior
Add a stimulus	Positive reinforcement	Positive punishment
Remove a stimulus	Negative reinforcement	Negative punishment

Transference and countertransference

Transference	Patient projects feelings about formative or other important persons onto physician (eg, psychiatrist is seen as parent).
Countertransference	Doctor projects feelings about formative or other important persons onto patient (eg, patient reminds physician of younger sibling).

Ego defenses	Mental processes (unconscious or conscious) used to resolve conflict and prevent undesirable feelings (eg, anxiety, depression).

IMMATURE DEFENSES	DESCRIPTION	EXAMPLE
Acting out	Expressing unacceptable feelings and thoughts through actions.	A young boy throws a temper tantrum when he does not get the toy he wants.
Denial	Avoiding the awareness of some painful reality.	A patient with cancer plans a full-time work schedule despite being warned of significant fatigue during chemotherapy.
Displacement	Redirection of emotions or impulses to a neutral person or object (vs projection).	A teacher is yelled at by the principal. Instead of confronting the principal directly, the teacher goes home and criticizes her husband's dinner selection.
Dissociation	Temporary, drastic change in personality, memory, consciousness, or motor behavior to avoid emotional stress. Patient has incomplete or no memory of traumatic event.	A victim of sexual abuse suddenly appears numb and detached when she is exposed to her abuser.

Ego defenses *(continued)*

IMMATURE DEFENSES	DESCRIPTION	EXAMPLE
Fixation	Partially remaining at a more childish level of development (vs regression).	A surgeon throws a tantrum in the operating room because the last case ran very late.
Idealization	Expressing extremely positive thoughts of self and others while ignoring negative thoughts.	A patient boasts about his physician and his accomplishments while ignoring any flaws.
Identification	Largely unconscious assumption of the characteristics, qualities, or traits of another person or group.	A resident starts putting his stethoscope in his pocket like his favorite attending, instead of wearing it around his neck like before.
Intellectualization	Using facts and logic to emotionally distance oneself from a stressful situation.	In a therapy session, patient diagnosed with cancer focuses only on rates of survival.
Isolation (of affect)	Separating feelings from ideas and events.	Describing murder in graphic detail with no emotional response.
Passive aggression	Demonstrating hostile feelings in a nonconfrontational manner; showing indirect opposition.	Disgruntled employee is repeatedly late to work, but won't admit it is a way to get back at the manager.
Projection	Attributing an unacceptable internal impulse to an external source (vs displacement).	A man who wants to cheat on his wife accuses his wife of being unfaithful.
Rationalization	Proclaiming logical reasons for actions actually performed for other reasons, usually to avoid self-blame.	After getting fired, claiming that the job was not important anyway.
Reaction formation	Replacing a warded-off idea or feeling with an (unconsciously derived) emphasis on its opposite (vs sublimation).	A patient with lustful thoughts enters a monastery.
Regression	**Involuntarily** turning back the maturational clock and going back to earlier modes of dealing with the world (vs fixation).	Seen in children under stress such as illness, punishment, or birth of a new sibling (eg, bedwetting in a previously toilet-trained child).
Repression	Involuntarily withholding an idea or feeling from conscious awareness (vs suppression).	A 20-year-old does not remember going to counseling during his parents' divorce 10 years earlier.
Splitting	Believing that people are either all good or all bad at different times due to intolerance of ambiguity. Commonly seen in borderline personality disorder.	A patient says that all the nurses are cold and insensitive but that the doctors are warm and friendly.
MATURE DEFENSES		
Sublimation	Replacing an unacceptable wish with a course of action that is similar to the wish but socially acceptable (vs reaction formation).	Teenager's aggressive urges toward his parents' high expectations are channeled into excelling in sports.
Altruism	Alleviating negative feelings via unsolicited generosity, which provides gratification (vs reaction formation).	Mafia boss makes large donation to charity.
Suppression	**Intentionally** withholding an idea or feeling from conscious awareness (vs repression); temporary.	Choosing to not worry about the big game until it is time to play.
Humor	Appreciating the amusing nature of an anxiety-provoking or adverse situation.	Nervous medical student jokes about the boards.
	Mature adults wear a **SASH**.	

▶ PSYCHIATRY—PATHOLOGY

Infant deprivation effects	Long-term deprivation of affection results in: ▪ Failure to thrive ▪ Poor language/socialization skills ▪ Lack of basic trust ▪ Reactive attachment disorder (infant withdrawn/unresponsive to comfort) ▪ Disinhibited social engagement (infant indiscriminately attaches to strangers)	Deprivation for > 6 months can lead to irreversible changes. Severe deprivation can result in infant death.

Child abuse

	Physical abuse	Sexual abuse
EVIDENCE	Fractures (eg, ribs, long bone spiral, multiple in different stages of healing), bruises (eg, trunk, ear, neck; in pattern of implement), burns (eg, cigarette, buttocks/thighs), subdural hematomas/retinal hemorrhages ("shaken baby syndrome"). During exam, children often avoid eye contact. Red flags include history inconsistent with degree or type of injury (eg, 2-month-old rolling out of bed or falling down stairs), delayed medical care, caregiver story changes with retelling.	Genital, anal, or oral trauma; STIs; UTIs.
ABUSER	Usually biological mother.	Known to victim, usually male.
EPIDEMIOLOGY	40% of deaths related to child abuse or neglect occur in children < 1 year old.	Peak incidence 9–12 years old.

Child neglect	Failure to provide a child with adequate food, shelter, supervision, education, and/or affection. Most common form of child maltreatment. Evidence: poor hygiene, malnutrition, withdrawal, impaired social/emotional development, failure to thrive. As with child abuse, suspected child neglect must be reported to local child protective services.
Vulnerable child syndrome	Parents perceive the child as especially susceptible to illness or injury. Usually follows a serious illness or life-threatening event. Can result in missed school or overuse of medical services.

Childhood and early-onset disorders

Attention-deficit hyperactivity disorder	Onset before age 12. At least 6 months of limited attention span and/or poor impulse control. Characterized by hyperactivity, impulsivity, and/or inattention in multiple settings (school, home, places of worship, etc). Normal intelligence, but commonly coexists with difficulties in school. Often persists into adulthood. Treatment: stimulants (eg, methylphenidate) +/– cognitive behavioral therapy (CBT); alternatives include atomoxetine, guanfacine, clonidine.
Autism spectrum disorder	Characterized by poor social interactions, social communication deficits, repetitive/ritualized behaviors, restricted interests. Must present in early childhood. May be accompanied by intellectual disability; rarely accompanied by unusual abilities (savants). More common in boys. Associated with ↑ head/brain size.
Conduct disorder	Repetitive and pervasive behavior violating the basic rights of others or societal norms (eg, aggression to people and animals, destruction of property, theft). After age 18, often reclassified as antisocial personality disorder. Treatment for both: psychotherapy such as CBT.
Disruptive mood dysregulation disorder	Onset before age 10. Severe and recurrent temper outbursts out of proportion to situation. Child is constantly angry and irritable between outbursts. Treatment: stimulants, antipsychotics, CBT.
Oppositional defiant disorder	Enduring pattern of hostile, defiant behavior toward authority figures in the absence of serious violations of social norms. Treatment: psychotherapy such as CBT.
Separation anxiety disorder	Overwhelming fear of separation from home or attachment figure lasting ≥ 4 weeks. Can be normal behavior up to age 3–4. May lead to factitious physical complaints to avoid school. Treatment: CBT, play therapy, family therapy.
Tourette syndrome	Onset before age 18. Characterized by sudden, rapid, recurrent, nonrhythmic, stereotyped motor and vocal tics that persist for > 1 year. Coprolalia (involuntary obscene speech) found in only 40% of patients. Associated with OCD and ADHD. Treatment: psychoeducation, behavioral therapy. For intractable and distressing tics, high-potency antipsychotics (eg, haloperidol, fluphenazine), tetrabenazine, α_2-agonists (eg, guanfacine, clonidine), or atypical antipsychotics may be used.

Orientation	Patient's ability to know who he or she is, where he or she is, and the date and time. Common causes of loss of orientation: alcohol, drugs, fluid/electrolyte imbalance, head trauma, hypoglycemia, infection, nutritional deficiencies, hypoxia.	Order of loss: time → place → person.

Amnesias

Retrograde amnesia	Inability to remember things that occurred **before** a CNS insult.
Anterograde amnesia	Inability to remember things that occurred **after** a CNS insult (↓ acquisition of new memory).
Korsakoff syndrome	Amnesia (anterograde > retrograde) caused by vitamin B_1 deficiency and associated destruction of mammillary bodies. Seen in alcoholics as a late neuropsychiatric manifestation of Wernicke encephalopathy. Confabulations are characteristic.

Dissociative disorders

Depersonalization/ derealization disorder	Persistent feelings of detachment or estrangement from one's own body, thoughts, perceptions, and actions (depersonalization) or one's environment (derealization). Intact reality testing (vs psychosis).
Dissociative amnesia	Inability to recall important personal information, usually subsequent to severe trauma or stress.
Dissociative identity disorder	Formerly known as multiple personality disorder. Presence of 2 or more distinct identities or personality states. More common in women. Associated with history of sexual abuse, PTSD, depression, substance abuse, borderline personality, somatoform conditions. May be accompanied by dissociative fugue (abrupt travel or wandering associated with traumatic circumstances).

Delirium	"Waxing and waning" level of consciousness with acute onset; rapid ↓ in attention span and level of arousal. Characterized by disorganized thinking, hallucinations (often visual), illusions, misperceptions, disturbance in sleep-wake cycle, cognitive dysfunction, agitation. Usually 2° to other illness (eg, CNS disease, infection, trauma, substance abuse/withdrawal, metabolic/electrolyte disturbances, hemorrhage, urinary/fecal retention). Most common presentation of altered mental status in inpatient setting, especially in the intensive care unit and with prolonged hospital stays. EEG may show diffuse slowing. Treatment is aimed at identifying and addressing underlying condition. Use antipsychotics acutely as needed. Avoid benzodiazepines.	Delirium = changes in sensorium. May be caused by medications (eg, anticholinergics), especially in the elderly. **Reversible**.

Psychosis	Distorted perception of reality characterized by delusions, hallucinations, and/or disorganized thought/speech. Can occur in patients with medical illness, psychiatric illness, or both.
Delusions	Unique, false, fixed, idiosyncratic beliefs that persist despite the facts and are not typical of a patient's culture or religion (eg, thinking aliens are communicating with you). Types include erotomanic, grandiose, jealous, persecutory, somatic, mixed, and unspecified.
Disorganized thought	Speech may be incoherent ("word salad"), tangential, or derailed ("loose associations").
Hallucinations	Perceptions in the absence of external stimuli (eg, seeing a light that is not actually present). Contrast with illusions, misperceptions of real external stimuli. Types include:

Perceptions in the absence of external stimuli (eg, seeing a light that is not actually present). Contrast with illusions, misperceptions of real external stimuli. Types include:

- Visual—more commonly a feature of medical illness (eg, drug intoxication) than psychiatric illness.
- Auditory—more commonly a feature of psychiatric illness (eg, schizophrenia) than medical illness.
- Olfactory—often occur as an aura of temporal lobe epilepsy (eg, burning rubber) and in brain tumors.
- Gustatory—rare, but seen in epilepsy.
- Tactile—common in alcohol withdrawal and stimulant use (eg, cocaine, amphetamines), delusional parasitosis, "cocaine crawlies."
- Hypnagogic—occurs while **going** to sleep. Sometimes seen in narcolepsy.
- Hypno**pomp**ic—occurs while waking from sleep ("**pomp**ous upon awakening"). Sometimes seen in narcolepsy.

Schizophrenia	Chronic mental disorder with periods of psychosis, disturbed behavior and thought, and decline in functioning lasting ≥ 6 months (including prodrome and residual symptoms). Associated with ↑ dopaminergic activity, ↓ dendritic branching. Diagnosis requires ≥ 2 of the following symptoms for ≥ 1 month, and at least 1 of these should include #1–3 (first 4 are "positive symptoms"): 1. Delusions 2. Hallucinations—often auditory 3. Disorganized speech 4. Disorganized or catatonic behavior 5. Negative symptoms (affective flattening, avolition, anhedonia, asociality, alogia) **Brief psychotic disorder**—≥ 1 positive symptom(s) lasting < 1 month, usually stress related. **Schizophreniform disorder**—≥ 2 symptoms, lasting 1–6 months. **Schizoaffective disorder**—Meets criteria for schizophrenia in addition to major mood disorder (major depressive or bipolar). To differentiate from a major mood disorder with psychotic features, patient must have > 2 weeks of psychotic symptoms without major mood episode.	Frequent cannabis use is associated with psychosis/schizophrenia in teens. Lifetime prevalence—1.5% (males > females, African Americans = Caucasians). Presents earlier in men (late teens to early 20s vs late 20s to early 30s in women). Patients at ↑ risk for suicide. Ventriculomegaly on brain imaging. Treatment: atypical antipsychotics (eg, risperidone) are first line. Negative symptoms often persist after treatment, despite resolution of positive symptoms.

Delusional disorder	Fixed, persistent, false belief system lasting > 1 month. Functioning otherwise not impaired (eg, a woman who genuinely believes she is married to a celebrity when, in fact, she is not). Can be shared by individuals in close relationships (folie à deux).

Mood disorder	Characterized by an abnormal range of moods or internal emotional states and loss of control over them. Severity of moods causes distress and impairment in social and occupational functioning. Includes major depressive, bipolar, dysthymic, and cyclothymic disorders. Episodic superimposed psychotic features (delusions, hallucinations, disorganized speech/behavior) may be present.

Manic episode	Distinct period of abnormally and persistently elevated, expansive, or irritable mood and abnormally and persistently ↑ activity or energy lasting ≥ 1 week. Often disturbing to patient and causes marked functional impairment and oftentimes hospitalization. Diagnosis requires hospitalization or at least 3 of the following (manics **DIG FAST**): ▪ **D**istractibility ▪ **I**mpulsivity/Indiscretion—seeks pleasure without regard to consequences (hedonistic) ▪ **G**randiosity—inflated self-esteem ▪ **F**light of ideas—racing thoughts ▪ ↑ goal-directed **A**ctivity/psychomotor Agitation ▪ ↓ need for **S**leep ▪ **T**alkativeness or pressured speech

Hypomanic episode

Similar to a manic episode except mood disturbance is not severe enough to cause marked impairment in social and/or occupational functioning or to necessitate hospitalization. No psychotic features. Lasts ≥ 4 consecutive days.

Bipolar disorder (manic depression)

Bipolar I defined by presence of at least 1 manic episode +/− a hypomanic or depressive episode (may be separated by any length of time).

Bipolar II defined by presence of a hypomanic and a depressive episode (no history of manic episodes).

Patient's mood and functioning usually normalize between episodes. Use of antidepressants can destabilize mood. High suicide risk. Treatment: mood stabilizers (eg, lithium, valproic acid, carbamazepine, lamotrigine), atypical antipsychotics.

Cyclothymic disorder—milder form of bipolar disorder lasting ≥ 2 years, fluctuating between mild depressive and hypomanic symptoms.

Major depressive disorder

Episodes characterized by at least 5 of the 9 diagnostic symptoms lasting ≥ 2 weeks (symptoms must include patient-reported depressed mood or anhedonia). Screen for history of manic episodes to rule out bipolar disorder.

Treatment: CBT and SSRIs are first line. SNRIs, mirtazapine, bupropion can also be considered. Electroconvulsive therapy (ECT) in treatment-resistant patients.

Persistent depressive disorder (dysthymia)— often milder, ≥ 2 depressive symptoms lasting ≥ 2 years, with no more than 2 months without depressive symptoms.

MDD with seasonal pattern—formerly known as seasonal affective disorder. Lasting ≥ 2 years with ≥ 2 major depressive episodes associated with seasonal pattern (usually winter) and absence of nonseasonal depressive episodes. Atypical symptoms common (eg, hypersomnia, hyperphagia, leaden paralysis).

Diagnostic symptoms (SIG E CAPS):
- Depressed mood
- Sleep disturbance
- Loss of Interest (anhedonia)
- Guilt or feelings of worthlessness
- Energy loss and fatigue
- Concentration problems
- Appetite/weight changes
- Psychomotor retardation or agitation
- Suicidal ideations

Patients with depression typically have the following changes in their sleep stages:
- ↓ slow-wave sleep
- ↓ REM latency
- ↑ REM early in sleep cycle
- ↑ total REM sleep
- Repeated nighttime awakenings
- Early-morning awakening (terminal insomnia)

Depression with atypical features

Characterized by mood reactivity (able to experience improved mood in response to positive events, albeit briefly), "reversed" vegetative symptoms (hypersomnia, hyperphagia), leaden paralysis (heavy feeling in arms and legs), long-standing interpersonal rejection sensitivity. Most common subtype of depression. Treatment: CBT and SSRIs are first line. MAO inhibitors are effective but not first line because of their risk profile.

Postpartum mood disturbances	Onset during pregnancy or within 4 weeks of delivery.
Maternal (postpartum) blues	50–85% incidence rate. Characterized by depressed affect, tearfulness, and fatigue starting 2–3 days after delivery. Usually resolves within 10 days. Treatment: supportive. Follow up to assess for possible postpartum depression.
Postpartum depression	10–15% incidence rate. Characterized by depressed affect, anxiety, and poor concentration for ≥ 2 weeks. Treatment: CBT and SSRIs are first line.
Postpartum psychosis	0.1–0.2% incidence rate. Characterized by mood-congruent delusions, hallucinations, and thoughts of harming the baby or self. Risk factors include history of bipolar or psychotic disorder, first pregnancy, family history, recent discontinuation of psychotropic medication. Treatment: hospitalization and initiation of atypical antipsychotic; if insufficient, ECT may be used.

Grief	The five stages of grief per the Kübler-Ross model are denial, anger, bargaining, depression, and acceptance (may occur in any order). Other normal grief symptoms include shock, guilt, sadness, anxiety, yearning, and somatic symptoms that usually occur in waves. Simple hallucinations of the deceased person are common (eg, hearing the deceased speaking). Any thoughts of dying are limited to joining the deceased (vs pathological grief). Duration varies widely; usually within 6–12 months. Pathologic grief is persistent and causes functional impairment. Can meet criteria for major depressive episode.

Electroconvulsive therapy	Rapid-acting method to treat resistant or refractory depression, depression with psychotic symptoms, and acute suicidality. Induces grand mal seizure while patient anesthetized. Adverse effects include disorientation, temporary headache, partial anterograde/retrograde amnesia usually resolving in 6 months. No absolute contraindications. Safe in pregnant and elderly individuals.

Risk factors for suicide completion	Sex (male) Age (young adult or elderly) Depression Previous attempt (highest risk factor) Ethanol or drug use Rational thinking loss (psychosis) Sickness (medical illness) Organized plan No spouse or other social support Stated future intent	**SAD PERSONS** are more likely to complete suicide. Most common method in US is firearms; access to guns ↑ risk of suicide completion. Women try more often; men complete more often. Family history of completed suicide is another well-known risk factor.

Anxiety disorder	Inappropriate experience of fear/worry and its physical manifestations (anxiety) incongruent with the magnitude of the perceived stressor. Symptoms interfere with daily functioning and are not attributable to another mental disorder, medical condition, or substance abuse. Includes panic disorder, phobias, generalized anxiety disorder, and selective mutism. Treatment: CBT, SSRIs, SNRIs.

Panic disorder	Recurrent unexpected panic attacks not associated with a known trigger. Periods of intense fear and discomfort peak in 10 minutes with at least 4 of the following: Palpitations, Paresthesias, dePersonalization or derealization, Abdominal distress or Nausea, Intense fear of dying, Intense fear of losing control or "going crazy," lIght-headedness, Chest pain, Chills, Choking, Sweating, Shaking, Shortness of breath. Strong genetic component. ↑ risk of suicide. Treatment: CBT, SSRIs, and venlafaxine are first line. Benzodiazepines occasionally used in acute setting.	PANICS. Diagnosis requires attack followed by ≥ 1 month of ≥ 1 of the following: ▪ Persistent concern of additional attacks ▪ Worrying about consequences of attack ▪ Behavioral change related to attacks Symptoms are the systemic manifestations of fear.

Specific phobia	Severe, persistent (≥ 6 months) fear or anxiety due to presence or anticipation of a specific object or situation. Person often recognizes fear is excessive. Can be treated with systematic desensitization.
	Social anxiety disorder—exaggerated fear of embarrassment in social situations (eg, public speaking, using public restrooms). Treatment: CBT, SSRIs, venlafaxine. For performance type (eg, anxiety restricted to public speaking), use β-blockers or benzodiazepines as needed.
	Agoraphobia—irrational fear/anxiety while facing or anticipating ≥ 2 specific situations (eg, open/closed spaces, lines, crowds, public transport). If severe, patients may refuse to leave their homes. Associated with panic disorder. Treatment: CBT, SSRIs.

Generalized anxiety disorder	Anxiety lasting > 6 months unrelated to a specific person, situation, or event. Associated with restlessness, irritability, sleep disturbance, fatigue, muscle tension, difficulty concentrating. Treatment: CBT, SSRIs, SNRIs are first line. Buspirone, TCAs, benzodiazepines are second line.
	Adjustment disorder—emotional symptoms (anxiety, depression) that occur within 3 months of an identifiable psychosocial stressor (eg, divorce, illness) lasting < 6 months once the stressor has ended. If symptoms persist > 6 months after stressor ends, it is GAD. Symptoms do not meet criteria for MDD. Treatment: CBT, SSRIs.

Obsessive-compulsive disorder	Recurring intrusive thoughts, feelings, or sensations (obsessions) that cause severe distress; relieved in part by the performance of repetitive actions (compulsions). Ego-dystonic: behavior inconsistent with one's own beliefs and attitudes (vs obsessive-compulsive personality disorder, ego-syntonic). Associated with Tourette syndrome. Treatment: CBT, SSRIs, venlafaxine, and clomipramine are first line.
	Body dysmorphic disorder—preoccupation with minor or imagined defect in appearance → significant emotional distress or impaired functioning; patients often repeatedly seek cosmetic treatment. Treatment: CBT.

Post-traumatic stress disorder	Experiencing a potentially life-threatening situation (eg, serious injury, rape, witnessing death) → persistent Hyperarousal, Avoidance of associated stimuli, intrusive Re-experiencing of the event (nightmares, flashbacks), changes in cognition or mood (fear, horror, Distress) (having PTSD is **HARD**). Disturbance lasts > 1 month with significant distress or impaired social-occupational functioning. Treatment: CBT, SSRIs, and venlafaxine are first line. Prazosin can reduce nightmares.
	Acute stress disorder—lasts between 3 days and 1 month. Treatment: CBT; pharmacotherapy is usually not indicated.

Diagnostic criteria by symptom duration

Personality

Personality trait	An enduring, repetitive pattern of perceiving, relating to, and thinking about the environment and oneself.
Personality disorder	Inflexible, maladaptive, and rigidly pervasive pattern of behavior causing subjective distress and/or impaired functioning; person is usually not aware of problem (ego-syntonic). Usually presents by early adulthood. Three clusters: **A, B, C**; remember as **Weird, Wild,** and **Worried,** respectively, based on symptoms.

Cluster A personality disorders	Odd or eccentric; inability to develop meaningful social relationships. No psychosis; genetic association with schizophrenia.	"Weird." Cluster **A**: **A**ccusatory, **A**loof, **A**wkward.
Paranoid	Pervasive distrust (**A**ccusatory) and suspiciousness of others and a profoundly cynical view of the world.	
Schizoid	Voluntary social withdrawal (**A**loof), limited emotional expression, content with social isolation (vs avoidant).	
Schizotypal	Eccentric appearance, odd beliefs or magical thinking, interpersonal **A**wkwardness.	Pronounce schizo-**type**-al: odd-**type** thoughts.

Cluster B personality disorders	Dramatic, emotional, or erratic; genetic association with mood disorders and substance abuse.	"Wild." Cluster **B**: **B**ad, **B**orderline, flam**B**oyant, must be the **B**est
Antisocial	Disregard for and violation of rights of others with lack of remorse, criminality, impulsivity; males > females; must be ≥ 18 years old and have history of conduct disorder before age 15. Conduct disorder if < 18 years old.	Antisocial = sociopath. **B**ad.
Borderline	Unstable mood and interpersonal relationships, impulsivity, self-mutilation, suicidality, sense of emptiness; females > males; splitting is a major defense mechanism.	Treatment: dialectical behavior therapy. **B**orderline.
Histrionic	Excessive emotionality and excitability, attention seeking, sexually provocative, overly concerned with appearance.	Flam**B**oyant.
Narcissistic	Grandiosity, sense of entitlement; lacks empathy and requires excessive admiration; often demands the "best" and reacts to criticism with rage.	Must be the **B**est.

Cluster C personality disorders	Anxious or fearful; genetic association with anxiety disorders.	"Worried." Cluster **C**: **C**owardly, obsessive-**C**ompulsive, **C**lingy.
Avoidant	Hypersensitive to rejection, socially inhibited, timid, feelings of inadequacy, desires relationships with others (vs schizoid).	**C**owardly.
Obsessive-Compulsive	Preoccupation with order, perfectionism, and control; ego-syntonic: behavior consistent with one's own beliefs and attitudes (vs OCD).	
Dependent	Excessive need for support, low self-confidence. Patients often get stuck in abusive relationships.	Submissive and **C**lingy.

Malingering	Symptoms are **intentional**, motivation is **intentional**. Patient **consciously** fakes, profoundly exaggerates, or claims to have a disorder in order to attain a specific 2° (**external**) **gain** (eg, avoiding work, obtaining compensation). Poor compliance with treatment or follow-up of diagnostic tests. Complaints cease after gain (vs factitious disorder).
Factitious disorders	Symptoms are **intentional**, motivation is **unconscious**. Patient **consciously** creates physical and/or psychological symptoms in order to assume "sick role" and to get medical attention and sympathy (1° [**internal**] **gain**).
Factitious disorder imposed on self	Also known as Munchausen syndrome. **Chronic** factitious disorder with predominantly physical signs and symptoms. Characterized by a history of multiple hospital admissions and willingness to undergo invasive procedures. More common in women and healthcare workers.
Factitious disorder imposed on another	Also known as Munchausen syndrome by proxy. Illness in a child or elderly patient is caused or fabricated by the caregiver. Motivation is to assume a sick role by proxy. Form of child/elder abuse.
Somatic symptom and related disorders	Symptoms are **unconscious**, motivation is **unconscious**. Category of disorders characterized by physical symptoms causing significant distress and impairment. Symptoms not intentionally produced or feigned. More common in women.
Somatic symptom disorder	Variety of bodily complaints (eg, pain, fatigue) lasting for months to years. Associated with excessive, persistent thoughts and anxiety about symptoms. May co-occur with medical illness. Treatment: regular office visits with the same physician in combination with psychotherapy.
Conversion disorder	Also known as functional neurologic symptom disorder. Loss of sensory or motor function (eg, paralysis, blindness, mutism), often following an acute stressor; patient may be aware of but indifferent toward symptoms ("la belle indifférence"); more common in females, adolescents, and young adults.
Illness anxiety disorder	Also known as hypochondriasis. Excessive preoccupation with acquiring or having a serious illness, often despite medical evaluation and reassurance; minimal somatic symptoms.
Eating disorders	Most common in young females.
Anorexia nervosa	Intense fear of weight gain and distortion or overvaluation of body image leading to restriction of caloric intake and severe weight loss (BMI < 18.5 kg/m^2). Restricting and binge/purge subtypes. Associated with ↓ bone density (often irreversible), amenorrhea (due to loss of pulsatile GnRH secretion), lanugo, anemia, electrolyte disturbances. Commonly coexists with depression. Psychotherapy and nutritional rehabilitation are first line; pharmacotherapy includes SSRIs for comorbid anxiety and/or depression. **Refeeding syndrome**—↑ insulin → hypophosphatemia, hypokalemia, hypomagnesemia → cardiac complications, rhabdomyolysis, seizures. Can occur in significantly malnourished patients.
Bulimia nervosa	Binge eating with recurrent inappropriate compensatory behaviors (eg, self-induced vomiting, using laxatives or diuretics, fasting, excessive exercise) occurring weekly for at least 3 months and overvaluation of body image. Body weight often maintained within normal range. Associated with parotitis, enamel erosion, electrolyte disturbances (eg, hypokalemia, hypochloremia), metabolic alkalosis, dorsal hand calluses from induced vomiting (Russell sign). Treatment: psychotherapy, nutritional rehabilitation, antidepressants (eg, SSRIs). Bupropion is contraindicated due to seizure risk.
Binge eating disorder	Regular episodes of excessive, uncontrollable eating without inappropriate compensatory behaviors. ↑ risk of diabetes. Treatment: psychotherapy such as CBT is first line; SSRIs, lisdexamfetamine.

Gender dysphoria	Persistent cross-gender identification that leads to persistent distress with sex assigned at birth. **Transsexualism**—desire to live as the opposite **sex**, often through surgery or hormone treatment. **Transvestism**—paraphilia, not gender dysphoria. Wearing clothes (eg, **vest**) of the opposite sex (cross-dressing).
Sexual dysfunction	Includes sexual desire disorders (hypoactive sexual desire or sexual aversion), sexual arousal disorders (erectile dysfunction), orgasmic disorders (anorgasmia, premature ejaculation), sexual pain disorders (dyspareunia, vaginismus). Differential diagnosis includes: ▪ Drug side effects (eg, antihypertensives, antipsychotics, SSRIs, ethanol) ▪ Medical disorders (eg, depression, diabetes, STIs) ▪ Psychological or performance anxiety (eg, nighttime erections [nocturnal tumescence])
Sleep terror disorder	Inconsolable periods of terror with screaming in the middle of the night; occurs during slow-wave/deep (stage N3) sleep. Most common in children. Occurs during non-REM sleep (no memory of the arousal episode) as opposed to nightmares that occur during **REM** sleep (**rem**embering a scary dream). Cause unknown, but triggers include emotional stress, fever, or lack of sleep. Usually self limited.
Enuresis	Urinary incontinence ≥ 2 times/week for ≥ 3 months in person > 5 years old. First-line treatment: behavioral modification (eg, scheduled voids) and positive reinforcement. For refractory cases: bedwetting alarm, oral desmopressin (ADH analog; preferred over imipramine due to more favorable side effect profile).
Narcolepsy	Disordered regulation of sleep-wake cycles characterized by excessive daytime sleepiness (despite feeling rested upon waking) and "sleep attacks" (rapid-onset, overwhelming sleepiness). Caused by ↓ hypocretin (orexin) production in lateral hypothalamus. Strong genetic component. Also associated with: ▪ Hypnagogic (just before going to sleep) or hypnopompic (just before awakening; "**pomp**ous upon awakening") hallucinations. ▪ Nocturnal and narcoleptic sleep episodes that start with REM sleep (sleep paralysis). ▪ Cataplexy (loss of all muscle tone following strong emotional stimulus, such as laughter) in some patients. Treatment: good sleep hygiene (scheduled naps, regular sleep schedule), daytime stimulants (eg, amphetamines, modafinil) and nighttime sodium oxybate (GHB).

Substance use disorder

Maladaptive pattern of substance use defined as 2 or more of the following signs in 1 year related specifically to substance use:

- Tolerance—need more to achieve same effect
- Withdrawal—manifesting as characteristic signs and symptoms
- Substance taken in larger amounts, or over longer time, than desired
- Persistent desire or unsuccessful attempts to cut down
- Significant energy spent obtaining, using, or recovering from substance
- Important social, occupational, or recreational activities reduced
- Continued use despite knowing substance causes physical and/or psychological problems
- Craving
- Recurrent use in physically dangerous situations
- Failure to fulfill major obligations at work, school, or home
- Social or interpersonal conflicts

Stages of change in overcoming substance addiction

1. **Precontemplation**—not yet acknowledging that there is a problem
2. **Contemplation**—acknowledging that there is a problem, but not yet ready or willing to make a change
3. **Preparation/determination**—getting ready to change behaviors
4. **Action/willpower**—changing behaviors
5. **Maintenance**—maintaining the behavioral changes
6. **Relapse**—returning to old behaviors and abandoning new changes. Does not always happen.

Psychiatric emergencies

	CAUSE	MANIFESTATION	TREATMENT
Serotonin syndrome	Any drug that ↑ 5-HT. Psychiatric drugs: MAO inhibitors, SSRIs, SNRIs, TCAs, vilazodone, vortioxetine. Nonpsychiatric drugs: tramadol, ondansetron, triptans, linezolid, MDMA, dextromethorphan, meperidine, St. John's wort	3 A's: ↑ Activity (neuromuscular) Autonomic stimulation Agitation. Symptoms of neuromuscular hyperactivity include clonus, hyperreflexia, hypertonia, tremor, seizure. Symptoms of autonomic stimulation include hyperthermia, diaphoresis, diarrhea	Cyproheptadine (5-HT$_2$ receptor antagonist)
Carcinoid syndrome[a]	Carcinoid tumor of GI tract, lung	Diarrhea, flushing, wheezing, right heart disease (if tumor is in the gut)	Octreotide

Psychiatric emergencies (continued)

	CAUSE	MANIFESTATION	TREATMENT
Hypertensive crisis	Eating tyramine-rich foods (eg, aged cheeses, cured meats, wine) while taking MAO inhibitor	Hypertensive crisis (tyramine displaces other neurotransmitters [eg, NE] in the synaptic cleft → ↑ sympathetic stimulation)	Phentolamine
Neuroleptic malignant syndrome	Antipsychotics + genetic predisposition	Malignant **FEVER**: **M**yoglobinuria **F**ever **E**ncephalopathy **V**itals unstable ↑ **E**nzymes (eg, ↑ CK) **R**igidity of muscles ("lead pipe")	Dantrolene, dopamine agonist (eg, bromocriptine), discontinue causative agent
Malignant hyperthermia[a]	Inhaled anesthetics, succinylcholine + genetic predisposition	Fever, severe muscle contractions	Dantrolene
Delirium tremens	Alcohol withdrawal; occurs 2–4 days after last drink Classically seen in hospital setting when inpatient cannot drink	Altered mental status (eg, hallucinations), autonomic hyperactivity, anxiety, seizures, tremors, psychomotor agitation, insomnia, nausea	Benzodiazepines (eg, chlordiazepoxide, lorazepam, diazepam)
Acute dystonia	Typical antipsychotics, anticonvulsants (eg, carbamazepine), metoclopramide	Sudden onset of muscle spasm, stiffness, oculogyric crisis that occurs within hours to days after medication use; can lead to laryngospasm requiring intubation	Benztropine or diphenhydramine
Lithium toxicity	Change in lithium dosage or health status (narrow therapeutic window), concurrent use of thiazides, ACE inhibitors, NSAIDs, or other nephrotoxic agents	Nausea, vomiting, slurred speech, hyperreflexia, seizures, ataxia, nephrogenic diabetes insipidus	Discontinue lithium, hydrate aggressively with isotonic sodium chloride, consider hemodialysis
Tricyclic antidepressant toxicity	TCA overdose	Respiratory depression, hyperpyrexia, prolonged QT interval Tri-C's: **C**onvulsions **C**oma **C**ardiotoxicity (arrhythmia due to Na^+ channel inhibition)	Supportive treatment, monitor ECG, $NaHCO_3$ (prevents arrhythmia), activated charcoal

[a]Carcinoid syndrome and malignant hyperthermia are not psychiatric emergencies, but are included for comparison with serotonin syndrome and neuroleptic malignant syndrome, respectively.

Psychoactive drug intoxication and withdrawal

DRUG	INTOXICATION	WITHDRAWAL
Depressants		
	Nonspecific: mood elevation, ↓ anxiety, sedation, behavioral disinhibition, respiratory depression.	Nonspecific: anxiety, tremor, seizures, insomnia.

Alcohol	Emotional lability, slurred speech, ataxia, coma, blackouts. Serum γ-glutamyltransferase (GGT)—sensitive indicator of alcohol use. **AST** value is 2× **ALT** value ("to**AST** 2 **AL**cohol").	Time from last drink:
		  3–36 hr: tremors, insomnia, GI upset, diaphoresis, mild agitation
		  6–48 hr: withdrawal seizures
		  12–48 hr: alcoholic hallucinosis (usually visual)
		  48–96 hr: delirium tremens (DTs)
		Treatment: benzodiazepines.

Opioids	Euphoria, respiratory and CNS depression, ↓ gag reflex, pupillary constriction (pinpoint pupils), seizures (overdose). Most common cause of drug overdose death. Treatment: naloxone.	Sweating, dilated pupils, piloerection ("cold turkey"), fever, rhinorrhea, lacrimation, yawning, nausea, stomach cramps, diarrhea ("flu-like" symptoms). Treatment: long-term support, methadone, buprenorphine.
Barbiturates	Low safety margin, marked respiratory depression. Treatment: symptom management (eg, assist respiration, ↑ BP).	Delirium, life-threatening cardiovascular collapse.
Benzodiazepines	Greater safety margin. Ataxia, minor respiratory depression. Treatment: flumazenil (benzodiazepine receptor antagonist, but rarely used as it can precipitate seizures).	Sleep disturbance, depression, rebound anxiety, seizure.
Stimulants		
	Nonspecific: mood elevation, psychomotor agitation, insomnia, cardiac arrhythmias, tachycardia, anxiety.	Nonspecific: post-use "crash," including depression, lethargy, ↑ appetite, sleep disturbance, vivid nightmares.
Amphetamines	Euphoria, grandiosity, pupillary dilation, prolonged wakefulness and attention, hypertension, tachycardia, anorexia, paranoia, fever. Skin excoriations with methamphetamine use. Severe: cardiac arrest, seizures. Treatment: benzodiazepines for agitation and seizures.	
Cocaine	Impaired judgment, pupillary dilation, hallucinations (including tactile), paranoid ideations, angina, sudden cardiac death. Chronic use may lead to perforated nasal septum due to vasoconstriction and resulting ischemic necrosis. Treatment: α-blockers, benzodiazepines. β-blockers not recommended.	
Caffeine	Restlessness, ↑ diuresis, muscle twitching.	Headache, difficulty concentrating, flu-like symptoms.
Nicotine	Restlessness.	Irritability, anxiety, restlessness, difficulty concentrating. Treatment: nicotine patch, gum, or lozenges; bupropion/varenicline.

Psychoactive drug intoxication and withdrawal *(continued)*

DRUG	INTOXICATION	WITHDRAWAL
Hallucinogens		
Phencyclidine (PCP)	Violence, impulsivity, psychomotor agitation, nystagmus, tachycardia, hypertension, analgesia, psychosis, delirium, seizures. Trauma is most common complication.	
Lysergic acid diethylamide	Perceptual distortion (visual, auditory), depersonalization, anxiety, paranoia, psychosis, possible flashbacks.	
Marijuana (cannabinoid)	Euphoria, anxiety, paranoid delusions, perception of slowed time, impaired judgment, social withdrawal, ↑ appetite, dry mouth, conjunctival injection, hallucinations. Pharmaceutical form is dro**nabinol**: used as antiemetic (chemotherapy) and appetite stimulant (in AIDS).	Irritability, anxiety, depression, insomnia, restlessness, ↓ appetite.
MDMA (ecstasy)	Hallucinogenic stimulant: euphoria, disinhibition, hyperactivity, distorted sensory and time perception, teeth clenching. Life-threatening effects include hypertension, tachycardia, hyperthermia, hyponatremia, serotonin syndrome.	Depression, fatigue, change in appetite, difficulty concentrating, anxiety.
Alcoholism	Physiologic tolerance and dependence on alcohol with symptoms of withdrawal when intake is interrupted. Complications: alcoholic cirrhosis, hepatitis, pancreatitis, peripheral neuropathy, testicular atrophy. Treatment: disulfiram (to condition the patient to abstain from alcohol use), acamprosate, naltrexone (reduces cravings), supportive care. Support groups such as Alcoholics Anonymous are helpful in sustaining abstinence and supporting patient and family.	
Wernicke-Korsakoff syndrome	Caused by vitamin B_1 deficiency. Triad of confusion, ophthalmoplegia, ataxia (Wernicke encephalopathy). May progress to irreversible memory loss, confabulation, personality change (Korsakoff syndrome). Symptoms may be precipitated by giving dextrose before administering vitamin B_1 to a patient with thiamine deficiency. Associated with periventricular hemorrhage/necrosis of mammillary bodies. Treatment: IV vitamin B_1.	

▶ PSYCHIATRY—PHARMACOLOGY

Preferred medications for selected psychiatric conditions

PSYCHIATRIC CONDITION	PREFERRED DRUGS
ADHD	Stimulants (methylphenidate, amphetamines)
Alcohol withdrawal	Benzodiazepines (eg, chlordiazepoxide, lorazepam, diazepam)
Bipolar disorder	Lithium, valproic acid, carbamazepine, lamotrigine, atypical antipsychotics
Bulimia nervosa	SSRIs
Depression	SSRIs
Generalized anxiety disorder	SSRIs, SNRIs
Obsessive-compulsive disorder	SSRIs, venlafaxine, clomipramine
Panic disorder	SSRIs, venlafaxine, benzodiazepines
PTSD	SSRIs, venlafaxine
Schizophrenia	Atypical antipsychotics
Social anxiety disorder	SSRIs, venlafaxine Performance only: β-blockers, benzodiazepines
Tourette syndrome	Antipsychotics (eg, fluphenazine, risperidone), tetrabenazine

Central nervous system stimulants

Methylphenidate, dextroamphetamine, methamphetamine.

MECHANISM	↑ catecholamines in the synaptic cleft, especially norepinephrine and dopamine.
CLINICAL USE	ADHD, narcolepsy.
ADVERSE EFFECTS	Nervousness, agitation, anxiety, insomnia, anorexia, tachycardia, hypertension, weight loss, tics.

Typical antipsychotics	Haloperidol, pimozide, trifluoperazine, fluphenazine, thioridazine, chlorpromazine.	
MECHANISM	Block dopamine D_2 receptor ($\uparrow$ cAMP).	
CLINICAL USE	Schizophrenia (1° positive symptoms), psychosis, bipolar disorder, delirium, Tourette syndrome, Huntington disease, OCD.	
POTENCY	High potency: Trifluoperazine, Fluphenazine, Haloperidol (Try to Fly High)—more neurologic side effects (eg, extrapyramidal symptoms [EPS]). Low potency: Chlorpromazine, Thioridazine (Cheating Thieves are low)—more anticholinergic, antihistamine, α_1-blockade effects.	
ADVERSE EFFECTS	Lipid soluble → stored in body fat → slow to be removed from body. Endocrine: dopamine receptor antagonism → hyperprolactinemia → galactorrhea, oligomenorrhea, gynecomastia. Metabolic: dyslipidemia, weight gain, hyperglycemia. Antimuscarinic: dry mouth, constipation. Antihistamine: sedation. α_1-blockade: orthostatic hypotension. Cardiac: QT prolongation. Ophthalmologic: Chlorpromazine—Corneal deposits; Thioridazine—reTinal deposits. Neuroleptic malignant syndrome. **EPS—ADAPT:** <ul><li>Hours to days: Acute Dystonia (muscle spasm, stiffness, oculogyric crisis). Treatment: benztropine, diphenhydramine.</li><li>Days to months:<ul><li>Akathisia (restlessness). Treatment: β-blockers, benztropine, benzodiazepines.</li><li>Parkinsonism (bradykinesia). Treatment: benztropine, amantadine.</li></ul></li><li>Months to years: Tardive dyskinesia (orofacial chorea). Treatment: switch to atypical antipsychotic (eg, clozapine), tetrabenazine, reserpine.</li></ul>	

Atypical antipsychotics	Aripiprazole, asenapine, clozapine, olanzapine, quetiapine, iloperidone, paliperidone, risperidone, lurasidone, ziprasidone.	
MECHANISM	Not completely understood. Most are D_2 antagonists; aripiprazole is D_2 partial agonist. Varied effects on 5-HT$_2$, dopamine, and α- and H$_1$-receptors.	
CLINICAL USE	Schizophrenia—both positive and negative symptoms. Also used for bipolar disorder, OCD, anxiety disorder, depression, mania, Tourette syndrome.	Use clozapine for treatment-resistant schizophrenia or schizoaffective disorder and for suicidality in schizophrenia.
ADVERSE EFFECTS	All—prolonged QT interval, fewer EPS and anticholinergic side effects than typical antipsychotics. "-pines"—metabolic syndrome (weight gain, diabetes, hyperlipidemia). Clozapine—agranulocytosis (monitor WBCs frequently) and seizures (dose related). Risperidone—hyperprolactinemia (amenorrhea, galactorrhea, gynecomastia).	Olanzapine, clOzapine → Obesity Must watch bone marrow clozely with clozapine.

Lithium

MECHANISM	Not established; possibly related to inhibition of phosphoinositol cascade.
CLINICAL USE	Mood stabilizer for bipolar disorder; treats acute manic episodes and prevents relapse.
ADVERSE EFFECTS	Tremor, hypothyroidism, polyuria (causes nephrogenic diabetes insipidus), teratogenesis. Causes Ebstein anomaly in newborn if taken by pregnant mother. Narrow therapeutic window requires close monitoring of serum levels. Almost exclusively excreted by kidneys; most is reabsorbed at PCT with Na$^+$. Thiazides (and other nephrotoxic agents) are implicated in lithium toxicity.

LiTHIUM:
Low Thyroid (hypothyroidism)
Heart (Ebstein anomaly)
Insipidus (nephrogenic diabetes insipidus)
Unwanted Movements (tremor)

Buspirone

MECHANISM	Stimulates 5-HT$_{1A}$ receptors.
CLINICAL USE	Generalized anxiety disorder. Does not cause sedation, addiction, or tolerance. Takes 1–2 weeks to take effect. Does not interact with alcohol (vs barbiturates, benzodiazepines).

I'm always anxious if the bus will be on time, so I take buspirone.

Antidepressants

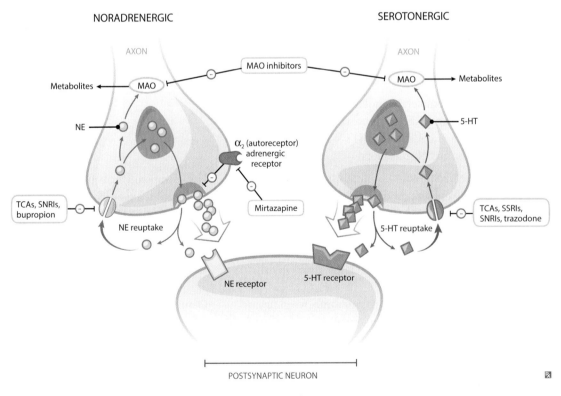

NORADRENERGIC

SEROTONERGIC

Selective serotonin reuptake inhibitors	Fluoxetine, fluvoxamine, paroxetine, sertraline, escitalopram, citalopram.	
MECHANISM	SSRIs inhibit 5-HT reuptake.	It normally takes 4–8 weeks for antidepressants to have an effect.
CLINICAL USE	Depression, generalized anxiety disorder, panic disorder, OCD, bulimia, social anxiety disorder, PTSD, premature ejaculation, premenstrual dysphoric disorder.	
ADVERSE EFFECTS	Fewer than TCAs. GI distress, SIADH, sexual dysfunction (anorgasmia, ↓ libido).	

Serotonin-norepinephrine reuptake inhibitors	Venlafaxine, desvenlafaxine, duloxetine, levomilnacipran, milnacipran.
MECHANISM	SNRIs inhibit 5-HT and NE reuptake.
CLINICAL USE	Depression, general anxiety disorder, diabetic neuropathy. Venlafaxine is also indicated for social anxiety disorder, panic disorder, PTSD, OCD. Duloxetine is also indicated for fibromyalgia.
ADVERSE EFFECTS	↑ BP, stimulant effects, sedation, nausea.

Tricyclic antidepressants	Amitriptyline, nortriptyline, imipramine, desipramine, clomipramine, doxepin, amoxapine.
MECHANISM	TCAs inhibit 5-HT and NE reuptake.
CLINICAL USE	Major depression, OCD (clomipramine), peripheral neuropathy, chronic pain, migraine prophylaxis. Nocturnal enuresis (imipramine, although adverse effects may limit use).
ADVERSE EFFECTS	Sedation, α_1-blocking effects including postural hypotension, and atropine-like (anticholinergic) side effects (tachycardia, urinary retention, dry mouth). 3° TCAs (amitriptyline) have more anticholinergic effects than 2° TCAs (nortriptyline). Can prolong QT interval. Tri-C's: Convulsions, Coma, Cardiotoxicity (arrhythmia due to Na^+ channel inhibition); also respiratory depression, hyperpyrexia. Confusion and hallucinations in the elderly due to anticholinergic side effects (nortriptyline better tolerated in the elderly). Treatment: $NaHCO_3$ to prevent arrhythmia.

Monoamine oxidase inhibitors	Tranylcypromine, Phenelzine, Isocarboxazid, Selegiline (selective MAO-B inhibitor). (**MAO** Takes Pride In Shanghai).
MECHANISM	Nonselective MAO inhibition ↑ levels of amine neurotransmitters (norepinephrine, 5-HT, dopamine).
CLINICAL USE	Atypical depression, anxiety. Parkinson disease (selegiline).
ADVERSE EFFECTS	CNS stimulation; hypertensive crisis, most notably with ingestion of tyramine. Contraindicated with SSRIs, TCAs, St. John's wort, meperidine, dextromethorphan (to prevent serotonin syndrome). Wait 2 weeks after stopping MAO inhibitors before starting serotonergic drugs or stopping dietary restrictions.

Atypical antidepressants

Bupropion	Inhibits NE and dopamine reuptake. Also used for smoking cessation. Toxicity: stimulant effects (tachycardia, insomnia), headache, seizures in anorexic/bulimic patients. Favorable sexual side effect profile.
Mirtazapine	α_2-antagonist (↑ release of NE and 5-HT), potent 5-HT$_2$ and 5-HT$_3$ receptor antagonist and H$_1$ antagonist. Toxicity: sedation (which may be desirable in depressed patients with insomnia), ↑ appetite, weight gain (which may be desirable in elderly or anorexic patients), dry mouth.
Trazodone	Primarily blocks 5-HT$_2$, α_1-adrenergic, and H$_1$ receptors; also weakly inhibits 5-HT reuptake. Used primarily for insomnia, as high doses are needed for antidepressant effects. Toxicity: sedation, nausea, priapism, postural hypotension. Called tra**ZZZ**obone due to sedative and male-specific side effects.
Varenicline	Nicotinic ACh receptor partial agonist. Used for smoking cessation. Toxicity: sleep disturbance, may depress mood. Vare**nic**line helps **nic**otine cravings de**cline**.
Vilazodone	Inhibits 5-HT reuptake; 5-HT$_{1A}$ receptor partial agonist. Used for major depressive disorder. Toxicity: headache, diarrhea, nausea, ↑ weight, anticholinergic effects. May cause serotonin syndrome if taken with other serotonergic agents.
Vortioxetine	Inhibits 5-HT reuptake; 5-HT$_{1A}$ receptor agonist and 5-HT$_3$ receptor antagonist. Used for major depressive disorder. Toxicity: nausea, sexual dysfunction, sleep disturbances (abnormal dreams), anticholinergic effects. May cause serotonin syndrome if taken with other serotonergic agents.

Opioid withdrawal and detoxification	Intravenous drug users at ↑ risk for hepatitis, HIV, abscesses, bacteremia, right-heart endocarditis.
Methadone	Long-acting oral opiate used for heroin detoxification or long-term maintenance therapy.
Buprenorphine + naloxone	Sublingual buprenorphine (partial agonist) is absorbed and used for maintenance therapy. Naloxone (antagonist, not orally bioavailable) is added to lower IV abuse potential.
Naltrexone	Long-acting opioid given IM or as nasal spray to treat acute overdose in unconscious individual. Also used for relapse prevention once detoxified. Use na**ltrex**one for the long **trex** back to sobriety.

Renal

"But I know all about love already. I know precious little still about kidneys."

—Aldous Huxley, *Antic Hay*

"This too shall pass. Just like a kidney stone."

—Hunter Madsen

"I drink too much. The last time I gave a urine sample it had an olive in it."

—Rodney Dangerfield

Being able to understand and apply renal physiology will be critical for the exam. Important topics include electrolyte disorders, acid-base derangements, glomerular disorders (including histopathology), kidney failure, urine casts, diuretics, ACE inhibitors, and AT-II receptor blockers. Renal anomalies linked to various congenital defects is also a high-yield association to think about when you encounter pediatric vignettes.

▶ **RENAL—EMBRYOLOGY**

Kidney embryology

Pronephros—week 4; then degenerates.
Mesonephros—functions as interim kidney for 1st trimester; later contributes to male genital system.
Metanephros—permanent; first appears in 5th week of gestation; nephrogenesis continues through weeks 32–36 of gestation.

- Ureteric bud—derived from caudal end of mesonephric duct; gives rise to ureter, pelvises, calyces, collecting ducts; fully canalized by 10th week
- Metanephric mesenchyme (ie, metanephric blastema)—ureteric bud interacts with this tissue; interaction induces differentiation and formation of glomerulus through to distal convoluted tubule (DCT)
- Aberrant interaction between these 2 tissues may result in several congenital malformations of the kidney (eg, renal agenesis, multicystic dysplastic kidney)

Ureteropelvic junction—last to canalize → most common site of obstruction (can be detected on prenatal ultrasound as hydronephrosis).

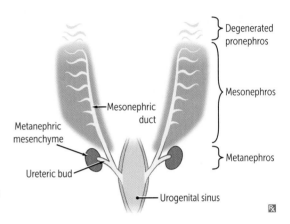

Potter sequence (syndrome)

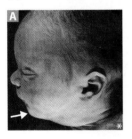

Oligohydramnios → compression of developing fetus → limb deformities, facial anomalies (eg, low-set ears and retrognathia A, flattened nose), compression of chest and lack of amniotic fluid aspiration into fetal lungs → pulmonary hypoplasia (cause of death).

Causes include ARPKD, obstructive uropathy (eg, posterior urethral valves), bilateral renal agenesis, chronic placental insufficiency.

Babies who can't "Pee" in utero develop Potter sequence.

POTTER sequence associated with:
Pulmonary hypoplasia
Oligohydramnios (trigger)
Twisted face
Twisted skin
Extremity defects
Renal failure (in utero)

Horseshoe kidney

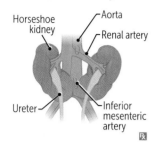

Horseshoe kidney — Aorta — Renal artery — Ureter — Inferior mesenteric artery

Inferior poles of both kidneys fuse abnormally 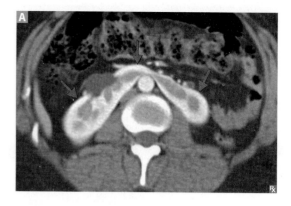. As they ascend from pelvis during fetal development, horseshoe kidneys get trapped under inferior mesenteric artery and remain low in the abdomen. Kidneys function normally. Associated with hydronephrosis (eg, ureteropelvic junction obstruction), renal stones, infection, chromosomal aneuploidy syndromes (eg, Turner syndrome; trisomies 13, 18, 21), and rarely renal cancer.

Congenital solitary functioning kidney	Condition of being born with only one functioning kidney. Majority asymptomatic with compensatory hypertrophy of contralateral kidney, but anomalies in contralateral kidney are common. Often diagnosed prenatally via ultrasound.
Unilateral renal agenesis	Ureteric bud fails to develop and induce differentiation of metanephric mesenchyme → complete absence of kidney and ureter.
Multicystic dysplastic kidney	Ureteric bud fails to induce differentiation of metanephric mesenchyme → nonfunctional kidney consisting of cysts and connective tissue. Predominantly nonhereditary and usually unilateral; bilateral leads to Potter sequence.

Duplex collecting system	Bifurcation of ureteric bud before it enters the metanephric blastema creates a Y-shaped bifid ureter. Duplex collecting system can alternatively occur through two ureteric buds reaching and interacting with metanephric blastema. Strongly associated with vesicoureteral reflux and/or ureteral obstruction, ↑ risk for UTIs.

Posterior urethral valves	Membrane remnant in the posterior urethra in males; its persistence can lead to urethral obstruction. Can be diagnosed prenatally by hydronephrosis and dilated or thick-walled bladder on ultrasound. Most common cause of bladder outlet obstruction in male infants.

▶ RENAL—ANATOMY

Kidney anatomy and glomerular structure

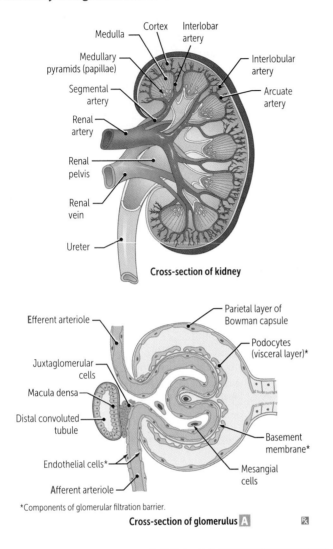

Cross-section of kidney

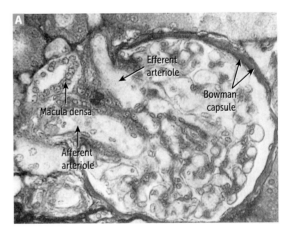

*Components of glomerular filtration barrier.

Cross-section of glomerulus A

Left kidney is taken during donor transplantation because it has a longer renal vein.

Afferent = Arriving.

Efferent = Exiting.

Renal blood flow: renal artery → segmental artery → interlobar artery → arcuate artery → interlobular artery → afferent arteriole → glomerulus → efferent arteriole → vasa recta/peritubular capillaries → venous outflow.

Course of ureters

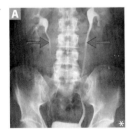

Course of ureter A: arises from renal pelvis, travels under gonadal arteries → **over common iliac artery** → **under uterine artery/vas deferens** (retroperitoneal).

Gynecologic procedures (eg, ligation of uterine or ovarian vessels) may damage ureter → ureteral obstruction or leak.

Muscle fibers within the intramural part of the ureter prevent urine reflux.

3 constrictions of ureter:
- Ureteropelvic junction
- Pelvic inlet
- Ureterovesical junction

Water (ureters) flows over the iliacs and under the bridge (uterine artery or vas deferens).

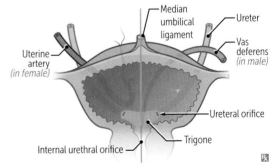

▶ RENAL—PHYSIOLOGY

Fluid compartments

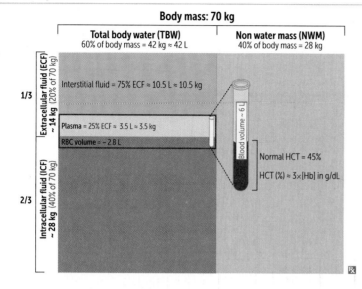

Body mass: 70 kg

| Total body water (TBW)
60% of body mass = 42 kg ≈ 42 L | Non water mass (NWM)
40% of body mass = 28 kg |

Extracellular fluid (ECF) ~ 14 kg (20% of 70 kg) — 1/3

Interstitial fluid = 75% ECF ≈ 10.5 L ≈ 10.5 kg

Plasma = 25% ECF ≈ 3.5 L ≈ 3.5 kg

RBC volume ≈ ~ 2.8 L

Intracellular fluid (ICF) ~ 28 kg (40% of 70 kg) — 2/3

Blood volume ~ 6 L

Normal HCT = 45%

HCT (%) ≈ 3×[Hb] in g/dL

HIKIN': HIgh K⁺ INtracellularly.

60–40–20 rule (% of body weight for average person):

- 60% total body water
- 40% ICF, mainly composed of K^+, Mg^{2+}, organic phosphates (eg, ATP)
- 20% ECF, mainly composed of Na^+, Cl^-, HCO_3^-, albumin

Plasma volume can be measured by radiolabeling albumin.

Extracellular volume can be measured by inulin or mannitol.

Osmolality = 285–295 mOsm/kg H_2O.

Glomerular filtration barrier

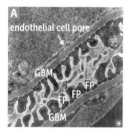

endothelial cell pore

GBM
FP
FP FP
GBM

Responsible for filtration of plasma according to size and charge selectivity.

Composed of:

- Fenestrated capillary endothelium
- Basement membrane with type IV collagen chains and heparan sulfate
- Epithelial layer consisting of podocyte foot processes A

Charge barrier—all 3 layers contain ⊖ charged glycoproteins that prevent entry of ⊖ charged molecules (eg, albumin).

Size barrier—fenestrated capillary endothelium (prevent entry of > 100 nm molecules/blood cells); podocyte foot processes interpose with basement membrane; slit diaphragm (prevent entry of molecules > 50–60 nm).

Renal clearance

$C_x = (U_x V)/P_x$ = volume of plasma from which the substance is completely cleared per unit time.

If $C_x <$ GFR: net tubular reabsorption of X.

If $C_x >$ GFR: net tubular secretion of X.

If $C_x =$ GFR: no net secretion or reabsorption.

C_x = clearance of X (mL/min).

U_x = urine concentration of X (eg, mg/mL).

P_x = plasma concentration of X (eg, mg/mL).

V = urine flow rate (mL/min).

Glomerular filtration rate

Inulin clearance can be used to calculate GFR because it is freely filtered and is neither reabsorbed nor secreted.

$$GFR = U_{inulin} \times V/P_{inulin} = C_{inulin}$$
$$= K_f [(P_{GC} - P_{BS}) - (\pi_{GC} - \pi_{BS})]$$

(GC = glomerular capillary; BS = Bowman space; π_{BS} normally equals zero; K_f = filtration coefficient).

Normal GFR ≈ 100 mL/min.

Creatinine clearance is an approximate measure of GFR. Slightly overestimates GFR because creatinine is moderately secreted by renal tubules.

Incremental reductions in GFR define the stages of chronic kidney disease.

Effective renal plasma flow

Effective renal plasma flow (eRPF) can be estimated using *para*-aminohippuric acid (PAH) clearance. Between filtration and secretion, there is nearly 100% excretion of all PAH that enters the kidney.

$eRPF = U_{PAH} \times V/P_{PAH} = C_{PAH}$.

Renal blood flow (RBF) = RPF/(1 − Hct). Usually 20–25% of cardiac output.

Plasma volume = TBV × (1 − Hct).

eRPF underestimates true renal plasma flow (RPF) slightly.

Filtration

Filtration fraction (FF) = GFR/RPF.
Normal FF = 20%.
Filtered load (mg/min) = GFR (mL/min) × plasma concentration (mg/mL).

GFR can be estimated with creatinine clearance.
RPF is best estimated with PAH clearance.
Prostaglandins Dilate Afferent arteriole (PDA)
Angiotensin II Constricts Efferent arteriole (ACE)

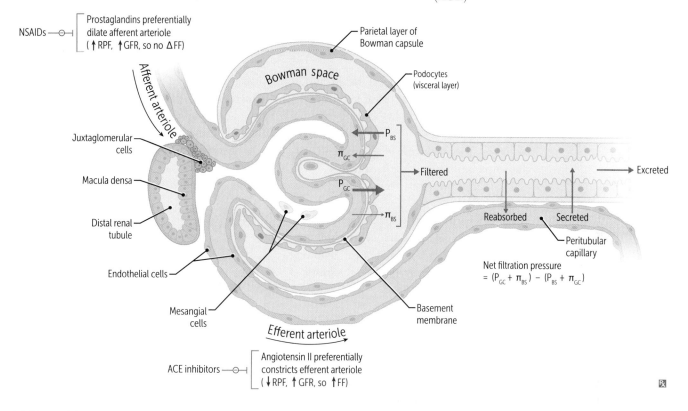

NSAIDs ─○┤ Prostaglandins preferentially dilate afferent arteriole (↑RPF, ↑GFR, so no ΔFF)

Parietal layer of Bowman capsule

Bowman space

Podocytes (visceral layer)

Afferent arteriole

Juxtaglomerular cells

Macula densa

Distal renal tubule

Endothelial cells

Mesangial cells

P_{BS}

π_{GC}

P_{GC}

π_{BS}

Filtered

Excreted

Reabsorbed   Secreted

Peritubular capillary

Net filtration pressure = $(P_{GC} + \pi_{BS}) - (P_{BS} + \pi_{GC})$

Basement membrane

Efferent arteriole

ACE inhibitors ─○┤ Angiotensin II preferentially constricts efferent arteriole (↓RPF, ↑GFR, so ↑FF)

Changes in glomerular dynamics

Effect	GFR	RPF	FF (GFR/RPF)
Afferent arteriole constriction	↓	↓	—
Efferent arteriole constriction	↑	↓	↑
↑ plasma protein concentration	↓	—	↓
↓ plasma protein concentration	↑	—	↑
Constriction of ureter	↓	—	↓
Dehydration	↓	↓↓	↑

| **Calculation of reabsorption and secretion rate** | Filtered load = GFR × P_x.
Excretion rate = V × U_x.
Reabsorption rate = filtered − excreted.
Secretion rate = excreted − filtered.
Fe_{Na} = fractional excretion of sodium. |

$$Fe_{Na} = \frac{Na^+ \text{ excreted}}{Na^+ \text{ filtered}} = \frac{V \times U_{Na}}{GFR \times P_{Na}} \quad \text{where GFR} = \frac{U_{Cr} \times V}{P_{Cr}} = \frac{P_{Cr} \times U_{Na}}{U_{Cr} \times P_{Na}}$$

| **Glucose clearance** | Glucose at a normal plasma level (range 60–120 mg/dL) is completely reabsorbed in proximal convoluted tubule (PCT) by Na^+/glucose cotransport.
In adults, at plasma glucose of ~ 200 mg/dL, glucosuria begins (threshold). At rate of ~ 375 mg/min, all transporters are fully saturated (T_m).
Normal pregnancy is associated with ↑ GFR. With ↑ filtration of all substances, including glucose, the glucose threshold occurs at lower plasma glucose concentrations → glucosuria at normal plasma glucose levels.
Sodium-glucose cotransporter 2 (SGLT2) inhibitors (eg, -flozin drugs) result in glucosuria at plasma concentrations < 200 mg/dL. | Glucosuria is an important clinical clue to diabetes mellitus.
Splay phenomenon—T_m for glucose is reached gradually rather than sharply due to the heterogeneity of nephrons (ie, different T_m points); represented by the portion of the titration curve between threshold and T_m.
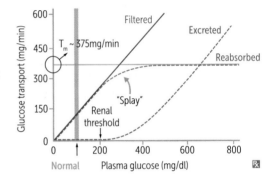 |

Nephron physiology

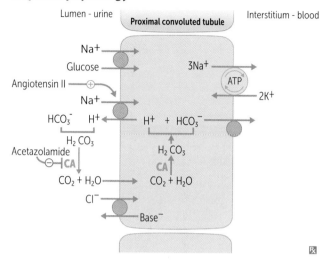

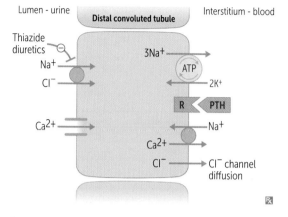

Early PCT—contains brush border. Reabsorbs all glucose and amino acids and most HCO_3^-, Na^+, Cl^-, PO_4^{3-}, K^+, H_2O, and uric acid. Isotonic absorption. Generates and secretes NH_3, which enables the kidney to secrete more H^+.
PTH—inhibits Na^+/PO_4^{3-} cotransport → PO_4^{3-} excretion.
AT II—stimulates Na^+/H^+ exchange → ↑ Na^+, H_2O, and HCO_3^- reabsorption (permitting contraction alkalosis).
65–80% Na^+ reabsorbed.

Thin descending loop of Henle—passively reabsorbs H_2O via medullary hypertonicity (impermeable to Na^+). Concentrating segment. Makes urine hypertonic.

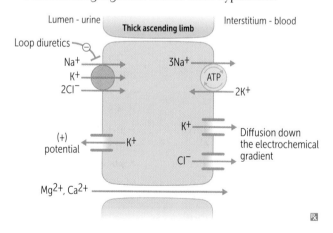

Thick ascending loop of Henle—reabsorbs Na^+, K^+, and Cl^-. Indirectly induces paracellular reabsorption of Mg^{2+} and Ca^{2+} through ⊕ lumen potential generated by K^+ backleak. Impermeable to H_2O. Makes urine less concentrated as it ascends.
10–20% Na^+ reabsorbed.

Early DCT—reabsorbs Na^+, Cl^-. Impermeable to H_2O. Makes urine fully dilute (hypotonic).
PTH—↑ Ca^{2+}/Na^+ exchange → Ca^{2+} reabsorption.
5–10% Na^+ reabsorbed.

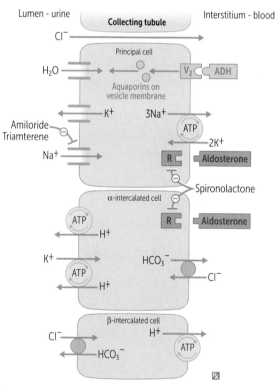

Collecting tubule—reabsorbs Na^+ in exchange for secreting K^+ and H^+ (regulated by aldosterone).
Aldosterone—acts on mineralocorticoid receptor → mRNA → protein synthesis. In principal cells: ↑ apical K^+ conductance, ↑ Na^+/K^+ pump, ↑ epithelial Na^+ channel (ENaC) activity → lumen negativity → K^+ secretion. In α-intercalated cells: lumen negativity → ↑ H^+ ATPase activity → ↑ H^+ secretion → ↑ HCO_3^-/Cl^- exchanger activity.
ADH—acts at V_2 receptor → insertion of aquaporin H_2O channels on apical side.
3–5% Na^+ reabsorbed.

Renal tubular defects The kidneys put out **FaB**ulous **G**littering **L**iquid**S** (from front to end of tube)

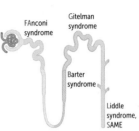

	DEFECTS	EFFECTS	CAUSES	NOTES
Fanconi syndrome	Generalized reabsorption defect in PCT → ↑ excretion of amino acids, glucose, HCO_3^-, and PO_4^{3-}, and all substances reabsorbed by the PCT	May lead to metabolic acidosis (proximal RTA), hypophosphatemia, osteopenia	Hereditary defects (eg, Wilson disease, tyrosinemia, glycogen storage disease), ischemia, multiple myeloma, nephrotoxins/drugs (eg, ifosfamide, cisplatin, expired tetracyclines), lead poisoning	
Bartter syndrome	Resorptive defect in thick ascending loop of Henle (affects $Na^+/K^+/2Cl^-$ cotransporter)	Metabolic alkalosis, hypokalemia, hypercalciuria	Autosomal recessive	Presents similarly to chronic loop diuretic use
Gitelman syndrome	Reabsorption defect of NaCl in DCT	Metabolic alkalosis, hypomagnesemia, hypokalemia, hypocalciuria	Autosomal recessive	Presents similarly to lifelong thiazide diuretic use Less severe than Bartter syndrome
Liddle syndrome	Gain of function mutation → ↑ activity of Na^+ channel → ↑ Na^+ reabsorption in collecting tubules	Metabolic alkalosis, hypokalemia, hypertension, ↓ aldosterone	Autosomal dominant	Presents similarly to hyperaldosteronism, but aldosterone is nearly undetectable Treat with amiloride
Syndrome of Apparent Mineralocorticoid Excess	In cells containing mineralocorticoid receptors, 11β-hydroxysteroid dehydrogenase converts cortisol (can activate these receptors) to cortisone (inactive on these receptors) Hereditary deficiency of 11β-hydroxysteroid dehydrogenase → excess cortisol → ↑ mineralocorticoid receptor activity	Metabolic alkalosis, hypokalemia, hypertension ↓ serum aldosterone level; cortisol tries to be the **SAME** as aldosterone	Autosomal recessive Can acquire disorder from glycyrrhetinic acid (present in licorice), which blocks activity of 11β-hydroxysteroid dehydrogenase	Treat with K^+-sparing diuretics (↓ mineralo-corticoid effects) or corticosteroids (exogenous cortico-steroid ↓ endogenous cortisol production → ↓ mineralocorticoid receptor activation)

Relative concentrations along proximal convoluted tubules

[TF/P] > 1 when solute is reabsorbed less quickly than water or when solute is secreted

[TF/P] = 1 when solute and water are reabsorbed at the same rate

[TF/P] < 1 when solute is reabsorbed more quickly than water

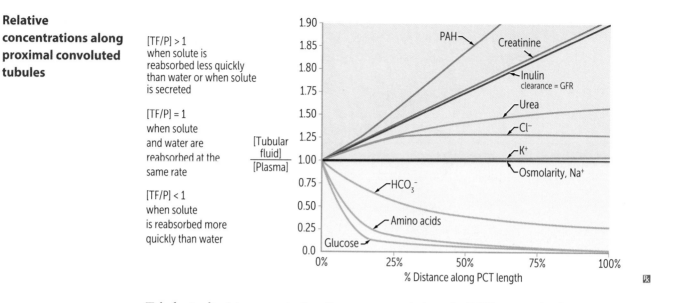

Tubular inulin ↑ in concentration (but not amount) along the PCT as a result of water reabsorption. Cl⁻ reabsorption occurs at a slower rate than Na⁺ in early PCT and then matches the rate of Na⁺ reabsorption more distally. Thus, its relative concentration ↑ before it plateaus.

Renin-angiotensin-aldosterone system

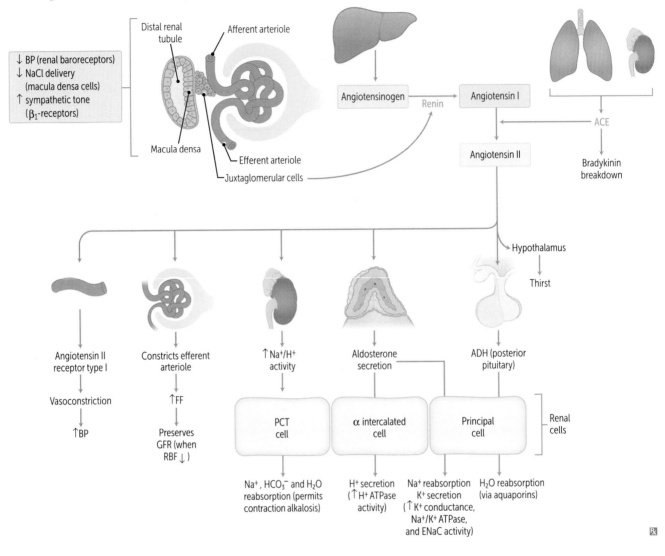

Renin	Secreted by JG cells in response to ↓ renal perfusion pressure (detected by renal baroreceptors in afferent arteriole), ↑ renal sympathetic discharge (β_1 effect), and ↓ NaCl delivery to macula densa cells.
AT II	Helps maintain blood volume and blood pressure. Affects baroreceptor function; limits reflex bradycardia, which would normally accompany its pressor effects.
ANP, BNP	Released from atria (ANP) and ventricles (BNP) in response to ↑ volume; may act as a "check" on renin-angiotensin-aldosterone system; relaxes vascular smooth muscle via cGMP → ↑ GFR, ↓ renin. Dilates afferent arteriole, constricts efferent arteriole, promotes natriuresis.
ADH	Primarily regulates serum osmolality; also responds to low blood volume states. Stimulates reabsorption of water in collecting ducts. Also stimulates reabsorption of urea in collecting ducts to maintain corticopapillary osmotic gradient.
Aldosterone	Primarily regulates ECF volume and Na^+ content; responds to low blood volume states. Responds to hyperkalemia by ↑ K^+ excretion.

| **Juxtaglomerular apparatus** | Consists of mesangial cells, JG cells (modified smooth muscle of afferent arteriole) and the macula densa (NaCl sensor, located at distal end of loop of Henle). JG cells secrete renin in response to ↓ renal blood pressure and ↑ sympathetic tone (β_1). Macula densa cells sense ↓ NaCl delivery to DCT → ↑ renin release → efferent arteriole vasoconstriction → ↑ GFR. | JGA maintains GFR via renin-angiotensin-aldosterone system.
In addition to vasodilatory properties, β-blockers can decrease BP by inhibiting β_1-receptors of the JGA → ↓ renin release. |

Kidney endocrine functions

Erythropoietin	Released by interstitial cells in peritubular capillary bed in response to hypoxia.	Stimulates RBC proliferation in bone marrow. Erythropoietin often supplemented in chronic kidney disease.
Calciferol (vitamin D)	PCT cells convert 25-OH vitamin D_3 to 1,25-$(OH)_2$ vitamin D_3 (calcitriol, active form).	$$25\text{-OH }D_3 \xrightarrow{1\alpha\text{-hydroxylase}} 1,25\text{-}(OH)_2\,D_3$$ ⊕ PTH
Prostaglandins	Paracrine secretion vasodilates the afferent arterioles to ↑ RBF.	NSAIDs block renal-protective prostaglandin synthesis → constriction of afferent arteriole and ↓ GFR; this may result in acute renal failure in low renal blood flow states.
Dopamine	Secreted by PCT cells, promotes natriuresis. At low doses, dilates interlobular arteries, afferent arterioles, efferent arterioles → ↑ RBF, little or no change in GFR. At higher doses, acts as vasoconstrictor.	

Hormones acting on kidney

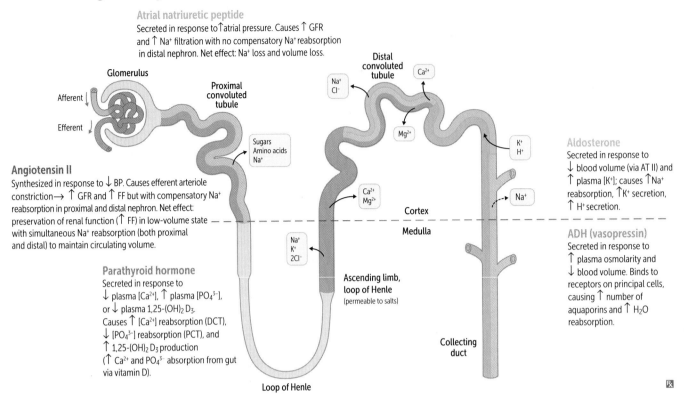

Atrial natriuretic peptide
Secreted in response to ↑atrial pressure. Causes ↑ GFR and ↑ Na$^+$ filtration with no compensatory Na$^+$ reabsorption in distal nephron. Net effect: Na$^+$ loss and volume loss.

Angiotensin II
Synthesized in response to ↓ BP. Causes efferent arteriole constriction → ↑ GFR and ↑ FF but with compensatory Na$^+$ reabsorption in proximal and distal nephron. Net effect: preservation of renal function (↑ FF) in low-volume state with simultaneous Na$^+$ reabsorption (both proximal and distal) to maintain circulating volume.

Parathyroid hormone
Secreted in response to ↓ plasma [Ca^{2+}], ↑ plasma [PO$_4$$^{3-}$], or ↓ plasma 1,25-(OH)$_2$ D$_3$. Causes ↑ [Ca^{2+}] reabsorption (DCT), ↓ [PO$_4$$^{3-}$] reabsorption (PCT), and ↑ 1,25-(OH)$_2$ D$_3$ production (↑ Ca^{2+} and PO$_4$$^{3-}$ absorption from gut via vitamin D).

Aldosterone
Secreted in response to ↓ blood volume (via AT II) and ↑ plasma [K$^+$]; causes ↑Na$^+$ reabsorption, ↑K$^+$ secretion, ↑ H$^+$ secretion.

ADH (vasopressin)
Secreted in response to ↑ plasma osmolarity and ↓ blood volume. Binds to receptors on principal cells, causing ↑ number of aquaporins and ↑ H$_2$O reabsorption.

Potassium shifts

SHIFTS K$^+$ INTO CELL (CAUSING HYPOKALEMIA)	SHIFTS K$^+$ OUT OF CELL (CAUSING HYPERKALEMIA)
	Digitalis (blocks Na$^+$/K$^+$ ATPase)
Hypo-osmolarity	HyperOsmolarity
	Lysis of cells (eg, crush injury, rhabdomyolysis, tumor lysis syndrome)
Alkalosis	Acidosis
β-adrenergic agonist (↑ Na$^+$/K$^+$ ATPase)	β-blocker
Insulin (↑ Na$^+$/K$^+$ ATPase)	High blood Sugar (insulin deficiency)
Insulin shifts K$^+$ into cells	Succinylcholine (↑ risk in burns/muscle trauma)
	Hyperkalemia? DO LAβSS

Electrolyte disturbances

ELECTROLYTE	LOW SERUM CONCENTRATION	HIGH SERUM CONCENTRATION
Na^+	Nausea and malaise, stupor, coma, seizures	Irritability, stupor, coma
K^+	U waves and flattened T waves on ECG, arrhythmias, muscle cramps, spasm, weakness	Wide QRS and peaked T waves on ECG, arrhythmias, muscle weakness
Ca^{2+}	Tetany, seizures, QT prolongation, twitching (Chvostek sign), spasm (Trousseau sign)	**Stones** (renal), **bones** (pain), **groans** (abdominal pain), **thrones** (↑ urinary frequency), **psychiatric overtones** (anxiety, altered mental status)
Mg^{2+}	Tetany, torsades de pointes, hypokalemia, hypocalcemia (when $[Mg^{2+}] < 1.2$ mg/dL)	↓ DTRs, lethargy, bradycardia, hypotension, cardiac arrest, hypocalcemia
PO_4^{3-}	Bone loss, osteomalacia (adults), rickets (children)	Renal stones, metastatic calcifications, hypocalcemia

Features of renal disorders

CONDITION	BLOOD PRESSURE	PLASMA RENIN	ALDOSTERONE	SERUM Mg^{2+}	URINE Ca^{2+}
Bartter syndrome	—	↑	↑		↑
Gitelman syndrome	—	↑	↑	↓	↓
Liddle syndrome, syndrome of apparent mineralocorticoid excess	↑	↓	↓		
SIADH	—/↑	↓	↓		
Primary hyperaldosteronism (Conn syndrome)	↑	↓	↑		
Renin-secreting tumor	↑	↑	↑		

↑ ↓ = important differentiating feature.

Acid-base physiology

	pH	Pco₂	[HCO₃⁻]	COMPENSATORY RESPONSE
Metabolic acidosis	↓	↓	↓	Hyperventilation (immediate)
Metabolic alkalosis	↑	↑	↑	Hypoventilation (immediate)
Respiratory acidosis	↓	↑	↑	↑ renal [HCO₃⁻] reabsorption (delayed)
Respiratory alkalosis	↑	↓	↓	↓ renal [HCO₃⁻] reabsorption (delayed)

Key: ↑ ↓ = 1° disturbance; ↓ ↑ = compensatory response.

Henderson-Hasselbalch equation: $pH = 6.1 + \log \dfrac{[HCO_3^-]}{0.03\ P_{CO_2}}$

Predicted respiratory compensation for a simple metabolic acidosis can be calculated using the Winters formula. If measured P_{CO_2} > predicted P_{CO_2} → concomitant respiratory acidosis; if measured P_{CO_2} < predicted P_{CO_2} → concomitant respiratory alkalosis:

$$P_{CO_2} = 1.5\ [HCO_3^-] + 8 \pm 2$$

Acidosis and alkalosis

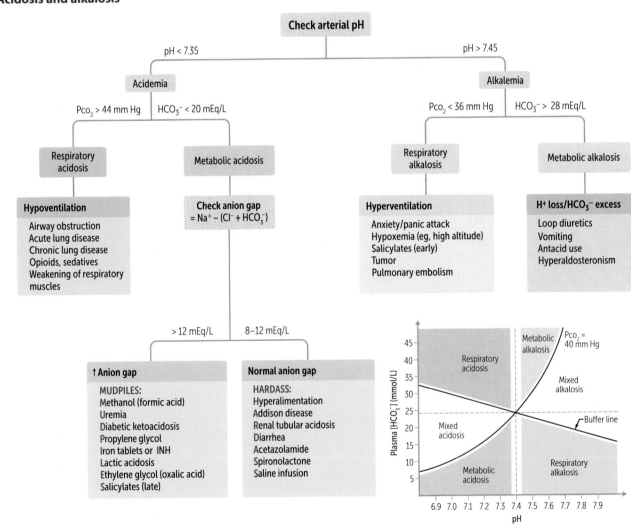

Renal tubular acidosis

Disorder of the renal tubules that causes normal anion gap (hyperchloremic) metabolic acidosis.

RTA TYPE	DEFECT	URINE PH	SERUM K$^+$	CAUSES	ASSOCIATIONS
Distal renal tubular acidosis (type 1)	Inability of α-intercalated cells to secrete H$^+$ → no new HCO$_3^-$ is generated → metabolic acidosis	> 5.5	↓	Amphotericin B toxicity, analgesic nephropathy, congenital anomalies (obstruction) of urinary tract, autoimmune diseases (eg, SLE)	↑ risk for calcium phosphate kidney stones (due to ↑ urine pH and ↑ bone turnover)
Proximal renal tubular acidosis (type 2)	Defect in PCT HCO$_3^-$ reabsorption → ↑ excretion of HCO$_3^-$ in urine → metabolic acidosis. Urine can be acidified by α-intercalated cells in collecting duct, but not enough to overcome the increased excretion of HCO$_3^-$ → metabolic acidosis	< 5.5	↓	Fanconi syndrome, multiple myeloma, carbonic anhydrase inhibitors	↑ risk for hypophosphatemic rickets (in Fanconi syndrome)
Hyperkalemic tubular acidosis (type 4)	Hypoaldosteronism or aldosterone resistance; hyperkalemia → ↓ NH$_3$ synthesis in PCT → ↓ NH$_4^+$ excretion	< 5.5 (or variable)	↑	↓ aldosterone production (eg, diabetic hyporeninism, ACE inhibitors, ARBs, NSAIDs, heparin, cyclosporine, adrenal insufficiency) or aldosterone resistance (eg, K$^+$-sparing diuretics, nephropathy due to obstruction, TMP-SMX)	

▶ RENAL—PATHOLOGY

Casts in urine	Presence of casts indicates that hematuria/pyuria is of glomerular or renal tubular origin. Bladder cancer, kidney stones → hematuria, no casts. Acute cystitis → pyuria, no casts.
RBC casts A	Glomerulonephritis, hypertensive emergency.
WBC casts B	Tubulointerstitial inflammation, acute pyelonephritis, transplant rejection.
Fatty casts ("oval fat bodies")	Nephrotic syndrome. Associated with "Maltese cross" sign.
Granular ("muddy brown") casts C	Acute tubular necrosis (ATN).
Waxy casts D	End-stage renal disease/chronic renal failure.
Hyaline casts E	Nonspecific, can be a normal finding, often seen in concentrated urine samples.

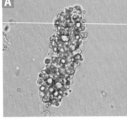 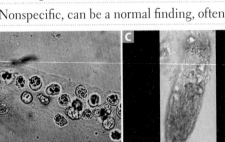 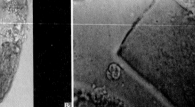 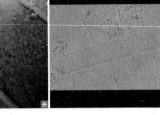

Nomenclature of glomerular disorders

TYPE	CHARACTERISTICS	EXAMPLE
Focal	< 50% of glomeruli are involved	Focal segmental glomerulosclerosis
Diffuse	> 50% of glomeruli are involved	Diffuse proliferative glomerulonephritis
Proliferative	Hypercellular glomeruli	Membranoproliferative glomerulonephritis
Membranous	Thickening of glomerular basement membrane (GBM)	Membranous nephropathy
Primary glomerular disease	1° disease of the kidney specifically impacting the glomeruli	Minimal change disease
Secondary glomerular disease	Systemic disease or disease of another organ system that also impacts the glomeruli	SLE, diabetic nephropathy

Glomerular diseases

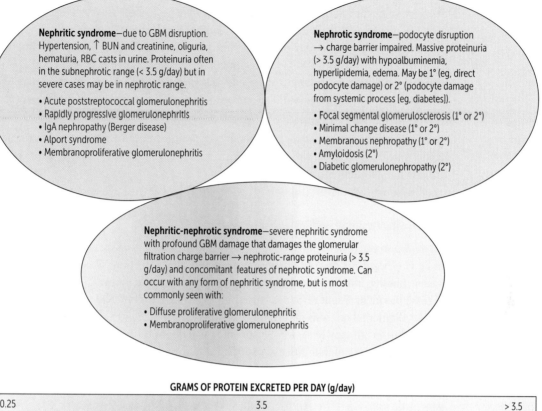

Nephritic syndrome—due to GBM disruption. Hypertension, ↑ BUN and creatinine, oliguria, hematuria, RBC casts in urine. Proteinuria often in the subnephrotic range (< 3.5 g/day) but in severe cases may be in nephrotic range.

- Acute poststreptococcal glomerulonephritis
- Rapidly progressive glomerulonephritis
- IgA nephropathy (Berger disease)
- Alport syndrome
- Membranoproliferative glomerulonephritis

Nephrotic syndrome—podocyte disruption → charge barrier impaired. Massive proteinuria (> 3.5 g/day) with hypoalbuminemia, hyperlipidemia, edema. May be 1° (eg, direct podocyte damage) or 2° (podocyte damage from systemic process [eg, diabetes]).

- Focal segmental glomerulosclerosis (1° or 2°)
- Minimal change disease (1° or 2°)
- Membranous nephropathy (1° or 2°)
- Amyloidosis (2°)
- Diabetic glomerulonephropathy (2°)

Nephritic-nephrotic syndrome—severe nephritic syndrome with profound GBM damage that damages the glomerular filtration charge barrier → nephrotic-range proteinuria (> 3.5 g/day) and concomitant features of nephrotic syndrome. Can occur with any form of nephritic syndrome, but is most commonly seen with:

- Diffuse proliferative glomerulonephritis
- Membranoproliferative glomerulonephritis

GRAMS OF PROTEIN EXCRETED PER DAY (g/day)

0.25	3.5	> 3.5

Nephrotic syndrome	NephrOtic syndrome—massive prOteinuria (> 3.5 g/day) with hypoalbuminemia, resulting edema, hyperlipidemia. Frothy urine with fatty casts. Disruption of glomerular filtration charge barrier may be 1° (eg, direct sclerosis of podocytes) or 2° (systemic process [eg, diabetes] secondarily damages podocytes). Severe nephritic syndrome may present with nephrotic syndrome features (nephritic-nephrotic syndrome) if damage to GBM is severe enough to damage charge barrier. Associated with hypercoagulable state due to antithrombin (AT) III loss in urine and ↑ risk of infection (loss of immunoglobulins in urine and soft tissue compromise by edema).
Minimal change disease (lipoid nephrosis)	Most common cause of nephrotic syndrome in children. Often 1° (idiopathic) and may be triggered by recent infection, immunization, immune stimulus. Rarely, may be 2° to lymphoma (eg, cytokine-mediated damage). 1° disease has excellent response to corticosteroids. ▪ LM—Normal glomeruli (lipid may be seen in PCT cells) ▪ IF—⊖ ▪ EM—effacement of podocyte foot processes **A**
Focal segmental glomerulosclerosis	Most common cause of nephrotic syndrome in African-Americans and Hispanics. Can be 1° (idiopathic) or 2° to other conditions (eg, HIV infection, sickle cell disease, heroin abuse, massive obesity, interferon treatment, or congenital malformations). 1° disease has inconsistent response to steroids. May progress to CKD. ▪ LM—segmental sclerosis and hyalinosis **B** ▪ IF—often ⊖ but may be ⊕ for nonspecific focal deposits of IgM, C3, C1 ▪ EM—effacement of foot processes similar to minimal change disease
Membranous nephropathy	Also known as membranous glomerulonephritis. Can be 1° (eg, antibodies to phospholipase A_2 receptor) or 2° to drugs (eg, NSAIDs, penicillamine, gold), infections (eg, HBV, HCV, syphilis), SLE, or solid tumors. 1° disease has poor response to steroids. May progress to CKD. ▪ LM—diffuse capillary and GBM thickening **C** ▪ IF—granular due to IC deposition ▪ EM—"Spike and dome" appearance of subepithelial deposits
Amyloidosis	Kidney is the most commonly involved organ (systemic amyloidosis). Associated with chronic conditions that predispose to amyloid deposition (eg, AL amyloid, AA amyloid). ▪ LM—Congo red stain shows apple-green birefringence under polarized light due to amyloid deposition in the mesangium
Diabetic glomerulo-nephropathy	Most common cause of ESRD in the United States. Hyperglycemia → nonenzymatic glycation of tissue proteins → mesangial expansion; GBM thickening and ↑ permeability. Hyperfiltration (glomerular HTN and ↑ GFR) → glomerular hypertrophy and glomerular scarring (glomerulosclerosis) leading to further progression of nephropathy. ▪ LM—Mesangial expansion, GBM thickening, eosinophilic nodular glomerulosclerosis (Kimmelstiel-Wilson lesions, arrows in **D**)

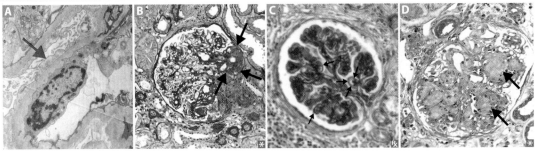

Nephritic syndrome	NephrItic syndrome = Inflammatory process. When glomeruli are involved, leads to hematuria and RBC casts in urine. Associated with azotemia, oliguria, hypertension (due to salt retention), proteinuria, hypercellular/inflamed glomeruli on biopsy.
Acute poststreptococcal glomerulonephritis	Most frequently seen in children. ~ 2–4 weeks after group A streptococcal infection of pharynx or skin. Resolves spontaneously in most children; may progress to renal insufficiency in adults. Type III hypersensitivity reaction. Presents with peripheral and periorbital edema, cola-colored urine, HTN. ⊕ strep titers/serologies, ↓ complement levels (C3) due to consumption. <ul><li>LM—glomeruli enlarged and hypercellular **A**</li><li>IF—("starry sky") granular appearance ("lumpy-bumpy") **B** due to IgG, IgM, and C3 deposition along GBM and mesangium</li><li>EM—subepithelial immune complex (IC) humps</li></ul>
Rapidly progressive (crescentic) glomerulonephritis	Poor prognosis, rapidly deteriorating renal function (days to weeks). <ul><li>LM—crescent moon shape **C**. Crescents consist of fibrin and plasma proteins (eg, C3b) with glomerular parietal cells, monocytes, macrophages</li></ul> Several disease processes may result in this pattern which may be delineated via IF pattern. <ul><li>Linear IF due to antibodies to GBM and alveolar basement membrane: **Goodpasture syndrome**—hematuria/hemoptysis; type II hypersensitivity reaction; Treatment: plasmapheresis</li><li>Negative IF/Pauci-immune (no Ig/C3 deposition): **Granulomatosis with polyangiitis (Wegener)**—PR3-ANCA/c-ANCA or **Microscopic polyangiitis**—MPO-ANCA/p-ANCA</li><li>Granular IF—PSGN or DPGN</li></ul>
Diffuse proliferative glomerulonephritis	Often due to SLE (think "wire lupus"). DPGN and MPGN often present as nephrotic syndrome and nephritic syndrome concurrently. <ul><li>LM—"wire looping" of capillaries</li><li>IF—granular; EM—subendothelial and sometimes intramembranous IgG-based ICs often with C3 deposition</li></ul>
IgA nephropathy (Berger disease)	Episodic hematuria that occurs concurrently with respiratory or GI tract infections (IgA is secreted by mucosal linings). Renal pathology of IgA vasculitis (HSP). <ul><li>LM—mesangial proliferation</li><li>IF—IgA-based IC deposits in mesangium; EM—mesangial IC deposition</li></ul>
Alport syndrome	Mutation in type IV collagen → thinning and splitting of glomerular basement membrane. Most commonly X-linked dominant. Eye problems (eg, retinopathy, lens dislocation), glomerulonephritis, sensorineural deafness; "can't see, can't pee, can't hear a bee." <ul><li>EM—"Basket-weave"</li></ul>
Membrano-proliferative glomerulonephritis	MPGN is a nephritic syndrome that often co-presents with nephrotic syndrome. Type I may be 2° to hepatitis B or C infection. May also be idiopathic. <ul><li>Subendothelial IC deposits with granular IF</li></ul> Type II is associated with C3 nephritic factor (IgG antibody that stabilizes C3 convertase → persistent complement activation → ↓ C3 levels). <ul><li>Intramembranous deposits, also called dense deposit disease</li></ul> In both types, mesangial ingrowth → GBM splitting → "tram-track" appearance on H&E **D** and PAS **E** stains.

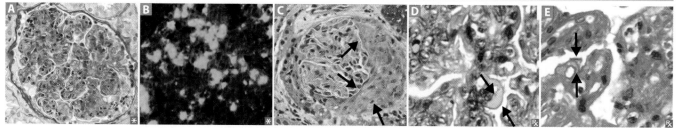

Kidney stones					
Can lead to severe complications such as hydronephrosis, pyelonephritis. Obstructed stone presents with unilateral flank tenderness, colicky pain radiating to groin, hematuria. Treat and prevent by encouraging fluid intake.
Most common kidney stone presentation: calcium oxalate stone in patient with hypercalciuria and normocalcemia.

CONTENT	PRECIPITATES WITH	X-RAY FINDINGS	CT FINDINGS	URINE CRYSTAL	NOTES
Calcium	Calcium oxalate: hypocitraturia	Radiopaque	Radiopaque	Shaped like envelope **A** or dumbbell	Calcium stones most common (80%); calcium oxalate more common than calcium phosphate stones. Hypocitraturia often associated with ↓ urine pH. Can result from ethylene glycol (antifreeze) ingestion, vitamin C abuse, hypocitraturia, malabsorption (eg, Crohn disease). Treatment: thiazides, citrate, low-sodium diet.
	Calcium phosphate: ↑ pH	Radiopaque	Radiopaque	Wedge-shaped prism	Treatment: low-sodium diet, thiazides.
Ammonium magnesium phosphate	↑ pH	Radiopaque	Radiopaque	Coffin lid **B**	Also known as struvite; account for 15% of stones. Caused by infection with urease ⊕ bugs (eg, *Proteus mirabilis*, *Staphylococcus saprophyticus*, *Klebsiella*) that hydrolyze urea to ammonia → urine alkalinization. Commonly form staghorn calculi **C**. Treatment: eradication of underlying infection, surgical removal of stone.
Uric acid	↓ pH	RadiolUcent	Minimally visible	Rhomboid **D** or rosettes	About 5% of all stones. Risk factors: ↓ urine volume, arid climates, acidic pH. Strong association with hyperuricemia (eg, gout). Often seen in diseases with ↑ cell turnover (eg, leukemia). Treatment: alkalinization of urine, allopurinol.
Cystine	↓ pH	Faintly radi-opaque	Moderately radiopaque	Hexagonal **E**	Hereditary (autosomal recessive) condition in which Cystine-reabsorbing PCT transporter loses function, causing cystinuria. Transporter defect also results in poor reabsorption of Ornithine, Lysine, Arginine (**COLA**). Cystine is poorly soluble, thus stones form in urine. Usually begins in childhood. Can form staghorn calculi. Sodium cyanide nitroprusside test ⊕. "SIXtine" stones have SIX sides. Treatment: low sodium diet, alkalinization of urine, chelating agents if refractory.

Hydronephrosis

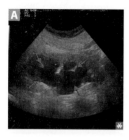

Distention/dilation of renal pelvis and calyces **A**. Usually caused by urinary tract obstruction (eg, renal stones, severe BPH, congenital obstructions, cervical cancer, injury to ureter); other causes include retroperitoneal fibrosis, vesicoureteral reflux. Dilation occurs proximal to site of pathology. Serum creatinine becomes elevated if obstruction is bilateral or if patient has an obstructed solitary kidney. Leads to compression and possible atrophy of renal cortex and medulla.

Renal cell carcinoma

Polygonal clear cells **A** filled with accumulated lipids and carbohydrate. Often golden-yellow **B** due to ↑ lipid content.

Originates from PCT → invades renal vein (may develop varicocele if left sided) → IVC → hematogenous spread → metastasis to lung and bone.

Manifests with hematuria, palpable masses, 2° polycythemia, flank pain, fever, weight loss.

Treatment: surgery/ablation for localized disease. Immunotherapy (eg, aldesleukin) or targeted therapy for metastatic disease, rarely curative. Resistant to chemotherapy and radiation therapy.

Most common 1° renal malignancy **C**.

Most common in men 50–70 years old, ↑ incidence with smoking and obesity.

Associated with paraneoplastic syndromes ("**PEAR**"-aneoplastic), eg, **P**THrP, **E**ctopic EPO, **A**CTH, **R**enin).

Associated with gene deletion on chromosome 3 (sporadic, or inherited as von Hippel-Lindau syndrome).

RCC = 3 letters = chromosome 3.

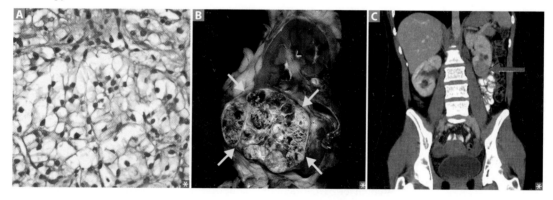

Renal oncocytoma

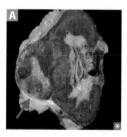

Benign epithelial cell tumor arising from collecting ducts (arrows in **A** point to well-circumscribed mass with central scar). Large eosinophilic cells with abundant mitochondria without perinuclear clearing **B** (vs chromophobe renal cell carcinoma). Presents with painless hematuria, flank pain, abdominal mass.

Often resected to exclude malignancy (eg, renal cell carcinoma).

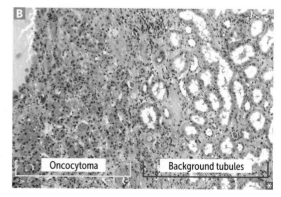

Oncocytoma   Background tubules

Nephroblastoma (Wilms tumor)

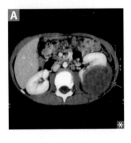

Most common renal malignancy of early childhood (ages 2–4). Contains embryonic glomerular structures. Presents with large, palpable, unilateral flank mass A and/or hematuria.

"Loss of function" mutations of tumor suppressor genes *WT1* or *WT2* on chromosome 11.

May be a part of several syndromes:

- **WAGR** complex: Wilms tumor, Aniridia (absence of iris), Genitourinary malformations, mental Retardation/intellectual disability (*WT1* deletion)
- **Denys-Drash** syndrome—Wilms tumor, Diffuse mesangial sclerosis (early-onset nephrotic syndrome), Dysgenesis of gonads (male pseudohermaphroditism), *WT1* mutation
- Beckwith-Wiedemann syndrome—Wilms tumor, macroglossia, organomegaly, hemihyperplasia (*WT2* mutation)

Transitional cell carcinoma

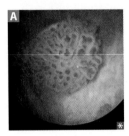

Also known as urothelial carcinoma. Most common tumor of urinary tract system (can occur in renal calyces, renal pelvis, ureters, and bladder) A B. Can be suggested by painless hematuria (no casts).

Associated with problems in your Pee SAC: Phenacetin, Smoking, Aniline dyes, and Cyclophosphamide.

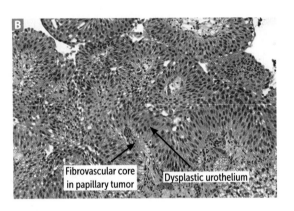

Fibrovascular core in papillary tumor   Dysplastic urothelium

Squamous cell carcinoma of the bladder

Chronic irritation of urinary bladder → squamous metaplasia → dysplasia and squamous cell carcinoma.

Risk factors include *Schistosoma haematobium* infection (Middle East), chronic cystitis, smoking, chronic nephrolithiasis. Presents with painless hematuria.

Urinary incontinence

Stress incontinence	Outlet incompetence (urethral hypermobility or intrinsic sphincteric deficiency) → leak with ↑ intra-abdominal pressure (eg, sneezing, lifting). ↑ risk with obesity, vaginal delivery, prostate surgery. ⊕ bladder stress test (directly observed leakage from urethra upon coughing or Valsalva maneuver). Treatment: pelvic floor muscle strengthening (Kegel) exercises, weight loss, pessaries.
Urgency incontinence	Overactive bladder (detrusor instability) → leak with urge to void immediately. Associated with UTI. Treatment: Kegel exercises, bladder training (timed voiding, distraction or relaxation techniques), antimuscarinics (eg, oxybutynin).
Mixed incontinence	Features of both stress and urgency incontinence.
Overflow incontinence	Incomplete emptying (detrusor underactivity or outlet obstruction) → leak with overfilling. Associated with polyuria (eg, diabetes), bladder outlet obstruction (eg, BPH), neurogenic bladder (eg, MS). ↑ post-void residual (urinary retention) on catheterization or ultrasound. Treatment: catheterization, relieve obstruction (eg, α-blockers for BPH).

Urinary tract infection (acute bacterial cystitis)	Inflammation of urinary bladder. Presents as suprapubic pain, dysuria, urinary frequency, urgency. Systemic signs (eg, high fever, chills) are usually absent.

Risk factors include female gender (short urethra), sexual intercourse ("honeymoon cystitis"), indwelling catheter, diabetes mellitus, impaired bladder emptying.

Causes:
- *E coli* (most common).
- *Staphylococcus saprophyticus*—seen in sexually active young women (*E coli* is still more common in this group).
- *Klebsiella*.
- *Proteus mirabilis*—urine has ammonia scent.

Lab findings: ⊕ leukocyte esterase. ⊕ nitrites (indicate gram ⊖ organisms). Sterile pyuria and ⊖ urine cultures suggest urethritis by *Neisseria gonorrhoeae* or *Chlamydia trachomatis*.

Pyelonephritis

Acute pyelonephritis

Neutrophils infiltrate renal interstitium A. Affects cortex with relative sparing of glomeruli/vessels. Presents with fevers, flank pain (costovertebral angle tenderness), nausea/vomiting, chills.

Causes include ascending UTI (*E coli* is most common), hematogenous spread to kidney. Presents with WBCs in urine +/– WBC casts. CT would show striated parenchymal enhancement B.

Risk factors include indwelling urinary catheter, urinary tract obstruction, vesicoureteral reflux, diabetes mellitus, pregnancy.

Complications include chronic pyelonephritis, renal papillary necrosis, perinephric abscess, urosepsis.

Treatment: antibiotics.

Chronic pyelonephritis

The result of recurrent episodes of acute pyelonephritis. Typically requires predisposition to infection such as vesicoureteral reflux or chronically obstructing kidney stones.

Coarse, asymmetric corticomedullary scarring, blunted calyx. Tubules can contain eosinophilic casts resembling thyroid tissue C (thyroidization of kidney).

Xanthogranulomatous pyelonephritis—rare; grossly orange nodules that can mimic tumor nodules; characterized by widespread kidney damage due to granulomatous tissue containing foamy macrophages. Associated with *Proteus* infection.

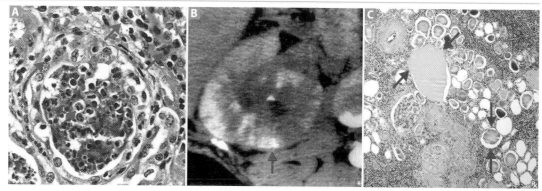

Acute kidney injury	Formerly known as acute renal failure. Acute kidney injury is defined as an abrupt decline in renal function as measured by ↑ creatinine and ↑ BUN or by oliguria/anuria.	
Prerenal azotemia	Due to ↓ RBF (eg, hypotension) → ↓ GFR. Na^+/H_2O and urea retained by kidney in an attempt to conserve volume → ↑ BUN/creatinine ratio (urea is reabsorbed, creatinine is not) and ↓ FE_{Na}.	
Intrinsic renal failure	Most commonly due to acute tubular necrosis (from ischemia or toxins); less commonly due to acute glomerulonephritis (eg, RPGN, hemolytic uremic syndrome) or acute interstitial nephritis. In ATN, patchy necrosis → debris obstructing tubule and fluid backflow across necrotic tubule → ↓ GFR. Urine has epithelial/granular casts. Urea reabsorption is impaired → ↓ BUN/creatinine ratio and ↑ FE_{Na}.	
Postrenal azotemia	Due to outflow obstruction (stones, BPH, neoplasia, congenital anomalies). Develops only with bilateral obstruction or in a solitary kidney.	

	Prerenal	Intrinsic renal	Postrenal
Urine osmolality (mOsm/kg)	> 500	< 350	< 350
Urine Na^+ (mEq/L)	< 20	> 40	Varies
FE_{Na}	< 1%	> 2%	Varies
Serum BUN/Cr	> 20	< 15	Varies

Consequences of renal failure	Decline in renal filtration can lead to excess retained nitrogenous waste products and electrolyte disturbances.
	Consequences (**MAD HUNGER**):
	▪ Metabolic Acidosis
	▪ Dyslipidemia (especially ↑ triglycerides)
	▪ Hyperkalemia
	▪ Uremia—clinical syndrome marked by:
	  ▪ Nausea and anorexia
	  ▪ Pericarditis
	  ▪ Asterixis
	  ▪ Encephalopathy
	  ▪ Platelet dysfunction
	▪ Na^+/H_2O retention (HF, pulmonary edema, hypertension)
	▪ Growth retardation and developmental delay
	▪ Erythropoietin failure (anemia)
	▪ Renal osteodystrophy
		2 forms of renal failure: acute (eg, ATN) and chronic (eg, hypertension, diabetes mellitus, congenital anomalies).

Renal osteodystrophy	Hypocalcemia, hyperphosphatemia, and failure of vitamin D hydroxylation associated with chronic renal disease → 2° hyperparathyroidism. High serum phosphate can bind with Ca^{2+} → tissue deposits → ↓ serum Ca^{2+}. ↓ 1,25-$(OH)_2D_3$ → ↓ intestinal Ca^{2+} absorption. Causes subperiosteal thinning of bones.	

Acute interstitial nephritis (tubulointerstitial nephritis)	Acute interstitial renal inflammation. Pyuria (classically eosinophils) and azotemia occurring after administration of drugs that act as haptens, inducing hypersensitivity (eg, diuretics, penicillin derivatives, proton pump inhibitors, sulfonamides, rifampin, NSAIDs). Less commonly may be 2° to other processes such as systemic infections (eg, *Mycoplasma*) or autoimmune diseases (eg, Sjögren syndrome, SLE, sarcoidosis).	Associated with fever, rash, hematuria, pyuria, and costovertebral angle tenderness, but can be asymptomatic. Remember these P's: ▪ Pee (diuretics) ▪ Pain-free (NSAIDs) ▪ Penicillins and cephalosporins ▪ Proton pump inhibitors ▪ RifamPin

Acute tubular necrosis

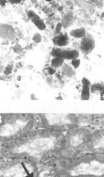

Most common cause of acute kidney injury in hospitalized patients. Spontaneously resolves in many cases. Can be fatal, especially during initial oliguric phase. ↑ FE_{Na}.

Key finding: granular ("muddy brown") casts A.

3 stages:

1. Inciting event
2. Maintenance phase—oliguric; lasts 1–3 weeks; risk of hyperkalemia, metabolic acidosis, uremia
3. Recovery phase—polyuric; BUN and serum creatinine fall; risk of hypokalemia and renal wasting of other electrolytes and minerals

Can be caused by ischemic or nephrotoxic injury:

▪ Ischemic—2° to ↓ renal blood flow (eg, hypotension, shock, sepsis, hemorrhage, HF). Results in death of tubular cells that may slough into tubular lumen B (PCT and thick ascending limb are highly susceptible to injury).

▪ Nephrotoxic—2° to injury resulting from toxic substances (eg, aminoglycosides, radiocontrast agents, lead, cisplatin, ethylene glycol), crush injury (myoglobinuria), hemoglobinuria. Proximal tubules are particularly susceptible to injury.

Diffuse cortical necrosis	Acute generalized cortical infarction of both kidneys. Likely due to a combination of vasospasm and DIC.	Associated with obstetric catastrophes (eg, abruptio placentae), septic shock.

Renal papillary necrosis

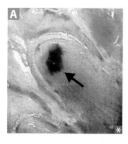

Sloughing of necrotic renal papillae A → gross hematuria and proteinuria. May be triggered by recent infection or immune stimulus. Associated with sickle cell disease or trait, acute pyelonephritis, NSAIDs, diabetes mellitus.

SAAD papa with papillary necrosis:
Sickle cell disease or trait
Acute pyelonephritis
Analgesics (NSAIDs)
Diabetes mellitus

Renal cyst disorders

Autosomal dominant polycystic kidney disease	Numerous cysts in cortex and medulla **A** causing bilateral enlarged kidneys ultimately destroy kidney parenchyma. Presents with flank pain, hematuria, hypertension, urinary infection, progressive renal failure in ~ 50% of individuals. Mutation in *PKD1* (85% of cases, chromosome 16) or *PKD2* (15% of cases, chromosome 4). Death from complications of chronic kidney disease or hypertension (caused by ↑ renin production). Associated with berry aneurysms, mitral valve prolapse, benign hepatic cysts, diverticulosis. Treatment: If hypertension or proteinuria develops, treat with ACE inhibitors or ARBs.
Autosomal recessive polycystic kidney disease	Cystic dilation of collecting ducts **B**. Often presents in infancy. Associated with congenital hepatic fibrosis. Significant oliguric renal failure in utero can lead to Potter sequence. Concerns beyond neonatal period include systemic hypertension, progressive renal insufficiency, and portal hypertension from congenital hepatic fibrosis.
Autosomal dominant tubulointerstitial kidney disease	Also known as medullary cystic kidney disease. Inherited disease causing tubulointerstitial fibrosis and progressive renal insufficiency with inability to concentrate urine. Medullary cysts usually not visualized; smaller kidneys on ultrasound. Poor prognosis.
Simple vs complex renal cysts	Simple cysts are filled with ultrafiltrate (anechoic on ultrasound **C**). Very common and account for majority of all renal masses. Found incidentally and typically asymptomatic. Complex cysts, including those that are septated, enhanced, or have solid components on imaging require follow-up or removal due to risk of renal cell carcinoma.

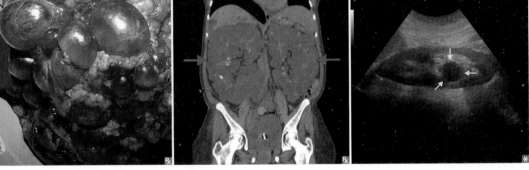

▶ RENAL—PHARMACOLOGY

Diuretics site of action

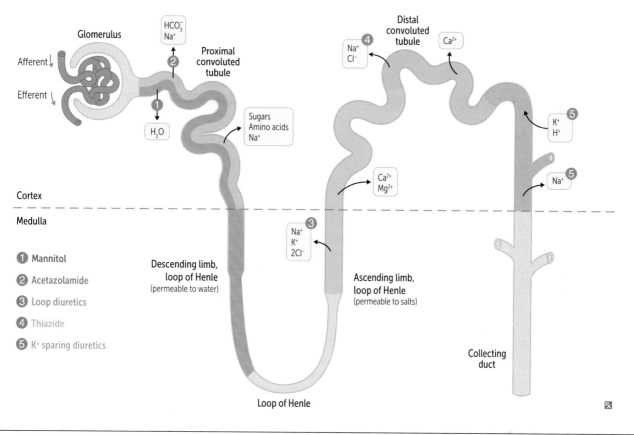

Afferent

Efferent

Glomerulus

Proximal convoluted tubule

HCO_3^-
Na^+

②

①

H_2O

Sugars
Amino acids
Na^+

Distal convoluted tubule

Na^+
Cl^-

④

Ca^{2+}

K^+
H^+

⑤

Ca^{2+}
Mg^{2+}

Na^+

⑤

Cortex

Medulla

Na^+
K^+
$2Cl^-$

③

① Mannitol

② Acetazolamide

③ Loop diuretics

④ Thiazide

⑤ K^+ sparing diuretics

Descending limb,
loop of Henle
(permeable to water)

Ascending limb,
loop of Henle
(permeable to salts)

Collecting
duct

Loop of Henle

℞

Mannitol

MECHANISM	Osmotic diuretic. ↑ tubular fluid osmolarity → ↑ urine flow, ↓ intracranial/intraocular pressure.
CLINICAL USE	Drug overdose, elevated intracranial/intraocular pressure.
ADVERSE EFFECTS	Pulmonary edema, dehydration, hypo- or hypernatremia. Contraindicated in anuria, HF.

Acetazolamide

MECHANISM	Carbonic anhydrase inhibitor. Causes self-limited $NaHCO_3$ diuresis and ↓ total body HCO_3^- stores.	
CLINICAL USE	Glaucoma, metabolic alkalosis, altitude sickness, pseudotumor cerebri. Alkalinizes urine.	
ADVERSE EFFECTS	Proximal renal tubular acidosis, paresthesias, NH_3 toxicity, sulfa allergy, hypokalemia. Promotes calcium phosphate stone formation (insoluble at high pH).	"ACID"azolamide causes ACIDosis.

Loop diuretics

Furosemide, bumetanide, torsemide

MECHANISM	Sulfonamide loop diuretics. Inhibit cotransport system ($Na^+/K^+/2Cl^-$) of thick ascending limb of loop of Henle. Abolish hypertonicity of medulla, preventing concentration of urine. Stimulate PGE release (vasodilatory effect on afferent arteriole); inhibited by NSAIDs. ↑ Ca^{2+} excretion. Loops Lose Ca^{2+}.	
CLINICAL USE	Edematous states (HF, cirrhosis, nephrotic syndrome, pulmonary edema), hypertension, hypercalcemia.	
ADVERSE EFFECTS	Ototoxicity, Hypokalemia, Hypomagnesemia, Dehydration, Allergy (sulfa), metabolic Alkalosis, Nephritis (interstitial), Gout.	OHH DAANG!

Ethacrynic acid

MECHANISM	Nonsulfonamide inhibitor of cotransport system ($Na^+/K^+/2Cl^-$) of thick ascending limb of loop of Henle.	
CLINICAL USE	Diuresis in patients allergic to sulfa drugs.	
ADVERSE EFFECTS	Similar to furosemide, but more ototoxic.	Loop earrings hurt your ears.

Thiazide diuretics	Hydrochlorothiazide, chlorthalidone, metolazone.	
MECHANISM	Inhibit NaCl reabsorption in early DCT → ↓ diluting capacity of nephron. ↓ Ca^{2+} excretion.	
CLINICAL USE	Hypertension, HF, idiopathic hypercalciuria, nephrogenic diabetes insipidus, osteoporosis.	HyperGLUC.
ADVERSE EFFECTS	Hypokalemic metabolic alkalosis, hyponatremia, hyperGlycemia, hyperLipidemia, hyperUricemia, hyperCalcemia. Sulfa allergy.	

Potassium-sparing diuretics	Spironolactone, Eplerenone, Amiloride, Triamterene.	TaKe a SEAT.
MECHANISM	Spironolactone and eplerenone are competitive aldosterone receptor antagonists in cortical collecting tubule. Triamterene and amiloride act at the same part of the tubule by blocking Na^+ channels in the cortical collecting tubule.	
CLINICAL USE	Hyperaldosteronism, K^+ depletion, HF, hepatic ascites (spironolactone), nephrogenic DI (amiloride), antiandrogen.	
ADVERSE EFFECTS	Hyperkalemia (can lead to arrhythmias), endocrine effects with spironolactone (eg, gynecomastia, antiandrogen effects).	

Diuretics: electrolyte changes

Urine NaCl	↑ with all diuretics (strength varies based on potency of diuretic effect). Serum NaCl may decrease as a result.
Urine K^+	↑ especially with loop and thiazide diuretics. Serum K^+ may decrease as a result.
Blood pH	↓ (**acidemia**): carbonic anhydrase inhibitors: ↓ HCO_3^- reabsorption. K^+ sparing: aldosterone blockade prevents K^+ secretion and H^+ secretion. Additionally, hyperkalemia leads to K^+ entering all cells (via H^+/K^+ exchanger) in exchange for H^+ exiting cells. ↑ (**alkalemia**): loop diuretics and thiazides cause alkalemia through several mechanisms: ▪ Volume contraction → ↑ AT II → ↑ Na^+/H^+ exchange in PCT → ↑ HCO_3^- reabsorption ("contraction alkalosis") ▪ K^+ loss leads to K^+ exiting all cells (via H^+/K^+ exchanger) in exchange for H^+ entering cells ▪ In low K^+ state, H^+ (rather than K^+) is exchanged for Na^+ in cortical collecting tubule → alkalosis and "paradoxical aciduria"
Urine Ca^{2+}	↑ with loop diuretics: ↓ paracellular Ca^{2+} reabsorption → hypocalcemia. ↓ with thiazides: enhanced Ca^{2+} reabsorption.

Angiotensin-converting enzyme inhibitors	Captopril, enalapril, lisinopril, ramipril.	
MECHANISM	Inhibit ACE → ↓ AT II → ↓ GFR by preventing constriction of efferent arterioles. ↑ renin due to loss of negative feedback. Inhibition of ACE also prevents inactivation of bradykinin, a potent vasodilator.	
CLINICAL USE	Hypertension, HF (↓ mortality), proteinuria, diabetic nephropathy. Prevent unfavorable heart remodeling as a result of chronic hypertension.	In chronic kidney disease (eg, diabetic nephropathy), ↓ intraglomerular pressure, slowing GBM thickening.
ADVERSE EFFECTS	Cough, Angioedema (both due to ↑ bradykinin; contraindicated in C1 esterase inhibitor deficiency), Teratogen (fetal renal malformations), ↑ Creatinine (↓ GFR), Hyperkalemia, and Hypotension. Used with caution in bilateral renal artery stenosis because ACE inhibitors will further ↓ GFR → renal failure.	Captopril's CATCHH.

Angiotensin II receptor blockers	Losartan, candesartan, valsartan.
MECHANISM	Selectively block binding of angiotensin II to AT_1 receptor. Effects similar to ACE inhibitors, but ARBs do not increase bradykinin.
CLINICAL USE	Hypertension, HF, proteinuria, or chronic kidney disease (eg, diabetic nephropathy) with intolerance to ACE inhibitors (eg, cough, angioedema).
ADVERSE EFFECTS	Hyperkalemia, ↓ GFR, hypotension; teratogen.

Aliskiren	
MECHANISM	Direct renin inhibitor, blocks conversion of angiotensinogen to angiotensin I.
CLINICAL USE	Hypertension.
ADVERSE EFFECTS	Hyperkalemia, ↓ GFR, hypotension, angioedema. Relatively contraindicated in patients already taking ACE inhibitors or ARBs and contraindicated in pregnancy.

Reproductive

> *"Artificial insemination is when the farmer does it to the cow instead of the bull."*
>
> —Student essay

> *"Whoever called it necking was a poor judge of anatomy."*
>
> —Groucho Marx

> *"See, the problem is that God gives men a brain and a penis, and only enough blood to run one at a time."*
>
> —Robin Williams

> *"I think you can say that life is a system in which proteins and nucleic acids interact in ways that allow the structure to grow and reproduce. It's that growth and reproduction, the ability to make more of yourself, that's important."*
>
> —Andrew H. Knoll

The reproductive system can be intimidating at first but is manageable once you organize the concepts into the pregnancy, endocrinologic, embryologic, and oncologic aspects of reproduction. Study the endocrine and reproductive chapters together, because mastery of the hypothalamic-pituitary-gonadal axis is key to answering questions on ovulation, menstruation, disorders of sexual development, contraception, and many pathologies.

Embryology is a nuanced subject that covers multiple organ systems. Approaching it from a clinical perspective will allow for better understanding. For instance, make the connection between the presentation of DiGeorge syndrome and the 3rd/4th branchial pouch, and between the Müllerian/Wolffian systems and disorders of sexual development.

As for oncology, don't worry about remembering screening or treatment guidelines. It is more important to know how these cancers present (eg, hormonal derangements, signs, and symptoms), their histologic pathology, and their underlying risk factors. In addition, some of the testicular and ovarian cancers have distinct patterns of hCG, AFP, LH, or FSH derangement that make good clues in exam questions.

▶ REPRODUCTIVE—EMBRYOLOGY

Important genes of embryogenesis

Sonic hedgehog gene	Produced at base of limbs in zone of polarizing activity. Involved in patterning along anteroposterior axis and CNS development; mutation can cause holoprosencephaly.
Wnt-7 gene	Produced at apical ectodermal ridge (thickened ectoderm at distal end of each developing limb). Necessary for proper organization along dorsal-ventral axis.
Fibroblast growth factor (*FGF*) gene	Produced at apical ectodermal ridge. Stimulates mitosis of underlying mesoderm, providing for lengthening of limbs. "Look at that Fetus, Growing Fingers."
Homeobox (Hox) genes	Involved in segmental organization of embryo in a craniocaudal direction. Code for transcription factors. Hox mutations → appendages in wrong locations.

Early fetal development

Early embryonic development		
Within week 1	hCG secretion begins around the time of implantation of blastocyst.	Blastocyst "sticks" at day 6.
Within week 2	Bilaminar disc (epiblast, hypoblast).	2 weeks = 2 layers.
Within week 3	Gastrulation forms trilaminar embryonic disc. Cells from epiblast invaginate → primitive streak → endoderm, mesoderm, ectoderm. Notochord arises from midline mesoderm; overlying ectoderm becomes neural plate.	3 weeks = 3 layers.
Weeks 3–8 (embryonic period)	Neural tube formed by neuroectoderm and closes by week 4. Organogenesis.	Extremely susceptible to teratogens.
Week 4	Heart begins to beat. Upper and lower limb buds begin to form.	4 weeks = 4 limbs and 4 heart chambers.
Week 6	Fetal cardiac activity visible by transvaginal ultrasound.	
Week 8	Fetal movements start.	Gait at week 8.
Week 10	Genitalia have male/female characteristics.	Tenitalia

Embryologic derivatives

Ectoderm		External/outer layer
Surface ectoderm	Epidermis; adenohypophysis (from Rathke pouch); lens of eye; epithelial linings of oral cavity, sensory organs of ear, and olfactory epithelium; anal canal below the pectinate line; parotid, sweat, mammary glands.	Craniopharyngioma—benign Rathke pouch tumor with cholesterol crystals, calcifications.
Neural tube	Brain (neurohypophysis, CNS neurons, oligo-dendrocytes, astrocytes, ependymal cells, pineal gland), retina, spinal cord.	Neuroectoderm—think CNS.
Neural crest	Melanocytes, Myenteric (Auerbach) plexus, Odontoblasts, Endocardial cushions, Laryngeal cartilage, Parafollicular (C) cells of the thyroid, PNS (dorsal root ganglia, cranial nerves, autonomic ganglia), Adrenal medulla and all ganglia, Spiral membrane (aorticopulmonary septum), Schwann cells, pia and arachnoid, bones of skull.	**MMOtEL PPASS** Neural crest—think PNS and non-neural structures nearby.
Mesoderm	Muscle, bone, connective tissue, serous linings of body cavities (eg, peritoneum, pericardium, pleura), spleen (derived from foregut mesentery), cardiovascular structures, lymphatics, blood, wall of gut tube, upper vagina, kidneys, adrenal cortex, dermis, testes, ovaries. Notochord induces ectoderm to form neuroectoderm (neural plate); its only postnatal derivative is the nucleus pulposus of the intervertebral disc.	Middle/"meat" layer. Mesodermal defects = **VACTERL**: Vertebral defects Anal atresia Cardiac defects Tracheo-Esophageal fistula Renal defects Limb defects (bone and muscle)
Endoderm	Gut tube epithelium (including anal canal above the pectinate line), most of urethra and lower vagina (derived from urogenital sinus), luminal epithelial derivatives (eg, lungs, liver, gallbladder, pancreas, eustachian tube, thymus, parathyroid, thyroid follicular cells).	"Enternal" layer.

Types of errors in morphogenesis

Agenesis	Absent organ due to absent primordial tissue.
Aplasia	Absent organ despite presence of primordial tissue.
Hypoplasia	Incomplete organ development; primordial tissue present.
Disruption	2° breakdown of previously normal tissue or structure (eg, amniotic band syndrome).
Deformation	Extrinsic disruption; occurs after embryonic period.
Malformation	Intrinsic disruption; occurs during embryonic period (weeks 3–8).
Sequence	Abnormalities result from a single 1° embryologic event (eg, oligohydramnios → Potter sequence).

Teratogens   Most susceptible in 3rd–8th weeks (embryonic period—organogenesis) of pregnancy. Before week 3, "all-or-none" effects. After week 8, growth and function affected.

TERATOGEN	EFFECTS ON FETUS	NOTES
Medications		
ACE inhibitors	Renal damage	
Alkylating agents	Absence of digits, multiple anomalies	
Aminoglycosides	Ototoxicity	A mean guy hit the baby in the ear.
Antiepileptic drugs	Neural tube defects, cardiac defects, cleft palate, skeletal abnormalities (eg, phalanx/nail hypoplasia, facial dysmorphism)	High-dose folate supplementation recommended. Most commonly valproate, carbamazepine, phenytoin, phenobarbital.
Diethylstilbestrol	Vaginal clear cell adenocarcinoma, congenital Müllerian anomalies	
Folate antagonists	Neural tube defects	Includes trimethoprim, methotrexate, antiepileptic drugs.
Isotretinoin	Multiple severe birth defects	Contraception mandatory. IsoTERATinoin.
Lithium	Ebstein anomaly (apical displacement of tricuspid valve)	
Methimazole	Aplasia cutis congenita	
Tetracyclines	Discolored teeth, inhibited bone growth	"Teethracyclines."
Thalidomide	Limb defects (phocomelia, micromelia— "flipper" limbs)	Limb defects with "tha-limb-domide."
Warfarin	Bone deformities, fetal hemorrhage, abortion, ophthalmologic abnormalities	Do not wage **warfare** on the baby; keep it heppy with **heparin** (does not cross placenta).
Substance abuse		
Alcohol	Common cause of birth defects and intellectual disability; fetal alcohol syndrome	
Cocaine	Low birth weight, preterm birth, IUGR, placental abruption	Cocaine → vasoconstriction.
Smoking (nicotine, CO)	Low birth weight (leading cause in developed countries), preterm labor, placental problems, IUGR, SIDS, ADHD	Nicotine → vasoconstriction. CO → impaired O_2 delivery.
Other		
Iodine (lack or excess)	Congenital goiter or hypothyroidism (cretinism)	
Maternal diabetes	Caudal regression syndrome (anal atresia to sirenomelia), congenital heart defects (eg, VSD, transposition of the great vessels), neural tube defects, macrosomia, neonatal hypoglycemia, polycythemia	
Methylmercury	Neurotoxicity	Highest in swordfish, shark, tilefish, king mackerel.
Vitamin A excess	Extremely high risk for spontaneous abortions and birth defects (cleft palate, cardiac)	
X-rays	Microcephaly, intellectual disability	Minimized by lead shielding.

Fetal alcohol syndrome	Leading cause of intellectual disability in the US. Newborns of alcohol-consuming mothers have ↑ incidence of congenital abnormalities, including pre- and postnatal developmental retardation, microcephaly, facial abnormalities 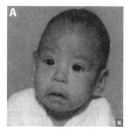 (eg, smooth philtrum, thin vermillion border [upper lip], small palpebral fissures), limb dislocation, heart defects. Heart-lung fistulas and holoprosencephaly in most severe form. Mechanism is failure of cell migration.

Neonatal abstinence syndrome	Complex disorder involving CNS, ANS, and GI systems. Secondary to maternal opiate use/abuse. Risk factors for maternal substance abuse during pregnancy include poor mental health, poor prenatal care, low SES, lack of family support, HCV. Universal screening for substance abuse is recommended in all pregnant patients.
	Newborns may present with uncoordinated sucking reflexes, irritability, high-pitched crying, tremors, tachypnea, sneezing, diarrhea, and possibly seizures.

Twinning

Dizygotic ("fraternal") twins arise from 2 eggs that are separately fertilized by 2 different sperm (always 2 zygotes) and will have 2 separate amniotic sacs and 2 separate placentas (chorions). Monozygotic ("identical") twins arise from 1 fertilized egg (1 egg + 1 sperm) that splits in early pregnancy. The timing of cleavage determines chorionicity (number of chorions) and amnionicity (number of amnions) (**SCAB**):

- Cleavage 0–4 days: **S**eparate chorion and amnion
- Cleavage 4–8 days: shared **C**horion
- Cleavage 8–12 days: shared **A**mnion
- Cleavage 13+ days: shared **B**ody (conjoined)

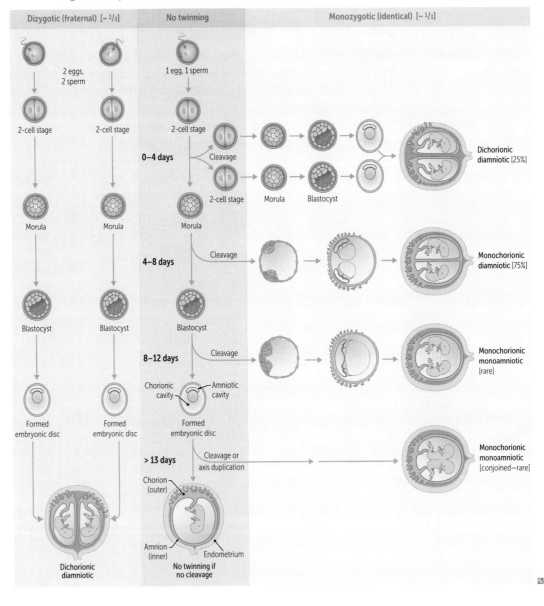

Placenta	1° site of nutrient and gas exchange between mother and fetus.	
Fetal component		
Cytotrophoblast	Inner layer of chorionic villi.	Cytotrophoblast makes Cells.
Syncytiotrophoblast	Outer layer of chorionic villi; synthesizes and secretes hormones, eg, hCG (structurally similar to LH; stimulates corpus luteum to secrete progesterone during first trimester).	Syncytiotrophoblast synthesizes hormones. Lacks MHC-I expression → ↓ chance of attack by maternal immune system.
Maternal component		
Decidua basalis	Derived from endometrium. Maternal blood in lacunae.	

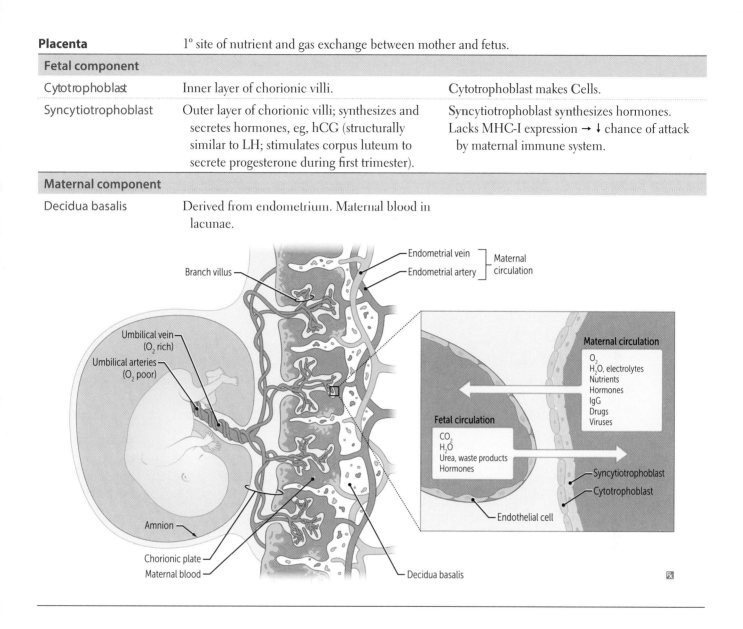

Umbilical cord	Umbilical arteries (2)—return deoxygenated blood from fetal internal iliac arteries to placenta 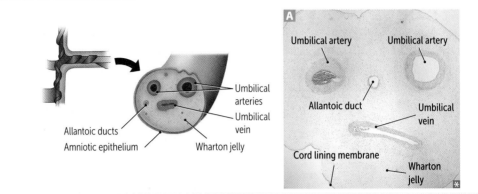. Umbilical vein (1)—supplies oxygenated blood from placenta to fetus; drains into IVC via liver or via ductus venosus.	Single umbilical artery (2-vessel cord) is associated with congenital and chromosomal anomalies. Umbilical arteries and vein are derived from allantois.

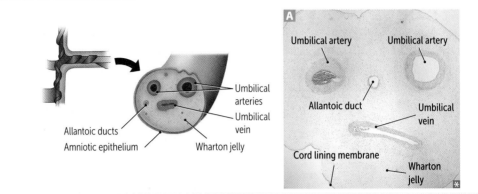

Urachus	In the 3rd week the yolk sac forms the allantois, which extends into urogenital sinus. Allantois becomes the urachus, a duct between fetal bladder and umbilicus. Failure of urachus to involute can lead to anomalies that may increase risk of infection and/or malignancy (eg, adenocarcinoma) if not treated. Obliterated urachus is represented by the median umbilical ligament after birth, which is covered by median umbilical fold of the peritoneum.
Patent urachus	Total failure of urachus to obliterate → urine discharge from umbilicus.
Urachal cyst	Partial failure of urachus to obliterate; fluid-filled cavity lined with uroepithelium, between umbilicus and bladder. Cyst can become infected and present as painful mass below umbilicus.
Vesicourachal diverticulum	Slight failure of urachus to obliterate → outpouching of bladder.

Umbilicus

Normal   Patent urachus   Urachal cyst   Vesicourachal diverticulum

Vitelline duct	7th week—obliteration of vitelline duct (omphalomesenteric duct), which connects yolk sac to midgut lumen.
Vitelline fistula	Vitelline duct fails to close → meconium discharge from umbilicus.
Meckel diverticulum	Partial closure of vitelline duct, with patent portion attached to ileum (true diverticulum). May have heterotopic gastric and/or pancreatic tissue → melena, hematochezia, abdominal pain.

Umbilicus

Normal   Vitelline fistula   Meckel diverticulum

Aortic arch derivatives	Develop into arterial system.	
1st	Part of maxillary artery (branch of external carotid).	1st arch is maximal.
2nd	Stapedial artery and hyoid artery.	Second = Stapedial.
3rd	Common Carotid artery and proximal part of internal Carotid artery.	C is 3rd letter of alphabet.
4th	On left, aortic arch; on right, proximal part of right subclavian artery.	4th arch (4 limbs) = systemic.
6th	Proximal part of pulmonary arteries and (on left only) ductus arteriosus.	6th arch = pulmonary and the pulmonary-to-systemic shunt (ductus arteriosus).

3rd — — 3rd
4th
Right recurrent laryngeal nerve loops around right subclavian artery — 4th — Left recurrent laryngeal nerve loops around aortic arch distal to ductus arteriosus
— 6th
6th
Truncus arteriosus —
6 months postnatal — Descending aorta

Branchial apparatus	Composed of branchial clefts, arches, pouches. Branchial clefts—derived from ectoderm. Also called branchial grooves. Branchial arches—derived from mesoderm (muscles, arteries) and neural crest (bones, cartilage). Branchial pouches—derived from endoderm.	CAP covers outside to inside:
		  Clefts = ectoderm
		  Arches = mesoderm + neural crest
		  Pouches = endoderm

— Pharyngeal floor
— Cartilage
I — Nerve
II — Artery
III
IV
◻ Cleft
◻ Arch VI
◻ Pouch

Branchial cleft derivatives	1st cleft develops into external auditory meatus. 2nd through 4th clefts form temporary cervical sinuses, which are obliterated by proliferation of 2nd arch mesenchyme. Persistent cervical sinus → branchial cleft cyst within lateral neck, anterior to sternocleidomastoid muscle.

Branchial arch derivatives

ARCH	CARTILAGE	MUSCLES	NERVES[a]	ABNORMALITIES/COMMENTS
1st branchial arch	Maxillary process → Maxilla, zygoMatic bone Mandibular process → Meckel cartilage → Mandible, Malleus and incus, sphenoMandibular ligament	Muscles of Mastication (temporalis, Masseter, lateral and Medial pterygoids), Mylohyoid, anterior belly of digastric, tensor tympani, anterior $\frac{2}{3}$ of tongue, tensor veli palatini	CN V$_3$ **chew**	Pierre Robin sequence—micrognathia, glossoptosis, cleft palate, airway obstruction Treacher Collins syndrome—neural crest dysfunction → mandibular hypoplasia, facial abnormalities
2nd branchial arch	Reichert cartilage: Stapes, Styloid process, lesser horn of hyoid, Stylohyoid ligament	Muscles of facial expression, Stapedius, Stylohyoid, platySma, posterior belly of digastric	CN VII (facial expression) **smile**	
3rd branchial arch	Greater horn of hyoid	Stylopharyngeus (think of stylopharyngeus innervated by glossopharyngeal nerve)	CN IX (stylopharyngeus) **swallow stylishly**	
4th–6th branchial arches	Arytenoids, Cricoid, Corniculate, Cuneiform, Thyroid (used to sing and ACCCT)	4th arch: most pharyngeal constrictors; cricothyroid, levator veli palatini 6th arch: all intrinsic muscles of larynx except cricothyroid	4th arch: CN X (superior laryngeal branch) **simply swallow** 6th arch: CN X (recurrent/inferior laryngeal branch) **speak**	Arches 3 and 4 form posterior $\frac{1}{3}$ of tongue; arch 5 makes no major developmental contributions

[a]These are the only CNs with both motor and sensory components (except V$_2$, which is sensory only).

When at the restaurant of the golden **arches**, children tend to first **chew** (1), then **smile** (2), then **swallow stylishly** (3) or **simply swallow** (4), and then **speak** (6).

Branchial pouch derivatives

POUCH	DERIVATIVES	NOTES	MNEMONIC
1st branchial pouch	Middle ear cavity, eustachian tube, mastoid air cells.	1st pouch contributes to endoderm-lined structures of ear.	Ear, tonsils, bottom-to-top: 1 (**ear**), 2 (**tonsils**), 3 dorsal (**bottom** for inferior parathyroids), 3 ventral (**to** = thymus), 4 (**top** = superior parathyroids).
2nd branchial pouch	Epithelial lining of palatine tonsil.		
3rd branchial pouch	Dorsal wings → **inferior** parathyroids. Ventral wings → thymus.	3rd pouch contributes to 3 structures (thymus, left and right inferior parathyroids). 3rd-pouch structures end up **below** 4th-pouch structures.	
4th branchial pouch	Dorsal wings → **superior** parathyroids. Ventral wings → ultimobranchial body → parafollicular (C) cells of thyroid.		
DiGeorge syndrome	Chromosome 22q11 deletion. Aberrant development of 3rd and 4th pouches → T-cell deficiency (thymic aplasia) and hypocalcemia (failure of parathyroid development). Associated with cardiac defects (conotruncal anomalies).		

Cleft lip and cleft palate

Cleft lip

Cleft lip—failure of fusion of the maxillary and merged medial nasal processes (formation of 1° palate).

Cleft palate—failure of fusion of the two lateral palatine shelves or failure of fusion of lateral palatine shelves with the nasal septum and/or median palatine shelf (formation of 2° palate).

Cleft lip and cleft palate have distinct, multifactorial etiologies, but often occur together.

Roof of mouth (1° palate) · Nasal cavity · Palatine shelves (2° palate) · Uvula

Cleft palate (partial)

Genital embryology

Female	Default development. Mesonephric duct degenerates and paramesonephric duct develops.
Male	SRY gene on Y chromosome—produces testis-determining factor → testes development. Sertoli cells secrete Müllerian inhibitory factor (MIF) that suppresses development of paramesonephric ducts. Leydig cells secrete androgens that stimulate development of mesonephric ducts.
Paramesonephric (Müllerian) duct	Develops into female internal structures—fallopian tubes, uterus, upper portion of vagina (lower portion from urogenital sinus). Male remnant is appendix testis. Müllerian agenesis (Mayer-Rokitansky-Küster-Hauser syndrome)—may present as 1° amenorrhea (due to a lack of uterine development) in females with fully developed 2° sexual characteristics (functional ovaries).
Mesonephric (Wolffian) duct	Develops into male internal structures (except prostate)—Seminal vesicles, Epididymis, Ejaculatory duct, Ductus deferens (SEED). Female remnant is Gartner duct.

Sexual differentiation

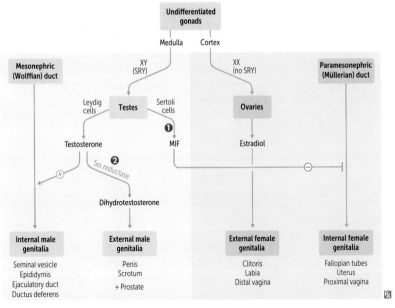

❶ No Sertoli cells or lack of Müllerian inhibitory factor → develop both male and female internal genitalia and male external genitalia

❷ 5α-reductase deficiency—inability to convert testosterone into DHT → male internal genitalia, ambiguous external genitalia until puberty (when ↑ testosterone levels cause masculinization)

In the testes:

Leydig Leads to male (internal and external) sexual differentiation.

Sertoli Shuts down female (internal) sexual differentiation.

Uterine (Müllerian duct) anomalies

Septate uterus	Common anomaly vs normal uterus **A**. Incomplete resorption of septum **B**. ↓ fertility and early miscarriage/pregnancy loss. Treat with septoplasty.
Bicornuate uterus	Incomplete fusion of Müllerian ducts **C**. ↑ risk of complicated pregnancy, early pregnancy loss, malpresentation, prematurity.
Uterus didelphys	Complete failure of fusion → double uterus, cervix, vagina **D**. Pregnancy possible.

Normal   Septate   Bicornuate   Didelphys

Male/female genital homologs

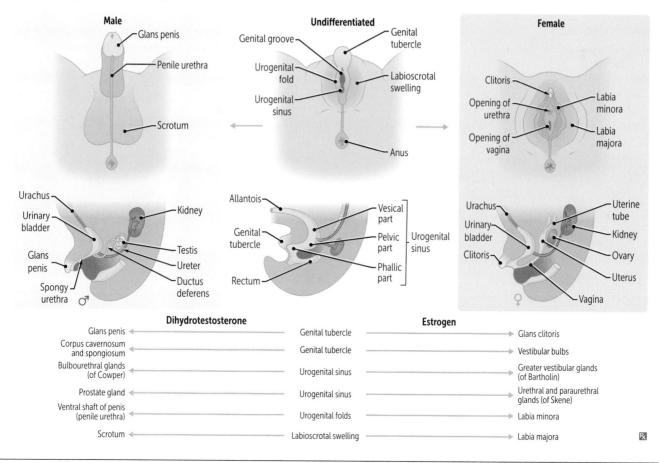

Dihydrotestosterone		Estrogen
Glans penis	Genital tubercle	Glans clitoris
Corpus cavernosum and spongiosum	Genital tubercle	Vestibular bulbs
Bulbourethral glands (of Cowper)	Urogenital sinus	Greater vestibular glands (of Bartholin)
Prostate gland	Urogenital sinus	Urethral and paraurethral glands (of Skene)
Ventral shaft of penis (penile urethra)	Urogenital folds	Labia minora
Scrotum	Labioscrotal swelling	Labia majora

Congenital penile abnormalities

Hypospadias 	Abnormal opening of penile urethra on ventral surface of penis due to failure of urethral folds to fuse.	Hypospadias is more common than epispadias. Associated with inguinal hernia and cryptorchidism. **Hypo** is **below.**
Epispadias 	Abnormal opening of penile urethra on dorsal surface of penis due to faulty positioning of genital tubercle.	Exstrophy of the bladder is associated with Epispadias. When you have Epispadias, you hit your Eye when you pEE.

Descent of testes and ovaries

	DESCRIPTION	MALE REMNANT	FEMALE REMNANT
Gubernaculum	Band of fibrous tissue.	Anchors testes within scrotum.	Ovarian ligament + round ligament of uterus.
Processus vaginalis	Evagination of peritoneum.	Forms tunica vaginalis.	Obliterated.

▶ REPRODUCTIVE—ANATOMY

Gonadal drainage

Venous drainage	Left ovary/testis → left gonadal vein → left renal vein → IVC. Right ovary/testis → right gonadal vein → IVC.	"Left gonadal vein takes the Longest way." Because the left spermatic vein enters the left renal vein at a 90° angle, flow is less laminar on left than on right → left venous pressure > right venous pressure → varicocele more common on the left.
Lymphatic drainage	Ovaries/testes → para-aortic lymph nodes. Body of uterus/superior bladder → external iliac nodes. Prostate/cervix/corpus cavernosum/proximal vagina → internal iliac nodes. Distal vagina/vulva/scrotum/distal anus → superficial inguinal nodes. Glans penis → deep inguinal nodes.	

Female reproductive anatomy

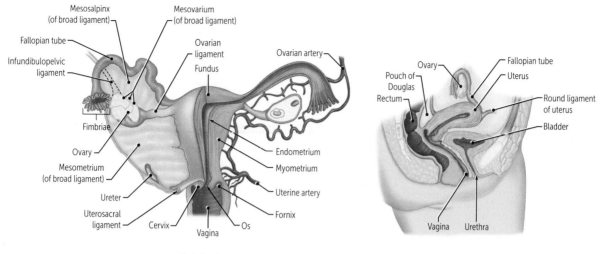

Posterior view

Sagittal view

LIGAMENT	CONNECTS	STRUCTURES CONTAINED	NOTES
Infundibulopelvic ligament	Ovaries to lateral pelvic wall	Ovarian vessels	Also called suspensory ligament of the ovary. Ligate vessels during oophorectomy to avoid bleeding. Ureter courses retroperitoneally, close to gonadal vessels → at risk of injury during ligation of ovarian vessels.
Cardinal ligament	Cervix to side wall of pelvis	Uterine vessels	Ureter at risk of injury during ligation of uterine vessels in hysterectomy. Not shown in diagram.
Round ligament of the uterus	Uterine horn to labia majora		Derivative of gubernaculum. Travels through **round** inguinal canal; above the artery of Sampson.
Broad ligament	Uterus, fallopian tubes, and ovaries to pelvic side wall	Ovaries, fallopian tubes, round ligaments of uterus	Fold of peritoneum that comprises the mesosalpinx, mesometrium, and mesovarium.
Ovarian ligament	Medial pole of ovary to uterine horn		Derivative of gubernaculum. Ovarian **L**igament **L**atches to **L**ateral uterus.

Female reproductive epithelial histology

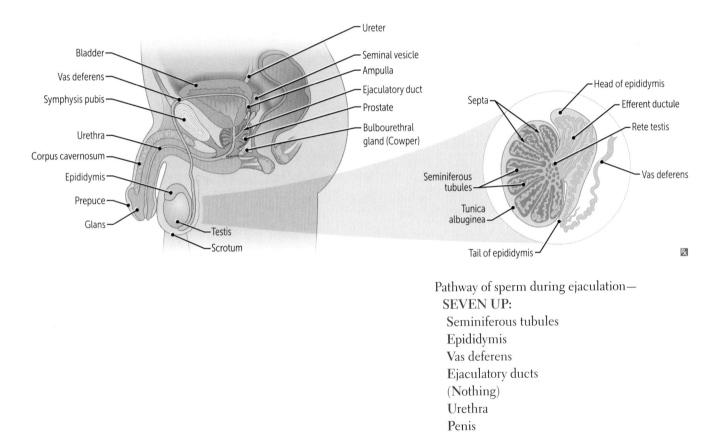

TISSUE	HISTOLOGY/NOTES
Vagina	Stratified squamous epithelium, nonkeratinized
Ectocervix	Stratified squamous epithelium, nonkeratinized
Transformation zone	Squamocolumnar junction A (most common area for cervical cancer)
Endocervix	Simple columnar epithelium
Uterus	Simple columnar epithelium with long tubular glands in proliferative phase; coiled glands in secretory phase
Fallopian tube	Simple columnar epithelium, ciliated
Ovary, outer surface	Simple cuboidal epithelium (germinal epithelium covering surface of ovary)

Male reproductive anatomy

Pathway of sperm during ejaculation—
SEVEN UP:
Seminiferous tubules
Epididymis
Vas deferens
Ejaculatory ducts
(Nothing)
Urethra
Penis

Urethral injury	Occurs almost exclusively in men. Suspect if blood seen at urethral meatus. Urethral catheterization is relatively contraindicated.	
	Anterior urethral injury	**Posterior urethral injury**
PART OF URETHRA	Bulbar (spongy) urethra	Membranous urethra
MECHANISM	Perineal straddle injury	Pelvic fracture
LOCATION OF URINE LEAK/BLOOD ACCUMULATION	Blood accumulates in scrotum If Buck fascia is torn, urine escapes into perineal space	Urine leaks into retropubic space
PRESENTATION	Blood at urethral meatus and scrotal hematoma	Blood at urethral meatus and high-riding prostate

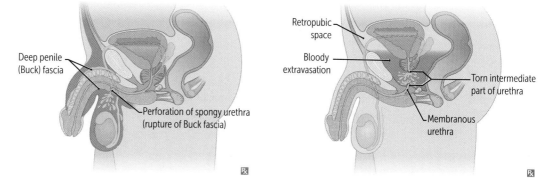

Autonomic innervation of male sexual response	Erection—Parasympathetic nervous system (pelvic splanchnic nerves, S2-S4): ■ NO → ↑ cGMP → smooth muscle relaxation → vasodilation → proerectile. ■ Norepinephrine → ↑ $[Ca^{2+}]_{in}$ → smooth muscle contraction → vasoconstriction → antierectile. Emission—Sympathetic nervous system (hypogastric nerve, T11-L2). Ejaculation—visceral and Somatic nerves (pudendal nerve).	Point, Squeeze, and Shoot. PDE-5 inhibitors (eg, sildenafil) ↓ cGMP breakdown.

Seminiferous tubules

CELL	FUNCTION	LOCATION/NOTES
Spermatogonia	Maintain germ cell pool and produce 1° spermatocytes.	Line seminiferous tubules 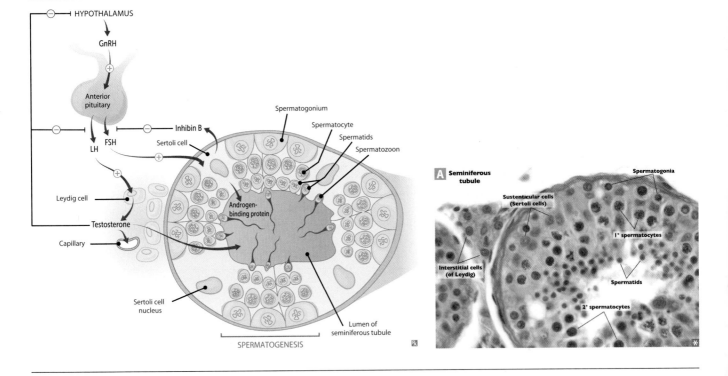 Germ cells
Sertoli cells	Secrete inhibin B → inhibit FSH. Secrete androgen-binding protein → maintain local levels of testosterone. Produce MIF. Tight junctions between adjacent Sertoli cells form blood-testis barrier → isolate gametes from autoimmune attack. Support and nourish developing spermatozoa. Regulate spermatogenesis. Temperature sensitive; ↓ sperm production and ↓ inhibin B with ↑ temperature.	Line seminiferous tubules Non-germ cells Convert testosterone and androstenedione to estrogens via aromatase Sertoli cells Support Sperm Synthesis and inhibit FSH Homolog of female granulosa cells ↑ temperature seen in varicocele, cryptorchidism
Leydig cells	Secrete testosterone in the presence of LH; testosterone production unaffected by temperature.	Interstitium Endocrine cells Homolog of female theca interna cells LH stimulates Leydig cells

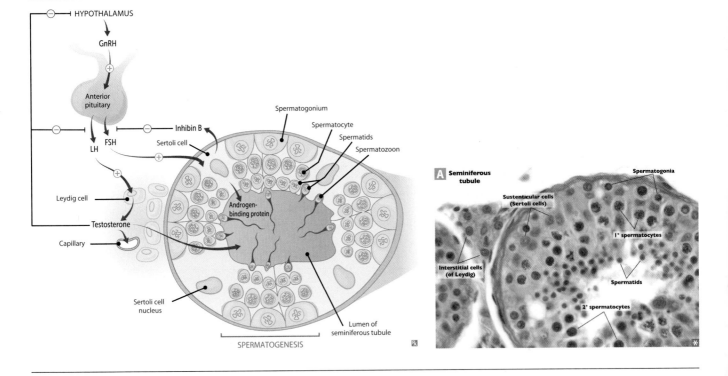

▶ REPRODUCTIVE—PHYSIOLOGY

Estrogen

SOURCE	Ovary (17β-estradiol), placenta (estriol), adipose tissue (estrone via aromatization).	Potency: estradiol > estrone > estriol
FUNCTION	Development of genitalia and breast, female fat distribution. Growth of follicle, endometrial proliferation, ↑ myometrial excitability. Upregulation of estrogen, LH, and progesterone receptors; feedback inhibition of FSH and LH, then LH surge; stimulation of prolactin secretion. ↑ transport proteins, SHBG; ↑ HDL; ↓ LDL.	Pregnancy: ▪ 50-fold ↑ in estradiol and estrone ▪ 1000-fold ↑ in estriol (indicator of fetal well-being) Estrogen receptors expressed in cytoplasm; translocate to nucleus when bound by estrogen

Progesterone

SOURCE	Corpus luteum, placenta, adrenal cortex, testes.	Fall in progesterone after delivery disinhibits prolactin → lactation. ↑ progesterone is indicative of ovulation. **Progesterone** is **pro-gest**ation. **Prolactin** is **pro-lactation.**
FUNCTION	Stimulation of endometrial glandular secretions and spiral artery development. Maintenance of pregnancy. ↓ myometrial excitability. Production of thick cervical mucus, which inhibits sperm entry into uterus. ↑ body temperature. Inhibition of gonadotropins (LH, FSH). Uterine smooth muscle relaxation (preventing contractions). ↓ estrogen receptor expression. Prevents endometrial hyperplasia.	

Oogenesis

1° oocytes begin meiosis I during fetal life and complete meiosis I just prior to ovulation.

Meiosis I is arrested in prOphase I for years until Ovulation (1° oocytes).

Meiosis II is arrested in **met**aphase II until fertilization (2° oocytes). "An egg **met** a sperm."

If fertilization does not occur within 1 day, the 2° oocyte degenerates.

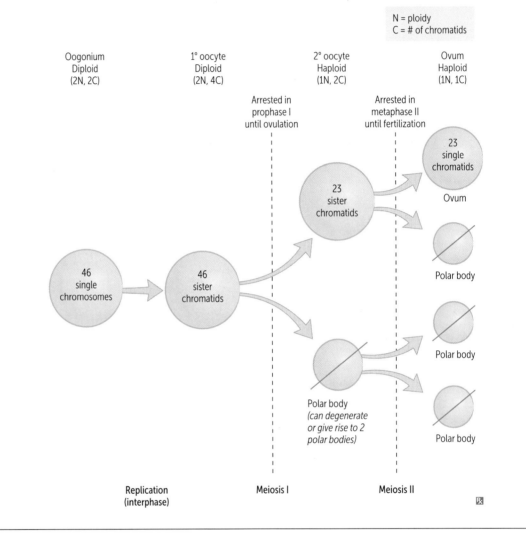

Ovulation

↑ estrogen, ↑ GnRH receptors on anterior pituitary. Estrogen surge then stimulates LH release → ovulation (rupture of follicle). ↑ temperature (progesterone induced).

Mittelschmerz—transient mid-cycle ovulatory pain ("Middle hurts"); classically associated with peritoneal irritation (eg, follicular swelling/rupture, fallopian tube contraction). Can mimic appendicitis.

Menstrual cycle

Follicular phase can vary in length. Luteal phase is 14 days. Ovulation day + 14 days = menstruation.

Follicular growth is fastest during 2nd week of the follicular phase.

Estrogen stimulates endometrial proliferation.

Progesterone maintains endometrium to support implantation.

↓ progesterone → ↓ fertility.

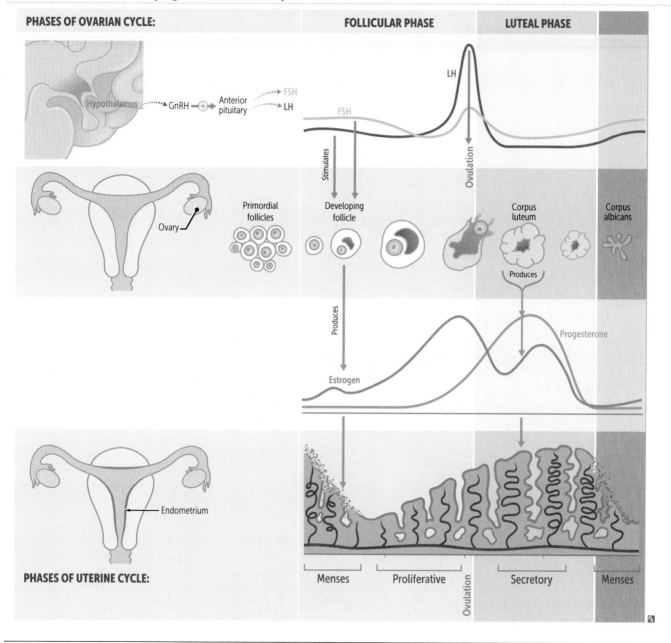

Abnormal uterine bleeding	Characterized as either heavy menstrual bleeding (AUB/HMB) or intermenstrual bleeding (AUB/IMB). These are further subcategorized by **PALM-COEIN**: ▪ Structural causes (**PALM**): Polyp, Adenomyosis, Leiomyoma, or Malignancy/hyperplasia ▪ Non-structural causes (**COEIN**): Coagulopathy, Ovulatory, Endometrial, Iatrogenic, Not yet classified	Terms such as dysfunctional uterine bleeding, menorrhagia, oligomenorrhea are no longer recommended.

Pregnancy	Fertilization most commonly occurs in upper end of fallopian tube (the ampulla). Occurs within 1 day of ovulation. Implantation within the wall of the uterus occurs 6 days after fertilization. Syncytiotrophoblasts secrete hCG, which is detectable in blood 1 week after conception and on home test in urine 2 weeks after conception. Gestational age—calculated from date of last menstrual period. Embryonic age—calculated from date of conception (gestational age minus 2 weeks). Physiologic adaptations in pregnancy: ▪ ↑ cardiac output (↑ preload, ↓ afterload, ↑ HR → ↑ placental and uterus perfusion) ▪ Anemia (↑↑ plasma, ↑ RBCs) ▪ Hypercoagulability (to ↓ blood loss at delivery) ▪ Hyperventilation (eliminate fetal CO_2)	 Placental hormone secretion generally increases over the course of pregnancy, but hCG peaks at 8–10 weeks.

Human chorionic gonadotropin

SOURCE	Syncytiotrophoblast of placenta.
FUNCTION	Maintains corpus luteum (and thus progesterone) for first 8–10 weeks of pregnancy by acting like LH (otherwise no luteal cell stimulation → abortion). After 8–10 weeks, placenta synthesizes its own estriol and progesterone and corpus luteum degenerates. Used to detect pregnancy because it appears early in urine (see above). Has identical α subunit as LH, FSH, TSH (states of ↑ hCG can cause hyperthyroidism). β subunit is unique (pregnancy tests detect β subunit). hCG is ↑ in multiple gestations, hydatidiform moles, choriocarcinomas, and Down syndrome; hCG is ↓ in ectopic/failing pregnancy, Edwards syndrome, and Patau syndrome.

Human placental lactogen	Also known as chorionic somatomammotropin.
SOURCE	Syncytiotrophoblast of placenta.
FUNCTION	Stimulates insulin production; overall ↑ insulin resistance. Maternal hypoglycemia from insulin resistance leads to lipolysis, which preserves available glucose and amino acids for the fetus. Gestational diabetes can occur if maternal pancreatic function cannot overcome the insulin resistance.

Apgar score

	Score 2	Score 1	Score 0
Appearance	Pink	Extremities blue	Pale or blue
Pulse	> 100 bpm	< 100 bpm	No pulse
Grimace	Cries and pulls away	Grimaces or weak cry	No response to stimulation
Activity	Active movement	Arms, legs flexed	No movement
Respiration	Strong cry	Slow, irregular	No breathing

Assessment of newborn vital signs following delivery via a 10-point scale evaluated at 1 minute and 5 minutes. **Apgar** score is based on Appearance, Pulse, Grimace, Activity, and Respiration. Apgar scores < 7 require further evaluation. If Apgar score remains low at later time points, there is ↑ risk the child will develop long-term neurologic damage.

Infant/child development	Milestone dates are ranges that have been approximated and vary by source. Children not meeting milestones may need assessment for potential developmental delay.		
AGE	MOTOR	SOCIAL	VERBAL/COGNITIVE
Infant	**Parents**	**Start**	**Observing,**
0–12 mo	Primitive reflexes disappear— Moro (by 3 mo), rooting (by 4 mo), palmar (by 6 mo), Babinski (by 12 mo) Posture—lifts head up prone (by 1 mo), rolls and sits (by 6 mo), crawls (by 8 mo), stands (by 10 mo), walks (by 12–18 mo) Picks—passes toys hand to hand (by 6 mo), Pincer grasp (by 10 mo) Points to objects (by 12 mo)	Social smile (by 2 mo) Stranger anxiety (by 6 mo) Separation anxiety (by 9 mo)	Orients—first to voice (by 4 mo), then to name and gestures (by 9 mo) Object permanence (by 9 mo) Oratory—says "mama" and "dada" (by 10 mo)
Toddler	**Child**	**Rearing**	**Working,**
12–36 mo	Cruises, takes first steps (by 12 mo) Climbs stairs (by 18 mo) Cubes stacked—number = age (yr) × 3 Cutlery—feeds self with fork and spoon (by 20 mo) Kicks ball (by 24 mo)	Recreation—parallel play (by 24–36 mo) Rapprochement—moves away from and returns to mother (by 24 mo) Realization—core gender identity formed (by 36 mo)	Words—200 words by age 2 (2 zeros), 2-word sentences
Preschool	**Don't**	**Forget, they're still**	**Learning!**
3–5 yr	Drive—tricycle (3 wheels at 3 yr) Drawings—copies line or circle, stick figure (by 4 yr) Dexterity—hops on one foot (by 4 yr), uses buttons or zippers, grooms self (by 5 yr)	Freedom—comfortably spends part of day away from mother (by 3 yr) Friends—cooperative play, has imaginary friends (by 4 yr)	Language—1000 words by age 3 (3 zeros), uses complete sentences and prepositions (by 4 yr) Legends—can tell detailed stories (by 4 yr)

Low birth weight	Defined as < 2500 g. Caused by prematurity or intrauterine growth restriction (IUGR). Associated with ↑ risk of sudden infant death syndrome (SIDS) and with ↑ overall mortality. Other problems include impaired thermoregulation and immune function, hypoglycemia, polycythemia, and impaired neurocognitive/emotional development. Complications include infections, respiratory distress syndrome, necrotizing enterocolitis, intraventricular hemorrhage, and persistent fetal circulation.

Lactation	After parturition and delivery of placenta, rapid ↓ in progesterone disinhibits and initiates lactation. Suckling is required to maintain milk production and ejection, since ↑ nerve stimulation → ↑ oxytocin and prolactin. Prolactin—induces and maintains lactation and ↓ reproductive function. Oxytocin—assists in milk letdown; also promotes uterine contractions. Breast milk is the ideal nutrition for infants < 6 months old. Contains maternal immunoglobulins (conferring passive immunity; mostly IgA), macrophages, lymphocytes. Breast milk reduces infant infections and is associated with ↓ risk for child to develop asthma, allergies, diabetes mellitus, and obesity. Guidelines recommend exclusively breastfed infants get vitamin D and possibly iron supplementation. Breastfeeding ↓ maternal risk of breast and ovarian cancer and facilitates mother-child bonding.

Menopause	Diagnosed by amenorrhea for 12 months. ↓ estrogen production due to age-linked decline in number of ovarian follicles. Average age at onset is 51 years (earlier in smokers). Usually preceded by 4–5 years of abnormal menstrual cycles. Source of estrogen (estrone) after menopause becomes peripheral conversion of androgens, ↑ androgens → hirsutism. ↑↑ FSH is specific for menopause (loss of negative feedback on FSH due to ↓ estrogen).	Hormonal changes: ↓ estrogen, ↑↑ FSH, ↑ LH (no surge), ↑ GnRH. Causes **HAVOCS**: **H**ot flashes, **A**trophy of the **V**agina, **O**steoporosis, **C**oronary artery disease, **S**leep disturbances. Menopause before age 40 suggests 1° ovarian insufficiency (premature ovarian failure).

Androgens	Testosterone, dihydrotestosterone (DHT), androstenedione.	
SOURCE	DHT and testosterone (testis), AnDrostenedione (ADrenal)	Potency: DHT > testosterone > androstenedione.
FUNCTION	Testosterone: <ul><li>Differentiation of epididymis, vas deferens, seminal vesicles (internal genitalia, except prostate).</li><li>Growth spurt: penis, seminal vesicles, sperm, muscle, RBCs.</li><li>Deepening of voice.</li><li>Closing of epiphyseal plates (via estrogen converted from testosterone).</li><li>Libido.</li></ul>DHT: <ul><li>Early—differentiation of penis, scrotum, prostate.</li><li>Late—prostate growth, balding, sebaceous gland activity.</li></ul>	Testosterone is converted to DHT by 5α-reductase, which is inhibited by finasteride. In the male, androgens are converted to estrogen by cytochrome P-450 aromatase (primarily in adipose tissue and testis). Aromatase is the key enzyme in conversion of androgens to estrogen. Exogenous testosterone → inhibition of hypothalamic–pituitary–gonadal axis → ↓ intratesticular testosterone → ↓ testicular size → azoospermia.

Spermatogenesis

Spermatogenesis begins at puberty with spermatogonia. Full development takes 2 months. Occurs in seminiferous tubules. Produces spermatids that undergo spermiogenesis (loss of cytoplasmic contents, gain of acrosomal cap) to form mature spermatozoon.

"Gonium" is going to be a sperm; "Zoon" is "Zooming" to egg.

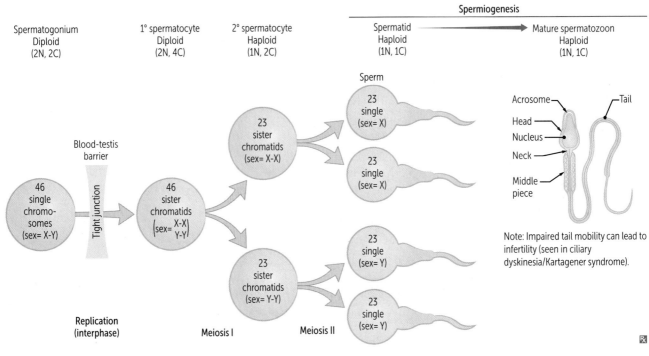

Note: Impaired tail mobility can lead to infertility (seen in ciliary dyskinesia/Kartagener syndrome).

Tanner stages of sexual development

Tanner stage is assigned independently to genitalia, pubic hair, and breast (eg, a person can have Tanner stage 2 genitalia, Tanner stage 3 pubic hair).

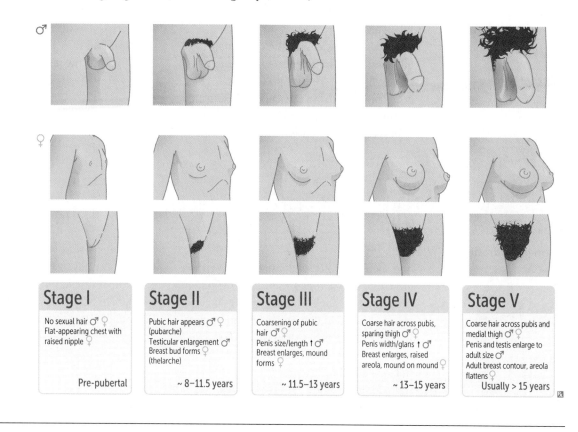

Stage I
No sexual hair ♂ ♀
Flat-appearing chest with raised nipple ♀

Pre-pubertal

Stage II
Pubic hair appears ♂ ♀ (pubarche)
Testicular enlargement ♂
Breast bud forms ♀ (thelarche)

~ 8–11.5 years

Stage III
Coarsening of pubic hair ♂ ♀
Penis size/length ↑ ♂
Breast enlarges, mound forms ♀

~ 11.5–13 years

Stage IV
Coarse hair across pubis, sparing thigh ♂ ♀
Penis width/glans ↑ ♂
Breast enlarges, raised areola, mound on mound ♀

~ 13–15 years

Stage V
Coarse hair across pubis and medial thigh ♂ ♀
Penis and testis enlarge to adult size ♂
Adult breast contour, areola flattens ♀

Usually > 15 years

▶ REPRODUCTIVE—PATHOLOGY

Sex chromosome disorders	Aneuploidy most commonly due to meiotic nondisjunction.	
Klinefelter syndrome	Male, 47,XXY. Testicular atrophy, eunuchoid body shape, tall, long extremities, gynecomastia, female hair distribution A. May present with developmental delay. Presence of inactivated X chromosome (Barr body). Common cause of hypogonadism seen in infertility work-up.	Dysgenesis of seminiferous tubules → ↓ inhibin B → ↑ FSH. Abnormal Leydig cell function → ↓ testosterone → ↑ LH → ↑ estrogen.
Turner syndrome	Female, 45,XO. Short stature (if untreated; preventable with growth hormone therapy), ovarian dysgenesis (streak ovary), shield chest B, bicuspid aortic valve, coarctation (femoral < brachial pulse), lymphatic defects (result in webbed neck or cystic hygroma; lymphedema in feet, hands), horseshoe kidney. Most common cause of 1° amenorrhea. No Barr body.	Menopause before menarche. ↓ estrogen leads to ↑ LH, FSH. Sometimes due to mitotic error → mosaicism (eg, 45,XO/46,XX). Pregnancy is possible in some cases (IVF, exogenous estradiol-17β and progesterone).
Double Y males	47, XYY. Phenotypically normal (usually undiagnosed), very tall. Normal fertility. May be associated with severe acne, learning disability, autism spectrum disorders.	
Ovotesticular disorder of sex development	46,XX > 46,XY. Both ovarian and testicular tissue present (ovotestis); ambiguous genitalia. Previously called true hermaphroditism.	

Diagnosing disorders of sex hormones	Testosterone	LH	Diagnosis
	↑	↑	Defective androgen receptor
	↑	↓	Testosterone-secreting tumor, exogenous steroids
	↓	↑	Hypergonadotropic hypogonadism (1°)
	↓	↓	Hypogonadotropic hypogonadism (2°)

Other disorders of sex development

Disagreement between the phenotypic sex (external genitalia, influenced by hormonal levels) and the gonadal sex (testes vs ovaries, corresponds with Y chromosome). Includes the terms pseudohermaphrodite, hermaphrodite, and intersex.

46,XX DSD

Ovaries present, but external genitalia are virilized or ambiguous. Due to excessive and inappropriate exposure to androgenic steroids during early gestation (eg, congenital adrenal hyperplasia or exogenous administration of androgens during pregnancy).

46,XY DSD

Testes present, but external genitalia are female or ambiguous. Most common form is androgen insensitivity syndrome (testicular feminization).

Disorders by physical characteristics	Uterus	Breasts	Disorders
	⊕	⊖	Hypergonadotropic hypogonadism (eg, Turner syndrome, genetic mosaicism, pure gonadal dysgenesis) Hypogonadotropic hypogonadism (eg, CNS lesions, Kallmann syndrome)
	⊖	⊕	Uterovaginal agenesis in genotypic female or androgen insensitivity in genotypic male
	⊖	⊖	Male genotype with insufficient production of testosterone

Placental aromatase deficiency

Inability to synthesize estrogens from androgens. Masculinization of female (46,XX DSD) infants (ambiguous genitalia), ↑ serum testosterone and androstenedione. Can present with maternal virilization during pregnancy (fetal androgens cross the placenta).

Androgen insensitivity syndrome

Defect in androgen receptor resulting in normal-appearing female (46,XY DSD); female external genitalia with scant axillary and pubic hair, rudimentary vagina; uterus and fallopian tubes absent. Patients develop normal functioning testes (often found in labia majora; surgically removed to prevent malignancy). ↑ testosterone, estrogen, LH (vs sex chromosome disorders).

5α-reductase deficiency

Autosomal recessive; sex limited to genetic males (46,XY DSD). Inability to convert testosterone to DHT. Ambiguous genitalia until puberty, when ↑ testosterone causes masculinization/↑ growth of external genitalia. Testosterone/estrogen levels are normal; LH is normal or ↑. Internal genitalia are normal.

Kallmann syndrome

Failure to complete puberty; a form of hypogonadotropic hypogonadism. Defective migration of GnRH-releasing neurons and subsequent failure of GnRH-releasing olfactory bulbs to develop → ↓ synthesis of GnRH in the hypothalamus; hyposmia/anosmia; ↓ GnRH, FSH, LH, testosterone. Infertility (low sperm count in males; amenorrhea in females).

Hydatidiform mole

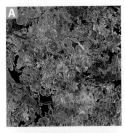

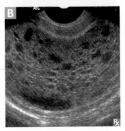

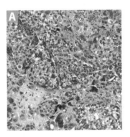

Cystic swelling of chorionic villi and proliferation of chorionic epithelium (only trophoblast).
Presents with vaginal bleeding, uterine enlargement more than expected, pelvic pressure/pain.
Associated with hCG-mediated sequelae: early preeclampsia (before 20 weeks), theca-lutein cysts,
hyperemesis gravidarum, hyperthyroidism.
Treatment: dilation and curettage and methotrexate. Monitor β-hCG.

	Complete mole	Partial mole
KARYOTYPE	46,XX; 46,XY	69,XXX; 69,XXY; 69,XYY
COMPONENTS	Most commonly enucleated egg + single sperm (subsequently duplicates paternal DNA)	2 sperm + 1 egg
FETAL PARTS	No	Yes (partial = fetal parts)
UTERINE SIZE	↑	—
hCG	↑↑↑↑	↑
IMAGING	"Honeycombed" uterus or "clusters of grapes" , "snowstorm" on ultrasound	Fetal parts
RISK OF MALIGNANCY (GESTATIONAL TROPHOBLASTIC NEOPLASIA)	15–20%	< 5%
RISK OF CHORIOCARCINOMA	2%	Rare

Choriocarcinoma

Rare; can develop during or after pregnancy in mother or baby. Malignancy of trophoblastic tissue **A** (cytotrophoblasts, syncytiotrophoblasts); **no** chorionic villi present. ↑ frequency of bilateral/multiple theca-lutein cysts. Presents with abnormal ↑ β-hCG, shortness of breath, hemoptysis. Hematogenous spread to lungs → "cannonball" metastases **B**.

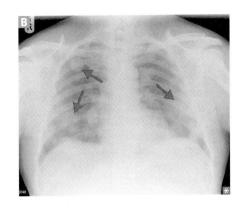

Pregnancy complications

Abruptio placentae	Premature separation (partial or complete) of placenta from uterine wall before delivery of infant. Risk factors: trauma (eg, motor vehicle accident), smoking, hypertension, preeclampsia, cocaine abuse. Presentation: **abrupt**, painful bleeding (concealed or apparent) in third trimester; possible DIC, maternal shock, fetal distress. Life threatening for mother and fetus.	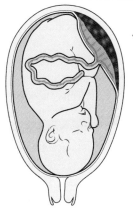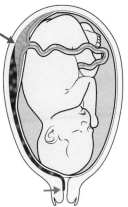 Complete abruption with concealed hemorrhage — Partial abruption (blue arrow) with apparent hemorrhage (red arrow)

Morbidly adherent placenta

Defective decidual layer → abnormal attachment and separation after delivery. Risk factors: prior C-section or uterine surgery involving myometrium, inflammation, placenta previa, advanced maternal age, multiparity. Three types distinguishable by the depth of penetration:

Placenta accreta—placenta **attaches** to myometrium without penetrating it; most common type.

Placenta increta—placenta penetrates **into** myometrium.

Placenta percreta—placenta penetrates ("**perforates**") through myometrium and into uterine serosa (invades entire uterine wall); can result in placental attachment to rectum or bladder (can result in hematuria).

Presentation: often detected on ultrasound prior to delivery. No separation of placenta after delivery → postpartum bleeding (can cause Sheehan syndrome).

Placenta previa

Attachment of placenta to lower uterine segment over (or < 2 cm from) internal cervical os. Risk factors: multiparity, prior C-section. Associated with painless third-trimester bleeding. A "**preview**" of the placenta is visible through cervix.

Partial placenta previa — Complete placenta previa

Pregnancy complications (continued)

Vasa previa	Fetal vessels run over, or in close proximity to, cervical os. May result in vessel rupture, exsanguination, fetal death. Presents with triad of membrane rupture, painless vaginal bleeding, fetal bradycardia (< 110 beats/min). Emergency C-section usually indicated. Frequently associated with velamentous umbilical cord insertion (cord inserts in chorioamniotic membrane rather than placenta → fetal vessels travel to placenta unprotected by Wharton jelly).	

Umbilical cord
Placenta (succenturiate lobe)
Placenta
Placenta
Velamentous attachment
Vasa previa

Postpartum hemorrhage	Due to 4 T's: Tone (uterine atony; most common), Trauma (lacerations, incisions, uterine rupture), Thrombin (coagulopathy), Tissue (retained products of conception).

Ectopic pregnancy	Implantation of fertilized ovum in a site other than the uterus, most often in ampulla of fallopian tube A. Suspect with history of amenorrhea, lower-than-expected rise in hCG based on dates, and sudden lower abdominal pain; confirm with ultrasound. Often clinically mistaken for appendicitis.	Pain +/– bleeding. Risk factors: ▪ Prior ectopic pregnancy ▪ History of infertility ▪ Salpingitis (PID) ▪ Ruptured appendix ▪ Prior tubal surgery ▪ Smoking ▪ Advanced maternal age

Amniotic fluid abnormalities

Polyhydramnios	Too much amniotic fluid. Often idiopathic, but associated with fetal malformations (eg, esophageal/duodenal atresia, anencephaly; both result in inability to swallow amniotic fluid), maternal diabetes, fetal anemia, multiple gestations.
Oligohydramnios	Too little amniotic fluid. Associated with placental insufficiency, bilateral renal agenesis, posterior urethral valves (in males) and resultant inability to excrete urine. Any profound oligohydramnios can cause Potter sequence.

Hypertension in pregnancy

Gestational hypertension	BP > 140/90 mm Hg after 20th week of gestation. No pre-existing hypertension. No proteinuria or end-organ damage.	Treatment: antihypertensives (Hydralazine, α-Methyldopa, Labetalol, Nifedipine), deliver at 37–39 weeks. Hypertensive Moms Love Nifedipine.
Preeclampsia	New-onset hypertension with either proteinuria or end-organ dysfunction after 20th week of gestation (< 20 weeks suggests molar pregnancy). Caused by abnormal placental spiral arteries → endothelial dysfunction, vasoconstriction, ischemia. Incidence ↑ in patients with pre-existing hypertension, diabetes, chronic renal disease, autoimmune disorders (eg, antiphospholipid antibody syndrome). Complications: placental abruption, coagulopathy, renal failure, pulmonary edema, uteroplacental insufficiency; may lead to eclampsia (+ seizures) and/or HELLP syndrome.	Treatment: antihypertensives, IV magnesium sulfate (to prevent seizure); definitive is delivery of fetus.
Eclampsia	Preeclampsia + maternal seizures. Maternal death due to stroke, intracranial hemorrhage, or ARDS.	Treatment: IV magnesium sulfate, antihypertensives, immediate delivery.
HELLP syndrome	Hemolysis, Elevated Liver enzymes, Low Platelets. A manifestation of severe preeclampsia. Blood smear shows schistocytes. Can lead to DIC and hepatic subcapsular hematomas → rupture → severe hypotension.	Treatment: immediate delivery.

Gynecologic tumor epidemiology	Incidence (US)—endometrial > ovarian > cervical; cervical cancer is more common worldwide due to lack of screening or HPV vaccination. Prognosis: Cervical (best prognosis, diagnosed < 45 years old) > Endometrial (middle-aged, about 55 years old) > Ovarian (worst prognosis, > 65 years).	CEOs often go from best to worst as they get older.

Vulvar pathology

Non-neoplastic	
Bartholin cyst and abscess	Due to blockage of Bartholin gland duct causing accumulation of gland fluid. May lead to abscess 2° to obstruction and inflammation **A**. Usually in reproductive-age females. Associated with *N gonorrhoeae* infections.
Lichen sclerosus	Thinning of epidermis with fibrosis/sclerosis of dermis. Presents with porcelain-white plaques with a red or violet border. Skin fragility with erosions can be observed **B**. Most common in postmenopausal women. Benign, but slightly increased risk for SCC.
Lichen simplex chronicus	Hyperplasia of vulvar squamous epithelium. Presents with leathery, thick vulvar skin with enhanced skin markings due to chronic rubbing or scratching. Benign, no risk of SCC.
Neoplastic	
Vulvar carcinoma	Carcinoma from squamous epithelial lining of vulva **C**. Rare. Presents with leukoplakia, biopsy often required to distinguish carcinoma from other causes. HPV-related vulvar carcinoma—associated with high-risk HPV types 16, 18. Risk factors: multiple partners, early coitarche. Usually in reproductive-age females. Non-HPV vulvar carcinoma—usually from long-standing lichen sclerosus. Females > 70 years old.
Extramammary Paget disease	Intraepithelial adenocarcinoma. Carcinoma in situ, low risk of underlying carcinoma. Presents with pruritus, erythema, crusting, ulcers **D**.

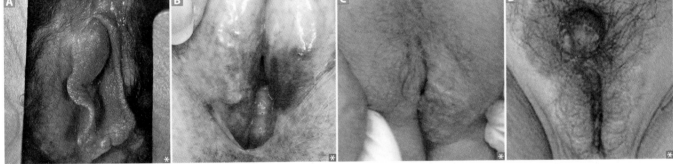

Vaginal tumors

Vaginal squamous cell carcinoma	Usually 2° to cervical SCC; 1° vaginal carcinoma rare.
Clear cell adenocarcinoma	Affects women who had exposure to DES in utero.
Sarcoma botryoides	Embryonal rhabdomyosarcoma variant. Affects girls < 4 years old; spindle-shaped cells; desmin ⊕. Presents with clear, grape-like, polypoid mass emerging from vagina.

Cervical pathology

Dysplasia and carcinoma in situ	Disordered epithelial growth; begins at basal layer of squamocolumnar junction (transformation zone) and extends outward. Classified as CIN 1, CIN 2, or CIN 3 (severe, irreversible dysplasia or carcinoma in situ), depending on extent of dysplasia. Associated with HPV-16 and HPV-18, which produce both the E6 gene product (inhibits $p53$) and E7 gene product (inhibits pRb); koilocytes **A** are pathognomonic of HPV infection. May progress slowly to invasive carcinoma if left untreated. Typically asymptomatic (detected with Pap smear) or presents as abnormal vaginal bleeding (often postcoital). Risk factors: multiple sexual partners (#1), smoking, early coitarche, DES exposure, immunocompromise (eg, HIV, transplant).
Invasive carcinoma	Often squamous cell carcinoma. Pap smear can detect cervical dysplasia before it progresses to invasive carcinoma. Diagnose via colposcopy and biopsy. Lateral invasion can block ureters → renal failure.
Primary ovarian insufficiency	Also known as premature ovarian failure. Premature atresia of ovarian follicles in women of reproductive age. Most often idiopathic; associated with chromosomal abnormalities (especially in females <30 years). Need karyotype screening. Patients present with signs of menopause after puberty but before age 40. ↓ estrogen, ↑ LH, ↑ FSH.
Most common causes of anovulation	Pregnancy, polycystic ovarian syndrome, obesity, HPO axis abnormalities, premature ovarian failure, hyperprolactinemia, thyroid disorders, eating disorders, competitive athletics, Cushing syndrome, adrenal insufficiency, chromosomal abnormalities (eg, Turner syndrome).
Polycystic ovarian syndrome	Also known as Stein-Leventhal syndrome. Hyperinsulinemia and/or insulin resistance hypothesized to alter hypothalamic hormonal feedback response → ↑ LH:FSH, ↑ androgens (eg, testosterone) from theca interna cells, ↓ rate of follicular maturation → unruptured follicles (cysts) + anovulation. Common cause of ↓ fertility in women. Enlarged, bilateral cystic ovaries **A**; presents with amenorrhea/oligomenorrhea, hirsutism, acne, ↓ fertility. Associated with obesity. ↑ risk of endometrial cancer 2° to unopposed estrogen from repeated anovulatory cycles. Treatment: cycle regulation via weight reduction (↓ peripheral estrone formation), OCPs (prevent endometrial hyperplasia due to unopposed estrogen); clomiphene, metformin to induce ovulation; spironolactone, ketoconazole (antiandrogens) to treat hirsutism.

Ovarian cysts

Follicular cyst	Distention of unruptured graafian follicle. May be associated with hyperestrogenism, endometrial hyperplasia. Most common ovarian mass in young women.
Theca-lutein cyst	Often bilateral/multiple. Due to gonadotropin stimulation. Associated with choriocarcinoma and hydatidiform moles.

Ovarian neoplasms

Most common adnexal mass in women > 55 years old. Can be benign or malignant. Arise from surface epithelium, germ cells, or sex cord stromal tissue.

Majority of malignant tumors are epithelial (serous cystadenocarcinoma most common). Risk ↑ with advanced age, infertility, endometriosis, PCOS, genetic predisposition *BRCA1* or *BRCA2* mutation, Lynch syndrome, strong family history. Risk ↓ with previous pregnancy, history of breastfeeding, OCPs, tubal ligation. Presents with adnexal mass, abdominal distension, bowel obstruction, pleural effusion. Monitor response to therapy/relapse by measuring CA 125 levels (not good for screening).

Surface epithelium tumors (benign)

Serous cystadenoma	Most common ovarian neoplasm. Lined with fallopian tube–like epithelium. Often bilateral.
Mucinous cystadenoma	Multiloculated, large. Lined by mucus-secreting epithelium A.
Endometrioma	Endometriosis within ovary with cyst formation. Presents with pelvic pain, dysmenorrhea, dyspareunia; symptoms may vary with menstrual cycle. "Chocolate cyst"—endometrioma filled with dark, reddish-brown blood. Complex mass on ultrasound.

Germ cell tumors (benign)

Mature cystic teratoma (dermoid cyst)	Germ cell tumor, most common ovarian tumor in females 10–30 years old. Cystic mass containing elements from all 3 germ layers (eg, teeth, hair, sebum) B. Can present with pain 2° to ovarian enlargement or torsion. A monodermal form with thyroid tissue (struma ovarii) uncommonly presents with hyperthyroidism C.

Sex cord stromal tumor (benign)

Fibroma	Bundles of spindle-shaped fibroblasts. Meigs syndrome—triad of ovarian fibroma, ascites, hydrothorax. "Pulling" sensation in groin.
Thecoma	Like granulosa cell tumors, may produce estrogen. Usually presents as abnormal uterine bleeding in a postmenopausal woman.

Other (benign)

Brenner tumor	Resembles bladder epithelium (transitional cell tumor). Solid tumor that is pale yellow-tan and appears encapsulated. "Coffee bean" nuclei on H&E stain. Usually benign.

Ovarian neoplasms *(continued)*

Surface epithelium tumors (malignant)	
Serous cystadenocarcinoma	Most common malignant ovarian neoplasm, frequently bilateral. Psammoma bodies.
Mucinous cystadenocarcinoma	Rare malignant mucinous ovarian epithelial tumor. May be metastatic from appendiceal or other GI tumors. Can result in pseudomyxoma peritonei—intraperitoneal accumulation of mucinous material.

Germ cell tumors (malignant)	
Dysgerminoma	Most common in adolescents. Equivalent to male seminoma but rarer. 1% of all ovarian tumors; 30% of germ cell tumors. Sheets of uniform "fried egg" cells **E**. hCG, LDH = tumor markers.
Immature teratoma	Aggressive, contains fetal tissue, neuroectoderm. Commonly diagnosed before age 20. Typically represented by immature/embryonic-like neural tissue.
Yolk sac tumor	Also known as ovarian endodermal sinus tumor. Aggressive, in ovaries or testes and sacrococcygeal area in young children. Most common tumor in male infants. Yellow, friable (hemorrhagic), solid mass. 50% have Schiller-Duval bodies (resemble glomeruli) **F**. AFP = tumor marker.

Sex cord stromal tumors (malignant)	
Granulosa cell tumor	Most common malignant stromal tumor. Predominantly women in their 50s. Often produces estrogen and/or progesterone and presents with postmenopausal bleeding, sexual precocity (in pre-adolescents), breast tenderness. Histology shows **Call-Exner bodies** **D** (granulosa cells arranged haphazardly around collections of eosinophilic fluid, resembling primordial follicles). "Give Granny a Call!"

Other (malignant)	
Krukenberg tumor	GI malignancy that metastasizes to ovaries → mucin-secreting signet cell adenocarcinoma. Commonly presents as bilateral ovarian masses.

Endometrial conditions

Polyp	Well-circumscribed collection of endometrial tissue within uterine wall. May contain smooth muscle cells. Can extend into endometrial cavity in the form of a polyp. May be asymptomatic or present with painless abnormal uterine bleeding.
Adenomyosis	Extension of endometrial tissue (glandular) into uterine myometrium. Caused by hyperplasia of basal layer of endometrium. Presents with dysmenorrhea, menorrhagia, uniformly enlarged, soft, globular uterus. Treatment: GnRH agonists, hysterectomy or excision of an organized adenomyoma.
Asherman syndrome	Adhesions and/or fibrosis of the endometrium. Presents with ↓ fertility, recurrent pregnancy loss, abnormal uterine bleeding, pelvic pain. Often associated with dilation and curettage of intrauterine cavity.
Leiomyoma (fibroid)	Most common tumor in females. Often presents with multiple discrete tumors **A**. ↑ incidence in African Americans. Benign smooth muscle tumor; malignant transformation to leiomyosarcoma is rare. Estrogen sensitive—tumor size ↑ with pregnancy and ↓ with menopause. Peak occurrence at 20–40 years old. May be asymptomatic, cause abnormal uterine bleeding, or result in miscarriage. Severe bleeding may lead to iron deficiency anemia. Whorled pattern of smooth muscle bundles with well-demarcated borders **B**.
Endometrial hyperplasia	Abnormal endometrial gland proliferation usually caused by excess estrogen stimulation. ↑ risk for endometrial carcinoma; nuclear atypia is greater risk factor than complex (vs simple) architecture. Presents as postmenopausal vaginal bleeding. Risk factors include anovulatory cycles, hormone replacement therapy, polycystic ovarian syndrome, granulosa cell tumor.
Endometrial carcinoma	Most common gynecologic malignancy **C**. Peak occurrence at 55–65 years old. Presents with vaginal bleeding. Typically preceded by endometrial hyperplasia. Risk factors include prolonged use of estrogen without progestins, obesity, diabetes, hypertension, nulliparity, late menopause, early menarche, Lynch syndrome.
Endometritis	Inflammation of endometrium **D** associated with retained products of conception following delivery, miscarriage, abortion, or with foreign body (eg, IUD). Retained material in uterus promotes infection by bacterial flora from vagina or intestinal tract. Chronic endometritis characterized by presence of plasma cells on histology. Treatment: gentamicin + clindamycin +/– ampicillin.
Endometriosis	Non-neoplastic endometrium-like glands/stroma outside endometrial cavity. Can be found anywhere; most common sites are ovary (frequently bilateral), pelvis, peritoneum. In ovary, appears as endometrioma (blood-filled "chocolate cysts" [oval structures above and below asterisks in **E**]). May be due to retrograde flow, metaplastic transformation of multipotent cells, transportation of endometrial tissue via lymphatic system. Characterized by cyclic pelvic pain, bleeding, dysmenorrhea, dyspareunia, dyschezia (pain with defecation), infertility; normal-sized uterus. Treatment: NSAIDs, continuous OCPs, progestins, GnRH agonists, danazol, laparoscopic removal.

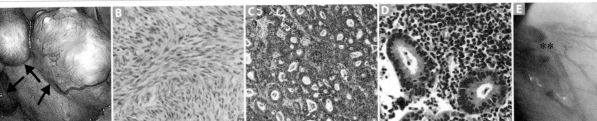

Breast pathology

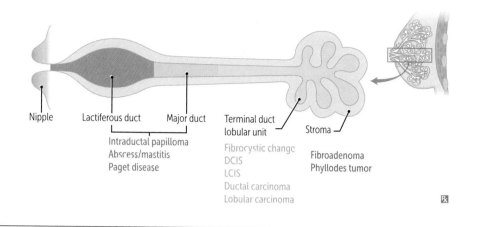

Nipple | Lactiferous duct | Major duct | Terminal duct lobular unit | Stroma

Intraductal papilloma
Abscess/mastitis
Paget disease

Fibrocystic change
DCIS
LCIS
Ductal carcinoma
Lobular carcinoma

Fibroadenoma
Phyllodes tumor

Benign breast disease

Fibrocystic changes	Most common in premenopausal women < 35 years old. Present with premenstrual breast pain or lumps; often bilateral and multifocal. Nonproliferative lesions include simple cysts (fluid-filled duct dilation, blue dome), papillary apocrine change/metaplasia, stromal fibrosis. Risk of cancer is usually not increased. Subtypes include: ▪ Sclerosing adenosis—acini and stromal fibrosis, associated with calcifications. Slight (1.5–2 ×) ↑ risk for cancer. ▪ Epithelial hyperplasia—cells in terminal ductal or lobular epithelium. ↑ risk of carcinoma with atypical cells.
Inflammatory processes	Fat necrosis—benign, usually painless, lump due to injury to breast tissue. Calcified oil cyst on mammography; necrotic fat and giant cells on biopsy. Up to 50% of patients may not report trauma. Lactational mastitis—occurs during breastfeeding, ↑ risk of bacterial infection through cracks in nipple. *S aureus* is most common pathogen. Treat with antibiotics and continue breastfeeding.
Benign tumors	Fibroadenoma—most common in women < 35 years old. Small, well-defined, mobile mass **A**. ↑ size and tenderness with ↑ estrogen (eg, pregnancy, prior to menstruation). Risk of cancer is usually not increased. Intraductal papilloma—small fibroepithelial tumor within lactiferous ducts, typically beneath areola. Most common cause of nipple discharge (serous or bloody). Slight (1.5–2 ×) ↑ risk for cancer. Phyllodes tumor—large mass **B** of connective tissue and cysts with "leaf-like" lobulations **C**. Most common in 5th decade. Some may become malignant.
Gynecomastia	Breast enlargement in males due to ↑ estrogen compared with androgen activity. Physiologic in newborn, pubertal, and elderly males, but may persist after puberty. Other causes include cirrhosis, hypogonadism (eg, Klinefelter syndrome), testicular tumors, and drugs (Spironolactone, Hormones, Cimetidine, Finasteride, Ketoconazole: "Some Hormones Create Funny Knockers").

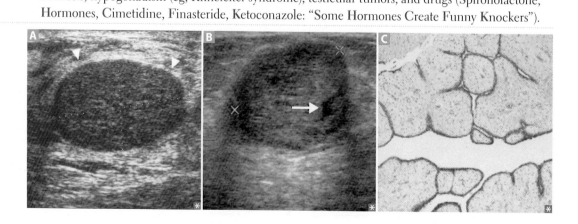

Malignant breast tumors	Commonly postmenopausal. Usually arise from terminal duct lobular unit. Amplification/ overexpression of estrogen/progesterone receptors or *c-erbB2* (HER-2, an EGF receptor) is common; triple negative (ER ⊖, PR ⊖, and Her2/Neu ⊖) more aggressive; type affects therapy and prognosis. Axillary lymph node involvement indicating metastasis is the most important prognostic factor in early-stage disease. Most often located in upper-outer quadrant of breast.	Risk factors: ↑ estrogen exposure, ↑ total number of menstrual cycles, older age at 1st live birth, obesity (↑ estrogen exposure as adipose tissue converts androstenedione to estrone), *BRCA1* or *BRCA2* gene mutations, African American ethnicity (↑ risk for triple ⊖ breast cancer).

TYPE	CHARACTERISTICS	NOTES
Noninvasive		
Ductal carcinoma in situ	Fills ductal lumen (black arrow in 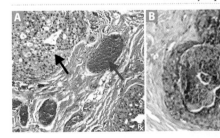 indicates neoplastic cells in duct; blue arrow shows engorged blood vessel). Arises from ductal atypia. Often seen early as microcalcifications on mammography.	Early malignancy without basement membrane penetration.
Comedocarcinoma	Ductal, central necrosis (arrow in B). Subtype of DCIS.	
Paget disease	Results from underlying DCIS or invasive breast cancer. Eczematous patches on nipple 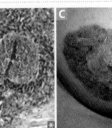. Paget cells = intraepithelial adenocarcinoma cells.	
Invasive		
Invasive ductal carcinoma	Firm, fibrous, "rock-hard" mass with sharp margins and small, glandular, duct-like cells. Tumor can deform suspensory ligaments → dimpling of skin. Classic morphology: "stellate" infiltration.	Most common (~ 75% of all breast cancers).
Invasive lobular carcinoma	Orderly row of cells ("single file" D), due to ↓ E-cadherin expression.	Often bilateral with multiple lesions in the same location. Lines of cells = Lobular.
Medullary carcinoma	Fleshy, cellular, lymphocytic infiltrate.	Good prognosis.
Inflammatory breast cancer	Dermal lymphatic invasion by breast carcinoma. Peau d'orange (skin texture resembles orange peel 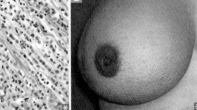 due to edema leading to tightening of Cooper's suspensory ligament); neoplastic cells block lymphatic drainage.	Poor prognosis (50% survival at 5 years). Often mistaken for mastitis or Paget disease.

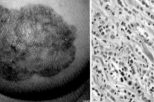

Penile pathology

Peyronie disease	Abnormal curvature of penis due to fibrous plaque within tunica albuginea. Associated with erectile dysfunction. Can cause pain, anxiety. Consider surgical repair once curvature stabilizes. Distinct from penile fracture (rupture of corpora cavernosa due to forced bending).
Ischemic priapism	Painful sustained erection lasting > 4 hours. Associated with sickle cell disease (sickled RBCs block venous drainage of corpus cavernosum vascular channels), medications (eg, sildenafil, trazodone). Treat immediately with corporal aspiration, intracavernosal phenylephrine, or surgical decompression to prevent ischemia.
Squamous cell carcinoma	More common in Asia, Africa, South America. Precursor in situ lesions: Bowen disease (in penile shaft, presents as leukoplakia), erythroplasia of Queyrat (carcinoma in situ of the glans, presents as erythroplakia), Bowenoid papulosis (carcinoma in situ of unclear malignant potential, presenting as reddish papules). Associated with uncircumcised males and HPV.

Cryptorchidism

Undescended testis (one or both); impaired spermatogenesis (since sperm develop best at temperatures < 37°C); can have normal testosterone levels (Leydig cells are mostly unaffected by temperature); associated with ↑ risk of germ cell tumors. Prematurity ↑ risk of cryptorchidism. ↓ inhibin B, ↑ FSH, ↑ LH; testosterone ↓ in bilateral cryptorchidism, normal in unilateral.

Testicular torsion

Rotation of testicle around spermatic cord and vascular pedicle. Commonly presents in males 12–18 years old. Characterized by acute, severe pain, high-riding testis, and absent cremasteric reflex.

Treatment: surgical correction (orchiopexy) within 6 hours, manual detorsion if surgical option unavailable in timeframe. If testis is not viable, orchiectomy. Orchiopexy, when performed, should be bilateral because the contralateral testis is at risk for subsequent torsion.

Varicocele

Dilated veins in pampiniform plexus due to ↑ venous pressure; most common cause of scrotal enlargement in adult males; most often on left side because of ↑ resistance to flow from left gonadal vein drainage into left renal vein; can cause infertility because of ↑ temperature; diagnosed by standing clinical exam/Valsalva maneuver (distension on inspection and "bag of worms" on palpation; augmented by Valsalva) or ultrasound with Doppler A; does not transilluminate.

Treatment: consider surgical ligation or embolization if associated with pain or infertility.

Extragonadal germ cell tumors

Arise in midline locations. In adults, most commonly in retroperitoneum, mediastinum, pineal, and suprasellar regions. In infants and young children, sacrococcygeal teratomas are most common.

Scrotal masses	Benign scrotal lesions present as testicular masses that can be transilluminated (vs solid testicular tumors).	
Congenital hydrocele	Common cause of scrotal swelling A in infants, due to incomplete obliteration of processus vaginalis. Most spontaneously resolve by 1 year old.	Transilluminating swelling.
Acquired hydrocele	Scrotal fluid collection usually 2° to infection, trauma, tumor. If bloody → hematocele.	
Spermatocele	Cyst due to dilated epididymal duct or rete testis.	Paratesticular fluctuant nodule.

Testicular germ cell tumors	~ 95% of all testicular tumors. Most often occur in young men. Risk factors: cryptorchidism, Klinefelter syndrome. Can present as a mixed germ cell tumor. Do not transilluminate. Usually not biopsied (risk of seeding scrotum), removed via radical orchiectomy.
Seminoma	Malignant; painless, homogenous testicular enlargement; most common testicular tumor. Does not occur in infancy. Large cells in lobules with watery cytoplasm and "fried egg" appearance. ↑ placental ALP. Highly radiosensitive. Late metastasis, excellent prognosis. Similar to dysgerminoma in females.
Yolk sac tumor	Also known as testicular endodermal sinus tumor. Yellow, mucinous. Aggressive malignancy of testes, analogous to ovarian yolk sac tumor. Schiller-Duval bodies resemble primitive glomeruli. ↑ AFP is highly characteristic. Most common testicular tumor in boys < 3 years old.
Choriocarcinoma	Malignant, ↑ hCG. Disordered syncytiotrophoblastic and cytotrophoblastic elements. Hematogenous metastases to lungs and brain. May produce gynecomastia, symptoms of hyperthyroidism (α-subunit of hCG is structurally similar to LH, FSH, TSH).
Teratoma	Unlike in females, mature teratoma in adult males may be malignant. Benign in children.
Embryonal carcinoma	Malignant, hemorrhagic mass with necrosis; painful; worse prognosis than seminoma. Often glandular/papillary morphology. "Pure" embryonal carcinoma is rare; most commonly mixed with other tumor types. May be associated with ↑ hCG and normal AFP levels when pure (↑ AFP when mixed).

Testicular non–germ cell tumors	5% of all testicular tumors. Mostly benign.
Leydig cell tumor	Golden brown color; contains Reinke crystals (eosinophilic cytoplasmic inclusions). Produces androgens or estrogens → gynecomastia in men, precocious puberty in boys.
Sertoli cell tumor	Androblastoma from sex cord stroma.
Testicular lymphoma	Most common testicular cancer in older men. Not a 1° cancer; arises from metastatic lymphoma to testes. Aggressive.

Benign prostatic hyperplasia	Common in men > 50 years old. Characterized by smooth, elastic, firm nodular enlargement (hyperplasia not hypertrophy) of periurethral (lateral and middle) lobes, which compress the urethra into a vertical slit. Not premalignant.

Often presents with ↑ frequency of urination, nocturia, difficulty starting and stopping urine stream, dysuria. May lead to distention and hypertrophy of bladder, hydronephrosis, UTIs. ↑ free prostate-specific antigen (PSA).

Treatment: α_1-antagonists (terazosin, tamsulosin), which cause relaxation of smooth muscle; 5α-reductase inhibitors (eg, finasteride); PDE-5 inhibitors (eg, tadalafil); surgical resection (eg, TURP, ablation).

Anterior lobe — Benign prostatic hyperplasia — Urethra — Lateral lobe — Middle lobe — Posterior lobe — Prostate cancer

---

Prostatitis

Characterized by dysuria, frequency, urgency, low back pain. Warm, tender, enlarged prostate.

Acute bacterial prostatitis—in older men most common bacterium is *E coli*; in young males consider *C trachomatis*, *N gonorrhoeae*.

Chronic prostatitis—either bacterial or nonbacterial (eg, 2° to previous infection, nerve problems, chemical irritation).

Prostatic adenocarcinoma

Common in men > 50 years old. Arises most often from posterior lobe (peripheral zone) of prostate gland and is most frequently diagnosed by ↑ PSA and subsequent needle core biopsies. Prostatic acid phosphatase (PAP) and PSA are useful tumor markers (↑ total PSA, with ↓ fraction of free PSA). Osteoblastic metastases in bone may develop in late stages, as indicated by lower back pain and ↑ serum ALP and PSA.

Control of reproductive hormones

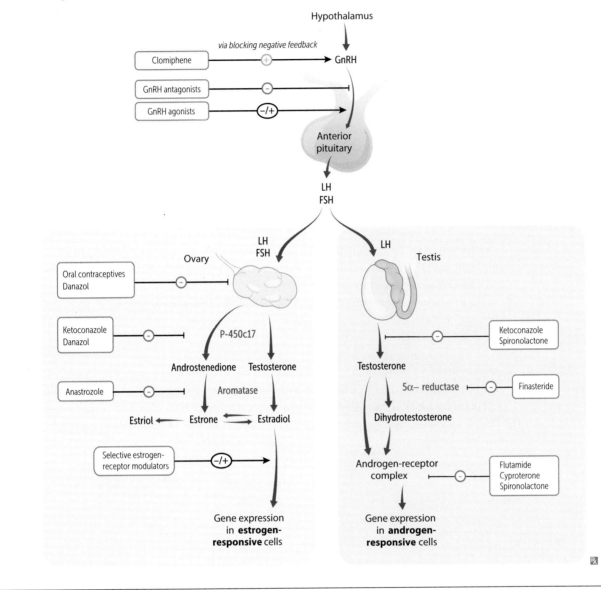

Leuprolide

MECHANISM	GnRH analog with agonist properties when used in pulsatile fashion; antagonist properties when used in continuous fashion (downregulates GnRH receptor in pituitary → ↓ FSH and ↓ LH).
CLINICAL USE	Uterine fibroids, endometriosis, precocious puberty, prostate cancer, infertility.
ADVERSE EFFECTS	Hypogonadism, ↓ libido, erectile dysfunction, nausea, vomiting.

Leuprolide can be used in lieu of GnRH.

Estrogens

Ethinyl estradiol, DES, mestranol.

MECHANISM	Bind estrogen receptors.
CLINICAL USE	Hypogonadism or ovarian failure, menstrual abnormalities (combined OCPs), hormone replacement therapy in postmenopausal women.
ADVERSE EFFECTS	↑ risk of endometrial cancer (when given without progesterone), bleeding in postmenopausal women, clear cell adenocarcinoma of vagina in females exposed to DES in utero, ↑ risk of thrombi. Contraindications—ER ⊕ breast cancer, history of DVTs, tobacco use in women > 35 years old.

Selective estrogen receptor modulators

Clomiphene	Antagonist at estrogen receptors in hypothalamus. Prevents normal feedback inhibition and ↑ release of LH and FSH from pituitary, which stimulates ovulation. Used to treat infertility due to anovulation (eg, PCOS). SERMs may cause hot flashes, ovarian enlargement, multiple simultaneous pregnancies, visual disturbances.
Tamoxifen	Antagonist at breast; agonist at bone, uterus; ↑ risk of thromboembolic events and endometrial cancer. Used to treat and prevent recurrence of ER/PR ⊕ breast cancer.
Raloxifene	Antagonist at breast, uterus; agonist at bone; ↑ risk of thromboembolic events but no increased risk of endometrial cancer (vs tamoxifen); used primarily to treat osteoporosis.

Aromatase inhibitors

Anastrozole, letrozole, exemestane.

MECHANISM	Inhibit peripheral conversion of androgens to estrogen.
CLINICAL USE	ER ⊕ breast cancer in postmenopausal women.

Hormone replacement therapy

Used for relief or prevention of menopausal symptoms (eg, hot flashes, vaginal atrophy), osteoporosis (↑ estrogen, ↓ osteoclast activity).

Unopposed estrogen replacement therapy ↑ risk of endometrial cancer, progesterone/progestin is added. Possible increased cardiovascular risk.

Progestins	Levonorgestrel, medroxyprogesterone, etonogestrel, norethindrone, megestrol, and many others when combined with estrogen.
MECHANISM	Bind progesterone receptors, ↓ growth and ↑ vascularization of endometrium, thicken cervical mucus.
CLINICAL USE	Contraception (forms include pill, intrauterine device, implant, depot injection), endometrial cancer, abnormal uterine bleeding. Progestin challenge: presence of withdrawal bleeding excludes anatomic defects (eg, Asherman syndrome) and chronic anovulation without estrogen.

Antiprogestins	Mifepristone, ulipristal.
MECHANISM	Competitive inhibitors of progestins at progesterone receptors.
CLINICAL USE	Termination of pregnancy (mifepristone with misoprostol); emergency contraception (ulipristal).

Combined contraception	Progestins and ethinyl estradiol; forms include pill, patch, vaginal ring. Estrogen and progestins inhibit LH/FSH and thus prevent estrogen surge. No estrogen surge → no LH surge → no ovulation. Progestins cause thickening of cervical mucus, thereby limiting access of sperm to uterus. Progestins also inhibit endometrial proliferation → endometrium is less suitable to the implantation of an embryo. Contraindications: smokers > 35 years old (↑ risk of cardiovascular events), patients with ↑ risk of cardiovascular disease (including history of venous thromboembolism, coronary artery disease, stroke), migraine (especially with aura), breast cancer, liver disease.

Copper intrauterine device	
MECHANISM	Produces local inflammatory reaction toxic to sperm and ova, preventing fertilization and implantation; hormone free.
CLINICAL USE	Long-acting reversible contraception. Most effective emergency contraception.
ADVERSE EFFECTS	Heavier or longer menses, dysmenorrhea. Risk of PID with insertion (contraindicated in active pelvic infection).

Tocolytics	Medications that relax the uterus; include terbutaline (β_2-agonist action), nifedipine (Ca^{2+} channel blocker), indomethacin (NSAID). Used to ↓ contraction frequency in preterm labor and allow time for administration of steroids (to promote fetal lung maturity) or transfer to appropriate medical center with obstetrical care.

Danazol	
MECHANISM	Synthetic androgen that acts as partial agonist at androgen receptors.
CLINICAL USE	Endometriosis, hereditary angioedema.
ADVERSE EFFECTS	Weight gain, edema, acne, hirsutism, masculinization, ↓ HDL levels, hepatotoxicity, pseudotumor cerebri.

Testosterone, methyltestosterone

MECHANISM	Agonists at androgen receptors.
CLINICAL USE	Treat hypogonadism and promote development of 2° sex characteristics; stimulate anabolism to promote recovery after burn or injury.
ADVERSE EFFECTS	Masculinization in females; ↓ intratesticular testosterone in males by inhibiting release of LH (via negative feedback) → gonadal atrophy. Premature closure of epiphyseal plates. ↑ LDL, ↓ HDL.

Antiandrogens

Finasteride	5α-reductase inhibitor (↓ conversion of testosterone to DHT). Used for BPH and male-pattern baldness. Adverse effects: gynecomastia and sexual dysfunction.	Testosterone $\xrightarrow{5\alpha\text{-reductase}}$ DHT (more potent).
Flutamide	Nonsteroidal competitive inhibitor at androgen receptors. Used for prostate carcinoma.	
Ketoconazole	Inhibits steroid synthesis (inhibits 17,20 desmolase/17α-hydroxylase).	Used in PCOS to reduce androgenic symptoms. Both can cause gynecomastia and amenorrhea.
Spironolactone	Inhibits steroid binding, 17,20 desmolase/17α-hydroxylase.	

Tamsulosin

α_1-antagonist used to treat BPH by inhibiting smooth muscle contraction. Selective for $\alpha_{1A/D}$ receptors (found on prostate) vs vascular α_{1B} receptors.

Phosphodiesterase type 5 inhibitors

Sildenafil, vardenafil, tadalafil.

MECHANISM	Inhibit PDE-5 → ↑ cGMP → prolonged smooth muscle relaxation in response to NO → ↑ blood flow in corpus cavernosum of penis, ↓ pulmonary vascular resistance.	Sildenafil, vardenafil, and tadalafil fill the penis.
CLINICAL USE	Erectile dysfunction, pulmonary hypertension, BPH (tadalafil only).	
ADVERSE EFFECTS	Headache, flushing, dyspepsia, cyanopia (blue-tinted vision). Risk of life-threatening hypotension in patients taking nitrates.	"Hot and sweaty," but then Headache, Heartburn, Hypotension.

Minoxidil

MECHANISM	Direct arteriolar vasodilator.
CLINICAL USE	Androgenetic alopecia (pattern baldness), severe refractory hypertension.

▶ NOTES

Respiratory

"There's so much pollution in the air now that if it weren't for our lungs, there'd be no place to put it all."

—Robert Orben

"Freedom is the oxygen of the soul."

—Moshe Dayan

"Whenever I feel blue, I start breathing again."

—L. Frank Baum

"Life is not the amount of breaths you take; it's the moments that take your breath away."

—Will Smith, *Hitch*

Group key respiratory, cardiovascular, and renal concepts together for study whenever possible. Know obstructive vs restrictive lung disorders, V̇/Q̇ mismatch, lung volumes, mechanics of respiration, and hemoglobin physiology. Lung cancers and other causes of lung masses are high yield. Be comfortable reading basic chest X-rays, CT scans, and PFTs.

▶ RESPIRATORY—EMBRYOLOGY

Lung development	Occurs in five stages. Initial development includes development of lung bud from distal end of respiratory diverticulum during week 4. Every Pulmonologist Can See Alveoli.	

STAGE	STRUCTURAL DEVELOPMENT	NOTES
Embryonic (weeks 4–7)	Lung bud → trachea → bronchial buds → mainstem bronchi → secondary (lobar) bronchi → tertiary (segmental) bronchi.	Errors at this stage can lead to tracheoesophageal fistula.
Pseudoglandular (weeks 5–17)	Endodermal tubules → terminal bronchioles. Surrounded by modest capillary network.	Respiration impossible, incompatible with life.
Canalicular (weeks 16–25)	Terminal bronchioles → respiratory bronchioles → alveolar ducts. Surrounded by prominent capillary network.	Airways increase in diameter. Respiration capable at 25 weeks. Pneumocytes develop starting at 20 weeks.
Saccular (week 26–birth)	Alveolar ducts → terminal sacs. Terminal sacs separated by 1° septae.	
Alveolar (week 36–8 years)	Terminal sacs → adult alveoli (due to 2° septation). In utero, "breathing" occurs via aspiration and expulsion of amniotic fluid → ↑ vascular resistance through gestation. At birth, fluid gets replaced with air → ↓ in pulmonary vascular resistance.	At birth: 20–70 million alveoli. By 8 years: 300–400 million alveoli.

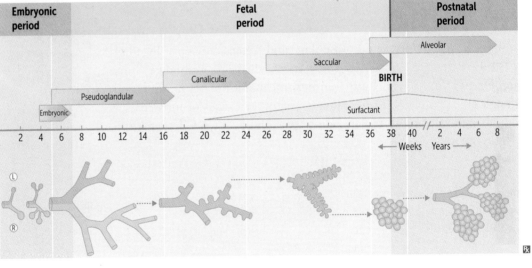

Congenital lung malformations

Pulmonary hypoplasia	Poorly developed bronchial tree with abnormal histology. Associated with congenital diaphragmatic hernia (usually left-sided), bilateral renal agenesis (Potter sequence).
Bronchogenic cysts	Caused by abnormal budding of the foregut and dilation of terminal or large bronchi. Discrete, round, sharply defined, fluid-filled densities on CXR (air-filled if infected). Generally asymptomatic but can drain poorly, causing airway compression and/or recurrent respiratory infections.

Club cells	Nonciliated; low columnar/cuboidal with secretory granules. Located in bronchioles. Degrade toxins; secrete component of surfactant; act as reserve cells.

Alveolar cell types

Type I pneumocytes	97% of alveolar surfaces. Line the alveoli. Squamous; thin for optimal gas diffusion.

$$\text{Collapsing pressure } (P) = \frac{2 \text{ (surface tension)}}{\text{radius}}$$

Alveoli have ↑ tendency to collapse on expiration as radius ↓ (law of Laplace).

Pulmonary surfactant is a complex mix of lecithins, the most important of which is dipalmitoylphosphatidylcholine (DPPC).

Surfactant synthesis begins around week 20 of gestation, but mature levels are not achieved until around week 35.

Corticosteroids important for fetus surfactant production and lung development.

Type II pneumocytes 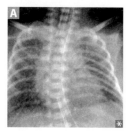	Secrete surfactant from lamellar bodies (arrow in A) → ↓ alveolar surface tension, prevents alveolar collapse, ↓ lung recoil, and ↑ compliance. Cuboidal and clustered B. Also serve as precursors to type I cells and other type II cells. Proliferate during lung damage.

Alveolar macrophages	Phagocytose foreign materials; release cytokines and alveolar proteases. Hemosiderin-laden macrophages may be seen in pulmonary hemorrhage.

Neonatal respiratory distress syndrome	Surfactant deficiency → ↑ surface tension → alveolar collapse ("ground-glass" appearance of lung fields) A.

Risk factors: prematurity, maternal diabetes (due to ↑ fetal insulin), C-section delivery (↓ release of fetal glucocorticoids; less stressful than vaginal delivery).

Complications: PDA, necrotizing enterocolitis.

Treatment: maternal steroids before birth; exogenous surfactant for infant.

Therapeutic supplemental O_2 can result in Retinopathy of prematurity, Intraventricular hemorrhage, Bronchopulmonary dysplasia (**RIB**).

Screening tests for fetal lung maturity: lecithin-sphingomyelin (L/S) ratio in amniotic fluid (≥ 2 is healthy; < 1.5 predictive of NRDS), foam stability index, surfactant-albumin ratio.

Persistently low O_2 tension → risk of PDA.

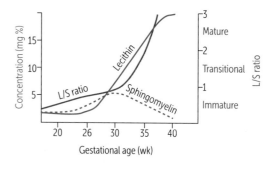

▸ RESPIRATORY—ANATOMY

Respiratory tree

Conducting zone	Large airways consist of nose, pharynx, larynx, trachea, and bronchi. Small airways consist of bronchioles that further divide into terminal bronchioles (large numbers in parallel → least airway resistance).
	Warms, humidifies, and filters air but does not participate in gas exchange → "anatomic dead space."
	Cartilage and goblet cells extend to the end of bronchi.
	Pseudostratified ciliated columnar cells primarily make up epithelium of bronchus and extend to beginning of terminal bronchioles, then transition to cuboidal cells. Clear mucus and debris from lungs (mucociliary escalator).
	Airway smooth muscle cells extend to end of terminal bronchioles (sparse beyond this point).
Respiratory zone	Lung parenchyma; consists of respiratory bronchioles, alveolar ducts, and alveoli. Participates in gas exchange.
	Mostly cuboidal cells in respiratory bronchioles, then simple squamous cells up to alveoli. Cilia terminate in respiratory bronchioles. Alveolar macrophages clear debris and participate in immune response.

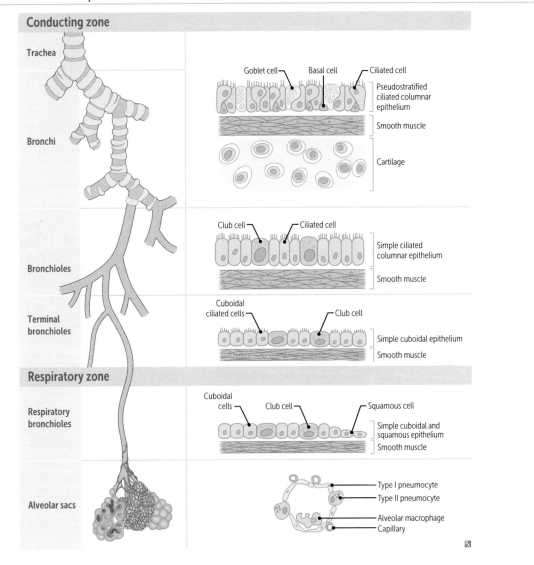

Lung anatomy

Right lung has 3 lobes; Left has Less Lobes (2) and Lingula (homolog of right middle lobe). Instead of a middle lobe, left lung has a space occupied by the heart **A**.

Relation of the pulmonary artery to the bronchus at each lung hilum is described by **RALS**—Right Anterior; Left Superior. Carina is posterior to ascending aorta and anteromedial to descending aorta **B**.

Right lung is a more common site for inhaled foreign bodies because right main stem bronchus is wider, more vertical, and shorter than the left. If you aspirate a peanut:

- While supine—usually enters right lower lobe.
- While lying on right side—usually enters right upper lobe.
- While upright—usually enters right lower lobe.

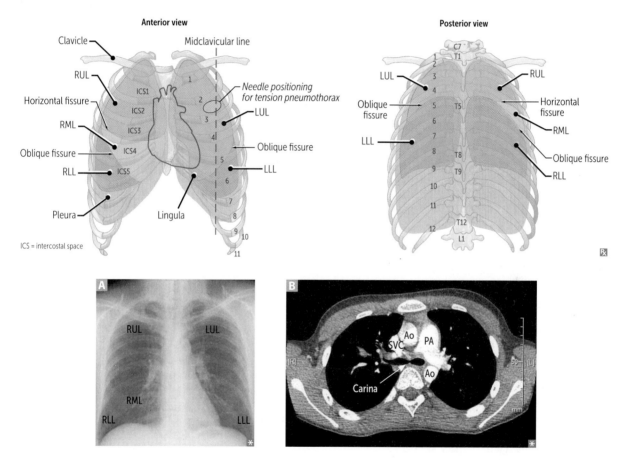

Diaphragm structures

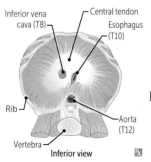

Structures perforating diaphragm:
- At T8: IVC, right phrenic nerve
- At T10: esophagus, vagus (CN 10; 2 trunks)
- At T12: aorta (red), thoracic duct (white), azygos vein (blue) ("At T-1-2 it's the red, white, and blue")

Diaphragm is innervated by C3, 4, and 5 (phrenic nerve). Pain from diaphragm irritation (eg, air, blood, or pus in peritoneal cavity) can be referred to shoulder (C5) and trapezius ridge (C3, 4).

Number of letters = T level:
- T8: vena cava
- T10: "oesophagus"
- T12: aortic hiatus

I (IVC) **ate** (8) **ten** (10) **eggs** (esophagus) **at** (aorta) **twelve** (12).

C3, 4, 5 keeps the diaphragm alive.

Other bifurcations:
- The common carotid bifurcates at C4.
- The trachea bifurcates at T4.
- The abdominal aorta bifurcates at L4.

▶ RESPIRATORY—PHYSIOLOGY

Lung volumes	Note: a **capacity** is a sum of ≥ 2 physiologic **volumes**.	
Inspiratory reserve volume	Air that can still be breathed in after normal inspiration	
Tidal volume	Air that moves into lung with each quiet inspiration, typically 500 mL	
Expiratory reserve volume	Air that can still be breathed out after normal expiration	
Residual volume	Air in lung after maximal expiration; RV and any lung capacity that includes RV cannot be measured by spirometry	
Inspiratory capacity	IRV + TV Air that can be breathed in after normal exhalation	
Functional residual capacity	RV + ERV Volume of gas in lungs after normal expiration	
Vital capacity	TV + IRV + ERV Maximum volume of gas that can be expired after a maximal inspiration	
Total lung capacity	IRV + TV + ERV + RV Volume of gas present in lungs after a maximal inspiration	

Lung volumes (LITER) · Lung capacities

Determination of physiologic dead space	$V_D = V_T \times \dfrac{Paco_2 - Peco_2}{Paco_2}$ V_D = physiologic dead space = anatomic dead space of conducting airways plus alveolar dead space; apex of healthy lung is largest contributor of alveolar dead space. Volume of inspired air that does not take part in gas exchange. V_T = tidal volume. $Paco_2$ = arterial Pco_2. $Peco_2$ = expired air Pco_2.	Taco, Paco, Peco, Paco (refers to order of variables in equation) Physiologic dead space—approximately equivalent to anatomic dead space in normal lungs. May be greater than anatomic dead space in lung diseases with $\dot{V}/\dot{Q}$ defects.

Ventilation

Minute ventilation	Total volume of gas entering lungs per minute $V_E = V_T \times RR$	Normal values: Respiratory rate (RR) = 12–20 breaths/min V_T = 500 mL/breath V_D = 150 mL/breath
Alveolar ventilation	Volume of gas that reaches alveoli each minute $V_A = (V_T - V_D) \times RR$	

Lung and chest wall

Elastic recoil—tendency for lungs to collapse inward and chest wall to spring outward.

At FRC, inward pull of lung is balanced by outward pull of chest wall, and system pressure is atmospheric.

At FRC, airway and alveolar pressures equal atmospheric pressure (called zero), and intrapleural pressure is negative (prevents atelectasis). The inward pull of the lung is balanced by the outward pull of the chest wall. System pressure is atmospheric. PVR is at a minimum.

Compliance—change in lung volume for a change in pressure; expressed as $\Delta V/\Delta P$ and is inversely proportional to wall stiffness. High compliance = lung easier to fill (emphysema, normal aging), lower compliance = lung harder to fill (pulmonary fibrosis, pneumonia, NRDS, pulmonary edema). Surfactant increases compliance.

Hysteresis—lung inflation curve follows a different curve than the lung deflation curve due to need to overcome surface tension forces in inflation.

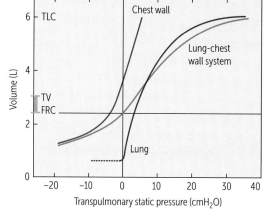

Compliant lungs comply (cooperate) and fill easily with air.

Respiratory system changes in the elderly

↑ lung compliance (loss of elastic recoil)

↓ chest wall compliance (↑ chest wall stiffness)

↑ RV

↓ FVC and FEV_1

Normal TLC

↑ ventilation/perfusion mismatch

↑ A-a gradient

↓ respiratory muscle strength

Hemoglobin

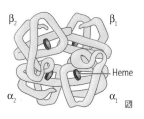

Hemoglobin (Hb) is composed of 4 polypeptide subunits (2 α and 2 β) and exists in 2 forms:
- Deoxygenated form has low affinity for O_2, thus promoting release/unloading of O_2.
- Oxygenated form has high affinity for O_2 (300×). Hb exhibits positive cooperativity and negative allostery.

↑ Cl^-, H^+, CO_2, 2,3-BPG, and temperature favor deoxygenated form over oxygenated form (shifts dissociation curve right → ↑ O_2 unloading).

Fetal Hb (2α and 2γ subunits) has a higher affinity for O_2 than adult Hb, driving diffusion of oxygen across the placenta from mother to fetus. ↑ O_2 affinity results from ↓ affinity of HbF for 2,3-BPG.

Hemoglobin acts as buffer for H^+ ions.

Myoglobin is composed of a single polypeptide chain associated with one heme moiety. Higher affinity for oxygen than Hb.

Hemoglobin modifications	Lead to tissue hypoxia from ↓ O_2 saturation and ↓ O_2 content.	
Methemoglobin	Oxidized form of Hb (ferric, Fe^{3+}), does not bind O_2 as readily as Fe^{2+}, but has ↑ affinity for cyanide. Fe^{2+} binds O_2. Iron in Hb is normally in a reduced state (ferrous, Fe^{2+}; "just the 2 of us"). Methemoglobinemia may present with cyanosis and chocolate-colored blood. Methemoglobinemia can be treated with methylene blue and vitamin C.	Nitrites (eg, from dietary intake or polluted/high altitude water sources) and benzocaine cause poisoning by oxidizing Fe^{2+} to Fe^{3+}.
Carboxyhemoglobin	Form of Hb bound to CO in place of O_2. Causes ↓ oxygen-binding capacity with left shift in oxygen-hemoglobin dissociation curve. ↓ O_2 unloading in tissues. CO binds competitively to Hb and with 200× greater affinity than O_2. CO poisoning can present with headaches, dizziness, and cherry red skin. May be caused by fires, car exhaust, or gas heaters. Treat with 100% O_2 and hyperbaric O_2.	

Cyanide poisoning	Usually due to inhalation injury (eg, fires). Inhibits aerobic metabolism via complex IV inhibition → hypoxia unresponsive to supplemental O_2 and ↑ anaerobic metabolism. Findings: almond breath odor, pink skin, cyanosis. Rapidly fatal if untreated. Treat with induced methemoglobinemia: first give nitrites (oxidize hemoglobin to methemoglobin, which can trap cyanide as cyanmethemoglobin), then thiosulfates (convert cyanide to thiocyanate, which is renally excreted).

Oxygen-hemoglobin dissociation curve

Sigmoidal shape due to positive cooperativity (ie, tetrameric Hb molecule can bind 4 O_2 molecules and has higher affinity for each subsequent O_2 molecule bound). Myoglobin is monomeric and thus does not show positive cooperativity; curve lacks sigmoidal appearance.

Shifting the curve to the right → ↓ Hb affinity for O_2 (facilitates unloading of O_2 to tissue) → ↑ P_{50} (higher P_{O_2} required to maintain 50% saturation).

Shifting the curve to the left → ↓ O_2 unloading → renal hypoxia → ↑ EPO synthesis → compensatory erythrocytosis.

Fetal Hb has higher affinity for O_2 than adult Hb (due to low affinity for 2,3-BPG), so its dissociation curve is shifted left.

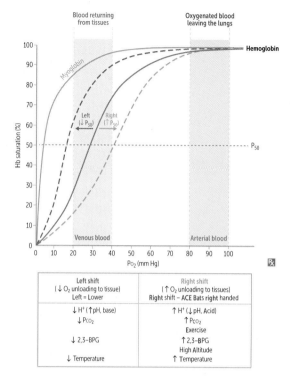

Left shift (↓ O_2 unloading to tissue) Left = Lower	Right shift (↑ O_2 unloading to tissues) Right shift – ACE Bats right handed
↓ H^+ (↑ pH, base)	↑ H^+ (↓ pH, Acid)
↓ P_{CO_2}	↑ P_{CO_2}
	Exercise
↓ 2,3–BPG	↑ 2,3–BPG
	High Altitude
↓ Temperature	↑ Temperature

Oxygen content of blood

O_2 content = $(1.34 \times Hb \times Sa_{O_2}) + (0.003 \times Pa_{O_2})$

Hb = hemoglobin level
Sa_{O_2} = arterial O_2 saturation
Pa_{O_2} = partial pressure of O_2 in arterial blood

Normally 1 g Hb can bind 1.34 mL O_2; normal Hb amount in blood is 15 g/dL.
O_2 binding capacity ≈ 20.1 mL O_2/dL of blood.
With ↓ Hb there is ↓ O_2 content of arterial blood, but no change in O_2 saturation and Pa_{O_2}.
O_2 delivery to tissues = cardiac output × O_2 content of blood.

	Hb CONCENTRATION	% O_2 SAT OF Hb	DISSOLVED O_2 (Pa_{O_2})	TOTAL O_2 CONTENT
CO poisoning	Normal	↓ (CO competes with O_2)	Normal	↓
Anemia	↓	Normal	Normal	↓
Polycythemia	↑	Normal	Normal	↑

Pulmonary circulation

Normally a low-resistance, high-compliance system. P_{O_2} and P_{CO_2} exert opposite effects on pulmonary and systemic circulation. A ↓ in P_{AO_2} causes a hypoxic vasoconstriction that shifts blood away from poorly ventilated regions of lung to well-ventilated regions of lung.

Perfusion limited—O_2 (normal health), CO_2, N_2O. Gas equilibrates early along the length of the capillary. Diffusion can be ↑ only if blood flow ↑.

Diffusion limited—O_2 (emphysema, fibrosis, exercise), CO. Gas does not equilibrate by the time blood reaches the end of the capillary.

A consequence of pulmonary hypertension is cor pulmonale and subsequent right ventricular failure.

Diffusion: $\dot{V}_{gas} = A \times D_k \times \dfrac{P_1 - P_2}{T}$ where

A = area, T = alveolar wall thickness, D_k = diffusion coefficient of gas, $P_1 - P_2$ = difference in partial pressures.

- A ↓ in emphysema.
- T ↑ in pulmonary fibrosis.

D_{LCO} is the extent to which CO, a surrogate for O_2, passes from air sacs of lungs into blood.

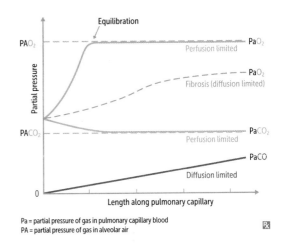

Pa = partial pressure of gas in pulmonary capillary blood
PA = partial pressure of gas in alveolar air

Pulmonary vascular resistance

$$PVR = \frac{P_{pulm\ artery} - P_{L\ atrium}}{cardiac\ output}$$

Remember: $\Delta P = Q \times R$, so $R = \Delta P / Q$

$R = 8\eta l / \pi r^4$

$P_{pulm\ artery}$ = pressure in pulmonary artery
$P_{L\ atrium}$ ≈ pulmonary capillary wedge pressure
Q = cardiac output (flow)
R = resistance
η = viscosity of blood
l = vessel length
r = vessel radius

Alveolar gas equation

$$P_{AO_2} = P_{IO_2} - \frac{P_{aCO_2}}{R}$$

$$\approx 150\ mm\ Hg^a - \frac{P_{aCO_2}}{0.8}$$

[a]At sea level breathing room air

P_{AO_2} = alveolar P_{O_2} (mm Hg)
P_{IO_2} = P_{O_2} in inspired air (mm Hg)
P_{aCO_2} = arterial P_{CO_2} (mm Hg)
R = respiratory quotient = CO_2 produced/O_2 consumed
A-a gradient = $P_{AO_2} - P_{aO_2}$. Normal range = 10–15 mm Hg
↑ A-a gradient may occur in hypoxemia; causes include shunting, $\dot{V}/\dot{Q}$ mismatch, fibrosis (impairs diffusion)

Oxygen deprivation

Hypoxia (↓ O_2 delivery to tissue)	Hypoxemia (↓ Pao_2)	Ischemia (loss of blood flow)
↓ cardiac output Hypoxemia Anemia CO poisoning	Normal A-a gradient • High altitude • Hypoventilation (eg, opioid use) ↑ A-a gradient • V̇/Q̇ mismatch • Diffusion limitation (eg, fibrosis) • Right-to-left shunt	Impeded arterial flow ↓ venous drainage

Ventilation/perfusion mismatch

Ideally, ventilation is matched to perfusion (ie, V̇/Q̇ = 1) for adequate gas exchange.

Lung zones:
- V̇/Q̇ at apex of lung = 3 (wasted ventilation)
- V̇/Q̇ at base of lung = 0.6 (wasted perfusion)

Both ventilation and perfusion are greater at the base of the lung than at the apex of the lung.

With exercise (↑ cardiac output), there is vasodilation of apical capillaries → V̇/Q̇ ratio approaches 1.

Certain organisms that thrive in high O_2 (eg, TB) flourish in the apex.

V̇/Q̇ = 0 = "oirway" obstruction (shunt). In shunt, 100% O_2 does not improve Pao_2 (eg, foreign body aspiration).

V̇/Q̇ = ∞ = blood flow obstruction (physiologic dead space). Assuming < 100% dead space, 100% O_2 improves Pao_2 (eg, pulmonary embolus).

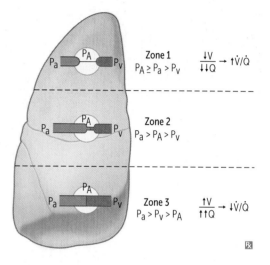

Carbon dioxide transport

CO_2 is transported from tissues to lungs in 3 forms:

1. HCO_3^- (70%).
2. Carbaminohemoglobin or $HbCO_2$ (21–25%). CO_2 bound to Hb at N-terminus of globin (not heme). CO_2 favors deoxygenated form (O_2 unloaded).
3. Dissolved CO_2 (5–9%).

In lungs, oxygenation of Hb promotes dissociation of H^+ from Hb. This shifts equilibrium toward CO_2 formation; therefore, CO_2 is released from ↑RBCs (Haldane effect).

In peripheral tissue, ↑ H^+ from tissue metabolism shifts curve to right, unloading O_2 (Bohr effect).

Majority of blood CO_2 is carried as HCO_3^- in the plasma.

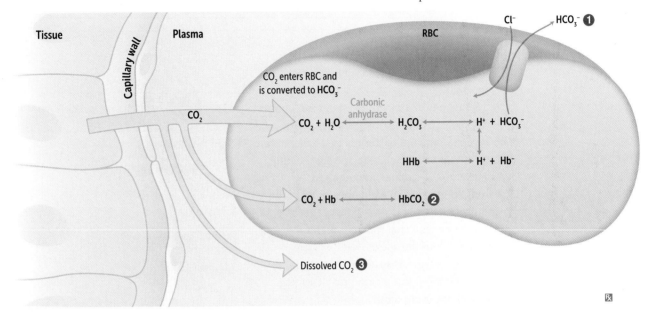

Response to high altitude

↓ atmospheric oxygen (PO_2) → ↓ PaO_2 → ↑ ventilation → ↓ $PaCO_2$ → respiratory alkalosis → altitude sickness.

Chronic ↑ in ventilation.

↑ erythropoietin → ↑ Hct and Hb (due to chronic hypoxia).

↑ 2,3-BPG (binds to Hb causing left shift so that Hb releases more O_2).

Cellular changes (↑ mitochondria).

↑ renal excretion of HCO_3^- to compensate for respiratory alkalosis (can augment with acetazolamide).

Chronic hypoxic pulmonary vasoconstriction results in pulmonary hypertension and RVH.

Response to exercise

↑ CO_2 production.

↑ O_2 consumption.

↑ ventilation rate to meet O_2 demand.

$\dot{V}/\dot{Q}$ ratio from apex to base becomes more uniform.

↑ pulmonary blood flow due to ↑ cardiac output.

↓ pH during strenuous exercise (2° to lactic acidosis).

No change in PaO_2 and $PaCO_2$, but ↑ in venous CO_2 content and ↓ in venous O_2 content.

▶ RESPIRATORY—PATHOLOGY

Rhinosinusitis

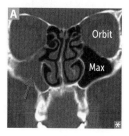

Obstruction of sinus drainage into nasal cavity → inflammation and pain over affected area. Typically affects maxillary sinuses, which drain against gravity due to ostia located superomedially (red arrow points to fluid-filled right maxillary sinus in A).

Most common acute cause is viral URI; may lead to superimposed bacterial infection, most commonly *S pneumoniae*, *H influenzae*, *M catarrhalis*.

Infections in sphenoid or ethmoid sinuses may extend to cavernous sinus and cause complications (eg, cavernous sinus syndrome).

Epistaxis

Nose bleed. Most commonly occurs in anterior segment of nostril (**Kiesselbach plexus**). Life-threatening hemorrhages occur in posterior segment (sphenopalatine artery, a branch of maxillary artery). Common causes include foreign body, trauma, allergic rhinitis, and nasal angiofibromas (common in adolescent males).

Kiesselbach drives his Lexus with his LEGS: superior Labial artery, anterior and posterior Ethmoidal arteries, Greater palatine artery, Sphenopalatine artery.

Head and neck cancer

Mostly squamous cell carcinoma. Risk factors include tobacco, alcohol, HPV-16 (oropharyngeal), EBV (nasopharyngeal). Field cancerization: carcinogen damages wide mucosal area → multiple tumors that develop independently after exposure.

Deep venous thrombosis

Blood clot within a deep vein → swelling, redness A, warmth, pain. Predisposed by Virchow triad (**SHE**):

- Stasis (eg, post-op, long drive/flight)
- Hypercoagulability (eg, defect in coagulation cascade proteins, such as factor V Leiden; oral contraceptive use)
- Endothelial damage (exposed collagen triggers clotting cascade)

D-dimer lab test used clinically to rule out DVT (high sensitivity, low specificity).

Most pulmonary emboli arise from proximal deep veins of lower extremity.

Use unfractionated heparin or low-molecular-weight heparins (eg, enoxaparin) for prophylaxis and acute management.

Use oral anticoagulants (eg, warfarin, rivaroxaban) for treatment (long-term prevention).

Imaging test of choice is compression ultrasound with Doppler.

Pulmonary emboli

V̇/Q̇ mismatch, hypoxemia, respiratory alkalosis. Sudden-onset dyspnea, pleuritic chest pain, tachypnea, tachycardia. Large emboli or saddle embolus A may cause sudden death due to electromechanical dissociation.

Lines of Zahn are interdigitating areas of pink (platelets, fibrin) and red (RBCs) found only in thrombi formed before death; help distinguish pre- and postmortem thrombi B.

Types: Fat, Air, Thrombus, Bacteria, Amniotic fluid, Tumor.

Fat emboli—associated with long bone fractures and liposuction; classic triad of hypoxemia, neurologic abnormalities, petechial rash.

Air emboli—nitrogen bubbles precipitate in ascending divers (caisson disease/ decompression sickness); treat with hyperbaric O_2; or, can be iatrogenic 2° to invasive procedures (eg, central line placement).

Amniotic fluid emboli—can lead to DIC, especially postpartum.

CT pulmonary angiography is imaging test of choice for PE (look for filling defects) C. May have S1Q3T3 abnormality on ECG.

An embolus moves like a **FAT BAT**.

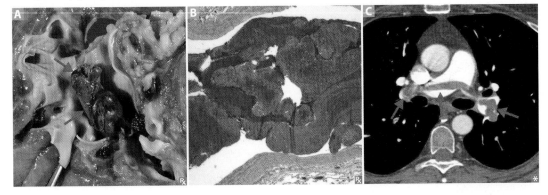

Flow-volume loops

FLOW-VOLUME PARAMETER	Obstructive lung disease	Restrictive lung disease
RV	↑	↓
FRC	↑	↓
TLC	↑	↓
FEV_1	↓↓	↓
FVC	↓	↓
FEV_1/FVC	↓	Normal or ↑
	FEV_1 decreased more than FVC	FEV_1 decreased proportionately to FVC

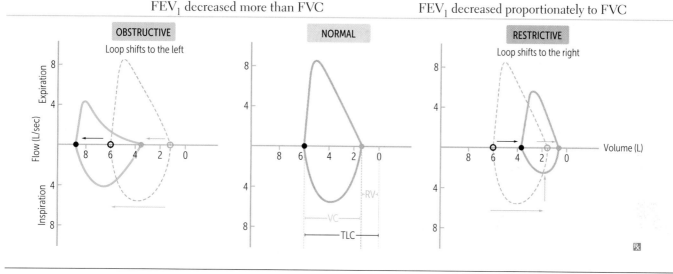

| **Obstructive lung diseases** | Obstruction of air flow → air trapping in lungs. Airways close prematurely at high lung volumes → ↑ FRC, ↑ RV, ↑ TLC. PFTs: ↓↓ FEV_1, ↓ FVC → ↓ FEV_1/FVC ratio (hallmark), V̇/Q̇ mismatch. Chronic, hypoxic pulmonary vasoconstriction can lead to cor pulmonale. Chronic obstructive pulmonary disease (COPD) includes chronic bronchitis and emphysema. "FRiCkin' RV needs some increased TLC, but it's hard with COPD!" | | |

TYPE	PRESENTATION	PATHOLOGY	OTHER
Chronic bronchitis ("blue bloater")	Findings: wheezing, crackles, cyanosis (hypoxemia due to shunting), dyspnea, CO_2 retention, 2° polycythemia.	Hypertrophy and hyperplasia of mucus-secreting glands in bronchi → Reid index (thickness of mucosal gland layer to thickness of wall between epithelium and cartilage) > 50%. D_{LCO} usually normal.	Diagnostic criteria: productive cough for > 3 months in a year for > 2 consecutive years.
Emphysema ("pink puffer")	Findings: barrel-shaped chest **D**, exhalation through pursed lips (increases airway pressure and prevents airway collapse).	Centriacinar—associated with smoking **A** **B**. Frequently in upper lobes (smoke rises up). Panacinar—associated with α_1-antitrypsin deficiency. Frequently in lower lobes. Enlargement of air spaces ↓ recoil, ↑ compliance, ↓ D_{LCO} from destruction of alveolar walls (arrow in **C**). Imbalance of proteases and antiproteases → ↑ elastase activity → ↑ loss of elastic fibers → ↑ lung compliance.	CXR: ↑ AP diameter, flattened diaphragm, ↑ lung field lucency.
Asthma	Findings: cough, wheezing, tachypnea, dyspnea, hypoxemia, ↓ inspiratory/ expiratory ratio, pulsus paradoxus, mucus plugging **E**. Triggers: viral URIs, allergens, stress. Diagnosis supported by spirometry and methacholine challenge.	Hyperresponsive bronchi → reversible bronchoconstriction. Smooth muscle hypertrophy and hyperplasia, Curschmann spirals **F** (shed epithelium forms whorled mucous plugs), and Charcot-Leyden crystals **G** (eosinophilic, hexagonal, double-pointed crystals formed from breakdown of eosinophils in sputum). D_{LCO} normal or ↑.	Type I hypersensitivity reaction. Aspirin-induced asthma is a combination of COX inhibition (leukotriene overproduction → airway constriction), chronic sinusitis with nasal polyps, and asthma symptoms.

Obstructive lung diseases *(continued)*

TYPE	PRESENTATION	PATHOLOGY	OTHER
Bronchiectasis	Findings: purulent sputum, recurrent infections, hemoptysis, digital clubbing.	Chronic necrotizing infection of bronchi or obstruction → permanently dilated airways.	Associated with bronchial obstruction, poor ciliary motility (eg, smoking, Kartagener syndrome), cystic fibrosis **H**, allergic bronchopulmonary aspergillosis.

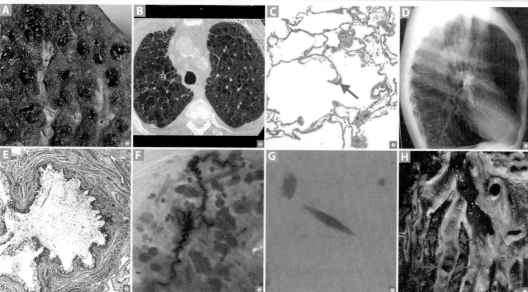

Restrictive lung diseases	Restricted lung expansion causes ↓ lung volumes (↓ FVC and TLC). PFTs: ↑ FEV_1/FVC ratio. Patient presents with short, shallow breaths.

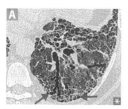

Types:

- Poor breathing mechanics (extrapulmonary, peripheral hypoventilation, normal A-a gradient):
    - Poor muscular effort—polio, myasthenia gravis, Guillain-Barré syndrome
    - Poor structural apparatus—scoliosis, morbid obesity
- Interstitial lung diseases (pulmonary ↓ diffusing capacity, ↑ A-a gradient):
    - Pneumoconioses (eg, coal workers' pneumoconiosis, silicosis, asbestosis)
    - Sarcoidosis: bilateral hilar lymphadenopathy, noncaseating granuloma; ↑ ACE and Ca^{2+}
    - Idiopathic pulmonary fibrosis **A** (repeated cycles of lung injury and wound healing with ↑ collagen deposition, "honeycomb" lung appearance and digital clubbing)
    - Goodpasture syndrome
    - Granulomatosis with polyangiitis (Wegener)
    - Pulmonary Langerhans cell histiocytosis (eosinophilic granuloma)
    - Hypersensitivity pneumonitis
    - Drug toxicity (bleomycin, busulfan, amiodarone, methotrexate)

Hypersensitivity pneumonitis—mixed type III/IV hypersensitivity reaction to environmental antigen. Causes dyspnea, cough, chest tightness, headache. Often seen in farmers and those exposed to birds. Reversible in early stages if stimulus is avoided.

Sarcoidosis

Characterized by immune-mediated, widespread noncaseating granulomas **A**, elevated serum ACE levels, and elevated CD4+/CD8+ ratio in bronchoalveolar lavage fluid. More common in African-American females. Often asymptomatic except for enlarged lymph nodes. Findings on CXR of bilateral adenopathy and coarse reticular opacities **B**; CT of the chest better demonstrates the extensive hilar and mediastinal adenopathy **C**.

Associated with **Bell palsy**, **U**veitis, **G**ranulomas (epithelioid, containing microscopic Schaumann and asteroid bodies), **L**upus pernio (skin lesions on face resembling lupus), **I**nterstitial fibrosis (restrictive lung disease), **E**rythema nodosum, **R**heumatoid arthritis-like arthropathy, hypercalcemia (due to ↑ 1α-hydroxylase–mediated vitamin D activation in macrophages). A **facial droop** is UGLIER.

Treatment: steroids (if symptomatic).

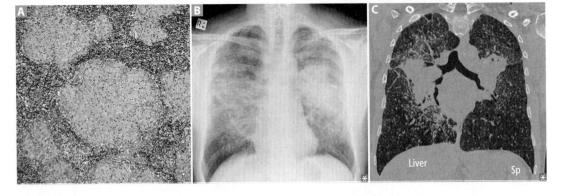

Inhalation injury and sequelae

Complication of smoke inhalation from fires or other noxious substances. Caused by heat, particulates (< 1 μm diameter), or irritants (eg, NH_3) → chemical tracheobronchitis, edema, pneumonia, ARDS. Many patients present 2° to burns, CO inhalation, cyanide poisoning, or arsenic poisoning. Singed nasal hairs common on exam.

Bronchoscopy shows severe edema, congestion of bronchus, and soot deposition (**A**, 18 hours after inhalation injury; **B**, resolution at 11 days after injury).

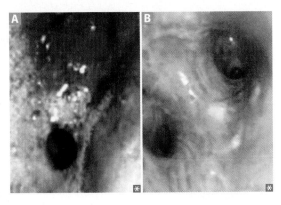

Pneumoconioses	Asbestos is from the **roof** (was common in insulation), but affects the **base** (lower lobes). **Silica and coal** are from the **base** (earth), but affect the **roof** (upper lobes).	
Asbestosis	Associated with shipbuilding, roofing, plumbing. "Ivory white," calcified, supradiaphragmatic 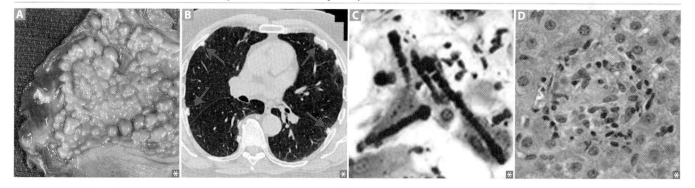 and pleural B plaques are pathognomonic of asbestosis. Risk of bronchogenic carcinoma > risk of mesothelioma.	Affects lower lobes. Asbestos (ferruginous) bodies are golden-brown fusiform rods resembling dumbbells C, found in alveolar sputum sample, visualized using Prussian blue stain, often obtained by bronchoalveolar lavage. ↑ risk of pleural effusions.
Berylliosis	Associated with exposure to beryllium in aerospace and manufacturing industries. Granulomatous (noncaseating) D on histology and therefore occasionally responsive to steroids. ↑ risk of cancer and cor pulmonale.	Affects upper lobes.
Coal workers' pneumoconiosis	Prolonged coal dust exposure → macrophages laden with carbon → inflammation and fibrosis. Also known as black lung disease. ↑ risk for Caplan syndrome (rheumatoid arthritis and pneumoconioses with intrapulmonary nodules).	Affects upper lobes. Small, rounded nodular opacities seen on imaging. Anthracosis—asymptomatic condition found in many urban dwellers exposed to sooty air.
Silicosis	Associated with **sand**blasting, **found**ries, **mines**. Macrophages respond to silica and release fibrogenic factors, leading to fibrosis. It is thought that silica may disrupt phagolysosomes and impair macrophages, increasing susceptibility to TB. ↑ risk of cancer, cor pulmonale, and Caplan syndrome.	Affects upper lobes. "**Eggshell**" calcification of hilar lymph nodes on CXR. The **silly egg sandwich I found is mine**!

Mesothelioma

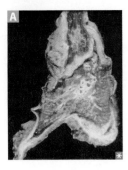

Malignancy of the pleura associated with asbestosis. May result in hemorrhagic pleural effusion (exudative), pleural thickening .

Psammoma bodies seen on histology.
Calretinin ⊕ in almost all mesotheliomas, ⊖ in most carcinomas.
Smoking not a risk factor.

Acute respiratory distress syndrome

PATHOPHYSIOLOGY	Alveolar insult → release of pro-inflammatory cytokines → neutrophil recruitment, activation, and release of toxic mediators (eg, reactive oxygen species, proteases, etc) → capillary endothelial damage and ↑ vessel permeability → leakage of protein-rich fluid into alveoli → formation of intra-alveolar hyaline membranes (arrows in A) and noncardiogenic pulmonary edema (normal PCWP). Loss of surfactant also contributes to alveolar collapse.
CAUSES	Sepsis (most common), aspiration, pneumonia, trauma, pancreatitis.
DIAGNOSIS	Diagnosis of exclusion with the following criteria (**ARDS**): ▪ Abnormal chest X-ray (bilateral lung opacities) B ▪ Respiratory failure within 1 week of alveolar insult ▪ Decreased Pa_{O_2}/Fi_{O_2} (ratio < 300, hypoxemia due to ↑ intrapulmonary shunting and diffusion abnormalities) ▪ Symptoms of respiratory failure are not due to HF/fluid overload
CONSEQUENCES	Impaired gas exchange ↓ lung compliance Pulmonary hypertension
MANAGEMENT	Treat the underlying cause Mechanical ventilation: ↓ tidal volumes, ↑ PEEP

Sleep apnea	Repeated cessation of breathing > 10 seconds during sleep → disrupted sleep → daytime somnolence. Diagnosis confirmed by sleep study. Normal Pa_{O_2} during the day. Nocturnal hypoxia → systemic/pulmonary hypertension, arrhythmias (atrial fibrillation/flutter), sudden death. Hypoxia → ↑ EPO release → ↑ erythropoiesis.
Obstructive sleep apnea	Respiratory effort against airway obstruction. Associated with obesity, loud snoring, daytime sleepiness. Caused by excess parapharyngeal tissue in adults, adenotonsillar hypertrophy in children. Treatment: weight loss, CPAP, surgery.
Central sleep apnea	Impaired respiratory effort due to CNS injury/toxicity, HF, opioids. May be associated with Cheyne-Stokes respirations (oscillations between apnea and hyperpnea). Treat with positive airway pressure.
Obesity hypoventilation syndrome	Obesity (BMI ≥ 30 kg/m^2) → hypoventilation → ↑ Pa_{CO_2} during waking hours (retention); ↓ Pa_{O_2} and ↑ Pa_{CO_2} during sleep. Also known as Pickwickian syndrome.

Pulmonary hypertension	Normal mean pulmonary artery pressure = 10–14 mm Hg; pulmonary hypertension ≥ 25 mm Hg at rest. Results in arteriosclerosis, medial hypertrophy, intimal fibrosis of pulmonary arteries, plexiform lesions. Course: severe respiratory distress → cyanosis and RVH → death from decompensated cor pulmonale.
ETIOLOGIES	
Pulmonary arterial hypertension	Often idiopathic. Heritable PAH can be due to an inactivating mutation in *BMPR2* gene (normally inhibits vascular smooth muscle proliferation); poor prognosis. Pulmonary vasculature endothelial dysfunction results in ↑ vasoconstrictors (eg, endothelin) and ↓ vasodilators (eg, NO and prostacyclins). Other causes include drugs (eg, amphetamines, cocaine), connective tissue disease, HIV infection, portal hypertension, congenital heart disease, schistosomiasis.
Left heart disease	Causes include systolic/diastolic dysfunction and valvular disease.
Lung diseases or hypoxia	Destruction of lung parenchyma (eg, COPD), lung inflammation/fibrosis (eg, interstitial lung diseases), hypoxemic vasoconstriction (eg, obstructive sleep apnea, living in high altitude).
Chronic thromboembolic	Recurrent microthrombi → ↓ cross-sectional area of pulmonary vascular bed.
Multifactorial	Causes include hematologic, systemic, and metabolic disorders, along with compression of the pulmonary vasculature by a tumor.

Lung—physical findings

ABNORMALITY	BREATH SOUNDS	PERCUSSION	FREMITUS	TRACHEAL DEVIATION
Pleural effusion	↓	Dull	↓	None if small Away from side of lesion if large
Atelectasis (bronchial obstruction)	↓	Dull	↓	Toward side of lesion
Simple pneumothorax	↓	Hyperresonant	↓	None
Tension pneumothorax	↓	Hyperresonant	↓	Away from side of lesion
Consolidation (lobar pneumonia, pulmonary edema)	Bronchial breath sounds; late inspiratory crackles, egophony, whispered pectoriloquy	Dull	↑	None

Pleural effusions

Excess accumulation of fluid A between pleural layers → restricted lung expansion during inspiration. Can be treated with thoracentesis to remove/reduce fluid B.

Transudate	↓ protein content. Due to ↑ hydrostatic pressure (eg, HF) or ↓ oncotic pressure (eg, nephrotic syndrome, cirrhosis).
Exudate	↑ protein content, cloudy. Due to malignancy, pneumonia, collagen vascular disease, trauma (occurs in states of ↑ vascular permeability). Must be drained due to risk of infection.
Lymphatic	Also known as chylothorax. Due to thoracic duct injury from trauma or malignancy. Milky-appearing fluid; ↑ triglycerides.

Pretreatment Pretreatment Post-treatment Post-treatment

Pneumothorax	Accumulation of air in pleural space A. Dyspnea, uneven chest expansion. Chest pain, ↓ tactile fremitus, hyperresonance, and diminished breath sounds, all on the affected side.
Primary spontaneous pneumothorax	Due to rupture of apical subpleural bleb or cysts. Occurs most frequently in tall, thin, young males and smokers.
Secondary spontaneous pneumothorax	Due to diseased lung (eg, bullae in emphysema, infections), mechanical ventilation with use of high pressures → barotrauma.
Traumatic pneumothorax	Caused by blunt (eg, rib fracture), penetrating (eg, gunshot), or iatrogenic (eg, central line placement, lung biopsy, barotrauma due to mechanical ventilation) trauma.
Tension pneumothorax	Can be from any of the above. Air enters pleural space but cannot exit. Increasing trapped air → tension pneumothorax. Trachea deviates away from affected lung B. Needs immediate needle decompression and chest tube placement. May lead to ↑ intrathoracic pressure → ↓ venous return → ↓ cardiac function.

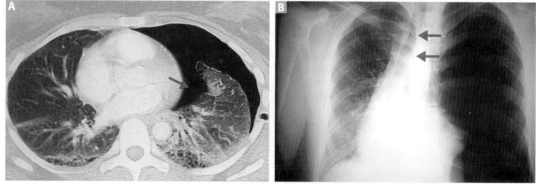

Pneumonia

TYPE	TYPICAL ORGANISMS	CHARACTERISTICS
Lobar pneumonia	*S pneumoniae* most frequently, also *Legionella*, *Klebsiella*	Intra-alveolar exudate → consolidation **A**; may involve entire lobe **B** or the whole lung.
Bronchopneumonia	*S pneumoniae*, *S aureus*, *H influenzae*, *Klebsiella*	Acute inflammatory infiltrates **C** from bronchioles into adjacent alveoli; patchy distribution involving ≥ 1 lobe **D**.
Interstitial (atypical) pneumonia	*Mycoplasma*, *Chlamydophila pneumoniae*, *Chlamydophila psittaci*, *Legionella*, viruses (RSV, CMV, influenza, adenovirus)	Diffuse patchy inflammation localized to interstitial areas at alveolar walls; diffuse distribution involving ≥ 1 lobe **E**. Generally follows a more indolent course ("walking" pneumonia).
Cryptogenic organizing pneumonia	Etiology unknown. Secondary organizing pneumonia caused by chronic inflammatory diseases (eg, rheumatoid arthritis) or medication side effects (eg, amiodarone). ⊖ sputum and blood cultures, no response to antibiotics.	Formerly known as bronchiolitis obliterans organizing pneumonia (BOOP). Noninfectious pneumonia characterized by inflammation of bronchioles and surrounding structure.

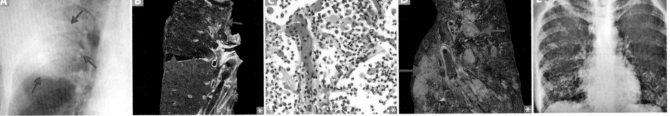

Natural history of lobar pneumonia

	Congestion	Red hepatization	Gray hepatization	Resolution
DAYS	1–2	3–4	5–7	8+
FINDINGS	Red-purple, partial consolidation of parenchyma Exudate with mostly bacteria	Red-brown, consolidated Exudate with fibrin, bacteria, RBCs, and WBCs	Uniformly gray Exudate full of WBCs, lysed RBCs, and fibrin	Enzymes digest components of exudate

Lung cancer

Leading cause of cancer death.

Presentation: cough, hemoptysis, bronchial obstruction, wheezing, pneumonic "coin" lesion on CXR or noncalcified nodule on CT.

Sites of metastases from lung cancer: adrenals, brain, bone (pathologic fracture), liver (jaundice, hepatomegaly).

In the lung, metastases (usually multiple lesions) are more common than 1° neoplasms. Most often from breast, colon, prostate, and bladder cancer.

SPHERE of complications:
Superior vena cava/thoracic outlet syndromes
Pancoast tumor
Horner syndrome
Endocrine (paraneoplastic)
Recurrent laryngeal nerve compression (hoarseness)
Effusions (pleural or pericardial)

Risk factors include smoking, secondhand smoke, radon, asbestos, family history.

Squamous and Small cell carcinomas are Sentral (central) and often caused by Smoking.

TYPE	LOCATION	CHARACTERISTICS	HISTOLOGY
Small cell			
Small cell (oat cell) carcinoma	Central	Undifferentiated → very aggressive. May produce ACTH (Cushing syndrome), SIADH, or Antibodies against presynaptic Ca^{2+} channels (Lambert-Eaton myasthenic syndrome) or neurons (paraneoplastic myelitis, encephalitis, subacute cerebellar degeneration). Amplification of *myc* oncogenes common. Managed with chemotherapy +/– radiation.	Neoplasm of neuroendocrine Kulchitsky cells → small dark blue cells 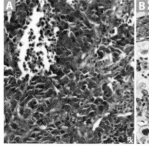. Chromogranin A ⊕, neuron-specific enolase ⊕, synaptophysin ⊕.
Non–small cell			
Adenocarcinoma	Peripheral	Most common 1° lung cancer. More common in women than men, most likely to arise in nonsmokers. Activating mutations include *KRAS*, *EGFR*, and *ALK*. Associated with hypertrophic osteoarthropathy (clubbing). Bronchioloalveolar subtype (adenocarcinoma in situ): CXR often shows hazy infiltrates similar to pneumonia; better prognosis. Bronchial carcinoid and bronchioloalveolar cell carcinoma have lesser association with smoking.	Glandular pattern on histology, often stains mucin ⊕ 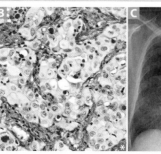. Bronchioloalveolar subtype: grows along alveolar septa → apparent "thickening" of alveolar walls. Tall, columnar cells containing mucus.
Squamous cell carcinoma	Central	Hilar mass 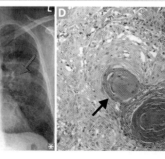 arising from bronchus; Cavitation; Cigarettes; hyperCalcemia (produces PTHrP).	Keratin pearls **D** and intercellular bridges.
Large cell carcinoma	Peripheral	Highly anaplastic undifferentiated tumor; poor prognosis. Less responsive to chemotherapy; removed surgically. Strong association with smoking.	Pleomorphic giant cells **E**.
Bronchial carcinoid tumor	Central or peripheral	Excellent prognosis; metastasis rare. Symptoms due to mass effect or carcinoid syndrome (flushing, diarrhea, wheezing).	Nests of neuroendocrine cells; chromogranin A ⊕.

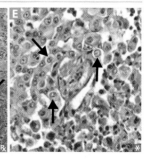

Lung abscess

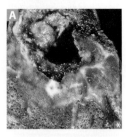

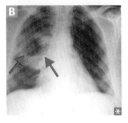

Localized collection of pus within parenchyma . Caused by aspiration of oropharyngeal contents (especially in patients predisposed to loss of consciousness [eg, alcoholics, epileptics]) or bronchial obstruction (eg, cancer).

Treatment: antibiotics.

Air-fluid levels often seen on CXR. Fluid levels common in cavities; presence suggests cavitation. Due to anaerobes (eg, *Bacteroides, Fusobacterium, Peptostreptococcus*) or *S aureus*.

Lung abscess 2° to aspiration is most often found in right lung. Location depends on patient's position during aspiration.

Pancoast tumor

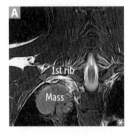

Also known as superior sulcus tumor. Carcinoma that occurs in the apex of lung may cause Pancoast syndrome by invading cervical sympathetic chain.

Compression of locoregional structures may cause array of findings:
- Recurrent laryngeal nerve → hoarseness
- Stellate ganglion → Horner syndrome (ipsilateral ptosis, miosis, anhidrosis)
- Superior vena cava → SVC syndrome
- Brachiocephalic vein → brachiocephalic syndrome (unilateral symptoms)
- Brachial plexus → sensorimotor deficits

Superior vena cava syndrome

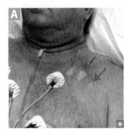

An obstruction of the SVC that impairs blood drainage from the head ("facial plethora"; note blanching after fingertip pressure in), neck (jugular venous distention), and upper extremities (edema). Commonly caused by malignancy (eg, mediastinal mass, Pancoast tumor) and thrombosis from indwelling catheters 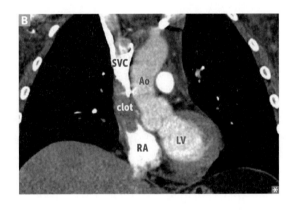. Medical emergency. Can raise intracranial pressure (if obstruction is severe) → headaches, dizziness, ↑ risk of aneurysm/rupture of intracranial arteries.

▶ RESPIRATORY—PHARMACOLOGY

Histamine-1 blockers	Reversible inhibitors of H_1 histamine receptors.	
First generation	Diphenhydramine, dimenhydrinate, chlorpheniramine.	Names contain "-en/-ine" or "-en/-ate."
CLINICAL USE	Allergy, motion sickness, sleep aid.	
ADVERSE EFFECTS	Sedation, antimuscarinic, anti-α-adrenergic.	
Second generation	Loratadine, fexofenadine, desloratadine, cetirizine.	Names usually end in "-adine."
CLINICAL USE	Allergy.	
ADVERSE EFFECTS	Far less sedating than 1st generation because of ↓ entry into CNS.	

Guaifenesin	Expectorant—thins respiratory secretions; does not suppress cough reflex.

N-acetylcysteine	Mucolytic—liquifies mucus in chronic bronchopulmonary diseases (eg, COPD, CF) by disrupting disulfide bonds. Also used as an antidote for acetaminophen overdose.

Dextromethorphan	Antitussive (antagonizes NMDA glutamate receptors). Synthetic codeine analog. Has mild opioid effect when used in excess. Naloxone can be given for overdose. Mild abuse potential. May cause serotonin syndrome if combined with other serotonergic agents.

Pseudoephedrine, phenylephrine

MECHANISM	α-adrenergic agonists, used as nasal decongestants.
CLINICAL USE	Reduce hyperemia, edema, nasal congestion; open obstructed eustachian tubes.
ADVERSE EFFECTS	Hypertension. Rebound congestion if used more than 4–6 days. Can also cause CNS stimulation/anxiety (pseudoephedrine).

Pulmonary hypertension drugs

DRUG	MECHANISM	CLINICAL NOTES
Endothelin receptor antagonists	Competitively antagonizes endothelin-1 receptors → ↓ pulmonary vascular resistance.	Hepatotoxic (monitor LFTs). Example: bosentan.
PDE-5 inhibitors	Inhibits PDE-5 → ↑ cGMP → prolonged vasodilatory effect of NO.	Also used to treat erectile dysfunction. Contraindicated when taking nitroglycerin or other nitrates. Example: sildenafil.
Prostacyclin analogs	PGI_2 (prostacyclin) with direct vasodilatory effects on pulmonary and systemic arterial vascular beds. Inhibits platelet aggregation.	Side effects: flushing, jaw pain. Examples: epoprostenol, iloprost.

Asthma drugs	Bronchoconstriction is mediated by (1) inflammatory processes and (2) parasympathetic tone; therapy is directed at these 2 pathways.
β_2-agonists	**Albuterol**—relaxes bronchial smooth muscle (short acting β_2-agonist). Used during acute exacerbation.
	Salmeterol, formoterol—long-acting agents for prophylaxis. Adverse effects are tremor and arrhythmia.
Inhaled corticosteroids	**Fluticasone, budesonide**—inhibit the synthesis of virtually all cytokines. Inactivate NF-κB, the transcription factor that induces production of TNF-α and other inflammatory agents. 1st-line therapy for chronic asthma. Use a spacer or rinse mouth after use to prevent oral thrush.
Muscarinic antagonists	**Tiotropium, ipratropium**—competitively block muscarinic receptors, preventing bronchoconstriction. Also used for COPD. Tiotropium is long acting.
Antileukotrienes	**Montelukast, zafirlukast**—block leukotriene receptors (CysLT1). Especially good for aspirin-induced and exercise-induced asthma. **Zileuton**—5-lipoxygenase pathway inhibitor. Blocks conversion of arachidonic acid to leukotrienes. Hepatotoxic.
Anti-IgE monoclonal therapy	**Omalizumab**—binds mostly unbound serum IgE and blocks binding to FcεRI. Used in allergic asthma with ↑ IgE levels resistant to inhaled steroids and long-acting β_2-agonists.
Methylxanthines	**Theophylline**—likely causes bronchodilation by inhibiting phosphodiesterase → ↑ cAMP levels due to ↓ cAMP hydrolysis. Usage is limited because of narrow therapeutic index (cardiotoxicity, neurotoxicity); metabolized by cytochrome P-450. Blocks actions of adenosine.
Mast cell stabilizers	**Cromolyn, nedocromil**—prevent release of inflammatory mediators from mast cells. Used for prevention of bronchospasm, not for acute bronchodilation.

Methacholine	Nonselective muscarinic receptor (M_3) agonist. Used in bronchial challenge test to help diagnose asthma.

Rapid Review

"Study without thought is vain: thought without study is dangerous."
—Confucius

"It is better, of course, to know useless things than to know nothing."
—Lucius Annaeus Seneca

"For every complex problem there is an answer that is clear, simple, and wrong."

—H. L. Mencken

The following tables represent a collection of high-yield associations of diseases with their clinical findings, treatments, and pathophysiology. They can be quickly reviewed in the days before the exam.

▶ **CLASSIC PRESENTATIONS**

CLINICAL PRESENTATION	DIAGNOSIS/DISEASE	PAGE
Gout, intellectual disability, self-mutilating behavior in a boy	Lesch-Nyhan syndrome (HGPRT deficiency, X-linked recessive)	37
Situs inversus, chronic sinusitis, bronchiectasis, infertility	Kartagener syndrome (dynein arm defect affecting cilia)	49
Blue sclera	Osteogenesis imperfecta (type I collagen defect)	51
Elastic skin, hypermobility of joints, ↑ bleeding tendency	Ehlers-Danlos syndrome (type V collagen defect, type III collagen defect seen in vascular subtype of ED)	51
Arachnodactyly, lens dislocation (upward), aortic dissection, hyperflexible joints	Marfan syndrome (fibrillin defect)	52
Café-au-lait spots (unilateral), polyostotic fibrous dysplasia, precocious puberty, multiple endocrine abnormalities	McCune-Albright syndrome (mosaic G-protein signaling mutation)	57
Calf pseudohypertrophy	Muscular dystrophy (most commonly Duchenne, due to X-linked recessive frameshift mutation of dystrophin gene)	61
Child uses arms to stand up from squat	Duchenne muscular dystrophy (Gowers sign)	61
Slow, progressive muscle weakness in boys	Becker muscular dystrophy (X-linked missense mutation in dystrophin; less severe than Duchenne)	61
Infant with cleft lip/palate, microcephaly or holoprosencephaly, polydactyly, cutis aplasia	Patau syndrome (trisomy 13)	63
Infant with microcephaly, rocker-bottom feet, clenched hands, and structural heart defect	Edwards syndrome (trisomy 18)	63
Single palmar crease	Down syndrome	63
Dilated cardiomyopathy, edema, alcoholism or malnutrition	Wet beriberi (thiamine [vitamin B_1] deficiency)	66
Dermatitis, dementia, diarrhea	Pellagra (niacin [vitamin B_3] deficiency)	67
Swollen gums, mucosal bleeding, poor wound healing, petechiae	Scurvy (vitamin C deficiency: can't hydroxylate proline/lysine for collagen synthesis)	69
Chronic exercise intolerance with myalgia, fatigue, painful cramps, myoglobinuria	McArdle disease (skeletal muscle glycogen phosphorylase deficiency)	87
Infant with hypoglycemia, hepatomegaly	Cori disease (debranching enzyme deficiency) or Von Gierke disease (glucose-6-phosphatase deficiency, more severe)	87
Myopathy (infantile hypertrophic cardiomyopathy), exercise intolerance	Pompe disease (lysosomal α-1,4-glucosidase deficiency)	87
"Cherry-red spots" on macula	Tay-Sachs (ganglioside accumulation) or Niemann-Pick (sphingomyelin accumulation), central retinal artery occlusion	88
Hepatosplenomegaly, pancytopenia, osteoporosis, aseptic necrosis of femoral head, bone crises	Gaucher disease (glucocerebrosidase deficiency)	88
Achilles tendon xanthoma	Familial hypercholesterolemia (↓ LDL receptor signaling)	94
Anaphylaxis following blood transfusion	IgA deficiency	116
Male child, recurrent infections, no mature B cells	Bruton disease (X-linked agammaglobulinemia)	116

CLINICAL PRESENTATION	DIAGNOSIS/DISEASE	PAGE
Recurrent cold (noninflamed) abscesses, unusual eczema, high serum IgE	Hyper-IgE syndrome (Job syndrome: neutrophil chemotaxis abnormality)	116
"Strawberry tongue"	Scarlet fever Kawasaki disease	136, 308
Adrenal hemorrhage, hypotension, DIC	Waterhouse-Friderichsen syndrome (meningococcemia)	142, 332
Red "currant jelly" sputum in alcoholic or diabetic patients	*Klebsiella pneumoniae* pneumonia	145
Large rash with bull's-eye appearance	Erythema chronicum migrans from *Ixodes* tick bite (Lyme disease: *Borrelia*)	146
Indurated, ulcerated genital lesion	Nonpainful: chancre (1° syphilis, *Treponema pallidum*) Painful, with exudate: chancroid (*Haemophilus ducreyi*)	147, 184
Pupil accommodates but doesn't react	Neurosyphilis (Argyll Robertson pupil)	147
Smooth, moist, painless, wart-like white lesions on genitals	Condylomata lata (2° syphilis)	147
Fever, chills, headache, myalgia following antibiotic treatment for syphilis	Jarisch-Herxheimer reaction (rapid lysis of spirochetes results in endotoxin-like release)	148
Dog or cat bite resulting in infection	*Pasteurella multocida* (cellulitis at inoculation site)	149
Rash on palms and soles	Coxsackie A, 2° syphilis, Rocky Mountain spotted fever	150
Black eschar on face of patient with diabetic ketoacidosis	*Mucor* or *Rhizopus* fungal infection	153
Chorioretinitis, hydrocephalus, intracranial calcifications	Congenital toxoplasmosis	156
Fever, cough, conjunctivitis, coryza, diffuse rash	Measles	170
Small, irregular red spots on buccal/lingual mucosa with blue-white centers	Koplik spots (measles [rubeola] virus)	170
Back pain, fever, night sweats	Pott disease (vertebral TB)	180
Child with fever later develops red rash on face that spreads to body	Erythema infectiosum/fifth disease ("slapped cheeks" appearance, caused by parvovirus B19)	183
Abdominal pain, diarrhea, leukocytosis, recent antibiotic use	*Clostridium difficile* infection	185
Bounding pulses, wide pulse pressure, diastolic heart murmur, head bobbing	Aortic regurgitation	285
Systolic ejection murmur (crescendo-decrescendo)	Aortic stenosis	285
Continuous "machine-like" heart murmur	PDA (close with indomethacin; keep open with PGE analogs)	285
Chest pain on exertion	Angina (stable: with moderate exertion; unstable: with minimal exertion or at rest)	299
Chest pain with ST depressions on ECG	Angina (⊖ troponins) or NSTEMI (⊕ troponins)	299
Chest pain, pericardial effusion/friction rub, persistent fever following MI	Dressler syndrome (autoimmune-mediated post-MI fibrinous pericarditis, 2 weeks to several months after acute episode)	302
Painful, raised red lesions on pads of fingers/toes	Osler nodes (infective endocarditis, immune complex deposition)	305
Painless erythematous lesions on palms and soles	Janeway lesions (infective endocarditis, septic emboli/microabscesses)	305

CLINICAL PRESENTATION	DIAGNOSIS/DISEASE	PAGE
Splinter hemorrhages in fingernails	Bacterial endocarditis	305
Retinal hemorrhages with pale centers	Roth spots (bacterial endocarditis)	305
Distant heart sounds, distended neck veins, hypotension	Beck triad of cardiac tamponade	307
Cervical lymphadenopathy, desquamating rash, coronary aneurysms, red conjunctivae and tongue, hand-foot changes	Kawasaki disease (treat with IVIG and aspirin)	308
Palpable purpura on buttocks/legs, joint pain, abdominal pain (child), hematuria	Henoch-Schönlein purpura (IgA vasculitis affecting skin and kidneys)	309
Telangiectasias, recurrent epistaxis, skin discoloration, arteriovenous malformations, GI bleeding, hematuria	Hereditary hemorrhagic telangiectasia (Osler-Weber-Rendu syndrome)	310
Skin hyperpigmentation, hypotension, fatigue	1° adrenocortical insufficiency (eg, Addison disease) causes ↑ ACTH and ↑ α-MSH production)	332
Cold intolerance	Hypothyroidism	335
Cutaneous/dermal edema due to deposition of mucopolysaccharides in connective tissue	Myxedema (caused by hypothyroidism, Graves disease [pretibial])	335
Facial muscle spasm upon tapping	Chvostek sign (hypocalcemia)	339
No lactation postpartum, absent menstruation, cold intolerance	Sheehan syndrome (postpartum hemorrhage leading to pituitary infarction)	343
Deep, labored breathing/hyperventilation	Diabetic ketoacidosis (Kussmaul respirations)	345
Cutaneous flushing, diarrhea, bronchospasm	Carcinoid syndrome (right-sided cardiac valvular lesions, ↑ 5-HIAA)	346
Pancreatic, pituitary, parathyroid tumors	MEN 1 (autosomal dominant)	347
Thyroid tumors, pheochromocytoma, ganglioneuromatosis, Marfanoid habitus	MEN 2B (autosomal dominant *RET* mutation)	347
Thyroid and parathyroid tumors, pheochromocytoma	MEN 2A (autosomal dominant *RET* mutation)	347
Jaundice, palpable distended non-tender gallbladder	Courvoisier sign (distal malignant obstruction of biliary tree)	362
Painless jaundice	Cancer of the pancreatic head obstructing bile duct	362
Vomiting blood following gastroesophageal lacerations	Mallory-Weiss syndrome (alcoholic and bulimic patients)	371
Dysphagia (esophageal webs), glossitis, iron deficiency anemia	Plummer-Vinson syndrome (may progress to esophageal squamous cell carcinoma)	371
Enlarged, hard left supraclavicular node	Virchow node (abdominal metastasis)	373
Weight loss, diarrhea, arthritis, fever, adenopathy	Whipple disease (*Tropheryma whipplei*)	375
Severe RLQ pain with palpation of LLQ	Rovsing sign (acute appendicitis)	377
Severe RLQ pain with deep tenderness	McBurney sign (acute appendicitis)	377
Hamartomatous GI polyps, hyperpigmentation of mouth/feet/hands/genitalia	Peutz-Jeghers syndrome (inherited, benign polyposis can cause bowel obstruction; ↑ cancer risk, mainly GI)	381
Multiple colon polyps, osteomas/soft tissue tumors, impacted/supernumerary teeth	Gardner syndrome (subtype of FAP)	381
Abdominal pain, ascites, hepatomegaly	Budd-Chiari syndrome (posthepatic venous thrombosis)	386
Severe jaundice in neonate	Crigler-Najjar syndrome (congenital unconjugated hyperbilirubinemia)	388

CLINICAL PRESENTATION	DIAGNOSIS/DISEASE	PAGE
Golden brown rings around peripheral cornea	Wilson disease (Kayser-Fleischer rings due to copper accumulation)	389
Fat, female, forty, fertile, familial	Cholelithiasis (gallstones)	390
Short stature, café-au-lait spots, thumb/radial defects, ↑ incidence of tumors/leukemia, aplastic anemia	Fanconi anemia (genetic loss of DNA crosslink repair; often progresses to AML)	409
Red urine in the morning, fragile RBCs	Paroxysmal nocturnal hemoglobinuria	410
Painful blue fingers/toes, hemolytic anemia	Cold agglutinin disease (autoimmune hemolytic anemia caused by *Mycoplasma pneumoniae*, infectious mononucleosis, CLL)	411
Mucosal bleeding and prolonged bleeding time	Glanzmann thrombasthenia (defect in platelet aggregation due to lack of GpIIb/IIIa)	415
Fever, night sweats, weight loss	B symptoms of lymphoma	417
Erythroderma, lymphadenopathy, hepatosplenomegaly, atypical T cells	Mycosis fungoides (cutaneous T-cell lymphoma) or Sézary syndrome (mycosis fungoides + malignant T cells in blood)	418
WBCs that look "smudged"	CLL	420
Athlete with polycythemia	2° to erythropoietin injection	421
Neonate with arm paralysis following difficult birth, arm in "waiter's tip" position	Erb-Duchenne palsy (superior trunk [C5–C6] brachial plexus injury)	438
Anterior "drawer sign" ⊕	Anterior cruciate ligament injury	440
Bone pain, bone enlargement, arthritis	Paget disease of bone (↑ osteoblastic and osteoclastic activity)	450
Swollen, hard, painful finger joints in an elderly individual, pain worse with activity	Osteoarthritis (osteophytes on PIP [Bouchard nodes], DIP [Heberden nodes])	454
Sudden swollen/painful big toe joint, tophi	Gout/podagra (hyperuricemia)	455
Dry eyes, dry mouth, arthritis	Sjögren syndrome (autoimmune destruction of exocrine glands)	456
Urethritis, conjunctivitis, arthritis in a male	Reactive arthritis associated with HLA-B27	457
"Butterfly" facial rash and Raynaud phenomenon in a young female	Systemic lupus erythematosus	458
Painful fingers/toes changing color from white to blue to red with cold or stress	Raynaud phenomenon (vasospasm in extremities)	459
Anticentromere antibodies	Scleroderma (CREST)	460
Dark purple skin/mouth nodules in a patient with AIDS	Kaposi sarcoma, associated with HHV-8	465
Anti-desmoglein (anti-desmosome) antibodies	Pemphigus vulgaris (blistering)	467
Pruritic, purple, polygonal planar papules and plaques (6 P's)	Lichen planus	468
↑ AFP in amniotic fluid/maternal serum	Dating error, anencephaly, spina bifida (open neural tube defects)	475
Toe extension/fanning upon plantar scrape	Babinski sign (UMN lesion)	494
Hyperphagia, hypersexuality, hyperorality, hyperdocility	Klüver-Bucy syndrome (bilateral amygdala lesion)	495

CLINICAL PRESENTATION	DIAGNOSIS/DISEASE	PAGE
Lucid interval after traumatic brain injury	Epidural hematoma (middle meningeal artery rupture)	497
"Worst headache of my life"	Subarachnoid hemorrhage	497
Resting tremor, rigidity, akinesia, postural instability, shuffling gait	Parkinson disease (loss of dopaminergic neurons in substantia nigra pars compacta)	504
Chorea, dementia, caudate degeneration	Huntington disease (autosomal dominant CAG repeat expansion)	504
Nystagmus, intention tremor, scanning speech, bilateral internuclear ophthalmoplegia	Multiple sclerosis	507
Rapidly progressive limb weakness that ascends following GI/upper respiratory infection	Guillain-Barré syndrome (acute inflammatory demyelinating polyradiculopathy subtype)	508
Café-au-lait spots, Lisch nodules (iris hamartoma), cutaneous neurofibromas, pheochromocytomas, optic gliomas	Neurofibromatosis type I	509
Vascular birthmark (port-wine stain) of the face	Nevus flammeus (benign, but associated with Sturge-Weber syndrome)	509
Renal cell carcinoma (bilateral), hemangioblastomas, angiomatosis, pheochromocytoma	von Hippel-Lindau disease (dominant tumor suppressor gene mutation)	509
Bilateral acoustic schwannomas	Neurofibromatosis type 2	509
Hyperreflexia, hypertonia, Babinski sign present	UMN damage	513
Hyporeflexia, hypotonia, atrophy, fasciculations	LMN damage	513
Unilateral facial drooping involving forehead	LMN facial nerve (CN VII) palsy; UMN lesions spare the forehead	516
Episodic vertigo, tinnitus, hearing loss	Meniere disease	518
Ptosis, miosis, anhidrosis	Horner syndrome (sympathetic chain lesion)	524
Conjugate horizontal gaze palsy, horizontal diplopia	Internuclear ophthalmoplegia (damage to MLF; may be unilateral or bilateral)	527
Polyuria, renal tubular acidosis type II, growth failure, electrolyte imbalances, hypophosphatemic rickets	Fanconi syndrome (multiple combined dysfunction of the proximal convoluted tubule)	570
Bluish line on gingiva	Burton line (lead poisoning)	576
Periorbital and/or peripheral edema, proteinuria (> 3.5g/day), hypoalbuminemia, hypercholesterolemia	Nephrotic syndrome	580
Hereditary nephritis, sensorineural hearing loss, cataracts	Alport syndrome (mutation in collagen IV)	581
Streak ovaries, congenital heart disease, horseshoe kidney, cystic hygroma at birth, short stature, webbed neck, lymphedema	Turner syndrome (45,XO)	620
Red, itchy, swollen rash of nipple/areola	Paget disease of the breast (sign of underlying neoplasm)	632
Fibrous plaques in soft tissue of penis with abnormal curvature	Peyronie disease (connective tissue disorder)	633
Hypoxemia, polycythemia, hypercapnia	Chronic bronchitis (hyperplasia of mucous cells, "blue bloater")	656

CLINICAL PRESENTATION	DIAGNOSIS/DISEASE	PAGE
Pink complexion, dyspnea, hyperventilation	Emphysema ("pink puffer," centriacinar [smoking] or panacinar [α_1-antitrypsin deficiency])	656
Bilateral hilar adenopathy, uveitis	Sarcoidosis (noncaseating granulomas)	658

▶ CLASSIC LABS/FINDINGS

LAB/DIAGNOSTIC FINDING	DIAGNOSIS/DISEASE	PAGE
↓ AFP in amniotic fluid/maternal serum	Down syndrome or other chromosomal abnormalities	63
Large granules in phagocytes, immunodeficiency	Chédiak-Higashi disease (congenital failure of phagolysosome formation)	117
Recurrent infections, eczema, thrombocytopenia	Wiskott-Aldrich syndrome	117
Branching gram ⊕ rods with sulfur granules	*Actinomyces israelii*	129
Optochin sensitivity	Sensitive: S *pneumoniae*; resistant: viridans streptococci (S *mutans*, S *sanguis*)	135
Novobiocin response	Sensitive: S *epidermidis*; resistant: S *saprophyticus*	135
Bacitracin response	Sensitive: S *pyogenes* (group A); resistant: S *agalactiae* (group B)	135
Streptococcus bovis bacteremia	Colon cancer	137
Hilar lymphadenopathy, peripheral granulomatous lesion in middle or lower lung lobes (can calcify)	Ghon complex (1° TB: *Mycobacterium* bacilli)	140
Bacteria-covered vaginal epithelial cells	"Clue cells" (*Gardnerella vaginalis*)	148
Ring-enhancing brain lesion on CT/MRI in AIDS	*Toxoplasma gondii*, CNS lymphoma	156
Cardiomegaly with apical atrophy	Chagas disease (*Trypanosoma cruzi*)	158
Heterophile antibodies	Infectious mononucleosis (EBV)	165
Intranuclear eosinophilic droplet-like bodies	Cowdry type A bodies (HSV or VZV)	166
Eosinophilic globule in liver	Councilman body (viral hepatitis, yellow fever), represents hepatocyte undergoing apoptosis	168
"Steeple" sign on frontal CXR	Croup (parainfluenza virus)	170
Eosinophilic inclusion bodies in cytoplasm of hippocampal and cerebellar neurons	Negri bodies of rabies	171
Atypical lymphocytes	EBV	177
Enlarged cells with intranuclear inclusion bodies	"Owl eye" appearance of CMV	177
"Thumb sign" on lateral neck x-ray	Epiglottitis (*Haemophilus influenzae*)	186
"Delta wave" on ECG, short PR interval, supraventricular tachycardia	Wolff-Parkinson-White syndrome (Bundle of Kent bypasses AV node)	289
"Boot-shaped" heart on x-ray	Tetralogy of Fallot (due to RVH)	294
Rib notching (inferior surface, on x-ray)	Coarctation of the aorta	295
Heart nodules (granulomatous)	Aschoff bodies (rheumatic fever)	306
Electrical alternans (alternating amplitude on ECG)	Pericardial tamponade	307
Hypertension, hypokalemia, metabolic alkalosis	1° hyperaldosteronism (Conn syndrome)	332

LAB/DIAGNOSTIC FINDING	DIAGNOSIS/DISEASE	PAGE
Enlarged thyroid cells with ground-glass nuclei with central clearing	"Orphan Annie" eyes nuclei (papillary carcinoma of the thyroid)	338
Antineutrophil cytoplasmic antibodies (ANCAs)	Microscopic polyangiitis and eosinophilic granulomatosis with polyangiitis (MPO-ANCA/p-ANCA); granulomatosis with polyangiitis (Wegener; PR3-ANCA/c-ANCA); primary sclerosing cholangitis (MPO-ANCA/p-ANCA)	340
Mucin-filled cell with peripheral nucleus	"Signet ring" (gastric carcinoma)	373
Anti-transglutaminase/anti-gliadin/anti-endomysial antibodies	Celiac disease (diarrhea, weight loss)	375
Narrowing of bowel lumen on barium x-ray	"String sign" (Crohn disease)	376
"Lead pipe" appearance of colon on abdominal imaging	Ulcerative colitis (loss of haustra)	376
Thousands of polyps on colonoscopy	Familial adenomatous polyposis (autosomal dominant, mutation of APC gene)	381
"Apple core" lesion on barium enema x-ray	Colorectal cancer (usually left-sided)	382
Eosinophilic cytoplasmic inclusion in liver cell	Mallory body (alcoholic liver disease)	385
Triglyceride accumulation in liver cell vacuoles	Fatty liver disease (alcoholic or metabolic syndrome)	385
"Nutmeg" appearance of liver	Chronic passive congestion of liver due to right heart failure or Budd-Chiari syndrome	386
Antimitochondrial antibodies (AMAs)	1° biliary cirrhosis (female, cholestasis, portal hypertension)	389
Low serum ceruloplasmin	Wilson disease (hepatolenticular degeneration; Kayser-Fleischer rings due to copper accumulation)	389
Migratory thrombophlebitis (leading to migrating DVTs and vasculitis)	Trousseau syndrome (adenocarcinoma of pancreas or lung)	391
Basophilic nuclear remnants in RBCs	Howell-Jolly bodies (due to splenectomy or nonfunctional spleen)	405
Hypochromic, microcytic anemia	Iron deficiency anemia, lead poisoning, thalassemia (fetal hemoglobin sometimes present)	406
Basophilic stippling of RBCs	Lead poisoning or sideroblastic anemia	407
"Hair on end" ("Crew-cut") appearance on x-ray	β-thalassemia, sickle cell disease (marrow expansion)	407
Hypersegmented neutrophils	Megaloblastic anemia (B_{12} deficiency: neurologic symptoms; folate deficiency: no neurologic symptoms)	408
Antiplatelet antibodies	Idiopathic thrombocytopenic purpura	415
High level of D-dimers	DVT, PE, DIC	416
Giant B cells with bilobed nuclei with prominent inclusions ("owl's eye")	Reed-Sternberg cells (Hodgkin lymphoma)	417
Sheets of medium-sized lymphoid cells with scattered pale, tingible body–laden macrophages ("starry sky" histology)	Burkitt lymphoma (t[8:14] c-*myc* activation, associated with EBV; "starry sky" made up of malignant cells)	418
Lytic ("punched-out") bone lesions on x-ray	Multiple myeloma	419

LAB/DIAGNOSTIC FINDING	DIAGNOSIS/DISEASE	PAGE
Monoclonal antibody spike	▪ Multiple myeloma (usually IgG or IgA) ▪ Monoclonal gammopathy of undetermined significance (MGUS consequence of aging) ▪ Waldenström (M protein = IgM) macroglobulinemia ▪ Primary amyloidosis	419
Stacks of RBCs	Rouleaux formation (high ESR, multiple myeloma)	419
Azurophilic peroxidase ⊕ granular inclusions in granulocytes and myeloblasts	Auer rods (AML, especially the promyelocytic [M3] type)	420
WBCs that look "smudged"	CLL (almost always B cell)	420
"Tennis racket"-shaped cytoplasmic organelles (EM) in Langerhans cells	Birbeck granules (Langerhans cell histiocytosis)	422
"Brown" tumor of bone	Hyperparathyroidism or osteitis fibrosa cystica (deposited hemosiderin from hemorrhage gives brown color)	451
Raised periosteum (creating a "Codman triangle")	Aggressive bone lesion (eg, osteosarcoma, Ewing sarcoma, osteomyelitis)	452
"Soap bubble" in femur or tibia on x-ray	Giant cell tumor of bone (generally benign)	452
"Onion skin" periosteal reaction	Ewing sarcoma (malignant small blue cell tumor)	453
Anti-IgG antibodies	Rheumatoid arthritis (systemic inflammation, joint pannus, boutonniere and swan neck deformities)	454
Rhomboid crystals, ⊕ birefringent	Pseudogout (calcium pyrophosphate dihydrate crystals)	455
Needle-shaped, ⊖ birefringent crystals	Gout (monosodium urate crystals)	455
↑ uric acid levels	Gout, Lesch-Nyhan syndrome, tumor lysis syndrome, loop and thiazide diuretics	455
"Bamboo spine" on x-ray	Ankylosing spondylitis (chronic inflammatory arthritis: HLA-B27)	457
Antinuclear antibodies (ANAs: anti-Smith and anti-dsDNA)	SLE (type III hypersensitivity)	458
Anti-topoisomerase antibodies	Diffuse systemic scleroderma	460
Keratin pearls on a skin biopsy	Squamous cell carcinoma	469
Antihistone antibodies	Drug-induced SLE (eg, hydralazine, isoniazid, phenytoin, procainamide)	472
Bloody or yellow tap on lumbar puncture	Subarachnoid hemorrhage	497
Yellowish CSF	Xanthochromia (eg, due to subarachnoid hemorrhage)	497
Eosinophilic cytoplasmic inclusion in neuron	Lewy body (Parkinson disease and Lewy body dementia)	504
Extracellular amyloid deposition in gray matter of brain	Senile plaques (Alzheimer disease)	504
Depigmentation of neurons in substantia nigra	Parkinson disease (basal ganglia disorder: rigidity, resting tremor, bradykinesia)	504
Protein aggregates in neurons from hyperphosphorylation of tau protein	Neurofibrillary tangles (Alzheimer disease) and Pick bodies (Pick disease)	504
Silver-staining spherical aggregation of tau proteins in neurons	Pick bodies (Pick disease: progressive dementia, changes in personality)	504
Pseudopalisading tumor cells on brain biopsy	Glioblastoma multiforme	510

LAB/DIAGNOSTIC FINDING	DIAGNOSIS/DISEASE	PAGE
Circular grouping of dark tumor cells surrounding pale neurofibrils	Homer-Wright rosettes (neuroblastoma, medulloblastoma)	512
"Waxy" casts with very low urine flow	Chronic end-stage renal disease	578
RBC casts in urine	Glomerulonephritis	578
"Tram-track" appearance of capillary loops of glomerular basement membranes on light microscopy	Membranoproliferative glomerulonephritis	578
Nodular hyaline deposits in glomeruli	Kimmelstiel-Wilson nodules (diabetic nephropathy)	578
Podocyte fusion or "effacement" on electron microscopy	Minimal change disease (child with nephrotic syndrome)	580
"Spikes" on basement membrane, "dome-like" subepithelial deposits	Membranous nephropathy (nephrotic syndrome)	580
Anti–glomerular basement membrane antibodies	Goodpasture syndrome (glomerulonephritis and hemoptysis)	581
Cellular crescents in Bowman capsule	Rapidly progressive crescentic glomerulonephritis	581
"Wire loop" glomerular capillary appearance on light microscopy	Diffuse proliferative glomerulonephritis (usually seen with lupus)	581
Linear appearance of IgG deposition on glomerular and alveolar basement membranes	Goodpasture syndrome	581
"Lumpy bumpy" appearance of glomeruli on immunofluorescence	Poststreptococcal glomerulonephritis (due to deposition of IgG, IgM, and C3)	581
Necrotizing vasculitis (lungs) and necrotizing glomerulonephritis	Granulomatosis with polyangiitis (Wegener; PR3-ANCA/ c-ANCA) and Goodpasture syndrome (anti–basement membrane antibodies)	581
Thyroid-like appearance of kidney	Chronic pyelonephritis (usually due to recurrent infections)	585
WBC casts in urine	Acute pyelonephritis	585
Renal epithelial casts in urine	Intrinsic renal failure (eg, ischemia or toxic injury)	586
hCG elevated	Choriocarcinoma, hydatidiform mole (occurs with and without embryo, and multiple pregnancy)	622
Dysplastic squamous cervical cells with "raisinoid" nuclei and hyperchromasia	Koilocytes (HPV: predisposes to cervical cancer)	627
Psammoma bodies	Meningiomas, papillary thyroid carcinoma, mesothelioma, papillary serous carcinoma of the endometrium and ovary	629
Disarrayed granulosa cells arranged around collections of eosinophilic fluid	Call-Exner bodies (granulosa cell tumor of the ovary)	629
"Chocolate cyst" of ovary	Endometriosis (frequently involves both ovaries)	630
Mammary gland ("blue domed") cyst	Fibrocystic change of the breast	631
Glomerulus-like structure surrounding vessel in germ cells	Schiller-Duval bodies (yolk sac tumor)	634
Rectangular, crystal-like, cytoplasmic inclusions in Leydig cells	Reinke crystals (Leydig cell tumor)	634
Thrombi made of white/red layers	Lines of Zahn (arterial thrombus, layers of platelets/ RBCs)	654

LAB/DIAGNOSTIC FINDING	DIAGNOSIS/DISEASE	PAGE
Hexagonal, double-pointed, needle-like crystals in bronchial secretions	Bronchial asthma (Charcot-Leyden crystals: eosinophilic granules)	656
Desquamated epithelium casts in sputum	Curschmann spirals (bronchial asthma; can result in whorled mucous plugs)	656
"Honeycomb lung" on x-ray or CT	Interstitial pulmonary fibrosis	657
Colonies of mucoid *Pseudomonas* in lungs	Cystic fibrosis (autosomal recessive mutation in *CFTR* gene → fat-soluble vitamin deficiency and mucous plugs)	657
Iron-containing nodules in alveolar septum	Ferruginous bodies (asbestosis: ↑ chance of lung cancer)	659
Bronchogenic apical lung tumor on imaging	Pancoast tumor (can compress cervical sympathetic chain and cause Horner syndrome)	666

▶ CLASSIC/RELEVANT TREATMENTS

CONDITION	COMMON TREATMENT(S)	PAGE
Ethylene glycol/methanol intoxication	Fomepizole (alcohol dehydrogenase inhibitor)	72
Neisseria meningitidis	Penicillin/ceftriaxone, rifampin (prophylaxis)	128
Clostridium botulinum	Antitoxin	132
Clostridium tetani	Antitoxin	132
Staphylococcus aureus	MSSA: nafcillin, oxacillin, dicloxacillin (antistaphylococcal penicillins); MRSA: vancomycin, daptomycin, linezolid, ceftaroline	133
Streptococcus pyogenes	Penicillin prophylaxis	135
Streptococcus pneumoniae	Penicillin/cephalosporin (systemic infection, pneumonia), vancomycin (meningitis)	136
Streptococcus bovis	Penicillin prophylaxis; evaluation for colon cancer if linked to endocarditis	137
Enterococci	Vancomycin, aminopenicillins/cephalosporins	137
Haemophilus influenzae (B)	Amoxicillin ± clavulanate (mucosal infections), ceftriaxone (meningitis), rifampin (prophylaxis)	142
Legionella pneumophila	Macrolides (eg, azithromycin)	143
Pseudomonas aeruginosa	Piperacillin/tazobactam, aminoglycosides, carbapenems	143
Treponema pallidum	Penicillin G	147
Chlamydia trachomatis	Doxycycline (+ ceftriaxone for gonorrhea coinfection), oral erythromycin to treat chlamydial conjunctivitis in infants	149
Rickettsia rickettsii	Doxycycline, chloramphenicol	150
Candida albicans	Topical azoles (vaginitis); nystatin, fluconazole, caspofungin (oral/esophageal); fluconazole, caspofungin, amphotericin B (systemic)	153
Cryptococcus neoformans	Induction with amphotericin B and flucytosine, maintenance with fluconazole (in AIDS patients)	153

CONDITION	COMMON TREATMENT(S)	PAGE
Sporothrix schenckii	Itraconazole, oral potassium iodide	154
Pneumocystis jirovecii	TMP-SMX (prophylaxis and treatment in immunosuppressed patients, CD4 < 200/mm^3)	154
Toxoplasma gondii	Sulfadiazine + pyrimethamine	156
Malaria	Chloroquine, mefloquine, atovaquone/proguanil (for blood schizont), primaquine (for liver hypnozoite)	157
Trichomonas vaginalis	Metronidazole (patient and partner)	158
Influenza	Oseltamivir, zanamivir	169
CMV	Ganciclovir, foscarnet, cidofovir	177
Neisseria gonorrhoeae	Ceftriaxone (add doxycycline to cover likely concurrent *C trachomatis*)	184
Clostridium difficile	Oral metronidazole; if refractory, oral vancomycin	185
Mycobacterium tuberculosis	RIPE (rifampin, isoniazid, pyrazinamide, ethambutol)	196
UTI prophylaxis	TMP-SMX	198
Chronic hepatitis B or C	IFN-α (HBV and HCV); ribavirin, simeprevir, sofosbuvir (HCV)	202
Patent ductus arteriosus	Close with indomethacin; keep open with PGE analogs	285
Stable angina	Sublingual nitroglycerin	299
Hypercholesterolemia	Statin (first-line)	299
Buerger disease	Smoking cessation	308
Granulomatosis with polyangiitis (Wegener)	Cyclophosphamide, corticosteroids	308
Kawasaki disease	IVIG, high-dose aspirin	308
Temporal arteritis	High-dose steroids	308
Arrhythmia in damaged cardiac tissue	Class IB antiarrhythmic (lidocaine, mexiletine)	315
Pheochromocytoma	α-antagonists (eg, phenoxybenzamine)	316
Prolactinoma	Cabergoline/bromocriptine (dopamine agonists)	324
Diabetes insipidus	Desmopressin (central); hydrochlorothiazide, indomethacin, amiloride (nephrogenic)	342
SIADH	Fluid restriction, IV hypertonic saline, conivaptan/tolvaptan, demeclocycline	342
Diabetes mellitus type 1	Dietary intervention (low carbohydrate) + insulin replacement	345
Diabetes mellitus type 2	Dietary intervention, oral hypoglycemics, and insulin (if refractory)	345
Diabetic ketoacidosis	Fluids, insulin, K$^+$	345
Carcinoid syndrome	Octreotide	365
Crohn disease	Corticosteroids, infliximab, azathioprine	376
Ulcerative colitis	5-ASA preparations (eg, mesalamine), 6-mercaptopurine, infliximab, colectomy	376
Hypertriglyceridemia	Fibrate	391

CONDITION	COMMON TREATMENT(S)	PAGE
Sickle cell disease	Hydroxyurea (↑ fetal hemoglobin)	410
Chronic myelogenous leukemia	Imatinib	420
Acute promyelocytic leukemia (M3)	All-*trans* retinoic acid	422
Drug of choice for anticoagulation during pregnancy	Heparin	423
Heparin reversal	Protamine sulfate	423
Immediate anticoagulation	Heparin	423
Long-term anticoagulation	Warfarin, dabigatran, rivaroxaban and apixaban	424
Warfarin reversal	Fresh frozen plasma (acute), vitamin K (non-acute)	424
Cyclophosphamide-induced hemorrhagic cystitis	Mesna	428
HER2/neu ⊕ breast cancer	Trastuzumab	431
Osteoporosis	Calcium/vitamin D supplementation (prophylaxis); bisphosphonates, PTH analogs, SERMs, calcitonin, denosumab (treatment)	449
Osteomalacia/rickets	Vitamin D supplementation	450
Chronic gout	Xanthine oxidase inhibitors (eg, allopurinol, febuxostat); pegloticase; probenecid	472
Acute gout attack	NSAIDs, colchicine, glucocorticoids	472
Neural tube defect prevention	Prenatal folic acid	475
Migraine	Abortive therapies (eg, sumatriptan, NSAIDs); prophylaxis (eg, propranolol, topiramate, CCBs, amitriptyline)	502
Trigeminal neuralgia (tic douloureux)z	Carbamazepine	502
Multiple sclerosis	Disease-modifying therapies (eg, β-interferon, natalizumab); for acute flares, use IV steroids	507
Degeneration of dorsal column fibers	Tabes dorsalis (3° syphilis), subacute combined degeneration (dorsal columns, lateral corticospinal, spinocerebellar tracts affected)	514
Tonic-clonic seizures	Levetiracetam, phenytoin, valproate, carbamazepine	528
Absence seizures	Ethosuximide	528
Malignant hyperthermia	Dantrolene	533
Anorexia	Nutrition, psychotherapy, mirtazapine	550
Bulimia nervosa	SSRIs	550
Alcoholism	Disulfiram, acamprosate, naltrexone, supportive care	555
ADHD	Methylphenidate, amphetamines, CBT, atomoxetine, guanfacine, clonidine	556
Alcohol withdrawal	Long-acting benzodiazepines	556
Bipolar disorder	Mood stabilizers (eg, lithium, valproic acid, carbamazepine), atypical antipsychotics	556
Depression	SSRIs (first-line)	556
Generalized anxiety disorder	SSRIs, SNRIs (first line); buspirone (second line)	556
Schizophrenia (positive symptoms)	Typical and atypical antipsychotics	556

CONDITION	COMMON TREATMENT(S)	PAGE
Schizophrenia (negative symptoms)	Atypical antipsychotics	557
Hyperaldosteronism	Spironolactone	591
Benign prostatic hyperplasia	α_1-antagonists, 5α-reductase inhibitors, PDE-5 inhibitors	635
Infertility	Leuprolide, GnRH (pulsatile), clomiphene	637
Breast cancer in postmenopausal woman	Aromatase inhibitor (anastrozole)	637
ER ⊕ breast cancer	Tamoxifen	637
Prostate adenocarcinoma/uterine fibroids	Leuprolide, GnRH (continuous)	637
Medical abortion	Mifepristone	638
Prostate adenocarcinoma	Flutamide	639
Erectile dysfunction	Sildenafil, tadalafil, vardenafil	639
Pulmonary arterial hypertension (idiopathic)	Sildenafil, bosentan, epoprostenol	667

▶ KEY ASSOCIATIONS

DISEASE/FINDING	MOST COMMON/IMPORTANT ASSOCIATIONS	PAGE
Mitochondrial inheritance	Disease occurs in both males and females, inherited through females only	59
Intellectual disability	Down syndrome, fragile X syndrome	62
Vitamin deficiency (USA)	Folate (pregnant women are at high risk; body stores only 3- to 4-month supply; prevents neural tube defects)	68
Lysosomal storage disease	Gaucher disease	88
Food poisoning (exotoxin mediated)	*S aureus, B cereus*	133
Osteomyelitis	*S aureus* (most common overall)	135
Bacterial meningitis (adults and elderly)	*S pneumoniae*	136
Bacterial meningitis (newborns and kids)	Group B streptococcus/*E coli*/*Listeria monocytogenes* (newborns), *S pneumoniae*/*N meningitidis* (kids/teens)	137
Bacteria associated with gastritis, peptic ulcer disease, and gastric malignancies (eg, adenocarcinoma, MALToma)	*H pylori*	146
Opportunistic infection in AIDS	*Pneumocystis jirovecii* pneumonia	154
Helminth infection (US)	*Ascaris lumbricoides*	159
Myocarditis	Coxsackie B	167
Infection 2° to blood transfusion	Hepatitis C	173
Osteomyelitis in sickle cell disease	*Salmonella*	180
Osteomyelitis with IV drug use	*Pseudomonas, Candida, S aureus*	180
UTI	*E coli, Staphylococcus saprophyticus* (young women)	181
Sexually transmitted disease	*C trachomatis* (usually coinfected with N *gonorrhoeae*)	184
Nosocomial pneumonia	*S aureus, Pseudomonas*, other enteric gram ⊖ rods	185
Pelvic inflammatory disease	*C trachomatis, N gonorrhoeae*	185

DISEASE/FINDING	MOST COMMON/IMPORTANT ASSOCIATIONS	PAGE
Infections in chronic granulomatous disease	S aureus, E coli, Aspergillus (catalase ⊕)	186
Metastases to bone	Prostate, breast > lung, thyroid, kidney	226
Metastases to brain	Lung > breast > prostate > melanoma > GI	226
Metastases to liver	Colon >> stomach > pancreas	226
S3 heart sound	↑ ventricular filling pressure (eg, mitral regurgitation, HF), common in dilated ventricles	282
S4 heart sound	Stiff/hypertrophic ventricle (aortic stenosis, restrictive cardiomyopathy)	282
Constrictive pericarditis	TB (developing world); idiopathic, viral illness (developed world)	282
Holosystolic murmur	VSD, tricuspid regurgitation, mitral regurgitation	285
Ejection click	Aortic stenosis	285
Mitral valve stenosis	Rheumatic heart disease	285
Opening snap	Mitral stenosis	285
Heart murmur, congenital	Mitral valve prolapse	285
Chronic arrhythmia	Atrial fibrillation (associated with high risk of emboli)	290
Cyanosis (early; less common)	Tetralogy of Fallot, transposition of great vessels, truncus arteriosus, total anomalous pulmonary venous return	294
Late cyanotic shunt (uncorrected left to right becomes right to left)	Eisenmenger syndrome (caused by ASD, VSD, PDA; results in pulmonary hypertension/polycythemia)	295
Congenital cardiac anomaly	VSD	295
Hypertension, 2°	Renal artery stenosis, chronic kidney disease (eg, polycystic kidney disease, diabetic nephropathy), hyperaldosteronism	296
Aortic aneurysm, thoracic	Marfan syndrome (idiopathic cystic medial degeneration)	296
Aortic dissection	Hypertension	296
Aortic aneurysm, abdominal	Atherosclerosis, smoking is major risk factor	298
Aortic aneurysm, ascending or arch	3° syphilis (syphilitic aortitis), vasa vasorum destruction	298
Sites of atherosclerosis	Abdominal aorta > coronary artery > popliteal artery > carotid artery	298
Cardiac manifestation of lupus	Marantic/thrombotic endocarditis (nonbacterial)	305
Heart valve in bacterial endocarditis	Mitral > aortic (rheumatic fever), tricuspid (IV drug abuse)	305
Endocarditis presentation associated with bacterium	S aureus (acute, IVDA, tricuspid valve), viridans stretococci (subacute, dental procedure), S bovis (colon cancer), culture negative (Coxiella, Bartonella, HACEK)	305
Temporal arteritis	Risk of ipsilateral blindness due to occlusion of ophthalmic artery; polymyalgia rheumatica	308
Recurrent inflammation/thrombosis of small/medium vessels in extremities	Buerger disease (strongly associated with tobacco)	308
Cardiac 1° tumor (kids)	Rhabdomyoma, often seen in tuberous sclerosis	309
Cardiac tumor (adults)	Metastasis, myxoma (90% in left atrium; "ball valve")	309

DISEASE/FINDING	MOST COMMON/IMPORTANT ASSOCIATIONS	PAGE
Congenital adrenal hyperplasia, hypotension	21-hydroxylase deficiency	326
Cushing syndrome	▪ Iatrogenic (from corticosteroid therapy) ▪ Adrenocortical adenoma (secretes excess cortisol) ▪ ACTH-secreting pituitary adenoma (Cushing disease) ▪ Paraneoplastic (due to ACTH secretion by tumors)	331
Tumor of the adrenal medulla (kids)	Neuroblastoma (malignant)	333
Tumor of the adrenal medulla (adults)	Pheochromocytoma (usually benign)	334
Cretinism	Iodine deficit/congenital hypothyroidism	336
HLA-DR3	Diabetes mellitus type 1, SLE, Graves disease, Hashimoto thyroiditis (also associated with HLA-DR5), Addison disease	337
Thyroid cancer	Papillary carcinoma (childhood irradiation)	338
Hypoparathyroidism	Accidental excision during thyroidectomy	339
1° hyperparathyroidism	Adenomas, hyperplasia, carcinoma	340
2° hyperparathyroidism	Hypocalcemia of chronic kidney disease	340
Hypopituitarism	Pituitary adenoma (usually benign tumor)	343
HLA-DR4	Diabetes mellitus type 1, rheumatoid arthritis, Addison disease	345
Refractory peptic ulcers and high gastrin levels	Zollinger-Ellison syndrome (gastrinoma of duodenum or pancreas), associated with MEN1	347
Esophageal cancer	Squamous cell carcinoma (worldwide); adenocarcinoma (US)	372
Acute gastric ulcer associated with CNS injury	Cushing ulcer (↑ intracranial pressure stimulates vagal gastric H^+ secretion)	373
Acute gastric ulcer associated with severe burns	Curling ulcer (greatly reduced plasma volume results in sloughing of gastric mucosa)	373
Bilateral ovarian metastases from gastric carcinoma	Krukenberg tumor (mucin-secreting signet ring cells)	373
Chronic atrophic gastritis (autoimmune)	Predisposition to gastric carcinoma (can also cause pernicious anemia)	373
Gastric cancer	Adenocarcinoma	373
Alternating areas of transmural inflammation and normal colon	Skip lesions (Crohn disease)	376
Diverticulum in pharynx	Zenker diverticulum (diagnosed by barium swallow)	378
Site of diverticula	Sigmoid colon	379
Hepatocellular carcinoma	Cirrhotic liver (associated with hepatitis B and C, alcoholism, and hemochromatosis)	383
Liver disease	Alcoholic cirrhosis	385
1° liver cancer	Hepatocellular carcinoma (chronic hepatitis, cirrhosis, hemochromatosis, α_1-antitrypsin deficiency, Wilson disease)	386
Congenital conjugated hyperbilirubinemia (black liver)	Dubin-Johnson syndrome (inability of hepatocytes to secrete conjugated bilirubin into bile)	388

DISEASE/FINDING	MOST COMMON/IMPORTANT ASSOCIATIONS	PAGE
Hereditary harmless jaundice	Gilbert syndrome (benign congenital unconjugated hyperbilirubinemia)	388
Hemochromatosis	Multiple blood transfusions or hereditary *HFE* mutation (can result in heart failure, "bronze diabetes," and ↑ risk of hepatocellular carcinoma)	389
Pancreatitis (acute)	Gallstones, alcohol	391
Pancreatitis (chronic)	Alcohol (adults), cystic fibrosis (kids)	391
Autosplenectomy (fibrosis and shrinkage)	Sickle cell disease (hemoglobin S)	410
Microcytic anemia	Iron deficiency	413
Bleeding disorder with GpIb deficiency	Bernard-Soulier syndrome (defect in platelet adhesion to von Willebrand factor)	415
Hereditary bleeding disorder	von Willebrand disease	416
DIC	Severe sepsis, obstetric complications, cancer, burns, trauma, major surgery, acute pancreatitis, APL	416
Malignancy associated with noninfectious fever	Hodgkin lymphoma	417
Type of Hodgkin lymphoma	Nodular sclerosing (vs mixed cellularity, lymphocytic predominance, lymphocytic depletion)	417
t(14;18)	Follicular lymphomas (*BCL-2* activation, anti-apoptotic oncogene)	418
t(8;14)	Burkitt lymphoma (c-*myc* fusion, transcription factor oncogene)	418
Type of non-Hodgkin lymphoma	Diffuse large B-cell lymphoma	418
1° bone tumor (adults)	Multiple myeloma	419
Age ranges for patient with ALL/CLL/AML/CML	ALL: child, CLL: adult > 60, AML: adult ~ 65, CML: adult 45–85	420
Malignancy (kids)	Leukemia, brain tumors	420, 512
Death in CML	Blast crisis	420
t(9;22)	Philadelphia chromosome, CML (*BCR-ABL* oncogene, tyrosine kinase activation), more rarely associated with ALL	422
Vertebral compression fracture	Osteoporosis (type I: postmenopausal woman; type II: elderly man or woman)	449
HLA-B27	Psoriatic arthritis, ankylosing spondylitis, IBD-associated arthritis, reactive arthritis (formerly Reiter syndrome)	457
Death in SLE	Lupus nephropathy	458
Tumor of infancy	Strawberry hemangioma (grows rapidly and regresses spontaneously by childhood)	465
Actinic (solar) keratosis	Precursor to squamous cell carcinoma	469
Cerebellar tonsillar herniation	Chiari I malformation	476
Atrophy of the mammillary bodies	Wernicke encephalopathy (thiamine deficiency causing ataxia, ophthalmoplegia, and confusion)	495

DISEASE/FINDING	MOST COMMON/IMPORTANT ASSOCIATIONS	PAGE
Viral encephalitis affecting temporal lobe	HSV-1	495
Hematoma—epidural	Rupture of middle meningeal artery (trauma; lentiform shaped)	497
Hematoma—subdural	Rupture of bridging veins (crescent shaped)	497
Dementia	Alzheimer disease, multiple infarcts (vascular dementia)	504
Demyelinating disease in young women	Multiple sclerosis	507
Brain tumor (adults)	Supratentorial: metastasis, astrocytoma (including glioblastoma multiforme), meningioma, schwannoma	510
Pituitary tumor	Prolactinoma, somatotropic adenoma	510
Brain tumor (kids)	Infratentorial: medulloblastoma (cerebellum) or supratentorial: craniopharyngioma	512
Mixed (UMN and LMN) motor neuron disease	Amyotrophic lateral sclerosis	514
1° hyperaldosteronism	Adrenal hyperplasia or adenoma	575
Nephrotic syndrome (adults)	Membranous nephropathy	580
Nephrotic syndrome (kids)	Minimal change disease	580
Glomerulonephritis (adults)	Berger disease (IgA nephropathy)	581
Kidney stones	▪ Calcium = radiopaque ▪ Struvite (ammonium) = radiopaque (formed by urease ⊕ organisms such as *Klebsiella*, *Proteus* species, and S *saprophyticus*) ▪ Uric acid = radiolucent ▪ Cystine = faintly radiopaque	582
Obstruction of male urinary tract	BPH	583
Renal tumor	Renal cell carcinoma: associated with von Hippel-Lindau and cigarette smoking; paraneoplastic syndromes (EPO, renin, PTHrP, ACTH)	583
1° amenorrhea	Turner syndrome (45,XO or 45,XO/46,XX mosaic)	620
Neuron migration failure	Kallmann syndrome (hypogonadotropic hypogonadism and anosmia)	621
Clear cell adenocarcinoma of the vagina	DES exposure in utero	626
Ovarian tumor (benign, bilateral)	Serous cystadenoma	628
Ovarian tumor (malignant)	Serous cystadenocarcinoma	628
Tumor in women	Leiomyoma (estrogen dependent, not precancerous)	630
Gynecologic malignancy	Endometrial carcinoma (most common in US); cervical carcinoma (most common worldwide)	630
Breast mass	Fibrocystic change, carcinoma (in postmenopausal women)	631
Breast tumor (benign, young woman)	Fibroadenoma	631
Breast cancer	Invasive ductal carcinoma	632
Testicular tumor	Seminoma (malignant, radiosensitive), ↑ placental ALP	634
Right heart failure due to a pulmonary cause	Cor pulmonale	650
Hypercoagulability, endothelial damage, blood stasis	Virchow triad (↑ risk of thrombosis)	653

DISEASE/FINDING	MOST COMMON/IMPORTANT ASSOCIATIONS	PAGE
Pulmonary hypertension	Idiopathic, heritable, left heart disease (eg, HF), lung disease (eg, COPD), hypoxemic vasoconstriction (eg, OSA), thromboembolic (eg, PE)	661
SIADH	Small cell carcinoma of the lung	665

▶ EQUATION REVIEW

TOPIC	EQUATION	PAGE
Volume of distribution	$V_d = \dfrac{\text{amount of drug in the body}}{\text{plasma drug concentration}}$	229
Half-life	$t_{1/2} = \dfrac{0.7 \times V_d}{CL}$	229
Drug clearance	$CL = \dfrac{\text{rate of elimination of drug}}{\text{plasma drug concentration}} = V_d \times K_e \text{ (elimination constant)}$	229
Loading dose	$LD = \dfrac{C_p \times V_d}{F}$	229
Maintenance dose	$D = \dfrac{C_p \times CL \times \tau}{F}$	229
Sensitivity	$\text{Sensitivity} = TP / (TP + FN)$	253
Specificity	$\text{Specificity} = TN / (TN + FP)$	253
Positive predictive value	$PPV = TP / (TP + FP)$	253
Negative predictive value	$NPV = TN / (FN + TN)$	253
Odds ratio (for case-control studies)	$OR = \dfrac{a/c}{b/d} = \dfrac{ad}{bc}$	254
Relative risk	$RR = \dfrac{a/(a + b)}{c/(c + d)}$	254
Attributable risk	$AR = \dfrac{a}{a + b} - \dfrac{c}{c + d}$	254
Relative risk reduction	$RRR = 1 - RR$	254
Absolute risk reduction	$ARR = \dfrac{c}{c + d} - \dfrac{a}{a + b}$	254
Number needed to treat	$NNT = 1/ARR$	254
Number needed to harm	$NNH = 1/AR$	254
Cardiac output	$CO = \dfrac{\text{rate of } O_2 \text{ consumption}}{\text{arterial } O_2 \text{ content} - \text{venous } O_2 \text{ content}}$	278
	$CO = \text{stroke volume} \times \text{heart rate}$	278

TOPIC	EQUATION	PAGE
Mean arterial pressure	$MAP = \text{cardiac output} \times \text{total peripheral resistance}$	278
	$MAP = \frac{2}{3}\text{ diastolic} + \frac{1}{3}\text{ systolic}$	278
Ejection fraction	$EF = \dfrac{SV}{EDV} = \dfrac{EDV - ESV}{EDV}$	279
Resistance	$\text{Resistance} = \dfrac{\text{driving pressure }(\Delta P)}{\text{flow }(Q)} = \dfrac{8\eta\ (\text{viscosity}) \times \text{length}}{\pi r^4}$	280
Stroke volume	$SV = EDV - ESV$	282
Capillary fluid exchange	$J_v = \text{net fluid flow} = K_f[(P_c - P_i) - \varsigma(\pi_c - \pi_i)]$	293
Renal clearance	$C_x = U_x V/P_x$	566
Glomerular filtration rate	$GFR = U_{inulin} \times V/P_{inulin} = C_{inulin}$	566
	$GFR = K_f[(P_{GC} - P_{BS}) - (\pi_{GC} - \pi_{BS})]$	
Effective renal plasma flow	$eRPF = U_{PAH} \times \dfrac{V}{P_{PAH}} = C_{PAH}$	566
Renal blood flow	$RBF = \dfrac{RPF}{1 - Hct}$	566
Filtration fraction	$FF = \dfrac{GFR}{RPF}$	567
Henderson-Hasselbalch equation (for extracellular pH)	$pH = 6.1 + \log \dfrac{[HCO_3^-]}{0.03\ P_{CO_2}}$	576
Winters formula	$P_{CO_2} = 1.5\ [HCO_3^-] + 8 \pm 2$	576
Physiologic dead space	$V_D = V_T \times \dfrac{P_{aCO_2} - P_{ECO_2}}{P_{aCO_2}}$	646
Pulmonary vascular resistance	$PVR = \dfrac{P_{pulm\ artery} - P_{L\ atrium}}{\text{cardiac output}}$	650
Alveolar gas equation	$P_{AO_2} = P_{IO_2} - \dfrac{P_{aCO_2}}{R}$	650

SECTION IV

Top-Rated Review Resources

"Some books are to be tasted, others to be swallowed, and some few to be chewed and digested."

—Sir Francis Bacon

"Always read something that will make you look good if you die in the middle of it."

—P.J. O'Rourke

"So many books, so little time."

—Frank Zappa

"If one cannot enjoy reading a book over and over again, there is no use in reading it at all."

—Oscar Wilde

▶ HOW TO USE THE DATABASE

This section is a database of top-rated basic science review books, sample examination books, software, websites, and apps that have been marketed to medical students studying for the USMLE Step 1. For each recommended resource, we list (where applicable) the **Title**, the **First Author** (or editor), the **Current Publisher**, the **Copyright Year**, the **Number of Pages**, the **Approximate List Price**, the **Format** of the resource, and the **Number of Test Questions**. Finally, each recommended resource receives a **Rating**. Within each section, resources are arranged first by Rating and then alphabetically by the first author within each Rating group.

For a complete list of resources, including summaries that describe their overall style and utility, go to www.firstaidteam.com/bonus.

A letter rating scale with six different grades reflects the detailed student evaluations for **Rated Resources**. Each rated resource receives a rating as follows:

A+	Excellent for boards review.
A A−	Very good for boards review; choose among the group.
B+ B	Good, but use only after exhausting better resources.
B−	Fair, but there are many better resources in the discipline; or low-yield subject material.

The Rating is meant to reflect the overall usefulness of the resource in helping medical students prepare for the USMLE Step 1. This is based on a number of factors, including:

- The cost
- The readability of the text or usability of the app
- The appropriateness and accuracy of the material
- The quality and number of sample questions
- The quality of written answers to sample questions
- The quality and appropriateness of the illustrations (eg, graphs, diagrams, photographs)
- The length of the text (longer is not necessarily better)
- The quality and number of other resources available in the same discipline
- The importance of the discipline for the USMLE Step 1

Please note that ratings do not reflect the quality of the resources for purposes other than reviewing for the USMLE Step 1. Many books with lower ratings are well written and informative but are not ideal for boards preparation. We have not listed or commented on general textbooks available in the basic sciences.

Evaluations are based on the cumulative results of formal and informal surveys of thousands of medical students at many medical schools across the country. The ratings represent a consensus opinion, but there may have been a broad range of opinion or limited student feedback on any particular resource.

Please note that the data listed are subject to change in that:

- Publishers' prices change frequently.
- Bookstores often charge an additional markup.
- New editions come out frequently, and the quality of updating varies.
- The same book may be reissued through another publisher.

We actively encourage medical students and faculty to submit their opinions and ratings of these basic science review materials so that we may update our database. (See p. xvii, How to Contribute.) In addition, we ask that publishers and authors submit for evaluation review copies of basic science review books, including new editions and books not included in our database. We also solicit reviews of new books or suggestions for alternate modes of study that may be useful in preparing for the examination, such as flash cards, computer software, commercial review courses, apps, and websites.

Disclaimer/Conflict of Interest Statement

No material in this book, including the ratings, reflects the opinion or influence of the publisher. All errors and omissions will gladly be corrected if brought to the attention of the authors through our blog at www.firstaidteam.com. Please note that USMLE-Rx and the entire *First Aid for the USMLE* series are publications by the senior authors of this book; the following ratings are based solely on recommendations from the student authors of this book as well as data from the student survey and feedback forms.

▶ TOP-RATED REVIEW RESOURCES

Question Banks

		AUTHOR	PUBLISHER	TYPE	PRICE
A⁺	*UWorld Qbank*	UWorld	www.uworld.com	Test/2400 q	$169–$599
A	*NBME Practice Exams*	National Board of Medical Examiners	https://nsas.nbme.org/home	Test/200 q	$60
A⁻	*USMLE-Rx Qmax*	USMLE-Rx	www.usmle-rx.com	Test/2300 q	$99–$299
B⁺	*Kaplan Qbank*	Kaplan	www.kaptest.com	Test/2200 q	$99–$299

Question Books

		AUTHOR	PUBLISHER	TYPE	PRICE
B⁺	*First Aid Q&A for the USMLE Step 1*	Le	McGraw-Hill, 2012, 784 pages	Test/1000 q	$46.00
B	*Kaplan USMLE Step 1 Qbook*	Kaplan	Kaplan, 2015, 456 pages	Test/850 q	$49.99

Web and Mobile Apps

		AUTHOR	PUBLISHER	TYPE	PRICE
A	*SketchyMedical*		www.SketchyMedical.com	Review	$169–$249
A⁻	*Anki*		www.ankisrs.net	Flash cards	Free/$24.99
A⁻	*Boards and Beyond*		https://www.boardsbeyond.com	Review	$89–$149
A⁻	*Cram Fighter*		www.cramfighter.com	Study plan	$29–$99
A⁻	*First Aid Step 1 Express*		www.usmle-rx.com	Review/Test	$99–$299
A⁻	*First Aid Step 1 Flash Facts*		https://www.usmle-rx.com	Flash cards	$49–$149
A⁻	*Physeo*		www.physeo.com	Review	$87–$110
A⁻	*WebPath: The Internet Pathology Laboratory*		http://library.med.utah.edu/WebPath/webpath.html	Review/Test/1300 q	Free
B⁺	*Dr. Najeeb Lectures*		www.drnajeeblectures.com	Review	$49–$199
B⁺	*Firecracker*	Firecracker Inc.	www.firecracker.me	Review/Test/1500 q	$100–$400
B⁺	*Medical School Pathology*		www.medicalschoolpathology.com	Review	Free
B⁺	*Osmosis*		www.osmosis.org	Test	$31–$599
B⁺	*The Whole Brain Atlas*	Johnson	www.med.harvard.edu/aanlib/	Review	Free
B⁺	*USMLE Step 1 Mastery*		usmle.usmlemastery.com	Test/1400 q	$49
B	*Blue Histology*		www.lab.anhb.uwa.edu.au/mb140	Review/Test	Free
B	*Digital Anatomist Project: Interactive Atlases*	University of Washington	www9.biostr.washington.edu/da.html	Review	Free
B	*Memorang*	Memorang Inc.	www.memorangapp.com	Flash cards	Free/$99
B	*The Pathology Guy*	Friedlander	www.pathguy.com	Review	Free
B	*Picmonic*		www.picmonic.com	Review	$24–$480
B	*Radiopaedia.org*		www.radiopaedia.org	Cases/Test	Free

Comprehensive

		AUTHOR	PUBLISHER	TYPE	PRICE
A⁻	*First Aid for the Basic Sciences: General Principles*	Le	McGraw-Hill, 2011, 576 pages	Review	$75.00
A⁻	*First Aid for the Basic Sciences: Organ Systems*	Le	McGraw-Hill, 2011, 880 pages	Review	$99.00
A⁻	*First Aid Cases for the USMLE Step 1*	Le	McGraw-Hill, 2012, 448 pages	Cases	$50.00
A⁻	*Crush Step 1: The Ultimate USMLE Step 1 Review*	O'Connell	Elsevier, 2013, 680 pages	Review	$41.95
B⁺	*USMLE Step 1 Secrets in Color*	Brown	Elsevier, 2016, 800 pages	Review	$42.99
B⁺	*Step-Up to USMLE Step 1 2015*	Jenkins	Lippincott Williams & Wilkins, 2014, 528 pages	Review	$54.99
B⁺	*medEssentials for the USMLE Step 1*	Manley	Kaplan, 2012, 588 pages	Review	$54.99
B⁺	*Cracking the USMLE Step 1*	Princeton Review	Princeton Review, 2013, 832 pages	Review	$44.99
B⁺	*USMLE Images for the Boards: A Comprehensive Image-Based Review*	Tully	Elsevier, 2012, 296 pages	Review	$42.95
B	*Déjà Review: USMLE Step 1*	Naheedy	McGraw-Hill, 2010, 416 pages	Review	$25.00
B⁻	*USMLE Step 1 Made Ridiculously Simple*	Carl	MedMaster, 2015, 416 pages	Review/Test 100 q	$29.95

Anatomy, Embryology, and Neuroscience

		AUTHOR	PUBLISHER	TYPE	PRICE
A⁻	*Clinical Anatomy Made Ridiculously Simple*	Goldberg	MedMaster, 2012, 175 pages	Review	$29.95
B⁺	*BRS Embryology*	Dudek	Lippincott Williams & Wilkins, 2014, 336 pages	Review/Test/220 q	$52.99
B⁺	*High-Yield Embryology*	Dudek	Lippincott Williams & Wilkins, 2013, 176 pages	Review	$39.99
B⁺	*High-Yield Gross Anatomy*	Dudek	Lippincott Williams & Wilkins, 2014, 320 pages	Review	$39.99
B⁺	*High-Yield Neuroanatomy*	Fix	Lippincott Williams & Wilkins, 2015, 208 pages	Review/Test/50 q	$37.99
B⁺	*Anatomy—An Essential Textbook*	Gilroy	Thieme, 2013, 504 pages	Text/Test/400 q	$44.99
B⁺	*Atlas of Anatomy*	Gilroy	Thieme, 2016, 760 pages	Text	$82.99
B⁺	*Clinical Neuroanatomy Made Ridiculously Simple*	Goldberg	MedMaster, 2014, 90 pages + CD-ROM	Review/Test/Few q	$25.95
B⁺	*Crash Course: Anatomy*	Stenhouse	Elsevier, 2015, 288 pages	Review	$44.99
B	*Anatomy Flash Cards: Anatomy on the Go*	Gilroy	Thieme, 2013, 565 flash cards	Flash cards	$59.99
B	*PreTest Neuroscience*	Siegel	McGraw-Hill, 2013, 412 pages	Test/500 q	$39.00

Anatomy, Embryology, and Neuroscience *(continued)*

		AUTHOR	PUBLISHER	TYPE	PRICE
B⁻	*Netter's Anatomy Flash Cards*	Hansen	Saunders, 2014, 674 flash cards	Flash cards	$39.95
B⁻	*Case Files: Anatomy*	Toy	McGraw-Hill, 2014, 416 pages	Cases	$35.00
B⁻	*Case Files: Neuroscience*	Toy	McGraw-Hill, 2014, 432 pages	Cases	$35.00

Behavioral Science

		AUTHOR	PUBLISHER	TYPE	PRICE
A⁻	*BRS Behavioral Science*	Fadem	Lippincott Williams & Wilkins, 2016, 384 pages	Review/Test/700 q	$51.99
A⁻	*High-Yield Behavioral Science*	Fadem	Lippincott Williams & Wilkins, 2012, 144 pages	Review	$37.99
A⁻	*Clinical Biostatistics and Epidemiology Made Ridiculously Simple*	Weaver	MedMaster, 2011, 104 pages	Review	$22.95
B⁺	*USMLE Medical Ethics*	Fischer	Kaplan, 2012, 216 pages	Cases	Variable
B⁺	*High-Yield Biostatistics, Epidemiology, and Public Health*	Glaser	Lippincott Williams & Wilkins, 2013, 168 pages	Review	$42.99
B⁺	*Jekel's Epidemiology, Biostatistics, Preventive Medicine, and Public Health*	Katz	Saunders, 2013, 420 pages	Review/Test/477 q	$59.95

Biochemistry

		AUTHOR	PUBLISHER	TYPE	PRICE
B⁺	*Lippincott's Illustrated Reviews: Biochemistry*	Ferrier	Lippincott Williams & Wilkins, 2013, 560 pages	Review/Test/500 q	$75.99
B⁺	*Medical Biochemistry—An Illustrated Review*	Panini	Thieme, 2013, 441 pages	Review/Test/400 q	$39.99
B⁺	*Rapid Review: Biochemistry*	Pelley	Elsevier, 2010, 208 pages	Review/Test/350 q	$42.95
B⁺	*PreTest Biochemistry and Genetics*	Wilson	McGraw-Hill, 2013, 592 pages	Test/500 q	$38.00
B	*Lange Flash Cards Biochemistry and Genetics*	Baron	McGraw-Hill, 2013, 184 flash cards	Flash cards	$40.00
B	*Clinical Biochemistry Made Ridiculously Simple*	Goldberg	MedMaster, 2010, 95 pages + foldout	Review	$24.95
B	*BRS Biochemistry, Molecular Biology, and Genetics*	Lieberman	Lippincott Williams & Wilkins, 2013, 432 pages	Review/Test	$52.99
B	*Case Files: Biochemistry*	Toy	McGraw-Hill, 2014, 480 pages	Cases	$35.00

Cell Biology and Histology

		AUTHOR	PUBLISHER	TYPE	PRICE
B⁺	*BRS Cell Biology and Histology*	Gartner	Lippincott Williams & Wilkins, 2014, 432 pages	Review/Test/320 q	$51.99
B⁺	*Crash Course: Cell Biology and Genetics*	Stubbs	Elsevier, 2015, 216 pages	Review/Print + online	$46.99

Cell Biology and Histology *(continued)*

		AUTHOR	PUBLISHER	TYPE	PRICE
B	*Elsevier's Integrated Review: Genetics*	Adkison	Elsevier, 2011, 272 pages	Review	$42.95
B⁻	*Wheater's Functional Histology*	Young	Elsevier, 2013, 464 pages	Text	$82.95

Microbiology and Immunology

		AUTHOR	PUBLISHER	TYPE	PRICE
A⁻	*Clinical Microbiology Made Ridiculously Simple*	Gladwin	MedMaster, 2016, 400 pages	Review	$36.95
A⁻	*Medical Microbiology and Immunology Flash Cards*	Rosenthal	Elsevier, 2016, 192 flash cards	Flash cards	$39.99
B⁺	*Basic Immunology*	Abbas	Elsevier, 2015, 352 pages	Review	$69.99
B⁺	*Elsevier's Integrated Review: Immunology and Microbiology*	Actor	Elsevier, 2011, 192 pages	Review	$42.95
B⁺	*Déjà Review: Microbiology & Immunology*	Chen	McGraw-Hill, 2010, 432 pages	Review	$25.00
B⁺	*Lippincott's Illustrated Reviews: Immunology*	Doan	Lippincott Williams & Wilkins, 2012, 384 pages	Reference/ Test/Few q	$69.99
B⁺	*Microcards: Microbiology Flash Cards*	Harpavat	Lippincott Williams & Wilkins, 2015, 312 flash cards	Flash cards	$51.99
B⁺	*Case Files: Microbiology*	Toy	McGraw-Hill, 2014, 416 pages	Cases	$36.00
B	*Case Studies in Immunology: Clinical Companion*	Geha	Garland Science, 2016, 384 pages	Cases	$61.95
B	*Lippincott's Illustrated Reviews: Microbiology*	Harvey	Lippincott Williams & Wilkins, 2012, 448 pages	Review/Test/ Few q	$67.99
B	*Pretest: Microbiology*	Kettering	McGraw-Hill, 2013, 480 pages	Test/500 q	$38.00
B	*Review of Medical Microbiology and Immunology*	Levinson	McGraw-Hill, 2016, 832 pages	Review/ Test/654 q	$64.00
B⁻	*Rapid Review: Microbiology and Immunology*	Rosenthal	Elsevier, 2010, 240 pages	Review/ Test/400 q	$42.95

Pathology

		AUTHOR	PUBLISHER	TYPE	PRICE
A⁺	*Pathoma: Fundamentals of Pathology*	Sattar	Pathoma, 2016, 218 pages	Review/ Lecture	$84.95– $119.95
A⁻	*Lange Pathology Flash Cards*	Baron	McGraw-Hill, 2013, 300 flash cards	Flash cards	$41.00
A⁻	*Rapid Review: Pathology*	Goljan	Elsevier, 2013, 784 pages	Review/ Test/400 q	$55.95
A⁻	*Crash Course: Pathology*	Xiu	Elsevier, 2015, 356 pages	Review	$44.99
B⁺	*Déjà Review: Pathology*	Davis	McGraw-Hill, 2010, 474 pages	Review	$25.00
B⁺	*Lippincott's Illustrated Q&A Review of Rubin's Pathology*	Fenderson	Lippincott Williams & Wilkins, 2010, 336 pages	Test/1000 q	$61.99

Pathology (continued)

		AUTHOR	PUBLISHER	TYPE	PRICE
B⁺	*Robbins and Cotran Review of Pathology*	Klatt	Elsevier, 2014, 504 pages	Test/1100 q	$54.99
B⁺	*Pocket Companion to Robbins and Cotran Pathologic Basis of Disease*	Mitchell	Elsevier, 2016, 896 pages	Review	$39.99
B⁺	*BRS Pathology*	Schneider	Lippincott Williams & Wilkins, 2013, 480 pages	Review/Test/450 q	$52.99
B	*PreTest Pathology*	Brown	McGraw-Hill, 2010, 612 pages	Test/500 q	$39.00
B	*High-Yield Histopathology*	Dudek	Lippincott Williams & Wilkins, 2016, 350 pages	Review	$35.99
B	*Pathophysiology of Disease: Introduction to Clinical Medicine*	McPhee	McGraw-Hill, 2014, 784 pages	Text	$80.00
B	*Haematology at a Glance*	Mehta	Blackwell Science, 2014, 136 pages	Review	$48.95

Pharmacology

		AUTHOR	PUBLISHER	TYPE	PRICE
A⁻	*Lippincott's Illustrated Reviews: Pharmacology*	Harvey	Lippincott Williams & Wilkins, 2014, 680 pages	Review/Test/380 q	$72.99
B⁺	*Lange Pharmacology Flash Cards*	Baron	McGraw-Hill, 2013, 230 flash cards	Flash cards	$41.00
B⁺	*Crash Course: Pharmacology*	Battista	Elsevier, 2015, 236 pages	Review	$44.99
B⁺	*Pharmacology Flash Cards*	Brenner	Elsevier, 2012, 200 flash cards	Flash cards	$39.95
B⁺	*Master the Boards USMLE Step 1 Pharmacology Flashcards*	Fischer	Kaplan, 2015, 200 flash cards	Flash cards	$54.99
B⁺	*Elsevier's Integrated Pharmacology*	Kester	Elsevier, 2011, 264 pages	Review	$42.95
B⁺	*Rapid Review: Pharmacology*	Pazdernik	Elsevier, 2010, 360 pages	Review/Test/450 q	$42.95
B⁺	*BRS Pharmacology*	Rosenfeld	Lippincott Williams & Wilkins, 2013, 384 pages	Review/Test/200 q	$52.99
B⁺	*Case Files: Pharmacology*	Toy	McGraw-Hill, 2013, 464 pages	Cases	$35.00
B⁺	*Katzung & Trevor's Pharmacology: Examination and Board Review*	Trevor	McGraw-Hill, 2015, 592 pages	Review/Test/1000 q	$54.00
B	*PreTest Pharmacology*	Shlafer	McGraw-Hill, 2013, 624 pages	Test/500 q	$38.00

Physiology

		AUTHOR	PUBLISHER	TYPE	PRICE
A	*BRS Physiology*	Costanzo	Lippincott Williams & Wilkins, 2014, 328 pages	Review/Test/350 q	$53.99
A⁻	*Physiology*	Costanzo	Saunders, 2013, 520 pages	Text	$62.95
A⁻	*Acid-Base, Fluids, and Electrolytes Made Ridiculously Simple*	Preston	MedMaster, 2011, 156 pages	Review	$22.95
A⁻	*Color Atlas of Physiology*	Silbernagl	Thieme, 2015, 472 pages	Review	$49.99

Physiology *(continued)*

		AUTHOR	PUBLISHER	TYPE	PRICE
A⁻	*Pulmonary Pathophysiology: The Essentials*	West	Lippincott Williams & Wilkins, 2012, 208 pages	Review/ Test/50 q	$52.99
B⁺	*BRS Physiology Cases and Problems*	Costanzo	Lippincott Williams & Wilkins, 2012, 368 pages	Cases	$53.99
B⁺	*Déjà Review: Physiology*	Gould	McGraw-Hill, 2010, 298 pages	Review	$25.00
B⁺	*PreTest Physiology*	Metting	McGraw-Hill, 2013, 528 pages	Test/500 q	$38.00
B	*Rapid Review: Physiology*	Brown	Elsevier, 2011, 288 pages	Test/350 q	$42.95
B	*Vander's Renal Physiology*	Eaton	McGraw-Hill, 2013, 224 pages	Text	$47.00
B	*Endocrine Physiology*	Molina	McGraw-Hill, 2013, 320 pages	Review	$50.00
B⁻	*Netter's Physiology Flash Cards*	Mulroney	Saunders, 2015, 200+ flash cards	Flash cards	$39.99

▶ NOTES

SECTION IV

Abbreviations and Symbols

ABBREVIATION	MEANING
1st MC*	1st metacarpal
A-a	alveolar-arterial [gradient]
AA	Alcoholics Anonymous, amyloid A
AAMC	Association of American Medical Colleges
Aao*	ascending aorta
Ab	antibody
AC	adenylyl cyclase
ACA	anterior cerebral artery
Acetyl-CoA	acetyl coenzyme A
ACD	anemia of chronic disease
ACE	angiotensin-converting enzyme
ACh	acetylcholine
AChE	acetylcholinesterase
ACL	anterior cruciate ligament
ACom	anterior communicating [artery]
ACTH	adrenocorticotropic hormone
AD*	Alzheimer disease
ADA	adenosine deaminase, Americans with Disabilities Act
ADH	antidiuretic hormone
ADHD	attention-deficit hyperactivity disorder
ADP	adenosine diphosphate
ADPKD	autosomal-dominant polycystic kidney disease
AFP	α-fetoprotein
Ag	antigen, silver
AICA	anterior inferior cerebellar artery
AIDS	acquired immunodeficiency syndrome
AIHA	autoimmune hemolytic anemia
AKT	protein kinase B
AL	amyloid light [chain]
ALA	aminolevulinate
ALL	acute lymphoblastic (lymphocytic) leukemia
ALP	alkaline phosphatase
α_1, α_2	sympathetic receptors
ALS	amyotrophic lateral sclerosis
ALT	alanine transaminase
AMA	American Medical Association, antimitochondrial antibody
AML	acute myelogenous (myeloid) leukemia
AMP	adenosine monophosphate
ANA	antinuclear antibody
ANCA	antineutrophil cytoplasmic antibody
ANOVA	analysis of variance
ANP	atrial natriuretic peptide
ANS	autonomic nervous system

ABBREVIATION	MEANING
Ant*	anterior
anti-CCP	anti-cyclic citrullinated peptide
Ao*	aorta
AOA	American Osteopathic Association
AP	action potential, A & P [ribosomal binding sites]
APAF-1	apoptotic protease activating factor 1
APC	antigen-presenting cell, activated protein C
Apo	apolipoprotein
APP	amyloid precursor protein
APRT	adenine phosphoribosyltransferase
APSAC	anistreplase
aPTT	activated partial thromboplastin time
APUD	amine precursor uptake decarboxylase
AR	attributable risk, autosomal recessive, aortic regurgitation
ara-C	arabinofuranosyl cytidine (cytarabine)
ARB	angiotensin receptor blocker
ARDS	acute respiratory distress syndrome
Arg	arginine
ARPKD	autosomal-recessive polycystic kidney disease
AS	aortic stenosis
ASA	anterior spinal artery
ASD	atrial septal defect
ASO	anti–streptolysin O
AST	aspartate transaminase
AT	angiotensin, antithrombin
ATCase	aspartate transcarbamoylase
ATN	acute tubular necrosis
ATP	adenosine triphosphate
ATPase	adenosine triphosphatase
ATTR	transthyretin-mediated amyloidosis
AUB	Abnormal uterine bleeding
AV	atrioventricular
AZT	azidothymidine
β_1, β_2	sympathetic receptors
BAL	British anti-Lewisite [dimercaprol]
BCG	bacille Calmette-Guérin
BH_4	tetrahydrobiopterin
BIMS	Biometric Identity Management System
BM	basement membrane
BMR	basal metabolic rate
BOOP	bronchiolitis obliterans organizing pneumonia
BP	bisphosphate, blood pressure
BPG	bisphosphoglycerate
BPH	benign prostatic hyperplasia

*Image abbreviation only

ABBREVIATION	MEANING
BT	bleeding time
BUN	blood urea nitrogen
Ca*	capillary
Ca^{2+}	calcium ion
CAD	coronary artery disease
CAF	common application form
CALLA	common acute lymphoblastic leukemia antigen
cAMP	cyclic adenosine monophosphate
CBG	corticosteroid-binding globulin
Cbl	cobalamin
Cbm*	cerebellum
CBSE	Comprehensive Basic Science Examination
CBSSA	Comprehensive Basic Science Self-Assessment
CBT	computer-based test, cognitive behavioral therapy
CC*	corpus callosum
CCA*	common carotid artery
CCK	cholecystokinin
CCS	computer-based case simulation
CD	cluster of differentiation
CDK	cyclin-dependent kinase
cDNA	complementary deoxyribonucleic acid
CEA	carcinoembryonic antigen
CETP	cholesteryl-ester transfer protein
CF	cystic fibrosis
CFTR	cystic fibrosis transmembrane conductance regulator
CFX	circumflex [artery]
CGD	chronic granulomatous disease
cGMP	cyclic guanosine monophosphate
CGN	cis-Golgi network
$C_H1–C_H3$	constant regions, heavy chain [antibody]
ChAT	choline acetyltransferase
CHD*	common hepatic duct
χ^2	chi-squared
CI	confidence interval
CIN	candidate identification number, carcinoma in situ, cervical intraepithelial neoplasia
CIS	Communication and Interpersonal Skills
CK	clinical knowledge, creatine kinase
CK-MB	creatine kinase, MB fraction
C_L	constant region, light chain [antibody]
CL	clearance
Cl^-	chloride ion
CLL	chronic lymphocytic leukemia
CMC	carpometacarpal (joint)
CML	chronic myelogenous (myeloid) leukemia
CMV	cytomegalovirus
CN	cranial nerve
CN^-	cyanide ion
CNS	central nervous system
CNV	copy number variation
CO	carbon monoxide, cardiac output
CO_2	carbon dioxide
CoA	coenzyme A
COL1A1	collagen, type I, alpha 1

ABBREVIATION	MEANING
COL1A2	collagen, type I, alpha 2
COMT	catechol-O-methyltransferase
COOH	carboxyl group
COP	coat protein
COPD	chronic obstructive pulmonary disease
CoQ	coenzyme Q
COX	cyclooxygenase
C_p	plasma concentration
CPAP	continuous positive airway pressure
CPK	creatine phosphokinase
CPR	cardiopulmonary resuscitation
Cr	creatinine
CRC	colorectal cancer
CREST	calcinosis, Raynaud phenomenon, esophageal dysfunction, sclerosis, and telangiectasias [syndrome]
CRH	corticotropin-releasing hormone
CRP	C-reactive protein
CS	clinical skills
C-section	cesarean section
CSF	cerebrospinal fluid
CT	computed tomography
CTP	cytidine triphosphate
CVA	cerebrovascular accident
CVID	common variable immunodeficiency
CXR	chest x-ray
Cys	cysteine
DA	dopamine
DAF	decay-accelerating factor
DAG	diacylglycerol
dATP	deoxyadenosine triphosphate
DCIS	ductal carcinoma in situ
DCT	distal convoluted tubule
ddC	dideoxycytidine [zalcitabine]
ddI	didanosine
DES	diethylstilbestrol
DHAP	dihydroxyacetone phosphate
DHB	dihydrobiopterin
DHEA	dehydroepiandrosterone
DHF	dihydrofolic acid
DHS	Department of Homeland Security
DHT	dihydrotestosterone
DI	diabetes insipidus
DIC	disseminated intravascular coagulation
DIP	distal interphalangeal [joint]
DKA	diabetic ketoacidosis
D_{LCO}	diffusing capacity for carbon monoxide
DM	diabetes mellitus
DNA	deoxyribonucleic acid
DNR	do not resuscitate
dNTP	deoxynucleotide triphosphate
DO	doctor of osteopathy
DPGN	diffuse proliferative glomerulonephritis
DPM	doctor of podiatric medicine
DPP-4	dipeptidyl peptidase-4
DPPC	dipalmitoylphosphatidylcholine

*Image abbreviation only

ABBREVIATION	MEANING
DS	double stranded
dsDNA	double-stranded deoxyribonucleic acid
dsRNA	double-stranded ribonucleic acid
d4T	didehydrodeoxythymidine [stavudine]
dTMP	deoxythymidine monophosphate
DTR	deep tendon reflex
DTs	delirium tremens
dUDP	deoxyuridine diphosphate
dUMP	deoxyuridine monophosphate
DVT	deep venous thrombosis
E*	euthromatin, esophagus
EBV	Epstein-Barr virus
EC	ejection click
ECA*	external carotid artery
ECF	extracellular fluid
ECFMG	Educational Commission for Foreign Medical Graduates
ECG	electrocardiogram
ECL	enterochromaffin-like [cell]
ECM	extracellular matrix
ECT	electroconvulsive therapy
ED_{50}	median effective dose
EDRF	endothelium-derived relaxing factor
EDTA	ethylenediamine tetra-acetic acid
EDV	end-diastolic volume
EEG	electroencephalogram
EF	ejection fraction
EGF	epidermal growth factor
EHEC	enterohemorrhagic E coli
EIEC	enteroinvasive E coli
ELISA	enzyme-linked immunosorbent assay
EM	electron micrograph/microscopy
EMB	eosin–methylene blue
EPEC	eneteropathogenic E coli
Epi	epinephrine
EPO	erythropoietin
EPS	extrapyramidal system
ER	endoplasmic reticulum, estrogen receptor
ERAS	Electronic Residency Application Service
ERCP	endoscopic retrograde cholangiopancreatography
ERP	effective refractory period
eRPF	effective renal plasma flow
ERT	estrogen replacement therapy
ERV	expiratory reserve volume
ESR	erythrocyte sedimentation rate
ESRD	end-stage renal disease
ESV	end-systolic volume
ETEC	enterotoxigenic E coli
EtOH	ethyl alcohol
EV	esophageal vein
F	bioavailability
FA	fatty acid
Fab	fragment, antigen-binding
FAD	flavin adenine dinucleotide
FAD^+	oxidized flavin adenine dinucleotide

ABBREVIATION	MEANING
$FADH_2$	reduced flavin adenine dinucleotide
FAP	familial adenomatous polyposis
F1,6BP	fructose-1,6-bisphosphate
F2,6BP	fructose-2,6-bisphosphate
FBPase	fructose bisphosphatase
Fc	fragment, crystallizable
FcR	Fc receptor
5f-dUMP	5-fluorodeoxyuridine monophosphate
Fe^{2+}	ferrous ion
Fe^{3+}	ferric ion
Fem*	femur
FENa	excreted fraction of filtered sodium
FEV_1	forced expiratory volume in 1 second
FF	filtration fraction
FFA	free fatty acid
FGF	fibroblast growth factor
FGFR	fibroblast growth factor receptor
FISH	fluorescence in situ hybridization
FKBP	FK506 binding protein
FLAIR	fluid-attenuated inversion recovery
f-met	formylmethionine
FMG	foreign medical graduate
FMN	flavin mononucleotide
FN	false negative
FNHTR	febrile nonhemolytic transfusion reaction
FP, FP*	false positive, foot process
F1P	fructose-1-phosphate
F6P	fructose-6-phosphate
FRC	functional residual capacity
FSH	follicle-stimulating hormone
FSMB	Federation of State Medical Boards
FTA-ABS	fluorescent treponemal antibody—absorbed
FTD*	frontotemporal dementia
5-FU	5-fluorouracil
FVC	forced vital capacity
GABA	γ-aminobutyric acid
GAG	glycosaminoglycan
Gal	galactose
GBM	glomerular basement membrane
GC	glomerular capillary
G-CSF	granulocyte colony-stimulating factor
GERD	gastroesophageal reflux disease
GFAP	glial fibrillary acid protein
GFR	glomerular filtration rate
GGT	γ-glutamyl transpeptidase
GH	growth hormone
GHB	γ-hydroxybutyrate
GHRH	growth hormone–releasing hormone
G_I	G protein, I polypeptide
GI	gastrointestinal
GIP	gastric inhibitory peptide
GIST	gastrointestinal stromal tumor
GLUT	glucose transporter
GM	granulocyte macrophage

*Image abbreviation only

ABBREVIATION	MEANING
GM-CSF	granulocyte-macrophage colony stimulating factor
GMP	guanosine monophosphate
GnRH	gonadotropin-releasing hormone
GP	glycoprotein
G3P	glucose-3-phosphate
G6P	glucose-6-phosphate
G6PD	glucose-6-phosphate dehydrogenase
GPe	globus pallidus externa
CPi	globus pallidus interna
GPI	glycosyl phosphatidylinositol
GRP	gastrin-releasing peptide
G_S	G protein, S polypeptide
GS	glycogen synthase
GSH	reduced glutathione
GSSG	oxidized glutathione
GTP	guanosine triphosphate
GTPase	guanosine triphosphatase
GU	genitourinary
H*	heterochromatin
H^+	hydrogen ion
H_1, H_2	histamine receptors
H_2S	hydrogen sulfide
HAART	highly active antiretroviral therapy
HAV	hepatitis A virus
HAVAb	hepatitis A antibody
Hb	hemoglobin
Hb^+	oxidized hemoglobin
Hb^-	ionized hemoglobin
HBcAb/HBcAg	hepatitis B core antibody/antigen
HBeAb/HBeAg	hepatitis B early antibody/antigen
HBsAb/HBsAg	hepatitis B surface antibody/antigen
$HbCO_2$	carbaminohemoglobin
HBV	hepatitis B virus
HCC	hepatocellular carcinoma
hCG	human chorionic gonadotropin
HCO_3^-	bicarbonate
Hct	hematocrit
HCTZ	hydrochlorothiazide
HCV	hepatitis C virus
HDL	high-density lipoprotein
HDN	hemolytic disease of the newborn
HDV	hepatitis D virus
H&E	hematoxylin and eosin
HEV	hepatitis E virus
HF	heart failure
Hfr	high-frequency recombination [cell]
HGPRT	hypoxanthine-guanine phosphoribosyltransferase
HHb	human hemoglobin
HHV	human herpesvirus
5-HIAA	5-hydroxyindoleacetic acid
HIE	hypoxic ischemic encephalopathy
His	histidine
HIT	heparin-induced thrombocytopenia
HIV	human immunodeficiency virus

ABBREVIATION	MEANING
HL	hepatic lipase
HLA	human leukocyte antigen
HMG-CoA	hydroxymethylglutaryl-coenzyme A
HMP	hexose monophosphate
HMWK	high-molecular-weight kininogen
HNPCC	hereditary nonpolyposis colorectal cancer
hnRNA	heterogeneous nuclear ribonucleic acid
H_2O_2	hydrogen peroxide
HOCM	hypertrophic obstructive cardiomyopathy
HPA	hypothalamic-pituitary-adrenal [axis]
HPL	human placental lactogen
HPO	hypothalamic-pituitary-ovarian [axis]
HPV	human papillomavirus
HR	heart rate
HRE	hormone receptor element
HSV	herpes simplex virus
5-HT	5-hydroxytryptamine (serotonin)
HTLV	human T-cell leukemia virus
HTN	hypertension
HTR	hemolytic transfusion reaction
HUS	hemolytic-uremic syndrome
HVA	homovanillic acid
HZV	herpes zoster virus
IBD	inflammatory bowel disease
IBS	irritable bowel syndrome
IC	inspiratory capacity, immune complex
I_{Ca}	calcium current [heart]
I_f	funny current [heart]
ICA	internal carotid artery
ICAM	intercellular adhesion molecule
ICD	implantable cardioverter defibrillator
ICE	Integrated Clinical Encounter
ICF	intracellular fluid
ICP	intracranial pressure
ID	identification
ID_{50}	median infective dose
IDL	intermediate-density lipoprotein
I/E	inspiratory/expiratory [ratio]
IF	immunofluorescence, initiation factor
IFN	interferon
Ig	immunoglobulin
IGF	insulin-like growth factor
I_K	potassium current [heart]
IL	interleukin
IM	intramuscular
IMA	inferior mesenteric artery
IMED	International Medical Education Directory
IMG	international medical graduate
IMP	inosine monophosphate
IMV	inferior mesenteric vein
I_{Na}	sodium current [heart]
INH	isoniazid
INO	internuclear ophthalmoplegia
INR	International Normalized Ratio

*Image abbreviation only

ABBREVIATION	MEANING
IO	inferior oblique [muscle]
IOP	intraocular pressure
IP$_3$	inositol triphosphate
IPV	inactivated polio vaccine
IR	current × resistance [Ohm's law], inferior rectus [muscle]
IRV	inspiratory reserve volume
ITP	idiopathic thrombocytopenic purpura
IUD	intrauterine device
IUGR	intrauterine growth restriction
IV	intravenous
IVC	inferior vena cava
IVDU	intravenous drug use
IVIG	intravenous immunoglobulin
JAK/STAT	Janus kinase/signal transducer and activator of transcription [pathway]
JGA	juxtaglomerular apparatus
JVD	jugular venous distention
JVP	jugular venous pulse
K$^+$	potassium ion
KatG	catalase-peroxidase produced by M tuberculosis
K$_e$	elimination constant
K$_f$	filtration constant
KG	ketoglutarate
K$_m$	Michaelis-Menten constant
KOH	potassium hydroxide
L	left, liver
LA	left atrial, left atrium
LAD	left anterior descending coronary artery
LAF	left anterior fascicle
LAP	leukocyte alkaline phosphatase
Lat cond*	lateral condyle
Lb*	lamellar body
LCA	left coronary artery
LCAT	lecithin-cholesterol acyltransferase
LCC*	left common carotid artery
LCFA	long-chain fatty acid
LCL	lateral collateral ligament
LCME	Liaison Committee on Medical Education
LCMV	lymphocytic choriomeningitis virus
LCX	left circumflex coronary artery
LD	loading dose
LD$_{50}$	median lethal dose
LDH	lactate dehydrogenase
LDL	low-density lipoprotein
LES	lower esophageal sphincter
LFA	leukocyte function–associated antigen
LFT	liver function test
LGN	lateral geniculate nucleus
LGV	left gastric vein
LH	luteinizing hormone
LLL*	left lower lobe (of lung)
LLQ	left lower quadrant
LM	light microscopy, left main coronary artery
LMN	lower motor neuron

ABBREVIATION	MEANING
LOS	lipooligosaccharide
LP	lumbar puncture
LPA*	left pulmonary artery
LPL	lipoprotein lipase
LPS	lipopolysaccharide
LR	lateral rectus [muscle]
LT	labile toxin leukotriene
LUL*	left upper lobe (of lung)
LV	left ventricle, left ventricular
Lys	lysine
M$_1$-M$_5$	muscarinic (parasympathetic) ACh receptors
MAC	membrane attack complex, minimal alveolar concentration
MALT	mucosa-associated lymphoid tissue
MAO	monoamine oxidase
MAOI	monoamine oxidase inhibitor
MAP	mean arterial pressure, mitogen-activated protein
MASP	mannose-binding lectin–associated serine protease
Max*	maxillary sinus
MBL	mannose-binding lectin
MC	midsystolic click
MCA	middle cerebral artery
MCAT	Medical College Admissions Test
MCHC	mean corpuscular hemoglobin concentration
MCL	medial collateral ligament
MCP	metacarpophalangeal [joint]
MCV	mean corpuscular volume
MD	maintenance dose
MDD	major depressive disorder
Med cond*	medial condyle
MELAS syndrome	mitochondrial encephalopathy, lactic acidosis, and stroke-like episodes
MEN	multiple endocrine neoplasia
Mg^{2+}	magnesium ion
MGN	medial geniculate nucleus
MgSO$_4$	magnesium sulfate
MGUS	monoclonal gammopathy of undetermined significance
MHC	major histocompatibility complex
MI	myocardial infarction
MIF	müllerian inhibiting factor
MIRL	membrane inhibitor of reactive lysis
MLCK	myosin light-chain kinase
MLF	medial longitudinal fasciculus
MMC	migrating motor complex
MMR	measles, mumps, rubella [vaccine]
6-MP	6-mercaptopurine
MPGN	membranoproliferative glomerulonephritis
MPO	myeloperoxidase
MPO-ANCA/ p-ANCA	perinuclear antineutrophil cytoplasmic antibody
MR	medial rectus [muscle], mitral regurgitation
MRI	magnetic resonance imaging
miRNA	microribonucleic acid
mRNA	messenger ribonucleic acid
MRSA	methicillin-resistant S aureus

*Image abbreviation only

ABBREVIATION	MEANING
MS	mitral stenosis, multiple sclerosis
MSH	melanocyte-stimulating hormone
MSM	men who have sex with men
mtDNA	mitochondrial DNA
mtRNA	mitochondrial RNA
mTOR	mammalian target of rapamycin
MTP	metatarsophalangeal [joint]
MTX	methotrexate
MUA/P	Medically Underserved Area and Population
MVO_2	myocardial oxygen consumption
MVP	mitral valve prolapse
N*	nucleus
Na^+	sodium ion
NAD	nicotinamide adenine dinucleotide
NAD^+	oxidized nicotinamide adenine dinucleotide
NADH	reduced nicotinamide adenine dinucleotide
$NADP^+$	oxidized nicotinamide adenine dinucleotide phosphate
NADPH	reduced nicotinamide adenine dinucleotide phosphate
NBME	National Board of Medical Examiners
NBOME	National Board of Osteopathic Medical Examiners
NBPME	National Board of Podiatric Medical Examiners
NE	norepinephrine
NF	neurofibromatosis
NFAT	nuclear factor of activated T-cell
NH_3	ammonia
NH_4^+	ammonium
NIDDM	non-insulin-dependent diabetes mellitus
NK	natural killer [cells]
N_M	muscarinic ACh receptor in neuromuscular junction
NMDA	N-methyl-d-aspartate
NMJ	neuromuscular junction
NMS	neuroleptic malignant syndrome
N_N	nicotinic ACh receptor in autonomic ganglia
NRMP	National Residency Matching Program
NNRTI	non-nucleoside reverse transcriptase inhibitor
NO	nitric oxide
N_2O	nitrous oxide
NPH	neutral protamine Hagedorn, normal pressure hydrocephalus
NPV	negative predictive value
NRI	norepinephrine receptor inhibitor
NRTI	nucleoside reverse transcriptase inhibitor
NSAID	nonsteroidal anti-inflammatory drug
NSE	neuron-specific enolase
NSTEMI	non–ST-segment elevation myocardial infarction
Nu*	nucleolus
OAA	oxaloacetic acid
OCD	obsessive-compulsive disorder
OCP	oral contraceptive pill
OH	hydroxy
OH_2	dihydroxy
1,25-OH D_3	calcitriol (active form of vitamin D)
25-OH D_3	storage form of vitamin D
3' OH	hydroxyl

ABBREVIATION	MEANING
OMT	osteopathic manipulative technique
OPV	oral polio vaccine
OR	odds ratio
OS	opening snap
OTC	ornithine transcarbamoylase
OVLT	organum vasculosum of the lamina terminalis
P-body	processing body (cytoplasmic)
P-450	cytochrome P-450 family of enzymes
PA	posteroanterior, pulmonary artery
PABA	para-aminobenzoic acid
$Paco_2$	arterial Pco_2
$PAco_2$	alveolar Pco_2
PAH	para-aminohippuric acid
PAN	polyarteritis nodosa
Pao_2	partial pressure of oxygen in arterial blood
Pao_2	partial pressure of oxygen in alveolar blood
PAP	Papanicolaou [smear], prostatic acid phosphatase
PAPPA	pregnancy-associated plasma protein A
PAS	periodic acid–Schiff
Pat*	patella
PBP	penicillin-binding protein
PC	plasma colloid osmotic pressure, platelet count, pyruvate carboxylase
PCA	posterior cerebral artery
PCC	prothrombin complex concentrate
PCL	posterior cruciate ligament
Pco_2	partial pressure of carbon dioxide
PCom	posterior communicating [artery]
PCOS	polycystic ovarian syndrome
PCP	phencyclidine hydrochloride, Pneumocystis jirovecii pneumonia
PCR	polymerase chain reaction
PCT	proximal convoluted tubule
PCWP	pulmonary capillary wedge pressure
PD	posterior descending [artery]
PDA	patent ductus arteriosus, posterior descending artery
PDC	pyruvate dehydrogenase complex
PDE	phosphodiesterase
PDGF	platelet-derived growth factor
PDH	pyruvate dehydrogenase
PE	pulmonary embolism
PECAM	platelet–endothelial cell adhesion molecule
$Peco_2$	expired air Pco_2
PEP	phosphoenolpyruvate
PF	platelet factor
PFK	phosphofructokinase
PFT	pulmonary function test
PG	phosphoglycerate
P_i	plasma interstitial osmotic pressure, inorganic phosphate
PICA	posterior inferior cerebellar artery
PID	pelvic inflammatory disease
Pio_2	Po_2 in inspired air
PIP	proximal interphalangeal [joint]
PIP_2	phosphatidylinositol 4,5-bisphosphate

*Image abbreviation only

ABBREVIATION	MEANING
PIP_3	phosphatidylinositol 3,4,5-bisphosphate
PKD	polycystic kidney disease
PKR	interferon-α–induced protein kinase
PKU	phenylketonuria
PLP	pyridoxal phosphate
PLS	Personalized Learning System
PML	progressive multifocal leukoencephalopathy
PMN	polymorphonuclear [leukocyte]
P_{net}	net filtration pressure
PNET	primitive neuroectodermal tumor
PNS	peripheral nervous system
Po_2	partial pressure of oxygen
PO_4	salt of phosphoric acid
PO_4^{3-}	phosphate
Pop*	popliteal artery
Pop a*	popliteal artery
Post*	posterior
PPAR	peroxisome proliferator-activated receptor
PPD	purified protein derivative
PPI	proton pump inhibitor
PPV	positive predictive value
PR3-ANCA/ c-ANCA	cytoplasmic antineutrophil cytoplasmic antibody
PrP	prion protein
PRPP	phosphoribosylpyrophosphate
PSA	prostate-specific antigen
PSS	progressive systemic sclerosis
PT	prothrombin time
PTH	parathyroid hormone
PTHrP	parathyroid hormone–related protein
PTSD	post-traumatic stress disorder
PTT	partial thromboplastin time
PV	plasma volume, venous pressure
Pv*	pulmonary vein
PVC	polyvinyl chloride
PVR	pulmonary vascular resistance
R	correlation coefficient, right, R variable [group]
R_3	Registration, Ranking, & Results [system]
RA	right atrium
RAAS	renin-angiotensin-aldosterone system
RANK-L	receptor activator of nuclear factor-κ B ligand
RAS	reticular activating system
RBF	renal blood flow
RCA	right coronary artery
REM	rapid eye movement
RER	rough endoplasmic reticulum
Rh	*rhesus* antigen
RLL*	right lower lobe (of lungs)
RLQ	right lower quadrant
RML*	right middle lobe (of lung)
RNA	ribonucleic acid
RNP	ribonucleoprotein
ROS	reactive oxygen species
RPF	renal plasma flow

ABBREVIATION	MEANING
RPGN	rapidly progressive glomerulonephritis
RPR	rapid plasma reagin
RR	relative risk, respiratory rate
rRNA	ribosomal ribonucleic acid
RS	Reed-Sternberg [cells]
RSC*	right subclavian artery
RSV	respiratory syncytial virus
RTA	renal tubular acidosis
RUL*	right upper lobe (of lung)
RUQ	right upper quadrant
RV	residual volume, right ventricle, right ventricular
RVH	right ventricular hypertrophy
[S]	substrate concentration
SA	sinoatrial
SAA	serum amyloid–associated [protein]
SAM	S-adenosylmethionine
SARS	severe acute respiratory syndrome
SC	subcutaneous
SCC	squamous cell carcinoma
SCD	sudden cardiac death
SCID	severe combined immunodeficiency disease
SCJ	squamocolumnar junction
SCM	sternocleidomastoid muscle
SCN	suprachiasmatic nucleus
SD	standard deviation
SE	standard error of the mean
SEP	Spoken English Proficiency
SER	smooth endoplasmic reticulum
SERM	selective estrogen receptor modulator
SGLT	sodium-glucose transporter
SHBG	sex hormone–binding globulin
SIADH	syndrome of inappropriate [secretion of] antidiuretic hormone
SIDS	sudden infant death syndrome
SLE	systemic lupus erythematosus
SLL	small lymphocytic lymphoma
SLT	Shiga-like toxin
SMA	superior mesenteric artery
SMX	sulfamethoxazole
SNARE	soluble NSF attachment protein receptor
SNc	substantia nigra pars compacta
SNP	single nucleotide polymorphism
SNr	substantia nigra pars reticulata
SNRI	serotonin and norepinephrine receptor inhibitor
snRNP	small nuclear ribonucleoprotein
SO	superior oblique [muscle]
SOAP	Supplemental Offer and Acceptance Program
Sp*	spleen
spp	species
SR	superior rectus [muscle]
SS	single stranded
ssDNA	single-stranded deoxyribonucleic acid
SSPE	subacute sclerosing panencephalitis
SSRI	selective serotonin reuptake inhibitor

*Image abbreviation only

ABBREVIATION	MEANING
ssRNA	single-stranded ribonucleic acid
St*	stomach
ST	Shiga toxin
StAR	steroidogenic acute regulatory protein
STEMI	ST-segment elevation myocardial infarction
STI	sexually transmitted infection
STN	subthalamic nucleus
SV	splenic vein, stroke volume
SVC	superior vena cava
SVT	supraventricular tachycardia
T*	trachea
$t_{1/2}$	half-life
T_3	triiodothyronine
T_4	thyroxine
TAPVR	total anomalous pulmonary venous return
TB	tuberculosis
TBG	thyroxine-binding globulin
3TC	dideoxythiacytidine [lamivudine]
TCA	tricarboxylic acid [cycle], tricyclic antidepressant
Tc cell	cytotoxic T cell
TCR	T-cell receptor
TDF	tenofovir disoproxil fumarate
TdT	terminal deoxynucleotidyl transferase
TE	tracheoesophageal
TFT	thyroid function test
TG	triglyceride
TGA	*trans*-Golgi apparatus
TGF	transforming growth factor
TGN	*trans*-Golgi network
Th cell	helper T cell
THF	tetrahydrofolic acid
TI	therapeutic index
TIA	transient ischemic attack
Tib*	tibia
TIBC	total iron-binding capacity
TIPS	transjugular intrahepatic portosystemic shunt
TLC	total lung capacity
T_m	maximum rate of transport
TMP	trimethoprim
TN	true negative
TNF	tumor necrosis factor
TNM	tumor, node, metastases [staging]
TOP	topoisomerase
ToRCHeS	*Toxoplasma gondii*, rubella, CMV, HIV, HSV-2, syphilis
TP	true positive
tPA	tissue plasminogen activator
TPO	thyroid peroxidase, thrombopoietin
TPP	thiamine pyrophosphate
TPR	total peripheral resistance
TR	tricuspid regurgitation
TRAP	tartrate-resistant acid phosphatase

ABBREVIATION	MEANING
TRH	thyrotropin-releasing hormone
tRNA	transfer ribonucleic acid
TSH	thyroid-stimulating hormone
TSI	triple sugar iron
TSS	toxic shock syndrome
TSST	toxic shock syndrome toxin
TTP	thrombotic thrombocytopenic purpura
TTR	transthyretin
TV	tidal volume
Tx	translation [factor]
TXA_2	thromboxane A_2
UDP	uridine diphosphate
UMN	upper motor neuron
UMP	uridine monophosphate
UPD	uniparental disomy
URI	upper respiratory infection
USMLE	United States Medical Licensing Examination
UTI	urinary tract infection
UTP	uridine triphosphate
UV	ultraviolet
$\dot{V}_1, \dot{V}_2$	Vasopressin receptors
VC	vital capacity
V_d	volume of distribution
VD	physiologic dead space
V(D)J	heavy-chain hypervariable region [antibody]
VDRL	Venereal Disease Research Laboratory
VEGF	vascular endothelial growth factor
V_H	variable region, heavy chain [antibody]
VHL	von Hippel-Lindau [disease]
VIP	vasoactive intestinal peptide
VIPoma	vasoactive intestinal polypeptide-secreting tumor
VJ	light-chain hypervariable region [antibody]
VL	ventral lateral [nucleus]; variable region, light chain [antibody]
VLDL	very low density lipoprotein
VMA	vanillylmandelic acid
VMAT	vesicular monoamine transporter
V_{max}	maximum velocity
VPL	ventral posterior nucleus, lateral
VPM	ventral posterior nucleus, medial
VPN	vancomycin, polymyxin, nystatin [media]
$\dot{V}/\dot{Q}$	ventilation/perfusion [ratio]
VRE	vancomycin-resistant enterococcus
VSD	ventricular septal defect
V_T	tidal volume
vWF	von Willebrand factor
VZV	varicella-zoster virus
VMAT	vesicular monoamine transporter
XR	X-linked recessive
XX/XY	normal complement of sex chromosomes for female/male
ZDV	zidovudine [formerly AZT]

*Image abbreviation only

Image Acknowledgments

In this edition, in collaboration with MedIQ Learning, LLC, and a variety of other partners, we are pleased to include the following clinical images and diagrams for the benefit of integrative student learning.

Portions of this book identified with the symbol are copyright © USMLE-Rx.com (MedIQ Learning, LLC).

Portions of this book identified with the symbol are copyright © Dr. Richard Usatine and are provided under license through MedIQ Learning, LLC.

Portions of this book identified with the symbol are listed below by page number.

This symbol refers to material that is available in the public domain. The image may have been modified by cropping, labeling, and/or captions. All rights to this adaptation by MedIQ Learning, LLC are reserved.

This symbol refers to the Creative Commons Attribution license, full text at http://creativecommons.org/licenses/by/4.0/legalcode. The image may have been modified by cropping, labeling, and/or captions. All rights to this adaptation by MedIQ Learning, LLC are reserved.

This symbol refers to the Creative Commons Attribution-Share Alike license, full text at: http://creativecommons.org/licenses/by-sa/4.0/legalcode.

Biochemistry

34 **Chromatin structure.** Electron micrograph showing heterochromatin, euchromatin, and nucleolus. This image is a derivative work, adapted from the following source, available under . Courtesy of Roller RA, Rickett JD, Stickle WB. The hypobranchial gland of the estuarine snail *Stramonita haemastoma caniculata* (Gray) (Prosobranchia: Muricidae): a light and electron microscopical study. *Am Malac Bull.* 1995;11(2):177–190. Available at https://archive.org/details/americanm101119931994amer.

49 **Cilia structure: Image A.** Courtesy of Louisa Howard and Michael Binder. The image may have been modified by cropping, labeling, and/or captions. All rights to this adaptation by MedIQ Learning, LLC are reserved.

49 **Cilia structure: Image B.** Cilia structure of basal body. This image is a derivative work, adapted from the following source, available under : Riparbelli MG, Cabrera OA, Callaini G, et al. Unique properties of Drosophila spermatocyte primary cilia. *Biol Open.* 2013 Nov;15;2(11):1137–1147. DOI: 10.1242/bio.20135355.

49 **Cilia structure: Image C.** Dextrocardia. This image is a derivative work, adapted from the following source, available under : Oluwadare O, Ayoka AO, Akomolafe RO, et al. The role of electrocardiogram in the diagnosis of dextrocardia with mirror image atrial arrangement and ventricular position in a young adult Nigerian in Ile-Ife: a case report. *J Med Case Rep.* 2015;9:222. DOI: 10.1186/s13256-015-0695-4.

51 **Osteogenesis imperfecta: Image A.** Skeletal deformities in lower body of child. This image is a derivative work, adapted from the following source, available under : Vanakker OM, Hemelsoet D, De Paepe. Hereditary connective tissue diseases in young adult stroke: a comprehensive synthesis. *Stroke Res Treat.* 2011;712903. DOI: 10.4061/2011/712903. The image may have been modified by cropping, labeling, and/or captions. All rights to this adaptation by MedIQ Learning, LLC are reserved.

51 **Osteogenesis imperfecta: Image B.** Skeletal deformities in upper extremity of child. This image is a derivative work, adapted from the following source, available under : Vanakker OM, Hemelsoet D, De Paepe. Hereditary connective tissue diseases in young adult stroke: a comprehensive synthesis. *Stroke Res Treat.* 2011;712903. DOI: 10.4061/2011/712903. The image may have been modified by cropping, labeling, and/or captions. All rights to this adaptation by MedIQ Learning, LLC are reserved.

51 **Osteogenesis imperfects: Image C.** Blue sclera. This image is a derivative work, adapted from the following source, available under : Wheatley K et al. *J Clin Med Res.* 2010;2(4):198–200. DOI: 10.4021/jocmr369w.

51 **Ehlers-Danlos syndrome: Images A and B.** Hyperextensibility of skin and DIP joint hyperextensibility. This image is a derivative work, adapted from the following source, available under : Whitaker JK et al. *BMC Ophthalmol.* 2012;2:47. DOI: 10.1186/1471-2415-12-47.

55 **Karyotyping.** This image is a derivative work, adapted from the following source, available under : Paar C, Herber G, Voskova, et al. A case of acute myeloid leukemia (AML) with an unreported combination of chromosomal abnormalities: gain of isochromosome 5p, tetrasomy 8 and unbalanced translocation der(19)t(17;19)(q23;p13). *Mol Cytogenet.* 2013;6:40. DOI: 10.1186/1755-8166-6-40.

55 **Fluorescence in situ hybridization.** This image is a derivative work, adapted from the following source, available under : Paar C, Herber G, Voskova, et al. A case of acute myeloid leukemia (AML) with an unreported combination of chromosomal abnormalities: gain of isochromosome 5p, tetrasomy 8 and unbalanced translocation der(19)t(17;19)(q23;p13). *Mol Cytogenet.* 2013;6:40. DOI: 10.1186/1755-8166-6-40.

57 **Genetic terms.** Café-au-lait spots. This image is a derivative work, adapted from the following source, available under : Dumitrescu CE and Collins MT. *Orphanet J Rare Dis.* 2008;3:12. DOI: 10.1186/1750-1172-3-12.

61 **Muscular dystrophies.** Fibrofatty replacement of muscle. Courtesy of the US Department of Health and Human Services and Dr. Edwin P. Ewing, Jr. The image may have been modified by cropping, labeling, and/or captions. All rights to this adaptation by MedIQ Learning, LLC are reserved.

66 **Vitamin A.** Bitot spots on conjunctiva. This image is a derivative work, adapted from the following source, available under : Baiyeroju A, Bowman R, Gilbert C, et al. Managing eye health in young children. *Comm Eye Health.* 2010;23(72):4–11. Available at https://www.ncbi.nlm.nih.gov/pmc/articles/PMC2873666/.

67 **Vitamin B$_3$.** Pellagra.This image is a derivative work, adapted from the following source, available under : van Dijk HA, Fred H. Images of memorable cases: case 2. Connexions Web site. Dec 4, 2008. Available at: http://cnx.org/contents/3d3dcb2e-8e98-496f-91c2-fe94e93428a1@3@3/.

70 **Vitamin D.** X-ray of lower extremity in child with rickets. This image is a derivative work, adapted from the following source, available under . Courtesy of Dr. Michael L. Richardson. The image may have been modified by cropping, labeling, and/or captions. MedIQ Learning, LLC makes this image available under .

71 **Malnutrition: Image A.** Child with kwashiorkor. Courtesy of the US Department of Health and Human Services and Dr. Lyle Conrad.

71 **Malnutrition: Image B.** Child with marasmus. Courtesy of the US Department of Health and Human Services.

84 **Alkaptonuria.** Pigment granules on dorsum of hand. This image is a derivative work, adapted from the following source, available under : Vasudevan B, Sawhney MPS, Radhakrishnan S. Alkaptonuria associated with degenerative collagenous palmar plaques. *Indian J Dermatol.* 2009;54:299–301. DOI: 10.4103/0019-5154.55650.

85 **Cystinuria.** Hexagonal stones in urine. This image is a derivative work, adapted from the following source, available under : Courtesy of Cayla Devine.

88 **Lysosomal storage diseases: Image A.** "Cherry-red" spot on macula in Tay-Sachs disease. This image is a derivative work, adapted from the following source, available under : Courtesy of Dr. Jonathan Trobe.

88 **Lysosomal storage diseases: Image B.** Angiokeratomas. This image is a derivative work, adapted from the following source, available under : Burlina AP, Sims KB, Politei JM, et al. Early diagnosis of peripheral nervous system involvement in Fabry disease and treatment of neuropathic pain: the report of an expert panel. *BMC Neurol.* 2011;11:61. DOI: 10.1186/1471-2377-11-61. The image may have been modified by cropping, labeling, and/or captions. All rights to this adaptation by MedIQ Learning, LLC are reserved.

88 **Lysosomal storage diseases: Image C.** Gaucher cells in Gaucher disease. This image is a derivative work, adapted from the following source, available under : Sokołowska B, Skomra D, Czartoryska B, et al. Gaucher disease diagnosed after bone marrow trephine biopsy—a report of two cases. *Folia Histochem Cytobiol.* 2011;49:352–356. DOI: 10.5603/FHC.2011.0048. The image may have been modified by cropping, labeling, and/or captions. All rights to this adaptation by MedIQ Learning, LLC are reserved.

88 **Lysosomal storage diseases: Image D.** Foam cells in Niemann-Pick disease. This image is a derivative work, adapted from the following source, available under : Prieto-Potin I, Roman-Blas JA, Martinez-Calatrava MJ, et al. Hypercholesterolemia boosts joint destruction in chronic arthritis. An experimental model aggravated by foam macrophage infiltration. *Arthritis Res Ther.* 2013;15:R81. DOI: 10.1186/ar4261.

Immunology

98 **Spleen.** Red and white pulp. This image is a derivative work, adapted from the following source, available under : Heinrichs S, Conover LF, Bueso-Ramos CE, et al. MYBL2 is a sub-haploinsufficient tumor suppressor gene in myeloid malignancy. *eLife.* 2013;2:e00825. DOI: 10.7554/*eLife*.00825. The image may have been modified by cropping, labeling, and/or captions. All rights to this adaptation by MedIQ Learning, LLC are reserved.

98 **Thymus: Image A.** Hassall corpuscles. This image is a derivative work, adapted from the following source, available under : Minato H, Kinoshita E, Nakada S, et al. Thymic lymphoid hyperplasia with multilocular thymic cysts diagnosed before the Sjögren syndrome diagnosis. *Diagn Pathol.* 2015;10:103. DOI: 10.1186/s13000-015-0332-y.

98 **Thymus: Image B.** "Sail sign" on x-ray of normal thymus in neonate. This image is a derivative work, adapted from the following source, available under : Di Serafino M, Esposito F, Severino R, et al. Think thymus, think well: the chest x-ray thymic signs. *J Pediatr Moth Care.* 2016;1(2):108–109. DOI: 10.19104/japm.2016.108.

117 **Immunodeficiencies: Image A.** Spider angioma (telangiectasia). This image is a derivative work, adapted from the following source, available under : Liapakis IE, Englander M, Sinani R, et al. Management of facial telangiectasias with hand cautery. *World J Plast Surg.* 2015 Jul;4(2):127–133.

117 **Immunodeficiencies: Image B.** Giant granules in granulocytes in Chédiak-Higashi syndrome. This image is a derivative work, adapted from the following source, available under : Bharti S, Bhatia P, Bansal D, et al. The accelerated phase of Chediak-Higashi syndrome: the importance of hematological evaluation. *Turk J Haematol.* 2013;30:85–87. DOI: 10.4274/tjh.2012.0027. The image may have been modified by cropping, labeling, and/or captions. All rights to this adaptation by MedIQ Learning, LLC are reserved.

Microbiology

126 **Stains: Image A.** *Trypanosoma lewisi* on Giemsa stain. Courtesy of the US Department of Health and Human Services and Dr. Mae Melvin.

126 **Stains: Image B.** *Tropheryma whipplei* on periodic acid–Schiff stain. This image is a derivative work, adapted from the following source, available under : Courtesy of Dr. Ed Uthman.

126 **Stains: Image C.** *Mycobacterium tuberculosis* on Ziehl-Neelsen stain. Courtesy of the US Department of Health and Human Services and Dr. George P. Kubica.

126 **Stains: Image D.** *Cryptococcus neoformans* on India ink stain. Courtesy of the US Department of Health and Human Services.

126 Stains: Image E. *Coccidioides immitis* on silver stain. Courtesy of the US Department of Health and Human Services and Dr. Edwin P. Ewing, Jr.

128 Encapsulated bacteria. Capsular swelling of *Streptococcus pneumoniae* using the Neufeld-Quellung test. Courtesy of the US Department of Health and Human Services.

128 Catalase-positive organisms. Oxygen bubbles released during catalase reaction. This image is a derivative work, adapted from the following source, available under . Courtesy of Stefano Nase. The image may have been modified by cropping, labeling, and/or captions. MedIQ Learning, LLC makes this image available under .

131 Bacterial spores. This image is a derivative work, adapted from the following source, available under : Jones SW, Paredes CJ, Tracy B. The transcriptional program underlying the physiology of clostridial sporulation. *Genome Biol.* 2008;9:R114. DOI: 10.1186/gb-2008-9-7-r114.

135 α-hemolytic bacteria. α-hemolysis. This image is a derivative work, adapted from the following source, available under . Courtesy of Y. Tambe. The image may have been modified by cropping, labeling, and/or captions. MedIQ Learning, LLC makes this image available under .

135 β-hemolytic bacteria. β-hemolysis. This image is a derivative work, adapted from the following source, available under . Courtesy of Y. Tambe. The image may have been modified by cropping, labeling, and/or captions. MedIQ Learning, LLC makes this image available under .

135 *Staphylococcus aureus*. Courtesy of the US Department of Health and Human Services and Dr. Richard Facklam.

136 *Streptococcus pneumoniae*. Courtesy of the US Department of Health and Human Services and Dr. Mike Miller.

136 *Streptococcus pyogenes* (group A streptococci). Gram stain. This image is a derivative work, adapted from the following source, available under . Courtesy of Y. Tambe. The image may have been modified by cropping, labeling, and/or captions. MedIQ Learning, LLC makes this image available under .

137 *Bacillus anthracis*. Ulcer with black eschar. Courtesy of the US Department of Health and Human Services and James H. Steele.

138 Clostridia (with exotoxins): Image A. Gas gangrene due to *Clostridium perfringens* infection. This image is a derivative work, adapted from the following source, available under : Schröpfer E, Rauthe S, Meyer T. Diagnosis and misdiagnosis of necrotizing soft tissue infections: three case reports. *Cases J.* 2008;1:252. DOI: 10.1186/1757-1626-1-252.

138 Clostridia (with exotoxins): Image B. Pseudomembranous enterocolitis on colonoscopy. This image is a derivative work, adapted from the following source, available under . Courtesy of Klinikum Dritter Orden für die Überlassung des Bildes zur Veröffentlichu. The image may have been modified by cropping, labeling, and/or captions. MedIQ Learning, LLC makes this image available under .

139 *Corynebacterium diphtheriae*. Pseudomembranous pharyngitis. This image is a derivative work, adapted from the following source, available under . Courtesy of Wikimedia Commons. The image may have been modified by cropping, labeling, and/or captions. MedIQ Learning, LLC makes this image available under .

139 *Listeria monocytogenes*. Actin rockets. This image is a derivative work, adapted from the following source, available under : Schuppler M, Loessner MJ. The opportunistic pathogen *Listeria monocytogenes*: pathogenicity and interaction with the mucosal immune system. *Int J Inflamm.* 2010;2010:704321. DOI: 10.4061/2010/704321. The image may have been modified by cropping, labeling, and/or captions. All rights to this adaptation by MedIQ Learning, LLC are reserved.

139 *Nocardia* vs *Actinomyces*: Image A. *Nocardia* on acid-fast stain. This image is a derivative work, adapted from the following source, available under : Venkataramana K. Human *Nocardia* infections: a review of pulmonary nocardiosis. *Cereus.* 2015;7(8):e304. DOI: 10.7759/cureus.304.

139 *Nocardia* vs *Actinomyces*: Image B. *Actinomyces israelii* on Gram stain. Courtesy of the US Department of Health and Human Services.

140 Mycobacteria. Acid-fast stain. Courtesy of the US Department of Health and Human Services and Dr. Edwin P. Ewing, Jr.

140 Tuberculosis. Langhans giant cell in caseating granuloma. Courtesy of J. Hayman.

141 Leprosy (Hansen disease): Image A. "Glove and stocking" distribution. This image is a derivative work, adapted from the following source, available under : Courtesy of Bruno Jehle.

142 *Neisseria*: Image A. Intracellular *N gonorrhoeae*. Courtesy of the US Department of Health and Human Services and Dr. Mike Miller.

142 *Haemophilus influenzae*: Image A. Epiglottitis. This image is a derivative work, adapted from the following source, available under : Courtesy of Wikimedia Commons. The image may have been modified by cropping, labeling, and/or captions. All rights to this adaptation by MedIQ Learning, LLC are reserved.

143 *Legionella pneumophila*. Lung findings of unilateral and lobar infiltrate. This image is a derivative work, adapted from the following source, available under : Robbins NM, Kumar A, Blair BM. *Legionella pneumophila* infection presenting as headache, confusion and dysarthria in a human immunodeficiency virus-1 (HIV-1) positive patient: case report. *BMC Infect Dis.* 2012;12:225. DOI: 10.1186/1471-2334-12-225.

143 *Pseudomonas aeruginosa*: Image A. Blue-green pigment on centrimide agar. This image is a derivative work, adapted from the following source, available under . Courtesy of Hansen. The image may have been modified by cropping, labeling, and/or captions. MedIQ Learning, LLC makes this image available under .

143 *Pseudomonas aeruginosa*: Image B. Ecthyma gangrenosum. This image is a derivative work, adapted from the following source, available under : Uludokumaci S, Balkan II, Mete B, et al. Ecthyma gangrenosum-like lesions in a febrile neutropenic patient with simultaneous *Pseudomonas* sepsis and disseminated fusariosis. *Turk J Haematol.* 2013 Sep;30(3):321–324. DOI: 10.4274/Tjh.2012.0030.

145 *Klebsiella*. Courtesy of the US Department of Health and Human Services.

145 *Campylobacter jejuni.* ⬛ Courtesy of the US Department of Health and Human Services.

146 *Vibrio cholerae.* This image is a derivative work, adapted from the following source, available under ⬛: Phetsouvanh R, Nakatsu M, Arakawa E, et al. Fatal bacteremia due to immotile *Vibrio cholerae* serogroup O21 in Vientiane, Laos—a case report. *Ann Clin Microbiol Antimicrob.* 2008;7:10. DOI: 10.1186/1476-0711-7-10.

146 *Helicobacter pylori.* ⬛ Courtesy of the US Department of Health and Human Services, Dr. Patricia Fields, and Dr. Collette Fitzgerald.

146 **Spirochetes.** Appearance on dark field microscopy. ⬛ Courtesy of the US Department of Health and Human Services.

146 **Lyme disease: Image A.** *Ixodes* tick. ⬛ Courtesy of the US Department of Health and Human Services and Dr. Michael L. Levin.

146 **Lyme disease: Image B.** Erythema migrans. ⬛ Courtesy of the US Department of Health and Human Services and James Gathany.

147 **Syphilis: Image A.** Painless chancre in 1° syphilis. ⬛ Courtesy of the US Department of Health and Human Services and M. Rein.

147 **Syphilis: Image B.** Treponeme on dark-field microscopy. ⬛ Courtesy of the US Department of Health and Human Services and Renelle Woodall.

147 **Syphilis: Image D.** Rash on palms. This image is a derivative work, adapted from the following source, available under ⬛: Drahansky M, Dolezel M, Urbanek J, et al. Influence of skin diseases on fingerprint recognition. *J Biomed Biotechnol.* 2012;626148. DOI: 10.1155/2012/626148.

147 **Syphilis: Image E.** Condyloma lata. ⬛ Courtesy of the US Department of Health and Human Services and Susan Lindsley.

147 **Syphilis: Image F.** Gumma. This image is a derivative work, adapted from the following source, available under ⬛: Chakir K, Benchikhi H. Granulome centro-facial révélant une syphilis tertiaire. *Pan Afr Med J.* 2013;15:82. DOI: 10.11604/pamj.2013.15.82.3011.

147 **Syphilis: Image G.** Congenital syphilis. ⬛ Courtesy of the US Department of Health and Human Services and Dr. Norman Cole.

147 **Syphilis: Image H.** Hutchinson teeth. ⬛ Courtesy of the US Department of Health and Human Services and Susan Lindsley.

148 *Gardnerella vaginalis.* ⬛ Courtesy of the US Department of Health and Human Services and M. Rein.

150 **Rickettsial diseases and vector-borne illnesses: Image A.** Rash of Rocky Mountain spotted fever. ⬛ Courtesy of the US Department of Health and Human Services.

150 **Rickettsial diseases and vector-borne illnesses: Image B.** *Ehrlichia* morulae. This image is a derivative work, adapted from the following source, available under ⬛: Dantas-Torres F. Canine vector-borne diseases in Brazil. *Parasit Vectors.* 2008;1:25. DOI: 10.1186/1756-3305-1-25. The image may have been modified by cropping, labeling, and/or captions. All rights to this adaptation by MedIQ Learning, LLC are reserved.

150 **Rickettsial diseases and vector-borne illnesses: Image C.** *Anaplasma phagocytophilium* in neutrophil. ⬛ Courtesy of the US Department of Health and Human Services and Dumler JS, Choi K, Garcia-Garcia JC, et al. Human granulocytic anaplasmosis. *Emerg Infect Dis.* 2005. DOI: 10.3201/eid1112.050898.

150 *Mycoplasma pneumoniae.* This image is a derivative work, adapted from the following source, available under ⬛: Rottem S, Kosower ND, Kornspan JD. Contamination of tissue cultures by *Mycoplasma.* In: Ceccherini-Nelli L, ed: Biomedical tissue culture. 2016. DOI: 10.5772/51518.

151 **Systemic mycoses: Image A.** *Histoplasma.* ⬛ Courtesy of the US Department of Health and Human Services and Dr. D.T. McClenan.

151 **Systemic mycoses: Image B.** *Blastomyces dermatitidis* undergoing broad-base budding. ⬛ Courtesy of the US Department of Health and Human Services and Dr. Libero Ajello.

151 **Systemic mycoses: Image C.** Coccidiomycosis with endospheres. ⬛ Courtesy of the US Department of Health and Human Services.

151 **Systemic mycoses: Image D.** "Captain's wheel" shape of *Paracoccidioides.* ⬛ Courtesy of the US Department of Health and Human Services and Dr. Lucille K. Georg.

152 **Cutaneous mycoses: Image G.** Tinea versicolor. This image is a derivative work, adapted from the following source, available under ⬛. Courtesy of Sarah (Rosenau) Korf. The image may have been modified by cropping, labeling, and/or captions. MedIQ Learning, LLC makes this image available under ⬛.

153 **Opportunistic fungal infections: Image A.** Budding yeast of *Candida albicans.* This image is a derivative work, adapted from the following source, available under ⬛. Courtesy of Y. Tambe. The image may have been modified by cropping, labeling, and/or captions. MedIQ Learning, LLC makes this image available under ⬛.

153 **Opportunistic fungal infections: Image B.** Germ tubes of *Candida albicans.* This image is a derivative work, adapted from the following source, available under ⬛. Courtesy of Y. Tambe. The image may have been modified by cropping, labeling, and/or captions. MedIQ Learning, LLC makes this image available under ⬛.

153 **Opportunistic fungal infections: Image C.** Oral thrush. ⬛ Courtesy of the US Department of Health and Human Services and Dr. Sol Silverman, Jr.

153 **Opportunistic fungal infections: Image E.** Conidiophores of *Aspergillus fumigatus.* ⬛ Courtesy of the US Department of Health and Human Services.

153 **Opportunistic fungal infections: Image F.** Aspergilloma in left lung. This image is a derivative work, adapted from the following source, available under ⬛: Souilamas R, Souilamas JI, Alkhamees K, et al. Extra corporal membrane oxygenation in general thoracic surgery: a new single veno-venous cannulation. *J Cardiothorac Surg.* 2011;6:52. DOI: 10.1186/1749-8090-6-52.

153 **Opportunistic fungal infections: Image G.** *Cryptococcus neoformans* on India ink stain. ⬛ Courtesy of the US Department of Health and Human Services and Dr. Leanor Haley.

153 **Opportunistic fungal infections: Image H.** *Cryptococcus neoformans* on mucicarmine stain. Courtesy of the US Department of Health and Human Services and Dr. Leanor Haley.

153 **Opportunistic fungal infections: Image I.** Mucor. Courtesy of the US Department of Health and Human Services and Dr. Lucille K. Georg.

154 *Pneumocystis jirovecii:* **Image A.** Interstitial opacities in lung. This image is a derivative work, adapted from the following source, available under : Chuang C, Zhanhong X, Yinyin G, et al. Unsuspected *Pneumocystis* pneumonia in an HIV-seronegative patient with untreated lung cancer: circa case report. *J Med Case Rep.* 2007;1:15. DOI: 10.1186/1752-1947-1-115.

154 *Pneumocystis jirovecii:* **Image B.** This image is a derivative work, adapted from the following source, available under : Allen CM, Al-Jahdali HH, Irion KL, et al. Imaging lung manifestations of HIV/AIDS. *Ann Thorac Med.* 2010 Oct-Dec;5(4):201–216. DOI: 10.4103/1817-1737.69106.

154 *Pneumocystis jiroveci:* **Image C.** Disc-shaped yeast. This image is a derivative work, adapted from the following source, available under : Kirby S, Satoskar A, Brodsky S, et al. Histological spectrum of pulmonary manifestations in kidney transplant recipients on sirolimus inclusive immunosuppressive regimens. *Diagn Pathol.* 2012;7:25. DOI: 10.1186/1746-1596-7-25.

154 *Sporothrix schenckii.* Subcutaneous mycosis. This image is a derivative work, adapted from the following source, available under : Govender NP, Maphanga TG, Zulu TG, et al. An outbreak of lymphocutaneous sporotrichosis among mineworkers in South Africa. *PLoS Negl Trop Dis.* 2015 Sep;9(9): e0004096. DOI: 10.1371/journal.pntd.0004096.

155 **Protozoa—GI infections: Image A.** *Giardia lamblia* trophozoite. This image is a derivative work, adapted from the following source, available under : Lipoldová M. *Giardia* and Vilém Dušan Lambl. *PLoS Negl Trop Dis.* 2014;8:e2686. DOI: 10.1371/journal.pntd.0002686.

155 **Protozoa—GI infections: Image B.** *Giardia lamblia* cyst. Courtesy of the US Department of Health and Human Services.

155 **Protozoa—GI infections: Image C.** *Entamoeba histolytica* trophozoites. Courtesy of the US Department of Health and Human Services.

155 **Protozoa—GI infections. Image D.** *Entamoeba histolytica* cyst. Courtesy of the US Department of Health and Human Services.

155 **Protozoa—GI infections: Image E.** *Cryptosporidium* oocysts. Courtesy of the US Department of Health and Human Services.

156 **Protozoa—CNS infections: Image A.** Ring-enhancing lesions in *T gondii* infection. This image is a derivative work, adapted from the following source, available under : Agrawal A, Bhake A, Sangole VM, et al. Multiple-ring enhancing lesions in an immunocompetent adult. *J Glob Infect Dis.* 2010 Sep-Dec;2(3):313–324. DOI: 10.4103/0974-777X.68545.

156 **Protozoa—CNS infections: Image B.** *Toxoplasma gondii* tachyzoite. Courtesy of the US Department of Health and Human Services and Dr. L.L. Moore, Jr.

156 **Protozoa—CNS infections: Image C.** *Naegleria fowleri* amoebas. Courtesy of the US Department of Health and Human Services.

156 **Protozoa—CNS infections: Image D.** *Trypanosoma brucei gambiense.* Courtesy of the US Department of Health and Human Services and Dr. Mae Melvin.

157 **Protozoa—hematologic infections: Image A.** *Plasmodium* trophozoite ring form. Courtesy of the US Department of Health and Human Services.

157 **Protozoa—hematologic infections: Image B.** *Plasmodium* schizont containing merozoites. Courtesy of the US Department of Health and Human Services and Steven Glenn.

157 **Protozoa—hematologic infections: Image C.** *Babesia.* Courtesy of the US Department of Health and Human Services.

158 **Protozoa—others: Image A.** Trypanosoma cruzi. Courtesy of the US Department of Health and Human Services and Dr. Mae Melvin.

158 **Protozoa—others: Image B.** *Leishmania donovani.* Courtesy of the US Department of Health and Human Services and Dr. Francis W. Chandler. The image may have been modified by cropping, labeling, and/or captions. All rights to this adaptation by MedIQ Learning, LLC are reserved.

158 **Protozoa—others: Image C.** Cutaneous leishmaniasis. This image is a derivative work, adapted from the following source, available under : Sharara SL, Kanj SS. War and infectious diseases: challenges of the Syrian civil war. *PLoS Pathog.* 2014 Nov;10(11):e1004438. DOI: 10.1371/journal.ppat.1004438.

158 **Protozoa—others: Image D.** *Trichomonas vaginalis.* Courtesy of the US Department of Health and Human Services.

159 **Nematodes (roundworms): Image A.** *Enterobius vermicularis* eggs. Courtesy of the US Department of Health and Human Services, BG Partin, and Dr. Moore.

159 **Nematodes (roundworms): Image B.** *Ascaris lumbricoides* egg. Courtesy of the US Department of Health and Human Services.

159 **Nematodes (roundworms): Image C.** Elephantiasis. Courtesy of the US Department of Health and Human Services.

160 **Cestodes (tapeworms): Image A.** *Taenia solium* scolex. Courtesy of the US Department of Health and Human Services Robert J. Galindo. The image may have been modified by cropping, labeling, and/or captions. MedIQ Learning, LLC makes this image available under .

160 **Cestodes (tapeworms): Image B.** Neurocysticercosis. This image is a derivative work, adapted from the following source, available under : Coyle CM, Tanowitz HB. Diagnosis and treatment of neurocysticercosis. *Interdiscip Perspect Infect Dis.* 2009;2009:180742. DOI: 10.1155/2009/180742. The image may have been modified by cropping, labeling, and/or captions. All rights to this adaptation by MedIQ Learning, LLC are reserved.

160 **Cestodes (tapeworms): Image C.** *Echinococcus granulosus.* Courtesy of the US Department of Health and Human Services.

160 **Cestodes (tapeworms): Image D.** Hyatid cyst of *Echinococcus granulosus.* Courtesy of the US Department of Health and Human Services and Dr. I. Kagan.

160 **Cestodes (tapeworms): Image E.** *Echinococcus granulosus* cyst in liver. This image is a derivative work, adapted from the following source, available under : Ma Z, Yang W, Yao Y, et al. The adventitia resection in treatment of liver hydatid cyst: a case report of a 15-year-old boy. *Case Rep Surg.* 2014;2014:123149. DOI: 10.1155/2014/123149.

160 Trematodes (flukes): Image A. *Schistosoma mansoni* egg with lateral spine. ⊚▤ Courtesy of the US Department of Health and Human Services.

160 Trematodes (flukes): Image B. *Schistosoma mansoni* egg with terminal spine. ⊚▤ Courtesy of the US Department of Health and Human Services.

161 Ectoparasites: Image A. Scabies. ⊚▤ Courtesy of the US Department of Health and Human Services and J. Pledger.

161 Ectoparasites: Image B. Nit of a louse. ⊚▤ Courtesy of the US Department of Health and Human Services and Joe Miller.

165 Herpesviruses: Image A. Keratoconjunctivitis in HSV-1 infection. This image is a derivative work, adapted from the following source, available under ⊚▤: Yang HK, Han YK, Wee WR, et al. Bilateral herpetic keratitis presenting with unilateral neurotrophic keratitis in pemphigus foliaceus: a case report. *J Med Case Rep.* 2011;5:328. DOI: 10.1186/1752-1947-5-328.

165 Herpesviruses: Image B. Herpes labialis. ⊚▤ Courtesy of the US Department of Health and Human Services and Dr. Herrmann.

165 Herpesviruses: Image E. Shingles (varicella-zoster virus infection). This image is a derivative work, adapted from the following source, available under ⊚▤. Courtesy of Fisle. The image may have been modified by cropping, labeling, and/or captions. MedIQ Learning, LLC makes this image available under ⊚▤.

165 Herpesviruses: Image F. Hepatosplenomegaly due to EBV infection. This image is a derivative work, adapted from the following source, available under ⊚▤: Gow NJ, Davidson RN, Ticehurst R, et al. Case report: no response to liposomal daunorubicin in a patient with drug-resistant HIV-associated visceral leishmaniasis. *PLoS Negl Trop Dis.* 2015 Aug; 9(8):e0003983. DOI: 10.1371/journal.pntd.0003983.

165 Herpesviruses: Image G. Atypical lymphocytes in Epstein-Barr virus infection. This image is a derivative work, adapted from the following source, available under ⊚▤: Courtesy of Dr. Ed Uthman. The image may have been modified by cropping, labeling, and/or captions. All rights to this adaptation by MedIQ Learning, LLC are reserved.

165 Herpesviruses: Image I. Roseola. ⊚▤ Courtesy of Emiliano Burzagli.

165 Herpesvirus: Image J. Kaposi sarcoma. ⊚▤ Courtesy of the US Department of Health and Human Services.

166 HSV identification. Positive Tzanck smear in HSV-2 infection. This image is a derivative work, adapted from the following source, available under ⊚▤. Courtesy of Dr. Yale Rosen. The image may have been modified by cropping, labeling, and/or captions. MedIQ Learning, LLC makes this image available under ⊚▤.

168 Rotavirus. ⊚▤ Courtesy of the US Department of Health and Human Services and Erskine Palmer.

169 Rubella virus. Rubella rash. ⊚▤ Courtesy of the US Department of Health and Human Services.

170 Croup (acute laryngotracheobronchitis). Steeple sign. Reproduced, with permission, from Dr. Frank Gaillard and www.radiopaedia.org.

170 Measles (rubeola) virus: Image A. Koplik spots. ⊚▤ Courtesy of the US Department of Health and Human Services. The image may have been modified by cropping, labeling, and/or captions.

All rights to this adaptation by MedIQ Learning, LLC are reserved.

170 Measles (rubeola) virus: Image B. Rash of measles. ⊚▤ Courtesy of the US Department of Health and Human Services.

170 Mumps virus. Swollen neck and parotid glands. ⊚▤ Courtesy of the US Department of Health and Human Services.

171 Rabies virus: Image A. Transmission electron micrograph. ⊚▤ Courtesy of the US Department of Health and Human Services Dr. Fred Murphy, and Sylvia Whitfield.

171 Rabies virus: Image B. Negri bodies. ⊚▤ Courtesy of the US Department of Health and Human Services and Dr. Daniel P. Perl.

171 Ebola virus. ⊚▤ Courtesy of the US Department of Health and Human Services and Cynthia Goldsmith.

180 Osteomyelitis: Image A. X-ray (left) and MRI (right) views. This image is a derivative work, adapted from the following source, available under ⊚▤: Huang P-Y, Wu P-K, Chen C-F, et al. Osteomyelitis of the femur mimicking bone tumors: a review of 10 cases. *World J Surg Oncol.* 2013;11:283. DOI: 10.1186/1477-7819-11-283.

181 Common vaginal infections: Image C. *Candida* vulvovaginitis. ⊚▤ Courtesy of Mikael Häggström.

182 ToRCHeS infections: Image A. "Blueberry muffin" rash. This image is a derivative work, adapted from the following source, available under ⊚▤: Benmiloud S, Elhaddou G, Belghiti ZA, et al. Blueberry muffin syndrome. *Pan Afr Med J.* 2012;13:23.

182 ToRCHeS infections: Image B. Periventricular calcifications in congenital cytomegalovirus infection. This image is a derivative work, adapted from the following source, available under ⊚▤: Bonthius D, Perlman S. Congenital viral infections of the brain: lessons learned from lymphocytic choriomeningitis virus in the neonatal rat. *PLoS Pathog.* 2007;3:e149. DOI: 10.1371/journal.ppat.0030149. The image may have been modified by cropping, labeling, and/or captions. All rights to this adaptation by MedIQ Learning, LLC are reserved.

183 Red rashes of childhood: Image C. Child with scarlet fever. This image is a derivative work, adapted from the following source, available under ⊚▤: www.badobadop.co.uk.

183 Red rashes of childhood: Image D. Chicken pox. ⊚▤ Courtesy of the US Department of Health and Human Services.

184 Sexually transmitted infections. Donovanosis. ⊚▤ Courtesy of the US Department of Health and Human Services and Dr. Pinozzi.

185 Pelvic inflammatory disease: Image A. Purulent cervical discharge. This image is a derivative work, adapted from the following source, available under ⊚▤. Courtesy of SOS-AIDS Amsterdam. The image may have been modified by cropping, labeling, and/or captions. MedIQ Learning, LLC makes this image available under ⊚▤.

185 Pelvic inflammatory disease: Image B. Adhesions in Fitz-Hugh–Curtis syndrome. ⊚▤ Courtesy of Hic et nunc.

190 Vancomycin. Red man syndrome. This image is a derivative work, adapted from the following source, available under ⊚▤: O'Meara P, Borici-Mazi R, Morton R, et al. DRESS with delayed onset acute interstitial nephritis and profound refractory eosinophilia secondary to vancomycin. *Allergy Asthma Clin Immunol.* 2011;7:16. DOI: 10.1186/1710-1492-7-16.

Pathology

209   **Necrosis: Image A.** Coagulative necrosis. Courtesy of the US Department of Health and Human Services and Dr. Steven Rosenberg.

209   **Necrosis: Image B.** Liquefactive necrosis. Courtesy of Daftblogger.

209   **Necrosis: Image C.** Caseous necrosis. This image is a derivative work, adapted from the following source, available under . Courtesy of Dr. Yale Rosen. The image may have been modified by cropping, labeling, and/or captions. MedIQ Learning, LLC makes this image available under .

209   **Necrosis: Image D.** Fat necrosis. This image is a derivative work, adapted from the following source, available under . Courtesy of Patho. The image may have been modified by cropping, labeling, and/or captions. MedIQ Learning, LLC makes this image available under .

209   **Necrosis: Image E.** Fibrinoid necrosis. This image is a derivative work, adapted from the following source, available under . Courtesy of Dr. Yale Rosen. The image may have been modified by cropping, labeling, and/or captions. MedIQ Learning, LLC makes this image available under .

209   **Necrosis: Image F.** Acral gangrene. Courtesy of the US Department of Health and Human Services and William Archibald.

110   **Infarcts: red vs. pale: Image B.** Pale infarct. Courtesy of the US Department of Health and Human Services and the Armed Forces Institute of Pathology.

212   **Acute inflammation.** Courtesy of Dr. Douglas Mata.

214   **Granulomatous diseases.** Granuloma. Courtesy of Sanjay Mukhopadhyay.

215   **Types of calcification: Image A.** Dystrophic calcification. This image is a derivative work, adapted from the following source, available under : Chun J-S, Hong R, Kim J-A. Osseous metaplasia with mature bone formation of the thyroid gland: three case reports. *Oncol Lett.* 2013;6:977–979. DOI: 10.3892/ol.2013.1475. The image may have been modified by cropping, labeling, and/or captions. All rights to this adaptation by MedIQ Learning, LLC are reserved.

215   **Types of calcification: Image B.** Metastatic calcification. This image is a derivative work, adapted from the following source, available under . Courtesy of Dr. Yale Rosen. The image may have been modified by cropping, labeling, and/or captions. MedIQ Learning, LLC makes this image available under .

215   **Lipofuscin.** This image is a derivative work, adapted from the following source, available under . Courtesy of Nephron. The image may have been modified by cropping, labeling, and/or captions. MedIQ Learning, LLC makes this image available under .

216   **Scar formation: Image A.** Hypertrophic scar. This image is a derivative work, adapted from the following source, available under : Baker R, Urso-Baiarda F, Linge C, et al. Cutaneous scarring: a clinical review. *Dermatol Res Pract.* 2009;2009:625376. DOI: 10.1155/2009/625376.

216   **Scar formation: Image B.** Keloid scar. This image is a derivative work, adapted from the following source, available under . Courtesy of Dr. Andreas Settje. The image may have been modified by cropping, labeling, and/or captions. MedIQ Learning, LLC makes this image available under .

218   **Amyloidosis: Image A.** Amyloid deposits on Congo red stain. This image is a derivative work, adapted from the following source, available under : Courtesy of Dr. Ed Uthman.

218   **Amyloidosis: Image B.** Amyloid deposits on Congo red stain under polarized light. This image is a derivative work, adapted from the following source, available under . Courtesy of Dr. Ed Uthman. The image may have been modified by cropping, labeling, and/or captions. MedIQ Learning, LLC makes this image available under .

218   **Amyloidosis: Image C.** Amyloidosis on H&E stain. This image is a derivative work, adapted from the following source, available under : Mendoza JM, Peev V, Ponce MA, et al. Amyloid A amyloidosis with subcutaneous drug abuse. *J Renal Inj Prev.* 2014;3:11–16. DOI: 10.12861/jrip.2014.06.

219   **Neoplastic progression.** Cervical tissue. This image is a derivative work, adapted from the following source, available under : Courtesy of Dr. Ed Uthman. The image may have been modified by cropping, labeling, and/or captions. All rights to this adaptation by MedIQ Learning, LLC are reserved.

224   **Psammoma bodies.** Courtesy of the US Department of Health and Human Services and the Armed Forces Institute of Pathology.

226   **Common metastases: Image A.** Brain metastases from breast cancer. This image is a derivative work, adapted from the following source, available under . Courtesy of Jmarchn. The image may have been modified by cropping, labeling, and/or captions. MedIQ Learning, LLC makes this image available under .

226   **Common metastases: Image B.** Brain metastasis. Courtesy of the US Department of Health and Human Services and the Armed Forces Institute of Pathology.

226   **Common metastases: Image C.** Liver metastasis. This image is a derivative work, adapted from the following source, available under . Courtesy of Dr. James Heilman. The image may have been modified by cropping, labeling, and/or captions. MedIQ Learning, LLC makes this image available under .

226   **Common metastases: Image D.** Liver metastasis. Courtesy of J. Hayman.

226   **Common metastases: Image E.** Bone metastasis. This image is a derivative work, adapted from the following source, available under . Courtesy of Hellerhoff.

226   **Common metastases: Image F.** Bone metastasis. This image is a derivative work, adapted from the following source, available under : Courtesy of M. Emmanuel.

Cardiovascular

277   **Coronary artery anatomy.** This image is a derivative work, adapted from the following source, available under : Zhang J, Chen L, Wang X, et al. Compounding local invariant features and global deformable geometry for medical image registration. *PLoS One.* 2014;9(8):e105815. DOI: 10.1371/journal.pone.0105815.

294 Congenital heart diseases: Image A. Tetralogy of Fallot. This image is a derivative work, adapted from the following source, available under ⊚⊙⊜: Rashid AKM: Heart diseases in Down syndrome. In: Dey S, ed: *Down syndrome.* DOI: 10.5772/46009. The image may have been modified by cropping, labeling, and/or captions. All rights to this adaptation by MedIQ Learning, LLC are reserved.

295 Congenital heart diseases: Image B. Ventricular septal defect. This image is a derivative work, adapted from the following source, available under ⊚⊙⊜: Bardo DME, Brown P. Cardiac multidetector computed tomography: basic physics of image acquisition and clinical applications. *Curr Cardiol Rev.* 2008 Aug;4(3):231–243. DOI: 10.2174/157340308785160615.

295 Congenital heart diseases: Image C. Atrial septal defect. This image is a derivative work, adapted from the following source, available under ⊚⊙⊜: Teo KSL, Dundon BK, Molaee P, et al. Percutaneous closure of atrial septal defects leads to normalisation of atrial and ventricular volumes. *J Cardiovasc Magn Reson.* 2008;10(1):55. DOI: 10.1186/1532-429X-10-55.

295 Congenital heart diseases: Image D. Patent ductus arteriosus. This image is a derivative work, adapted from the following source, available under ⊚⊙⊜: Henjes CR, Nolte I, Wesfaedt P. Multidetector-row computed tomography of thoracic aortic anomalies in dogs and cats: patent ductus arteriosus and vascular rings. *BMC Vet Res.* 2011;7:57. DOI: 10.1186/1746-6148-7-57.

295 Congenital heart diseases: Image E. Clubbing of fingers. ⊚⊙⊜ Courtesy of Ann McGrath.

296 Hypertension: Image A. "String of beads" appearance in fibromuscular dysplasia. This image is a derivative work, adapted from the following source, available under ⊚⊙⊜: Plouin PF, Perdu J, LaBatide-Alanore A, et al. Fibromuscular dysplasia. *Orphanet J Rare Dis.* 2007;7:28. DOI: 10.1186/1750-1172-2-28. The image may have been modified by cropping, labeling, and/or captions. All rights to this adaptation by MedIQ Learning, LLC are reserved.

297 Hyperlipidemia signs: Image C. Tendinous xanthoma. This image is a derivative work, adapted from the following source, available under ⊚⊙⊜.

297 Arteriosclerosis: Image A. Hyaline type. This image is a derivative work, adapted from the following source, available under ⊚⊙⊜. Courtesy of Nephron. The image may have been modified by cropping, labeling, and/or captions. MedIQ Learning, LLC makes this image available under ⊚⊙⊜.

297 Arteriosclerosis: Image B. Hyperplastic type. This image is a derivative work, adapted from the following source, available under ⊚⊙⊜. Courtesy of Paco Larosa. The image may have been modified by cropping, labeling, and/or captions. MedIQ Learning, LLC makes this image available under ⊚⊙⊜.

297 Arteriosclerosis: Image C. Monckeberg sclerosis (medial calcific sclerosis). This image is a derivative work, adapted from the following source, available under ⊚⊙⊜: Courtesy of CE Couri, GA da Silva, JA Martinez, FA Pereira, and F de Paula. The image may have been modified by cropping, labeling, and/or captions. All rights to this adaptation by MedIQ Learning, LLC are reserved.

298 Atherosclerosis: Image A. Carotid plaque. This image is a derivative work, adapted from the following source, available under ⊚⊙⊜: Courtesy of Dr. Ed Uthman. The image may have been modified by cropping, labeling, and/or captions. All rights to this adaptation by MedIQ Learning, LLC are reserved.

299 Aortic dissection. This image is a derivative work, adapted from the following source, available under ⊚⊙⊜. Courtesy of Dr. James Heilman.

302 Myocardial infarction complications: Image A. Papillary muscle rupture. This image is a derivative work, adapted from the following source, available under ⊚⊙⊜: Routy B, Huynh T, Fraser R, et al. Vascular endothelial cell function in catastrophic antiphospholipid syndrome: a case report and review of the literature. *Case Rep Hematol.* 2013;2013:710365. DOI: 10.1155/2013/710365.

302 Myocardial infarction complications: Image B. Drawing of pseudoaneurysm. This image is a derivative work, adapted from the following source, available under ⊚⊙⊜: Courtesy of Patrick J. Lynch and Dr. C. Carl Jaffe.

302 Myocardial infarction complications: Image C. Free wall rupture of left ventricle. This image is a derivative work, adapted from the following source, available under ⊚⊙⊜: Zacarias ML, da Trindade H, Tsutsu J, et al. Left ventricular free wall impeding rupture in post-myocardial infarction period diagnosed by myocardial contrast echocardiography: case report. *Cardiovasc Ultrasound.* 2006;4:7. DOI: 10.1186/1476-7120-4-7.

303 Cardiomyopathies: Image A. Dilated cardiomyopathy. This image is a derivative work, adapted from the following source, available under ⊚⊙⊜: Gho JMIH, van Es R, Stathonikos N, et al. High resolution systematic digital histological quantification of cardiac fibrosis and adipose tissue in phospholamban p.Arg14del mutation associated cardiomyopathy. *PLoS One.* 2014;9:e94820. DOI: 10.1371/journal.pone.0094820.

304 Heart failure. Pedal edema. This image is a derivative work, adapted from the following source, available under ⊚⊙⊜. Courtesy of Dr. James Heilman. The image may have been modified by cropping, labeling, and/or captions. MedIQ Learning, LLC makes this image available under ⊚⊙⊜.

305 Bacterial endocarditis: Image B. Courtesy of Dr. Nicholas Mahoney.

305 Bacterial endocarditis: Image C. This image is a derivative work, adapted from the following source, available under ⊚⊙⊜: Yang ML, Chen YH, Lin WR, et al. Case report: infective endocarditis caused by Brevundimonas vesicularis. *BMC Infect Dis.* 2006;6:179. DOI: 10.1186/1471-2334-6-179.

305 Bacterial endocarditis: Image D. Janeway lesions on sole. This image is a derivative work, adapted from the following source, available under ⊚⊙⊜: Courtesy of DeNanneke.

306 Rheumatic fever. Aschoff body and Anitschkow cells. This image is a derivative work, adapted from the following source, available under ⊚⊙⊜: Courtesy of Dr. Ed Uthman. The image may have been modified by cropping, labeling, and/or captions. All rights to this adaptation by MedIQ Learning, LLC are reserved.

306 Acute pericarditis. This image is a derivative work, adapted from the following source, available under ⊚⊙⊜: Bogaert J, Francone M. Cardiovascular magnetic resonance in pericardial diseases. *J Cardiovasc Magn Reson.* 2009;11:14. DOI: 10.1186/1532-429X-11-14. The image may have been modified by cropping, labeling, and/or captions. All rights to this adaptation by MedIQ Learning, LLC are reserved.

307   **Cardiac tamponade.** This image is a derivative work, adapted from the following source, available under ⌾⌾: Yousuf T, Kramer J, Kopiec A, et al. A rare case of cardiac tamponade induced by chronic rheumatoid arthritis. *J Clin Med Res.* 2015 Sep;7(9):720–723. DOI: 10.14740/jocmr2226w.

309   **Vasculitides: Image A.** Temporal arteritis histology. This image is a derivative work, adapted from the following source, available under ⌾⌾. Courtesy of Marvin. The image may have been modified by cropping, labeling, and/or captions. MedIQ Learning, LLC makes this image available under ⌾⌾.

309   **Vasculitides: Image B.** Angiogram in patient with Takayasu arteritis. ⌾⌾ Courtesy of the US Department of Health and Human Services and Justin Ly.

309   **Vasculitides: Image C.** Microaneurysms in polyarteritis nodosa. Reproduced, with permission, from Dr. Frank Gaillard and www.radiopaedia.org.

309   **Vasculitides: Image D.** Strawberry tongue in patient with Kawasaki disease. This image is a derivative work, adapted from the following source, available under ⌾⌾: Courtesy of Natr.

309   **Vasculitides: Image E.** Coronary artery aneurysm in Kawasaki disease. This image is a derivative work, adapted from the following source, available under ⌾⌾: Courtesy of Wikimedia Commons. The image may have been modified by cropping, labeling, and/or captions. All rights to this adaptation by MedIQ Learning, LLC are reserved.

309   **Vasculitides: Image F.** Gangrene as a consequence of Buerger disease. This image is a derivative work, adapted from the following source, available under ⌾⌾: Afsjarfard A, Mozaffar M, Malekpour F, et al. The wound healing effects of iloprost in patients with Buerger's disease: claudication and prevention of major amputations. *Iran Red Crescent Med J.* 2011;13:420–423.

309   **Vasculitides: Image G.** Granulomatosis with polyangiitis (formerly Wegener) and PR3-ANCA/c-ANCA. ⌾⌾ Courtesy of M.A. Little.

309   **Vasculitides: Image I.** Churg-Strauss syndrome histology. This image is a derivative work, adapted from the following source, available under ⌾⌾. Courtesy of Dr. Michael Bonert. The image may have been modified by cropping, labeling, and/or captions. MedIQ Learning, LLC makes this image available under ⌾⌾.

309   **Vasculitides: Image J.** Henoch-Schönlein purpura. ⌾⌾ Courtesy of Okwikikim.

Endocrine

320   **Thyroid development.** Thyroglossal duct cyst. This image is a derivative work, adapted from the following source, available under ⌾⌾: Adelchi C, Mara P, Melissa L, et al. Ectopic thyroid tissue in the head and neck: a case series. *BMC Res Notes.* 2014;7:790. DOI: 10.1186/1756-0500-7-790.

320   **Adrenal cortex and medulla.** Courtesy of Dr. Kristine Krafts.

332   **Adrenal insufficiency.** Mucosal hyperpigmentation in 1° adrenal insufficiency. ⌾⌾ Courtesy of FlatOut. The image may have been modified by cropping, labeling, and/or captions. All rights to this adaptation by MedIQ Learning, LLC are reserved.

333   **Neuroblastoma: Image A.** CT scan of abdomen. This image is a derivative work, adapted from the following source, available under ⌾⌾: Koumarianou A, Oikonomopoulou P, Baka M, et al. Implications of the incidental finding of a MYCN amplified adrenal tumor: a case report and update of a pediatric disease diagnosed in adults. *Case Rep Oncol Med.* 2013;2013:393128. DOI: 10.1155/2013/393128. The image may have been modified by cropping, labeling, and/or captions. All rights to this adaptation by MedIQ Learning, LLC are reserved.

333   **Neuroblastoma: Image B.** Neuroblastoma, Homer-Write rosettes. Courtesy of Dr. Kristine Krafts.

334   **Pheochromocytoma.** This image is a derivative work, adapted from the following source, available under ⌾⌾: Courtesy of Dr. Michael Feldman.

335   **Hypothyroidism vs hyperthyroidism.** Onycholysis. This image is a derivative work, adapted from the following source, available under ⌾⌾: Rajebi MR, Shahrokni A, Chaisson M. Uncommon osseous involvement in multisystemic sarcoidosis. *Ann Saudi Med.* 2009 Nov-Dec;29(6):485–486.

336   **Hypothyroidism: Image A.** Hashimoto thyroiditis, Hurthle cells. Courtesy of Dr. Kristine Krafts.

336   **Hypothyroidism: Image B.** Before and after treatment of congenital hypothyroidism. ⌾⌾ Courtesy of the US Department of Health and Human Services.

336   **Hypothyroidism: Image C.** Congenital hypothyroidism. This image is a derivative work, adapted from the following source, available under ⌾⌾: Courtesy of Sadasiv Swain. The image may have been modified by cropping, labeling, and/or captions. All rights to this adaptation by MedIQ Learning, LLC are reserved.

336   **Hypothyroidism: Image D.** Reidel thyroiditis histology. Courtesy of Dr. Kristine Krafts.

337   **Hyperthyroidism: Image B.** Scalloped colloid. Courtesy of Dr. Kristine Krafts.

338   **Thyroid adenoma.** Courtesy of Dr. Kristine Krafts.

339   **Hypoparathyroidism.** Shortened 4th and 5th digits. This image is a derivative work, adapted from the following source, available under ⌾⌾: Ferrario C, Gastaldi G, Portmann L, et al. Bariatric surgery in an obese patient with Albright hereditary osteodystrophy: a case report. *J Med Case Rep.* 2013;7:111. DOI: 10.1186/1752-1947-7-111.

340   **Hyperparathyroidism.** Multiple lytic lesions. This image is a derivative work, adapted from the following source, available under ⌾⌾: Khaoula BA, Kaouther BA, Ines C, et al. An unusual presentation of primary hyperparathyroidism: pathological fracture. *Case Rep Orthop.* 2011;2011:521578. DOI: 10.1155/2011/521578. The image may have been modified by cropping, labeling, and/or captions. All rights to this adaptation by MedIQ Learning, LLC are reserved.

346   **Carcinoid syndrome.** ⌾⌾ Courtesy of the US Department of Health and Human Services and the Armed Forces Institute of Pathology.

347   **Multiple endocrine neoplasias.** Mucosal neuroma. This image is a derivative work, adapted from the following source, available under ⌾⌾: Martucciello G, Lerone M, Bricco L, et al. Multiple endocrine neoplasias type 2B and RET proto-oncogene. *Ital J Pediatr.* 2012;38:9. DOI: 10.1186/1824-7288-38-9.

Gastrointestinal

352 Ventral wall defects. Drawings of gastroschisis (left) and omphalocele (right). ⊚ Courtesy of the US Department of Health and Human Services.

353 Intestinal atresia. "Double bubble" sign of duodenal atresia. This image is a derivative work, adapted from the following source, available under ⊚: Alorainy IA, Barlas NB, Al-Boukai AA. Pictorial essay: infants of diabetic mothers. *Indian J Radiol Imaging.* 2010;20:174–181. DOI: 0.4103/0971-3026.69349.

353 Hypertrophic pyloric stenosis. This image is a derivative work, adapted from the following source, available under ⊚: Hassan RAA, Choo YU, Noraida R, et al. Infantile hypertrophic pyloric stenosis in postoperative esophageal atresia with tracheoesophageal fistula. *J Neonatal Surg.* 2015 Jul-Sep;4(3):32.

353 Pancreas and spleen embryology. Annular pancreas. This image is a derivative work, adapted from the following source, available under ⊚: Mahdi B, Selim S, Hassen T, et al. A rare cause of proximal intestinal obstruction in adults—annular pancreas: a case report. *Pan Afr Med J.* 2011;10:56. The image may have been modified by cropping, labeling, and/or captions. All rights to this adaptation by MedIQ Learning, LLC are reserved.

354 Retroperitoneal structures. This image is a derivative work, adapted from the following source, available under ⊚: Sammut J, Ahiaku E, Williams DT. Complete regression of renal tumour following ligation of an accessory renal artery during repair of an abdominal aortic aneurysm. *Ann R Coll Surg Engl.* 2012 Sep;94(6):e198–e200. DOI: 10.1308/003588412X13 373405384972.

361 Liver tissue architecture: Image A. Portal triad of liver tissue. This image is a derivative work, adapted from the following source, available under ⊚: Liver development. In: Zorn AM. Stem book. Cambridge: Harvard Stem Cell Institute, 2008.

361 Liver tissue architecture: Image B. Kupffer cells. This image is a derivative work, adapted from the following source, available under ⊚. Courtesy of Dr. Michael Bonert. The image may have been modified by cropping, labeling, and/or captions. MedIQ Learning, LLC makes this image available under ⊚.

362 Biliary structures. Gallstones. This image is a derivative work, adapted from the following source, available under ⊚. Courtesy of J. Guntau. The image may have been modified by cropping, labeling, and/or captions. MedIQ Learning, LLC makes this image available under ⊚.

364 Hernias. Congenital diaphragmatic hernia. This image is a derivative work, adapted from the following source, available under ⊚: Tovar J. Congenital diaphragmatic hernia. *Orphanet J Rare Dis.* 2012;7:1. DOI: 10.1186/1750-1172-7-1.

368 Peyer patches. This image is a derivative work, adapted from the following source, available under ⊚. Courtesy of Plainpaper. The image may have been modified by cropping, labeling, and/or captions. MedIQ Learning, LLC makes this image available under ⊚.

370 Sialolithiasis. This image is a derivative work, adapted from the following source, available under ⊚: Pastor-Ramos V, Cuervo-Diaz A, Aracil-Kessler L. Sialolithiasis. Proposal for a new minimally invasive procedure: piezoelectric surgery. *J Clin Exp Dent.* 2014 Jul;6(3):e295–e298. DOI: 10.4317/jced.51253.

370 Salivary gland tumors. Pleomorphic adenoma histology. This image is a derivative work, adapted from the following source, available under ⊚. Courtesy of Wikimedia Commons. The image may have been modified by cropping, labeling, and/or captions. MedIQ Learning, LLC makes this image available under ⊚.

370 Achalasia. This image is a derivative work, adapted from the following source, available under ⊚: Courtesy of Farnoosh Farrokhi and Michael F. Vaezi. The image may have been modified by cropping, labeling, and/or captions. All rights to this adaptation by MedIQ Learning, LLC are reserved.

371 Esophageal pathologies. Pneumomediastinum in Boerhaave syndrome. This image is a derivative work, adapted from the following source, available under ⊚. Courtesy of Wikimedia Commons. The image may have been modified by cropping, labeling, and/or captions. MedIQ Learning, LLC makes this image available under ⊚.

371 Esophageal pathologies: Image B. Esophageal varices on endoscopy. This image is a derivative work, adapted from the following source, available under ⊚: Costaguta A, Alvarez F. Etiology and management of hemorrhagic complications of portal hypertension in children. *Int J Hepatol.* 2012;2012:879163. DOI: 10.1155/2012/879163.

371 Esophageal pathologies: Image C. Esophageal varices on CT. This image is a derivative work, adapted from the following source, available under ⊚. Courtesy of Hellerhoff. The image may have been modified by cropping, labeling, and/or captions. MedIQ Learning, LLC makes this image available under ⊚.

372 Barrett esophagus: Image A. Endoscopy. This image is a derivative work, adapted from the following source, available under ⊚: Coda S, Thillainayagam AV. State of the art in advanced endoscopic imaging for the detection and evaluation of dysplasia and early cancer of the gastrointestinal tract. *Clin Exp Gastroenterol.* 2014;7:133–150. DOI: 10.2147/CEG. S58157. The image may have been modified by cropping, labeling, and/or captions. All rights to this adaptation by MedIQ Learning, LLC are reserved.

372 Barrett esophagus: Image B. Goblet cells. This image is a derivative work, adapted from the following source, available under ⊚. Courtesy of Dr. Michael Bonert. The image may have been modified by cropping, labeling, and/or captions. MedIQ Learning, LLC makes this image available under ⊚.

373 Ménétriere disease. This image is a derivative work, adapted from the following source, available under ⊚. Courtesy of Hellerhoff. The image may have been modified by cropping, labeling, and/or captions. MedIQ Learning, LLC makes this image available under ⊚.

374 Ulcer complications. Free air under diaphragm in perforated ulcer. Reproduced, with permission, from Dr. Frank Gaillard and www.radiopaedia.org.

375 Malabsorption syndromes: Image B. *Tropheryma whippeli* on PAS stain. This image is a derivative work, adapted from the following source, available under ⊚: Tran HA. Reversible hypothyroidism and Whipple's disease. *BMC Endocr Disord.* 2006;6:3. DOI: 10.1186/1472-6823-6-3.

376 Inflammatory bowel disease: Image A. "String sign" on barium swallow in Crohn disease. This image is a derivative work, adapted from the following source, available under ⊚: Al-Mofarreh MA, Al Mofleh IA, Al-Teimi IN, et al. Crohn's disease in a Saudi outpatient population: is it still rare? *Saudi*

J Gastroenterol. 2009;15:111–116. DOI: 10.4103/1319-3767.45357. The image may have been modified by cropping, labeling, and/or captions. All rights to this adaptation by MedIQ Learning, LLC are reserved.

376 **Inflammatory bowel diseases: Images B** (normal mucosa) and **C** (punched-out ulcers) in ulcerative colitis. This image is a derivative work, adapted from the following source, available under ⊚⊚: Ishikawa D, Ando T, Watanabe O, et al. Images of colonic real-time tissue sonoelastography correlate with those of colonoscopy and may predict response to therapy in patients with ulcerative colitis. *BMC Gastroenterol.* 2011;11:29. DOI: 10.1186/1471-230X-11-29.

377 **Appendicitis.** Fecalith. This image is a derivative work, adapted from the following source, available under ⊚⊚: Courtesy of Dr. James Heilman. The image may have been modified by cropping, labeling, and/or captions. MedIQ Learning, LLC makes this image available under ⊚⊚.

377 **Diverticula of the GI tract: Image B.** Diverticulosis. This image is a derivative work, adapted from the following source, available under ⊚⊚: Sartelli M, Moore FA, Ansaloni L, et al. A proposal for a CT driven classification of left colon acute diverticulitis. *World J Emerg Surg.* 2015;10:3. DOI: 10.1186/1749-7922-10-3.

377 **Diverticula of the GI tract: Image C.** Diverticulitis. This image is a derivative work, adapted from the following source, available under ⊚⊚: Mazzei MA, Squitieri NC, Guerrini S, et al. Sigmoid diverticulitis: US findings. *Crit Ultrasound J.* 2013;5(Suppl 1):S5. DOI: 10.1186/2036-7902-5-S1-S5.

378 **Zenker diverticulum.** This image is a derivative work, adapted from the following source, available under ⊚⊚: Courtesy of Bernd Brägelmann.

379 **Maltotation.** This image is a derivative work, adapted from the following source, available under ⊚⊚: Mathews R, Thenabadu S, Jaiganesh T. Abdominal pain with a twist. *Int J Emerg Med.* 2011;4:21. DOI: 10.1186/1865-1380-4-21.

379 **Volvulus.** Coffee bean sign. This image is a derivative work, adapted from the following source, available under ⊚⊚: Yigit M, Turkdogan KA. Coffee bean sign, whirl sign and bird's beak sign in the diagnosis of sigmoid volvulus. *Pan Afr Med J.* 1014;19:56. DOI: 10.11604/pamj.2014.19.56.5142.

379 **Intussusception.** Interoperative image of intussusception. This image is a derivative work, adapted from the following source, available under ⊚⊚: Vasiliadis K, Kogopoulos E, Katsamakas M, et al. Ileoileal intussusception induced by a gastrointestinal stromal tumor. *World J Surg Oncol.* 2008;6:133. DOI: 10.1186/1477-7819-6-133.

380 **Other intestinal disorders: Image A.** Necrosis due to occlusion of SMA. This image is a derivative work, adapted from the following source, available under ⊚⊚: Van De Winkel N, Cheragwandi A, Nieboer K, et al. Superior mesenteric arterial branch occlusion causing partial jejunal ischemia: a case report. *J Med Case Rep.* 2012;6:48. DOI: 10.1186/1752-1947-6-48.

380 **Other intestinal disorders: Image B.** Endoscopy showing dilated vessels. This image is a derivative work, adapted from the following source, available under ⊚⊚: Gunjan D, Sharma V, Rana SS, et al. Small bowel bleeding: a comprehensive review. *Gastroenterol Rep.* 2014 Nov;2(4):262–275. DOI: 10.1093/gastro/gou025.

380 **Other intestinal disorders: Image C.** Loops of dilated bowel suggestive of small bowel obstruction. This image is a derivative work, adapted from the following source, available under ⊚⊚: Welte FJ, Crosso M. Left-sided appendicitis in a patient with congenital gastrointestinal malrotation: a case report. *J Med Case Rep.* 2007;1:92. DOI: 10.1186/1752-1947-1-92.

380 **Other intestinal disorders: Image D.** Pneumatosis intestinalis. This image is a derivative work, adapted from the following source, available under ⊚⊚: Pelizzo G, Nakib G, Goruppi I, et al. Isolated colon ischemia with norovirus infection in preterm babies: a case series. *J Med Case Rep.* 2013;7:108. DOI: 10.1186/1752-1947-7-108.

381 **Colonic polyps: Image A.** Colonic polyps and cancer. This image is a derivative work, adapted from the following source, available under ⊚⊚: Courtesy of M. Emannuel.

382 **Colorectal cancer: Image A.** Polyp on endoscopy. This image is a derivative work, adapted from the following source, available under ⊚⊚: Chen C-W, Hsiao K-H, Yue C-T, et al. Invasive adenocarcinoma arising from a mixed hyperplastic/adenomatous polyp and synchronous transverse colon cancer. *World J Surg Oncol.* 2013;11:214. DOI: 10.1186/1477-7819-11-214.

383 **Cirrhosis and portal hypertension.** Splenomegaly and liver nodularity in cirrhosis. This image is a derivative work, adapted from the following source, available under ⊚⊚. Courtesy of Inversitus. The image may have been modified by cropping, labeling, and/or captions. MedIQ Learning, LLC makes this image available under ⊚⊚.

385 **Alcoholic liver disease: Image B.** Mallory bodies. This image is a derivative work, adapted from the following source, available under ⊚⊚. Courtesy of Dr. Michael Bonert. The image may have been modified by cropping, labeling, and/or captions. MedIQ Learning, LLC makes this image available under ⊚⊚.

385 **Alcoholic liver disease: Image C.** Sclerosis in alcoholic cirrhosis. This image is a derivative work, adapted from the following source, available under ⊚⊚. Courtesy of Dr. Michael Bonert. The image may have been modified by cropping, labeling, and/or captions. MedIQ Learning, LLC makes this image available under ⊚⊚.

385 **Non-alcoholic fatty liver disease.** This image is a derivative work, adapted from the following source, available under ⊚⊚: El-Karaksy HM, El-Koofy NM, Anwar GM, et al. Predictors of non-alcoholic fatty liver disease in obese and overweight Egyptian children: single center study. *Saudi J Gastroenterol.* 2011;17:40–46. DOI: 10.4103/1319-3767.74476.

386 **Hepatocellular carcinoma/hepatoma: Image A.** Gross specimen. Reproduced, with permission, from Jean-Christophe Fournet and Humpath.

386 **Other liver tumors.** Cavernous liver hemangioma. This image is a derivative work, adapted from the following source, available under ⊚⊚. Courtesy of Dr. Michael Bonert. The image may have been modified by cropping, labeling, and/or captions. MedIQ Learning, LLC makes this image available under ⊚⊚.

386 **α_1-antitrypsin deficiency.** Liver histology. This image is a derivative work, adapted from the following source, available under ⊚⊚. Courtesy of Dr. Jerad M. Gardner. The image may have been modified by cropping, labeling, and/or captions. MedIQ Learning, LLC makes this image available under ⊚⊚.

387 **Jaundice.** Yellow sclera. ▣ Courtesy of the US Department of Health and Human Services and Dr. Thomas F. Sellers.

389 **Hemochromatosis.** Hemosiderin deposits. This image is a derivative work, adapted from the following source, available under ▣: Mathew J, Leong MY, Morley N, et al. A liver fibrosis cocktail? Psoriasis, methotrexate and genetic hemochromatosis. *BMC Dermatol.* 2005;5:12. DOI: 10.1186/1471-5945-5-12.

390 **Gallstones (cholelithiasis): Image A.** Gross specimen. This image is a derivative work, adapted from the following source, available under ▣: Courtesy of M. Emmanuel.

390 **Gallstones (cholelithiasis): Image B.** This image is a derivative work, adapted from the following source, available under ▣: Spangler R, Van Pham T, Khoujah D, et al. Abdominal emergencies in the geriatric patient. *Int J Emerg Med.* 2014;7: 43. DOI: 10.1186/s12245-014-0043-2.

390 **Gallstones (cholelithiasis): Image C.** Porcelain gallbladder. This image is a derivative work, adapted from the following source, available under ▣: Fred H, van Dijk H. Images of memorable cases: case 19. Connexions Web site. December 4, 2008. Available at: http://cnx.org/content/m14939/1.3/. The image may have been modified by cropping, labeling, and/or captions. All rights to this adaptation by MedIQ Learning, LLC are reserved.

391 **Acute pancreatitis: Image A.** Acute exudative pancreatitis. This image is a derivative work, adapted from the following source, available under ▣. Courtesy of Hellerhoff. The image may have been modified by cropping, labeling, and/or captions. MedIQ Learning, LLC makes this image available under ▣.

391 **Acute pancreatitis: Image B.** Pancreatic pseudocyst. This image is a derivative work, adapted from the following source, available under ▣. Courtesy of Thomas Zimmerman. The image may have been modified by cropping, labeling, and/or captions. MedIQ Learning, LLC makes this image available under ▣.

391 **Chronic pancreatitis.** This image is a derivative work, adapted from the following source, available under ▣. Courtesy of Hellerhoff. The image may have been modified by cropping, labeling, and/or captions. MedIQ Learning, LLC makes this image available under ▣.

391 **Pancreatic adenocarcinoma: Image A.** Histology. This image is a derivative work, adapted from the following source, available under ▣. Courtesy of KGH. The image may have been modified by cropping, labeling, and/or captions. MedIQ Learning, LLC makes this image available under ▣.

391 **Pancreatic adenocarcinoma: Image B.** CT scan. ▣ Courtesy of MBq. The image may have been modified by cropping, labeling, and/or captions. All rights to this adaptation by MedIQ Learning, LLC are reserved.

Hematology and Oncology

396 **Erythrocytes.** ▣ Courtesy of the US Department of Health and Human Services and Drs. Noguchi, Rodgers, and Schechter.

396 **Thrombocytes (platelets).** This image is a derivative work, adapted from the following source, available under ▣. Courtesy of Dr. Ed Uthman. The image may have been modified by cropping, labeling, and/or captions. MedIQ Learning, LLC makes this image available under ▣.

396 **Neutrophils.** ▣ Courtesy of B. Lennert.

397 **Monocytes.** This image is a derivative work, adapted from the following source, available under ▣. Courtesy of Dr. Graham Beards. The image may have been modified by cropping, labeling, and/or captions. MedIQ Learning, LLC makes this image available under ▣.

397 **Macrophages.** This image is a derivative work, adapted from the following source, available under ▣: De Tommasi AS, Otranto D, Furlanello T, et al. Evaluation of blood and bone marrow in selected canine vector-borne diseases. *Parasit Vectors.* 2014;7:534. DOI: 10.1186/s13071-014-0534-2.

397 **Eosinophils.** This image is a derivative work, adapted from the following source, available under ▣: Courtesy of Dr. Ed Uthman.

397 **Basophils.** This image is a derivative work, adapted from the following source, available under ▣. Courtesy of Dr. Erhabor Osaro. The image may have been modified by cropping, labeling, and/or captions. MedIQ Learning, LLC makes this image available under ▣.

398 **Mast cells.** ▣ Courtesy of Wikimedia Commons.

398 **Dendritic cells.** This image is a derivative work, adapted from the following source, available under ▣: Cheng J-H, Lee S-Y, Lien Y-Y, et al. Immunomodulating activity of *Nymphaea rubra* roxb. extracts: activation of rat dendritic cells and improvement of the TH1 immune response. *Int J Mol Sci.* 2012;13:10722–10735. DOI: 10.3390/ijms130910722.

398 **Lymphocytes.** This image is a derivative work, adapted from the following source, available under ▣: Courtesy of Fickleandfreckled.

399 **Plasma cells.** ▣ Courtesy of the US Department of Health and Human Services and Dr. Francis W. Chandler. The image may have been modified by cropping, labeling, and/or captions. All rights to this adaptation by MedIQ Learning, LLC are reserved.

404 **Pathologic RBC forms: Image A.** Acanthocyte ("spur cell"). Courtesy of Dr. Kristine Krafts.

404 **Pathologic RBC forms: Image B.** Basophilic stippling. This image is a derivative work, adapted from the following source, available under ▣: van Dijk HA, Fred HL. Images of memorable cases: case 81. Connexions Web site. December 3, 2008. Available at http://cnx.org/contents/3196bf3e-1e1e-4c4d-a1ac-d4fc9ab65443@4@4.

404 **Pathologic RBC forms: Image C.** Dacrocyte ("teardrop cell"). Courtesy of Dr. Kristine Krafts.

404 **Pathologic RBC forms: Image D.** Degmacyte ("bite cell"). Courtesy of Dr. Kristine Krafts.

404 **Pathologic RBC forms: Image E.** Echinocyte ("burr cell"). Courtesy of Dr. Kristine Krafts.

404 **Pathologic RBC forms: Image F.** Elliptocyte. Courtesy of Dr. Kristine Krafts.

404 **Pathologic RBC forms: Image G.** Macro-ovalocyte. Courtesy of Dr. Kristine Krafts.

405 **Pathologic RBC forms: Image H.** Ringed sideroblast. This image is a derivative work, adapted from the following source, available under ▣. Courtesy of Paulo Henrique Orlandi Mourao. The image may have been modified by cropping, labeling, and/or captions. MedIQ Learning, LLC makes this image available under ▣.

405 Pathologic RBC forms: Image I. Schistocyte. Courtesy of Dr. Kristine Krafts.

405 Pathologic RBC forms: Image J. Sickle cell. ⬛ Courtesy of the US Department of Health and Human Services and the Sickle Cell Foundation of Georgia, Jackie George, and Beverly Sinclair.

405 Pathologic RBC forms: Image K. Spherocyte. Courtesy of Dr. Kristine Krafts.

405 Pathologic RBC forms: Image L. Target cell. Courtesy of Dr. Kristine Krafts.

405 Other RBC abnormalities: Image A. Heinz bodies. Courtesy of Dr. Kristine Krafts.

405 Other RBC abnormalities: Image B. Howell-Jolly bodies. This image is a derivative work, adapted from the following source, available under ⬛: Serio B, Pezzullo L, Giudice V, et al. OPSI threat in hematological patients. *Transl Med UniSa.* 2013 May-Aug;62–10.

407 Microcytic, hypochromic anemia: Image C. β-thalassemia. Courtesy of Dr. Kristine Krafts.

407 Microcytic, hypochromic anemia: Image D. Lead lines in lead poisoning. Reproduced, with permission, from Dr. Frank Gaillard and www.radiopaedia.org.

407 Microcytic, hypochromic anemia: Image E. Sideroblastic anemia. This image is a derivative work, adapted from the following source, available under ⬛. Courtesy of Paulo Henrique Orlandi Moura. The image may have been modified by cropping, labeling, and/or captions. MedIQ Learning, LLC makes this image available under ⬛.

408 Macrocytic anemia. Megaloblastic anemia. This image is a derivative work, adapted from the following source, available under ⬛: Courtesy of Dr. Ed Uthman.

410 Intrinsic hemolytic anemia: Image B. Dactylitis. This image is a derivative work, adapted from the following source, available under ⬛: Pedram M, Jaseb K, Haghi S, et al. First presentation of sickle cell anemia in a 3.5-year-old girl: a case report. *Iran Red Crescent Med J.* 2012;14:184–185.

411 Extrinsic hemolytic anemia. Autoimmune hemolytic anemia. Courtesy of Dr. Kristine Krafts.

413 Heme synthesis, porphyrias, and lead poisoning: Image A. Basophilic stippling in lead poisoning. This image is a derivative work, adapted from the following source, available under ⬛: van Dijk HA, Fred HL. Images of memorable cases: case 81. Connexions Web site. December 3, 2008. Available at http://cnx. org/contents/3196bf3e-1e1e-4c4d-a1ac-d4fc9ab65443@4@4.

413 Heme synthesis, porphyrias, and lead poisoning: Image B. Porphyria cutanea tarda. This image is a derivative work, adapted from the following source, available under ⬛: Bovenschen HJ, Vissers WHPM. Primary hemochromatosis presented by porphyria cutanea tarda: a case report. *Cases J,* 2009;2:7246. DOI: 10.4076/1757-1626-2-7246.

414 Coagulation disorders. Hemarthrosis. This image is a derivative work, adapted from the following source, available under ⬛: Benajiba N, El Boussaadni Y, Aljabri M, et al. Hémophilie: état des lieux dans un service de pédiatrie dans la région de l'oriental du Maroc. *Pan Afr Med J.* 2014;18:126. DOI: 10.11604/pamj.2014.18.126.4007.

418 Non-Hodgkin lymphoma: Image C. Primary central nervous system lymphoma. This image is a derivative work, adapted from the following source, available under ⬛: Mansour A, Qandeel M, Abdel-Razeq H, et al. MR imaging features of intracranial primary CNS lymphoma in immune competent patients. *Cancer Imaging.* 2014;14(1):22. DOI: 10.1186/1470-7330-14-22.

419 Multiple myeloma: Image B. RBC rouleaux formation. Courtesy of Dr. Kristine Krafts.

419 Multiple myeloma: Image C. Plasma cells. This image is a derivative work, adapted from the following source, available under ⬛: Sharma A, Kaushal M, Chaturvedi NK, et al. Cytodiagnosis of multiple myeloma presenting as orbital involvement: a case report. *Cytojournal.* 2006;3:19. DOI: 10.1186/1742-6413-3-19.

420 Leukemias: Image C. Hairy cell leukemia. This image is a derivative work, adapted from the following source, available under ⬛: Chan SM, George T, Cherry AM, et al. Complete remission of primary plasma cell leukemia with bortezomib, doxorubicin, and dexamethasone: a case report. *Cases J.* 2009;2:121. DOI: 10.1186/1757-1626-2-121.

420 Leukemias: Image E. Chronic myelogenous leukemia. Courtesy of Dr. Kristine Krafts.

421 Chronic myeloproliferative disorders: Image A. Erythromelalgia in polycythemia vera. This image is a derivative work, adapted from the following source, available under ⬛: Fred H, van Dijk H. Images of memorable cases: case 151. Connexions Web site. December 4, 2008. Available at http://cnx.org/content/m14932/1.3/.

421 Chronic myeloproliferative disorders: Image B. Essential thrombocytosis with enlarged megakaryocytes. Courtesy of Dr. Kristine Krafts.

421 Chronic myeloproliferative disorders: Image C. Myelofibrosis. This image is a derivative work, adapted from the following source, available under ⬛: Courtesy of Dr. Ed Uthman.

422 Langerhans cell histiocytosis: Image A. Lytic bone lesion. This image is a derivative work, adapted from the following source, available under ⬛: Dehkordi NR, Rajabi P, Naimi A, et al. Langerhans cell histiocytosis following Hodgkin lymphoma: a case report from Iran. *J Res Med Sci* 2010;15:58–61. PMCID PMC3082786.

422 Langerhans cell histiocytosis: Image B. Birbeck granules. This image is a derivative work, adapted from the following source, available under ⬛. Courtesy of Dr. Yale Rosen. The image may have been modified by cropping, labeling, and/or captions. MedIQ Learning, LLC makes this image available under ⬛.

424 Warfarin. Skin necrosis. This image is a derivative work, adapted from the following source, available under ⬛: Fred H, van Dijk H. Images of memorable cases: cases 84 and 85. Connexions Web site. December 2, 2008. Available at http://cnx.org/content/m15024/latest/.

Musculoskeletal, Skin, and Connective Tissue

434 Rotator cuff muscles. Glenohumeral instability. This image is a derivative work, adapted from the following source, available under ⬛: Koike Y, Sano H, Imamura I, et al. Changes with time in skin temperature of the shoulders in healthy controls and a patient with shoulder-hand syndrome. *Ups J Med Sci*

435   Wrist region: Image B. Anatomic snuff box. This image is a derivative work, adapted from the following source, available under ▣◉▣: Rhemrev SJ, Ootes D, Beeres FJP, et al. Current methods ofdiagnosis and treatment of scaphoid fractures. *Int J Emerg Med.* 2011;4:4. DOI: 10.1186/1865-1380-4-4.

435   Wrist regions: Image C. Thenar eminence atrophy in carpal tunnel syndrome. ▣◉▣ Courtesy of Dr. Harry Gouvas.

436   Common pediatric fractures: Image A. Greenstick fracture. This image is a derivative work, adapted from the following source, available under ▣◉▣: Randsborg PH, Sivertsen EA. Classification of distal radius fractures in children: good inter- and intraobserver reliability, which improves with clinical experience. *BMC Musculoskelet Disord.* 2013;13:6. DOI: 10.1186/1471-2474-13-6.

436   Common pediatric fractures: Image B. Buckle fracture. This image is a derivative work, adapted from the following source, available under ▣◉▣: Randsborg PH, Sivertsen EA. Classification of distal radius fractures in children: good inter- and intraobserver reliability, which improves with clinical experience. *BMC Musculoskelet Disord.* 2012;13:6. DOI: 10.1186/1471-2474-13-6.

438   Brachial plexus lesions: Image A. Cervical rib. This image is a derivative work, adapted from the following source, available under ▣◉▣: Dahlin LB, Backman C, Duppe H, et al. Compression of the lower trunk of the brachial plexus by a cervical rib in two adolescent girls: case reports and surgical treatment. *J Brachial Plex Peripher Nerve Inj.* 2009;4:14. DOI: 10.1186/1749-7221-4-14.

438   Brachial plexus lesions: Image B. Winged scapula. This image is a derivative work, adapted from the following source, available under ▣◉▣: Boukhris J, Boussouga M, Jaafar A, et al. Stabilisation dynamique d'un winging scapula (à propos d'un cas avec revue de la littérature). *Pan Afr Med J.* 2014;19:331. DOI: 10.11604/pamj.2014.19.331.3429.

441   Common hip and knee conditions: Image A. ACL tear. This image is a derivative work, adapted from the following source, available under ▣◉▣: Chang MJ, Chang CB, Choi J-Y, et al. Can magnetic resonance imaging findings predict the degree of knee joint laxity in patients undergoing anterior cruciate ligament reconstruction? *BMC Musculoskelet Disord.* 2014;15:214. DOI: 10.1186/1471-2474-15-214. The image may have been modified by cropping, labeling, and/or captions. All rights to this adaptation by MedIQ Learning, LLC are reserved.

441   Common hip and knee conditions: Images B (prepatellar bursitis) and **C** (Baker cyst). This image is a derivative work, adapted from the following source, available under ▣◉▣: Hirji Z, Hunhun JS, Choudur HN. Imaging of the bursae. *J Clin Imaging Sci.* 2011;1:22. DOI: 10.4103/2156-7514.80374. The image may have been modified by cropping, labeling, and/or captions. All rights to this adaptation by MedIQ Learning, LLC are reserved.

449   Osteoporosis. Vertebral compression fractures of spine. This image is a derivative work, adapted from the following source, available under ▣◉▣: Imani F, Gharaei H, Rahimzadeh P, et al. Management of painful vertebral compression fracture with kyphoplasty in a sever cardio-respiratory compromised patient.

Anesth Pain Med. 2012 summer;2(1):42–45. DOI: 10.5812/aapm.5030.

449   Osteopetrosis (marble bone disease). This image is a derivative work, adapted from the following source, available under ▣◉▣: Kant P, Sharda N, Bhowate RR. Clinical and radiological findings of autosomal dominant osteopetrosis type II: a case report. *Case Rep Dent.* 2013;2013:707343. DOI: 10.1155/2013/707343.

450   Osteomalacia/rickets: Image A, left. Clinical photo. This image is a derivative work, adapted from the following source, available under ▣◉▣: Linglart A, Biosse-Duplan M, Briot K, et al. Therapeutic management of hypophosphatemic rickets from infancy to adulthood. *Endocr Connect.* 2014;3:R13–R30. DOI: 10.1530/EC-13-0103.

450   Osteomalacia/rickets: Image B. Rachitic rosary on chest X-ray. This image is a derivative work, adapted from the following source, available under ▣◉▣: Essabar L, Meskini T, Ettair S, et al. Malignant infantile osteopetrosis: case report with review of literature. *Pan Afr Med J.* 2014;17:63. DOI: 10.11604/pamj.2014.17.63.3759.

450   Paget disease of bone (osteitis deformans). Thickened calvarium. This image is a derivative work, adapted from the following source, available under ▣◉▣: Dawes L. Paget's disease. [Radiology Picture of the Day Website]. Published June 21, 2007. Available at http://www.radpod.org/2007/06/21/pagets-disease/.

450   Osteonecrosis (avascular necrosis). Bilateral necrosis of femoral head. This image is a derivative work, adapted from the following source, available under ▣◉▣: Ding H, Chen S-B, Lin S, et al. The effect of postoperative corticosteroid administration on free vascularized fibular grafting for treating osteonecrosis of the femoral head. *Sci World J.* 2013;708014. DOI: 10.1155/2013/708014. The image may have been modified by cropping, labeling, and/or captions. All rights to this adaptation by MedIQ Learning, LLC are reserved.

453   Primary bone tumors: Image A. Osteochondroma. This image is a derivative work, adapted from the following source, available under ▣◉▣. Courtesy of Lucien Monfils. The image may have been modified by cropping, labeling, and/or captions. MedIQ Learning, LLC makes this image available under ▣◉▣.

453   Primary bone tumors: Image B. Giant cell tumor. Reproduced, with permission, from Dr. Frank Gaillard and www.radiopaedia.org.

453   Primary bone tumors: Image C. Osteosarcoma. Reproduced, with permission, from Dr. Frank Gaillard and www.radiopaedia.org.

454   Osteoarthritis and rheumatoid arthritis: Image A. Histology of rheumatoid nodule. This image is a derivative work, adapted from the following source, available under ▣◉▣: Gomez-Rivera F, El-Naggar AK, Guha-Thakurta N, et al. Rheumatoid arthritis mimicking metastatic squamous cell carcinoma. *Head Neck Oncol.* 2011;3:26. DOI: 10.1186/1758-3284-3-26.

455   Gout: Image B. Uric acid crystals under polarized light. This image is a derivative work, adapted from the following source, available under ▣◉▣. Courtesy of Robert J. Galindo. The image may have been modified by cropping, labeling, and/or captions. MedIQ Learning, LLC makes this image available under ▣◉▣.

455   Gout: Image C. Podagra. This image is a derivative work, adapted from the following source, available under ▣◉▣: Roddy E.

Revisiting the pathogenesis of podagra: why does gout target the foot? *J Foot Ankle Res.* 2011;4:13. DOI: 10.1186/1757-1146-4-13.

455 **Calcium pyrophosphate deposition disease.** Calcium phosphate crystals. This image is a derivative work, adapted from the following source, available under ![cc]: Dieppe P, Swan A. Identification of crystals in synovial fluid. *Ann Rheum Dis.* 1999 May;58(5):261–263.

456 **Sjögren syndrome: Image A.** Lymphocytic infiltration. ![cc] Courtesy of the US Department of Health and Human Services.

456 **Sjögren syndrome: Image B.** Dry tongue. This image is a derivative work, adapted from the following source, available under ![cc]: Negrato CA, Tarzia O. Buccal alterations in diabetes mellitus. Diabetol Metab Syndr. 2010;2:3. DOI: 10.1186/1758-5996-2-3.

456 **Septic arthritis.** Joint effusion. This image is a derivative work, adapted from the following source, available under ![cc]. Courtesy of Dr. James Heilman. The image may have been modified by cropping, labeling, and/or captions. MedIQ Learning, LLC makes this image available under ![cc].

457 **Seronegative spondyloarthropathies: Image C, left.** Bamboo spine. This image is a derivative work, adapted from the following source, available under ![cc]. Courtesy of Stevenfruitsmaak. The image may have been modified by cropping, labeling, and/or captions. MedIQ Learning, LLC makes this image available under ![cc].

457 **Seronegative spondyloarthropathies: Image C, right.** Bamboo spine. ![cc] Courtesy of Heather Hawker.

458 **Systemic lupus erythematosus: Image B.** Discoid rash. Courtesy of Dr. Kachiu Lee.

459 **Raynaud phenomenon.** This image is a derivative work, adapted from the following source, available under ![cc]. Courtesy of Jamclaassen. The image may have been modified by cropping, labeling, and/or captions. MedIQ Learning, LLC makes this image available under ![cc].

461 **Epithelial cell junctions: Image A.** Large, electron-dense actin structures within adherens junction. This image is a derivative work, adapted from the following source, available under ![cc]: Taylor RR, Jagger DJ, Saeed SR, et al. Characterizing human vestibular sensory epithelia for experimental studies: new hair bundles on old tissue and implications for therapeutic interventions in ageing. *Neurobiol Aging.* 2015 Jun;36(6):2068–2084. DOI: 10.1016/j.neurobiolaging.2015.02.013.

461 **Epithelial cell junctions: Image B.** Desmosome. This image is a derivative work, adapted from the following source, available under ![cc]: Massa F, Devader C, Lacas-Gervais S, et al. Impairement of HT29 cancer cells cohesion by the soluble form of neurotensin receptor-3. *Genes Cancer.* 2014 Jul;5(7-8):240–249. DOI: 10.18632/genesandcancer.22.

463 **Seborrheic dermatitis.** This image is a derivative work, adapted from the following source, available under ![cc]. Courtesy of Roymishali.

464 **Common skin disorders: Image O.** Urticaria. This image is a derivative work, adapted from the following source, available under ![cc]. Courtesy of Dr. James Heilman. The image may have been modified by cropping, labeling, and/or captions. MedIQ Learning, LLC makes this image available under ![cc].

465 **Vascular tumors of skin: Image C.** Cystic hygroma. This image is a derivative work, adapted from the following source, available under ![cc]: Sharif M, Elsiddig IE, Atwan F. Complete resolution of cystic hygroma with single session of intralesional bleomycin. *J Neonatal Surg.* 2012 Jul-Sep;1(3):44.

465 **Vascular tumors of skin: Image D.** Glomus tumor under fingernail. This image is a derivative work, adapted from the following source, available under ![cc]: Hazani R, Houle JM, Kasdan ML, et al. Glomus tumors of the hand. *Eplasty.* 2008;8:e48. The image may have been modified by cropping, labeling, and/or captions. All rights to this adaptation by MedIQ Learning, LLC are reserved.

466 **Skin infections: Image C.** Erysipelas. This image is a derivative work, adapted from the following source, available under ![cc]: Courtesy of Klaus D. Peter.

467 **Blistering skin disorders: Image D.** Bullous pemphigoid on immunofluorescence. This image is a derivative work, adapted from the following source, available under ![cc]: Courtesy of M. Emmanuel.

469 **Skin cancer: Image D.** Basal cell carcinoma histopathology. This image is a derivative work, adapted from the following source, available under ![cc]. Courtesy of Wikimedia Commons. The image may have been modified by cropping, labeling, and/or captions. MedIQ Learning, LLC makes this image available under ![cc].

Neurology and Special Senses

475 **Holoprosencephaly.** This image is a derivative work, adapted from the following source, available under ![cc]: Alorainy IA, Barlas NB, Al-Boukai AA. Pictorial essay: infants of diabetic mothers. *Indian J Radiol Imaging.* 2010 Aug;20(3):174–181. DOI: 10.4103/0971-3026.69349.

476 **Posterior fossa malformations: Image A.** Chiari I malformation. This image is a derivative work, adapted from the following source, available under ![cc]: Toldo I, De Carlo D, Mardari R, et al. Short lasting activity-related headaches with sudden onset in children: a case-based reasoning on classification and diagnosis. *J Headache Pain.* 2013;14(1):3. DOI: 10.1186/1129-2377-14-3.

476 **Posterior fossa malformations: Image B.** Dandy-Walker malformation. This image is a derivative work, adapted from the following source, available under ![cc]: Krupa K, Bekiesinska-Figatowska M. Congenital and acquired abnormalities of the corpus callosum: a pictorial essay. *Biomed Res Int.* 2013;2013:265619. DOI: 10.1155/2013/265619.

476 **Syringomyelia.** Reproduced, with permission, from Dr. Frank Gaillard and www.radiopaedia.org.

478 **Myelin.** Myelinated neuron. ![cc] Courtesy of the Electron Microscopy Facility at Trinity College.

479 **Chromatolysis.** This image is a derivative work, adapted from the following source, available under ![cc]. Courtesy of Dr. Michael Bonnert. The image may have been modified by cropping, labeling, and/or captions. MedIQ Learning, LLC makes this image available under ![cc].

482 **Limbic system.** This image is a derivative work, adapted from the following source, available under ![cc]: Schopf V, Fischmeister FP, Windischberger C, et al. Effects of individual glucose levels

on the neuronal correlates of emotions. *Front Hum Neurosci.* 2013 May;21;7:212. DOI: 10.3389/fnhum.2013.00212.

483 Cerebellum. This image is a derivative work, adapted from the following source, available under [cc]: Jarius S, Wandinger KP, Horn S, et al. A new Purkinje cell antibody (anti-Ca) associated with subacute cerebellar ataxia: immunological characterization. *J Neuroinflammation.* 2010;7: 21. DOI: 10.1186/1742-2094-7-21.

486 Cerebral arteries—cortical distribution. Cortical watershed areas. This image is a derivative work, adapted from the following source, available under [cc]: Isabel C, Lecler A, Turc G, et al. Relationship between watershed infarcts and recent intra plaque haemorrhage in carotid atherosclerotic plaque. *PLoS One.* 2014;9(10):e108712. DOI: 10.1371/journal.pone.0108712.

487 Dural venous sinuses. This image is a derivative work, adapted from the following source, available under [cc]: Cikla U, Aagaard-Kienitz B, Turski PA, et al. Familial perimesencephalic subarachnoid hemorrhage: two case reports. *J Med Case Rep.* 2014;8. DOI: 10.1186/1752-1947-8-380. The image may have been modified by cropping, labeling, and/or captions. All rights to this adaptation by MedIQ Learning, LLC are reserved.

492 Spinal cord and associated tracts. Spinal cord cross-section. This image is a derivative work, adapted from the following source, available under [cc]: Courtesy of Regents of University of Michigan Medical School.

496 Neonatal interventricular hemorrhage. This image is a derivative work, adapted from the following source, available under [cc]: Shooman D, Portess H, Sparrow O. A review of the current treatment methods for posthaemorrhagic hydrocephalus of infants. *Cerebrospinal Fluid Res.* 2009;6:1. DOI: 10.1186/1743-8454-6-1.

497 Intracranial hemorrhage: Image A. Axial CT of brain showing epidural blood. This image is a derivative work, adapted from the following source, available under [cc]. Courtesy of Hellerhoff. The image may have been modified by cropping, labeling, and/or captions. MedIQ Learning, LLC makes this image available under [cc].

497 Intracranial hemorrhage: Image B. Axial CT of brain showing skull fracture and scalp hematoma. This image is a derivative work, adapted from the following source, available under [cc]. Courtesy of Hellerhoff. The image may have been modified by cropping, labeling, and/or captions. MedIQ Learning, LLC makes this image available under [cc].

497 Intracranial hemorrhage: Image C. Subdural hematoma. This image is a derivative work, adapted from the following source, available under [cc]. Courtesy of Dr. James Heilman. The image may have been modified by cropping, labeling, and/or captions. MedIQ Learning, LLC makes this image available under [cc].

497 Intracranial hemorrhage: Image E. Subarachnoid hemorrhage. This image is a derivative work, adapted from the following source, available under [cc]: Hakan T, Turk CC, Celik H. Intra-operative real time intracranial subarachnoid haemorrhage during glial tumour resection: a case report. *Cases J.* 2008;1:306. DOI: 10.1186/1757-1626-1-306. The image may have been modified by cropping, labeling, and/or captions. All rights to this adaptation by MedIQ Learning, LLC are reserved.

499 Effects of strokes: Image A. Large abnormality of the left MCA territory. This image is a derivative work, adapted from the

following source, available under [cc]: Hakimelahi R, Yoo AJ, He J, et al. Rapid identification of a major diffusion/perfusion mismatch in distal internal carotid artery or middle cerebral artery ischemic stroke. *BMC Neurol.* 2012 Nov;5;12:132. DOI: 10.1186/1471-2377-12-132. The image may have been modified by cropping, labeling, and/or captions. All rights to this adaptation by MedIQ Learning, LLC are reserved.

499 Effects of strokes: Image B. MRI diffusion weighted image shows a hypersensitive lesion on posterior limb of internal capsular. This image is a derivative work, adapted from the following source, available under [cc]: Zhou L, Ni J, Yao M, et al. High-resolution MRI findings in patients with capsular warning syndrome. *BMC Neurol.* 2014;14:16. DOI: 10.1186/1471-2377-14-16.

499 Effects of strokes: Image C. Infarct of posterior inferior cerebellar artery. This image is a derivative work, adapted from the following source, available under [cc]: Nouh A, Remke J, Ruland S. Ischemic posterior circulation stroke: a review of anatomy, clinical presentations, diagnosis, and current management. *Front Neurol.* 2014 Apr;7;5:30. DOI: 10.3389/fneur.2014.00030.

499 Effects of strokes: Image D. Infarct of posterior cerebral artery. This image is a derivative work, adapted from the following source, available under [cc]: Nakao Y, Terai H. Embolic brain infarction related to posttraumatic occlusion of vertebral artery resulting from cervical spine injury: a case report. *J Med Case Rep.* 2014;8:344. DOI: 10.1186/1752-1947-8-344.

499 Diffuse axonal injury. Moenninghoff C, Kraff O, Maderwald S, et al. Diffuse axonal injury at ultra-high field MRI. *PLoS One.* 2015;10(3):e0122329. DOI: 10.1371/journal.pone.0122329.

505 Neurodegenerative disorders: Image A. Lewy body in substantia nigra. This image is a derivative work, adapted from the following source, available under [cc]: Werner CJ, Heyny-von Haussen R, Mall G, et al. Parkinson's disease. *Proteome Sci.* 2008;6:8. DOI: 10.1186/1477-5956-6-8. The image may have been modified by cropping, labeling, and/or captions. All rights to this adaptation by MedIQ Learning, LLC are reserved.

505 Neurodegenerative disorders: Image B. Gross specimen of normal brain. This image is a derivative work, adapted from the following source, available under [cc]: Niedowicz DM, Nelson PT, Murphy MP. Alzheimer's disease: pathological mechanisms and recent insights. *Curr Neuropharmacol.* 2011 Dec;9(4):674–84. DOI: 10.2174/157015911798376181.

505 Neurodegenerative disorders: Images C (brain atrophy in Alzheimer disease) and **F** (atrophy in frontotemporal dementia). This image is a derivative work, adapted from the following source, available under [cc]: Niedowicz DM, Nelson PT, Murphy MP. Alzheimer's disease: pathological mechanisms and recent insights. *Curr Neuropharmacol.* 2011 Dec;9(4):674–684. DOI: 10.2174/157015911798376181.

505 Neurodegenerative disorders: Image D. Neurofibrillary tangles in Alzheimer disease. Courtesy of Dr. Kristine Krafts

505 Neurodegenerative disorders: Image G. Pick bodies in frontotemporal dementia. This image is a derivative work, adapted from the following source, available under [cc]: Niedowicz DM, Nelson PT, Murphy MP. Alzheimer's disease: pathological mechanisms and recent insights. *Curr Neuropharmacol.* 2011;9:674–684. DOI: 10.2174/157015911798376181.

505 **Neurodegenerative disorders: Image H.** Spongiform changes in brain in Creutzfeld-Jacob disease. This image is a derivative work, adapted from the following source, available under [cc]. Courtesy of DRdoubleB. The image may have been modified by cropping, labeling, and/or captions. MedIQ Learning, LLC makes this image available under [cc].

506 **Hydrocephalus: Image B.** Communicating hydrocephalus. This image is a derivative work, adapted from the following source, available under [cc]: Torres-Martin M, Pena-Granero C, Carceller F, et al. Homozygous deletion of *TNFRSF4*, *TP73*, *PPAP2B* and *DPYD* at 1p and *PDCD5* at 19q identified by multiplex ligation-dependent probe amplification (MLPA) analysis in pediatric anaplastic glioma with questionable oligodendroglial component. *Mol Cytogenet.* 2014;7:1. DOI: 10.1186/1755-8166-7-1.

506 **Hydrocephalus: Image C.** Ex vacuo ventriculomegaly. This image is a derivative work, adapted from the following source, available under [cc]: Ghetti B, Oblak AL, Boeve BF, et al. Frontotemporal dementia caused by microtubule-associated protein tau gene (*MAPT*) mutations: a chameleon for neuropathology and neuroimaging. *Neurophathol Appl Neurobiol.* 2015 Feb;41(1):24–46. DOI: 10.1111/nan.12213.

507 **Multiple sclerosis.** Periventricular plaques. This image is a derivative work, adapted from the following source, available under [cc]: Dooley MC, Foroozan R. Optic neuritis. *J Ophthalmic Vis Res.* 2010 Jul;5(3):182–187.

508 **Other demyelinated and dysmyelinating disorders: Image A.** Central pontine myelinolysis. This image is a derivative work, adapted from the following source, available under [cc]. Courtesy of Wikimedia Commons. The image may have been modified by cropping, labeling, and/or captions. MedIQ Learning, LLC makes this image available under [cc].

508 **Other demyelinating and dysmyelinating disorders: Image B.** Progressive multifocal leukoencephalopathy. This image is a derivative work, adapted from the following source, available under [cc]: Garrote H, de la Fuente A, Ona R, et al. Long-term survival in a patient with progressive multifocal leukoencephalopathy after therapy with rituximab, fludarabine and cyclophosphamide for chronic lymphocytic leukemia. *Exp Hematol Oncol.* 2015;4:8. DOI: 10.1186/s40164-015-0003-4.

509 **Neurocutaneous disorders: Image A.** Sturge-Weber syndrome and port wine stain. This image is a derivative work, adapted from the following source, available under [cc]: Babaji P, Bansal A, Krishna G, et al. Sturge-Weber syndrome with osteohypertrophy of maxilla. *Case Rep Pediatr* 2013. DOI: 10.1155/2013/964596.

509 **Neurocutaneous disorders: Image B.** Leptomeningeal angioma in Sturge-Weber syndrome. Reproduced, with permission, from Dr. Frank Gaillard and www.radiopaedia.org.

509 **Neurocutaneous disorders: Image C.** Tuberous sclerosis. This image is a derivative work, adapted from the following source, available under [cc]: Fred H, van Dijk H. Images of memorable cases: case 143. Connexions Web site. December 4, 2008. Available at: http://cnx.org/content/m14923/1.3/.

509 **Neurocutaneous disorders: Image D.** Ash leaf spots in tuberous sclerosis. This image is a derivative work, adapted from the following source, available under [cc]: Tonekaboni SH, Tousi P, Ebrahimi A, et al. Clinical and para clinical manifestations of tuberous sclerosis: a cross sectional study on 81 pediatric patients. *Iran J Child Neurol.* 2012;6:25–31. PMCID PMC3943027.

509 **Neurocutaneous disorders: Image E.** Angiomyolipoma in tuberous sclerosis. This image is a derivative work, adapted from the following source, available under [cc]. Courtesy of KGH. The image may have been modified by cropping, labeling, and/or captions. MedIQ Learning, LLC makes this image available under [cc].

509 **Neurocutaneous disorders: Image F.** Café-au-lait spots in neurofibromatosis. This image is a derivative work, adapted from the following source, available under [cc]. Courtesy of Wikimedia Commons. The image may have been modified by cropping, labeling, and/or captions. MedIQ Learning, LLC makes this image available under [cc].

509 **Neurocutaneous disorders: Image G.** Lisch nodules in neurofibromatosis. [cc] Courtesy of the US Department of Health and Human Services.

509 **Neurocutaneous disorders: Image H.** Cutaneous neurofibromas. This image is a derivative work, adapted from the following source, available under [cc]: Kim BK, Choi YS, Gwoo S, et al. Neurofibromatosis type 1 associated with papillary thyroid carcinoma incidentally detected by thyroid ultrasonography: a case report. *J Med Case Rep.* 2012;6:179. DOI: 10.1186/1752-1947-6-179.

509 **Neurocutaneous disorders: Image I.** Cerebellar hemangioblastoma histology. This image is a derivative work, adapted from the following source, available under [cc]. Courtesy of Dr. Michael Bonert. The image may have been modified by cropping, labeling, and/or captions. MedIQ Learning, LLC makes this image available under [cc].

509 **Neurocutaneous disorders: Image J.** Brainstem and spinal cord hemangioblastomas in von Hippel-Lindau disease. This image is a derivative work, adapted from the following source, available under [cc]: Park DM, Zhuang Z, Chen L, et al. von Hippel-Lindau disease-associated hemangioblastomas are derived from embryologic multipotent cells. *PLoS Med.* 2007 Feb;4(2):e60. DOI: 10.1371/journal.pmed.0040060.

511 **Adult primary brain tumors: Image A.** Glioblastoma multiforme. [cc] Courtesy of the US Department of Health and Human Services and the Armed Forces Institute of Pathology.

511 **Adult primary brain tumors: Image B.** Glioblastoma multiforme histology. This image is a derivative work, adapted from the following source, available under [cc]. Courtesy of Wikimedia Commons. The image may have been modified by cropping, labeling, and/or captions. MedIQ Learning, LLC makes this image available under [cc].

511 **Adult primary brain tumors: Image C.** Oligodendroglioma in frontal lobes. This image is a derivative work, adapted from the following source, available under [cc]: Celzo FG, Venstermans C, De Belder F, et al. Brain stones revisited—between a rock and a hard place. *Insights Imaging.* 2013 Oct;4(5):625–35. DOI: 10.1007/s13244-013-0279-z.

511 **Adult primary brain tumors: Image D.** Oligodendroglioma, "fried egg" cells. This image is a derivative work, adapted from the following source, available under [cc]. Courtesy of Nephron. The image may have been modified by cropping, labeling, and/or captions. MedIQ Learning, LLC makes this image available under [cc].

511 **Adult primary brain tumors: Image E.** Meningioma with dural tail. This image is a derivative work, adapted from the following source, available under [cc]: Smits A, Zetterling M, Lundin M, et al. Neurological impairment linked with cortico-subcortical infiltration of diffuse low-grade gliomas at initial diagnosis supports early brain plasticity. *Front Neurol.* 2015;6:137. DOI: 10.3389/fneur.2015.00137.

511 **Adult primary brain tumors: Image F.** Meningioma, psammoma bodies. This image is a derivative work, adapted from the following source, available under [cc]. Courtesy of Nephron. The image may have been modified by cropping, labeling, and/or captions. MedIQ Learning, LLC makes this image available under [cc].

511 **Adult primary brain tumors: Image G.** Cerebellar hemangioblastoma. This image is a derivative work, adapted from the following source, available under [cc]: Park DM, Zhengping Z, Chen L, et al. von Hippel-Lindau disease-associated hemangioblastomas are derived from embryologic multipotent cells. *PLoS Med.* 2007 Feb;4(2):e60. DOI: 10.1371/journal.pmed.0040060.

511 **Adult primary brain tumors: Image H.** Minimal parenchyma in hemangioblastoma. This image is a derivative work, adapted from the following source, available under [cc]. Courtesy of Marvin 101. The image may have been modified by cropping, labeling, and/or captions. MedIQ Learning, LLC makes this image available under [cc].

511 **Adult primary brain tumors: Image I.** Prolactinoma. This image is a derivative work, adapted from the following source, available under [cc]: Wang CS, Yeh TC, Wu TC, et al. Pituitary macroadenoma co-existent with supraclinoid internal carotid artery cerebral aneurysm: a case report and review of the literature. *Cases J.* 2009;2:6459. DOI: 10.4076/1757-1626-2-6459.

511 **Adult primary brain tumors: Image J.** Field of vision in bitemporal hemianopia. This image is a derivative work, adapted from the following source, available under [cc]. Courtesy of Wikimedia Commons. The image may have been modified by cropping, labeling, and/or captions. MedIQ Learning, LLC makes this image available under [cc].

511 **Adult primary brain tumors: Image K.** Schwannoma at cerebellopontine angle. [cc] Courtesy of MRT-Bild.

511 **Adult primary brain tumors: Image L.** Schwann cell origin of schwannoma. This image is a derivative work, adapted from the following source, available under [cc]. Courtesy of Nephron. The image may have been modified by cropping, labeling, and/or captions. MedIQ Learning, LLC makes this image available under [cc].

512 **Childhood primary brain tumors: Image A.** MRI of pilocytic astrocytoma. This image is a derivative work, adapted from the following source, available under [cc]: Hafez RFA. Stereotaxic gamma knife surgery in treatment of critically located pilocytic astrocytoma: preliminary result. *World J Surg Oncol.* 2007;5:39. DOI: 10.1186/1477-7819-5-39.

512 **Childhood primary brain tumors: Image C.** CT of medulloblastoma. [cc] Courtesy of the US Department of Health and Human Services and the Armed Forces Institute of Pathology.

512 **Childhood primary brain tumors: Image D.** Medulloblastoma histology. This image is a derivative work, adapted from the following source, available under [cc]. Courtesy of KGH. The image may have been modified by cropping, labeling, and/or captions. MedIQ Learning, LLC makes this image available under [cc].

512 **Childhood primary brain tumors: Image E.** MRI of ependymoma. This image is a derivative work, adapted from the following source, available under [cc]. Courtesy of Hellerhoff. The image may have been modified by cropping, labeling, and/or captions. MedIQ Learning, LLC makes this image available under [cc].

512 **Childhood primary brain tumors: Image F.** Ependymoma histology. This image is a derivative work, adapted from the following source, available under [cc]. Courtesy of Nephron. The image may have been modified by cropping, labeling, and/or captions. MedIQ Learning, LLC makes this image available under [cc].

512 **Childhood primary brain tumors: Image G.** CT of craniopharyngioma. This image is a derivative work, adapted from the following source, available under [cc]: Garnet MR, Puget S, Grill J, et al. Craniopharyngioma. *Orphanet J Rare Dis.* 2007;2:18. DOI: 10.1186/1750-1172-2-18.

512 **Childhood primary brain tumors: Image H.** Craniopharyngioma histology. This image is a derivative work, adapted from the following source, available under [cc]. Courtesy of Nephron. The image may have been modified by cropping, labeling, and/or captions. MedIQ Learning, LLC makes this image available under [cc].

515 **Friedreich ataxia: Image A.** Clinical kyphoscoliosis. This image is a derivative work, adapted from the following source, available under [cc]: Axelrod FB, Gold-von Simson. Hereditary sensory and autonomic neuropathies: types II, III, and IV. *Orphanet J Rare Dis.* 2007;2:39. DOI: 10.1186/1750-1172-2-39.

515 **Friedreich ataxia: Image B.** Radiograph showing kyphoscoliosis. This image is a derivative work, adapted from the following source, available under [cc]: Bounakis N, Karampalis C, Tsirikos AI. Surgical treatment of scoliosis in Rubinstein-Taybi syndrome type 2: a case report. *J Med Case Rep.* 2015;9:10. DOI: 10.1186/1752-1947-9-10.

516 **Facial nerve lesions.** Facial nerve palsy. This image is a derivative work, adapted from the following source, available under [cc]: Socolovsky M, Paez MD, Di Masi G, et al. Bell's palsy and partial hypoglossal to facial nerve transfer: Case presentation and literature review. *Surg Neurol Int.* 2012;3:46. DOI:10.4103/2152-7806.95391.

517 **Cholesteatoma.** This image is a derivative work, adapted from the following source, available under [cc]. Courtesy of Welleschik. The image may have been modified by cropping, labeling, and/or captions. MedIQ Learning, LLC makes this image available under [cc].

518 **Normal eye.** This image is a derivative work, adapted from the following source, available under [cc]. Courtesy of Jan Kaláb. The image may have been modified by cropping, labeling, and/or captions. MedIQ Learning, LLC makes this image available under [cc].

518 **Conjunctivitis.** This image is a derivative work, adapted from the following source, available under [cc]: Baiyeroju A, Bowman R, Gilbert C, et al. Managing eye health in young children. *Community Eye Health.* 2010;23:4–11.

519 **Cataract.** Juvenile cataract. This image is a derivative work, adapted from the following source, available under [icon]: Roshan M, Vijaya PH, Lavanya GR, et al. A novel human CRYGD mutation in a juvenile autosomal dominant cataract. *Mol Vis.* 2010;16:887–896. PMCID PMC2875257.

520 **Glaucoma: Images A** (normal optic cup) and **B** (optic cup in glaucoma). Courtesy of Dr. Nicholas Mahoney.

520 **Glaucoma: Image C.** Closed/narrow angle glaucoma. This image is a derivative work, adapted from the following source, available under [icon]: Low S, Davidson AE, Holder GE, et al. Autosomal dominant Best disease with an unusual electrooculographic light rise and risk of angle-closure glaucoma: a clinical and molecular genetic study. *Mol Vis.* 2011;17:2272–2282. PMCID PMC3171497. The image may have been modified by cropping, labeling, and/or captions. All rights to this adaptation by MedIQ Learning, LLC are reserved.

520 **Glaucoma: Image D.** Acute angle closure glaucoma. This image is a derivative work, adapted from the following source, available under [icon]. Courtesy of Dr. Jonathan Trobe.

520 **Uveitis.** This image is a derivative work, adapted from the following source, available under [icon]: Weber AC, Levison AL, Srivastava, et al. A case of *Listeria monocytogenes* endophthalmitis with recurrent inflammation and novel management. *J Ophthalmic Inflamm Infect.* 2015;5(1):28. DOI: 10.1186/s12348-015-0058-8.

520 **Age-related macular degeneration.** [icon] Courtesy of the US Department of Health and Human Services.

521 **Diabetic retinopathy.** This image is a derivative work, adapted from the following source, available under [icon]: Sundling V, Gulbrandsen P, Straand J. Sensitivity and specificity of Norwegian optometrists' evaluation of diabetic retinopathy in single-field retinal images—a cross-sectional experimental study. *BMC Health Services Res.* 2013;13:17. DOI: 10.1186/1472-6963-13-17.

521 **Hypertensive retinopathy.** This image is a derivative work, adapted from the following source, available under [icon]: Diallo JW, Méda N, Tougouma SJB, et al. Intérêts de l'examen du fond d'œil en pratique de ville: bilan de 438 cas. *Pan Afr Med J.* 2015;20:363. DOI: 10.11604/pamj.2015.20.363.6629.

521 **Retinal vein occlusion.** This image is a derivative work, adapted from the following source, available under [icon]: Alasil T, Rauser ME. Intravitreal bevacizumab in the treatment of neovascular glaucoma secondary to central retinal vein occlusion: a case report. *Cases J.* 2009;2:176. DOI: 10.1186/1757-1626-2-176. The image may have been modified by cropping, labeling, and/or captions. All rights to this adaptation by MedIQ Learning, LLC are reserved.

521 **Retinal detachment.** Courtesy of EyeRounds.

522 **Retinitis pigmentosa.** Courtesy of EyeRounds.

522 **Retinitis.** [icon] Courtesy of the US Department of Health and Human Services.

522 **Papilledema.** Courtesy of Dr. Nicholas Mahoney.

524 **Ocular motility.** Testing ocular muscles. This image is a derivative work, adapted from the following source, available under [icon]. Courtesy of Au.yousef. The image may have been modified by cropping, labeling, and/or captions. MedIQ Learning, LLC makes this image available under [icon].

525 **Cranial nerve III, IV, VI palsies: Image A.** Cranial nerve III damage. This image is a derivative work, adapted from the following source, available under [icon]: Hakim W, Sherman R, Rezk T, et al. An acute case of herpes zoster ophthalmicus with ophthalmoplegia. *Case Rep Ophthalmol Med.* 1012; 2012:953910. DOI: 10.1155/2012/953910.

525 **Cranial nerve III, IV, VI palsies: Image B.** Cranial nerve IV damage. This image is a derivative work, adapted from the following source, available under [icon]: Mendez JA, Arias CR, Sanchez D, et al. Painful ophthalmoplegia of the left eye in a 19-year-old female, with an emphasis in Tolosa-Hunt syndrome: a case report. *Cases J.* 2009;2:8271. DOI: 10.4076/1757-1626-2-8271.

525 **Cranial nerve III, IV, VI palsies: Image C.** Cranial nerve VI damage. This image is a derivative work, adapted from the following source, available under [icon]. Courtesy of Jordi March i Nogué. The image may have been modified by cropping, labeling, and/or captions. MedIQ Learning, LLC makes this image available under [icon].

Renal

562 **Potter sequence (syndrome).** [icon] Courtesy of the US Department of Health and Human Services and the Armed Forces Institute of Pathology.

564 **Course of ureters.** This image is a derivative work, adapted from the following source, available under [icon]. Courtesy of Wikimedia Commons. The image may have been modified by cropping, labeling, and/or captions. MedIQ Learning, LLC makes this image available under [icon].

565 **Glomerular filtration barrier.** This image is a derivative work, adapted from the following source, available under [icon]: Feng J, Wei H, Sun Y, et al. Regulation of podocalyxin expression in the kidney of streptozotocin-induced diabetic rats with Chinese herbs (Yishen capsule). *BMC Complement Altern Med.* 2013;13:76. DOI: 10.1186/1472-6882-13-76.

578 **Casts in urine: Image A.** RBC casts. Courtesy of Dr. Adam Weinstein.

578 **Casts in urine: Image B.** This image is a derivative work, adapted from the following source, available under [icon]: Perazella MA. Diagnosing drug-induced AIN in the hospitalized patient: a challenge for the clinician. *Clin Nephrol.* 2014 Jun;81(6):381-8. DOI: 10.5414/CN108301.

578 **Casts in urine: Image C.** Granular cysts. Courtesy of Dr. Adam Weinstein.

578 **Casts in urine: Image D.** Waxy casts. This image is a derivative work, adapted from the following source, available under [icon]: Courtesy of Iqbal Osman.

578 **Casts in urine: Image E.** Hyaline casts. Courtesy of Dr. Adam Weinstein.

580 **Nephrotic syndrome: Image B.** Histology of focal segmental glomerulosclerosis. This image is a derivative work, adapted from the following source, available under [icon]. Courtesy of Dr. Michael Bonert. The image may have been modified by cropping, labeling, and/or captions. MedIQ Learning, LLC makes this image available under [icon].

580 **Nephrotic syndrome: Image D.** Diabetic glomerulosclerosis with Kimmelstiel-Wilson lesions. This image is a derivative work, adapted from the following source, available under [icon].

581 Nephritic syndrome: Image A. Histology of acute poststreptococcal glomerulonephritis. This image is a derivative work, adapted from the following source, available under ⊜⊙⊚. Courtesy of Dr. Michael Bonert. The image may have been modified by cropping, labeling, and/or captions. MedIQ Learning, LLC makes this image available under ⊜⊙⊚.

581 Nephritic syndrome: Image B. This image is a derivative work, adapted from the following source, available under ⊜⊙⊚: Immunofluorescence of acute poststreptococcal glomerulonephritis. Oda T, Yoshizawa N, Yamakami K, et al. The role of nephritis-associated plasmin receptor (naplr) in glomerulonephritis associated with streptococcal infection. *Biomed Biotechnol.* 2012;2012:417675. DOI: 10.1155/2012/417675.

581 Nephritic syndrome: Image C. Histology of rapidly progressive glomerulonephritis. ⊜⊙⊚ Courtesy of the US Department of Health and Human Services and Uniformed Services University of the Health Sciences.

581 Nephritic syndrome: Image E. Membranoproliferative glomerulonephritis with "tram tracks" appearance on H&E stain. Courtesy of Dr. Adam Weinstein.

581 Nephritic syndrome: Image E. Membranoproliferative glomerulonephritis with "tram tracks" appearance on PAS. Courtesy of Dr. Adam Weinstein.

582 Kidney stones: Image D. Uric acid crystals. Courtesy of Dr. Adam Weinstein.

583 Hydronephrosis. Ultrasound. This image is a derivative work, adapted from the following source, available under ⊜⊙⊚. Courtesy of Wikimedia Commons. The image may have been modified by cropping, labeling, and/or captions. MedIQ Learning, LLC makes this image available under ⊜⊙⊚.

583 Renal cell carcinoma: Image A. Histoilogy. This image is a derivative work, adapted from the following source, available under ⊜⊙⊚. Courtesy of Dr. Yale Rosen. The image may have been modified by cropping, labeling, and/or captions. MedIQ Learning, LLC makes this image available under ⊜⊙⊚.

583 Renal cell carcinoma: Image B. Gross specimen. ⊜⊙⊚ Courtesy of Dr. Ed Uthman.

583 Renal cell carcinoma: Image C. CT scan. This image is a derivative work, adapted from the following source, available under ⊜⊙⊚: Behnes CL, Schlegel C, Shoukier M, et al. Hereditary papillary renal cell carcinoma primarily diagnosed in a cervical lymph node: a case report of a 30-year-old woman with multiple metastases. *BMC Urol.* 2013;13:3. DOI: 10.1186/1471-2490-13-3.

583 Renal oncocytoma: Image A. Gross specimen. This image is a derivative work, adapted from the following source, available under ⊜⊙⊚: Courtesy of M. Emmanuel.

583 Renal oncocytoma: Image B. Histology. This image is a derivative work, adapted from the following source, available under ⊜⊙⊚. Courtesy of Dr. Michael Bonert. The image may have been modified by cropping, labeling, and/or captions. MedIQ Learning, LLC makes this image available under ⊜⊙⊚.

584 Nephroblastoma (Wilms tumor). This image is a derivative work, adapted from the following source, available under ⊜⊙⊚: Refaie H, Sarhan M, Hafez A. Role of CT in assessment of unresectable Wilms tumor response after preoperative chemotherapy in pediatrics. *Sci World J.* 2008;8:661–669. DOI: 10.1100/tsw.2008.96.

584 Transitional cell carcinoma: Image A. This image is a derivative work, adapted from the following source, available under ⊜⊙⊚: Geavlete B, Stanescu F, Moldoveanu C, et al. NBI cystoscopy and bipolar electrosurgery in NMIBC management—an overview of daily practice. *J Med Life.* 2013;6:140–145. PMCID PMC3725437.

585 Pyelonephritis: Image B. CT scan in acute pyelonephritis. ⊜⊙⊚ Courtesy of the US Department of Health and Human Services and the Armed Forces Institute of Pathology.

587 Acute tubular necrosis: Image A. Muddy brown casts. This image is a derivative work, adapted from the following source, available under ⊜⊙⊚. Courtesy of Dr. Serban Nicolescu.

587 Renal papillary necrosis. ⊜⊙⊚ Courtesy of the US Department of Health and Human Services and William D. Craig, Dr. Brent J. Wagner, and Mark D. Travis.

588 Renal cyst disorders: Image C. Ultrasound of simple cyst. This image is a derivative work, adapted from the following source, available under ⊜⊙⊚. Courtesy of Nevit Dilmen. The image may have been modified by cropping, labeling, and/or captions. MedIQ Learning, LLC makes this image available under ⊜⊙⊚.

Reproductive

597 Fetal alcohol syndrome. Characteristic facies. This image is a derivative work, adapted from the following source, available under ⊜⊙⊚. Courtesy of Teresa Kellerman. The image may have been modified by cropping, labeling, and/or captions. MedIQ Learning, LLC makes this image available under ⊜⊙⊚.

600 Umbilical cord. Cross-section of normal umbilical cord. This image is a derivative work, adapted from the following source, available under ⊜⊙⊚. Courtesy of Dr. Ed Uthman. The image may have been modified by cropping, labeling, and/or captions. MedIQ Learning, LLC makes this image available under ⊜⊙⊚.

605 Uterine (Müllerian) duct anomalies: Images A-D. This image is a derivative work, adapted from the following source, available under ⊜⊙⊚: Ahmadi F, Zafarani F, Haghighi H, et al. Application of 3D ultrasonography in detection of uterine abnormalities. *Int J Fertil Steril.* 2011;4:144–147. PMCID PMC4023499.

608 Female reproductive epithelial histology. Transformation zone. This image is a derivative work, adapted from the following source, available under ⊜⊙⊚: Courtesy of Dr. Ed Uthman. The image may have been modified by cropping, labeling, and/or captions. All rights to this adaptation by MedIQ Learning, LLC are reserved.

610 Seminiferous tubules. This image is a derivative work, adapted from the following source, available under ⊜⊙⊚. Courtesy of Dr. Anlt Rao. The image may have been modified by cropping, labeling, and/or captions. MedIQ Learning, LLC makes this image available under ⊜⊙⊚.

622 Choriocarcinoma: Image B. "Cannonball" metastases. This image is a derivative work, adapted from the following source, available under ©®: Lekanidi K, Vlachou PA, Morgan B, et al. Spontaneous regression of metastatic renal cell carcinoma: case report. *J Med Case Rep.* 2007;1:89. DOI: 10.1186/1752-1947-1-89.

623 **Pregnancy complications.** Ectopic pregnancy. This image is a derivative work, adapted from the following source, available under ©®: Li W, Wang G, Lin T, et al. Misdiagnosis of bilateral tubal pregnancy: a case report. *J Med Case Rep.* 2014;8:342. DOI: 10.1186/1752-1947-8-342.

626 **Vulvar pathology: Image A.** Bartholin cyst. ©®: Courtesy of the US Department of Health and Human Services and Susan Lindsley.

626 **Vulvar pathology: Image B.** Lichen sclerosis. This image is a derivative work, adapted from the following source, available under ©®: Lambert J. Pruritus in female patients. *Biomed Res Int.* 2014;2014:541867. DOI: 10.1155/2014/541867.

626 **Vulvar pathology: Image C.** Vulvar carcinoma. This image is a derivative work, adapted from the following source, available under ©®: Ramli I, Hassam B. Carcinome épidermoïde vulvaire: pourquoi surveiller un lichen scléro-atrophique. *Pan Afr Med J.* 2015;21:48. DOI: 10.11604/pamj.2015.21.48.6018.

626 **Vulvar pathology: Image D.** Extramallary Paget disease. This image is a derivative work, adapted from the following source, available under ©®: Wang X, Yang W, Yang J. Extramammary Paget's disease with the appearance of a nodule: a case report. *BMC Cancer.* 2010;10:405. DOI: 10.1186/1471-2407-10-405.

627 **Polycystic ovarian syndrome (Stein-Leventhal syndrome).** This image is a derivative work, adapted from the following source, available under ©®: Lujan ME, Chizen DR, Peppin AK, et al. Improving inter-observer variability in the evaluation of ultrasonographic features of polycystic ovaries. *Reprod Biol Endocrinol.* 2008;6:30. DOI: 10.1186/1477-7827-6-30.

628 **Ovarian neoplasms: Image C.** Mature cystic teratoma. This image is a derivative work, adapted from the following source, available under ©®. Courtesy of Dr. Michael Bonert. The image may have been modified by cropping, labeling, and/or captions. MedIQ Learning, LLC makes this image available under ©®.

628 **Ovarian neoplasms: Image D.** Call-Exner bodies. This image is a derivative work, adapted from the following source, available under ©®: Katoh T, Yasuda M, Hasegawa K, et al. Estrogen-producing endometrioid adenocarcinoma resembling sex cord-stromal tumor of the ovary: a review of four postmenopausal cases. *Diagn Pathol.* 2012;7:164. DOI: 10.1186/1746-1596-7-164.

628 **Ovarian neoplasms: Image E.** Dysgerminoma. This image is a derivative work, adapted from the following source, available under ©®: Montesinos L, Acien P, Martinez-Beltran M, et al. Ovarian dysgerminoma and synchronic contralateral tubal pregnancy followed by normal intra-uterine gestation: a case report. *J Med Rep.* 2012;6:399. DOI: 10.1186/1752-1947-6-399.

628 **Ovarian neoplasms: Image F.** Yolk sac tumor. This image is a derivative work, adapted from the following source, available under ©®. Courtesy of Jensflorian. The image may have been modified by cropping, labeling, and/or captions. MedIQ Learning, LLC makes this image available under ©®.

630 **Endometrial conditions: Image A.** Leiomyoma (fibroid), gross specimen. This image is a derivative work, adapted from the following source, available under ©®: Courtesy of Hic et nunc.

630 **Endometrial conditions: Image B.** Leiomyoma (fibroid) histology. This image is a derivative work, adapted from the following source, available under ©®: Londero AP, Perego P, Mangioni C, et al. Locally relapsed and metastatic uterine leiomyoma: a case report. *J Med Case Rep.* 2008;2:308. DOI: 10.1186/1752-1947-2-308. The image may have been modified by cropping, labeling, and/or captions. All rights to this adaptation by MedIQ Learning, LLC are reserved.

630 **Endometrial conditions: Image D.** Endometritis with inflammation of the endometrium. This image is a derivative work, adapted from the following source, available under ©®: Montesinos L, Acien P, Martinez-Beltran M, et al. Ovarian dysgerminoma and synchronic contralateral tubal pregnancy followed by normal intra-uterine gestation: a case report. *J Med Rep.* 2012;6:399. DOI: 10.1186/1752-1947-6-399.

630 **Endometrial conditions: Image E.** Endometrial tissue found outside the uterus. This image is a derivative work, adapted from the following source, available under ©®: Hastings JM, Fazleabas AT. A baboon model for endometriosis: implications for fertility. *Reprod Biol Endocrinol.* 2006;4(suppl 1):S7. DOI: 10.1186/1477-7827-4-S1-S7.

631 **Benign breast disease: Image A.** Fibroadenomas. This image is a derivative work, adapted from the following source, available under ©®: Gokhale S. Ultrasound characterization of breast masses. *Indian J Radiol Imaging.* 2009 Aug;19(3):242–247. DOI: 10.4103/0971-3026.54878.

631 **Benign breast disease: Images B** (phyllodes tumor on ultrasound) and **C** (phyllodes cyst). This image is a derivative work, adapted from the following source, available under ©®: Muttarak MD, Lerttumnongtum P, Somwangjaroen A, et al. Phyllodes tumour of the breast. *Biomed Imaging Interv J.* 2006 Apr-Jun;2(2):e33. DOI: 10.2349/biij.2.2.e33.

632 **Malignant breast tumors: Image B.** Comedocarcinoma. This image is a derivative work, adapted from the following source, available under ©®: Costarelli L, Campagna D, Mauri M, et al. Intraductal proliferative lesions of the breast—terminology and biology matter: premalignant lesions or preinvasive cancer? *Int J Surg Oncol.* 2012;501904. DOI: 10.1155/2012/501904. The image may have been modified by cropping, labeling, and/or captions. All rights to this adaptation by MedIQ Learning, LLC are reserved.

632 **Malignant breast tumors: Image C.** Paget disease of breast. This image is a derivative work, adapted from the following source, available under ©®: Muttarak M, Siriya B, Kongmebhol P, et al. Paget's disease of the breast: clinical, imaging and pathologic findings: a review of 16 patients. *Biomed Imaging Interv J.* 2011;7:e16. DOI: 10.2349/biij.7.2.e16.

632 **Malignant breast tumors: Image D.** Invasive lobular carcinoma. This image is a derivative work, adapted from the following source, available under ©®: Franceschini G, Manno A, Mule A, et al. Gastro-intestinal symptoms as clinical manifestation of peritoneal and retroperitoneal spread of an invasive lobular breast cancer: report of a case and review of the literature. *BMC Cancer.* 2006;6:193. DOI: 10.1186/1471-2407-6-193.

632 **Malignant breast tumors: Image E.** Peau d'orange of inflammatory breast cancer. This image is a derivative work, adapted from the following source, available under ©®: Levine PH, Zolfaghari L, Young H, et al. What Is inflammatory breast cancer? Revisiting the case definition. *Cancers (Basel).* 2010 Mar;2(1):143–152. DOI: 10.3390/cancers2010143.

633 **Varicocele.** Dilated pampiniform veins. Courtesy of Dr. Bruce R. Gilbert.

634 **Scrotal masses.** Congenital hydrocele. This image is a derivative work, adapted from the following source, available under 😐: Leonardi S, Barone P, Gravina G, et al. Severe Kawasaki disease in a 3-month-old patient: a case report. *BMC Res Notes.* 2013;6:500. DOI: 10.1186/1756-0500-6-500.

Respiratory

643 **Alveolar cell types: Image A.** Electron micrograph of type II pneumocyte. This image is a derivative work, adapted from the following source, available under 😐: Fehrenbach H, Tews S, Fehrenbach A, et al. Improved lung preservation relates to an increase in tubular myelin-associated surfactant protein A. *Respir Res.* 2005 Jun;21;6:60. The image may have been modified by cropping, labeling, and/or captions. All rights to this adaptation by MedIQ Learning, LLC are reserved.

643 **Alveolar cell types: Image B.** Micrograph of type II pneumocyte. This image is a derivative work, adapted from the following source, available under 😐: Courtesy of Dr. Thomas Caceci.

643 **Neonatal respiratory distress syndrome.** This image is a derivative work, adapted from the following source, available under 😐: Alorainy IA, Balas NB, Al-Boukai AA. Pictorial essay: infants of diabetic mothers. *Indian J Radiol Imaging.* 2010;20:174–181. DOI: 10.4103/0971-3026.69349.

645 **Lung relations: Image A.** X-ray of normal lung. This image is a derivative work, adapted from the following source, available under 😐: Namkoong H, Fujiwara H, Ishii M, et al. Immune reconstitution inflammatory syndrome due to *Mycobacterium avium* complex successfully followed up using 18 F-fluorodeoxyglucose positron emission tomography-computed tomography in a patient with human immunodeficiency virus infection: A case report. *BMC Med Imaging.* 2015;15:24. DOI: 10.1186/s12880-015-0063-2.

645 **Lung relations: Image B.** This image is a derivative work, adapted from the following source, available under 😐: Wang JF, Wang B, Jansen JA, et al. Primary squamous cell carcinoma of lung in a 13-year-old boy: a case report. *Cases J.* 2008 Aug;22;1(1):123. DOI: 10.1186/1757-1626-1-123. The image may have been modified by cropping, labeling, and/or captions. All rights to this adaptation by MedIQ Learning, LLC are reserved.

653 **Rhinosinusitis.** This image is a derivative work, adapted from the following source, available under 😐: Strek P, Zagolski O, Sktadzien J. Fatty tissue within the maxillary sinus: a rare finding. *Head Face Med.* 2006;2:28. DOI: 10.1186/1746-160X-2-28.

653 **Deep venous thrombosis.** This image is a derivative work, adapted from the following source, available under 😐. Courtesy of Dr. James Heilman. The image may have been modified by cropping, labeling, and/or captions. MedIQ Learning, LLC makes this image available under 😐.

654 **Pulmonary emboli: Image C.** CT scan. This image is a derivative work, adapted from the following source, available under 😐. Courtesy of Dr. Carl Chartrand-Lefebvre. The image may have been modified by cropping, labeling, and/or captions. MedIQ Learning, LLC makes this image available under 😐.

657 **Obstructive lung diseases: Image A.** Lung tissue with enlarged alveoli in emphysema. This image is a derivative work, adapted

from the following source, available under 😐. Courtesy of Dr. Michael Bonnert.

657 **Obstructive lung diseases: Image B.** CT of centriacinar emphysema. 😐 Courtesy of the US Department of Health and Human Services and Dr. Edwin P. Ewing, Jr.

657 **Obstructive lung diseases: Image C.** Emphysema histology. This image is a derivative work, adapted from the following source, available under 😐. Courtesy of Dr. Michael Bonert. The image may have been modified by cropping, labeling, and/or captions. MedIQ Learning, LLC makes this image available under 😐.

657 **Obstructive lung diseases: Image D.** Barrel-shaped chest in emphysema. This image is a derivative work, adapted from the following source, available under 😐. Courtesy of Dr. James Heilman. The image may have been modified by cropping, labeling, and/or captions. MedIQ Learning, LLC makes this image available under 😐.

657 **Obstructive lung disease: Image E.** Curschmann spirals. The image may have been modified by cropping, labeling, and/or captions. MedIQ Learning, LLC makes this image available under 😐. Dr. James Heilman.

657 **Obstructive lung diseases: Image F.** Mucus plugs in asthma. This image is a derivative work, adapted from the following source, available under 😐. Courtesy of Courtesy of Dr. Yale Rosen. The image may have been modified by cropping, labeling, and/or captions. MedIQ Learning, LLC makes this image available under 😐.

657 **Obstructive lung diseases: Image G.** Charcot-Leyden crystals on bronchalverolar lavage. This image is a derivative work, adapted from the following source, available under 😐: Gholamnejad M, Rezaie N. Unusual presentation of chronic eosinophilic pneumonia with "reversed halo sign": a case report. *Iran J Radiol.* 2014 May;11(2):e7891. DOI: 10.5812/iranjradiol.7891.

657 **Obstructive lung disease: Image H.** Bronchiectasis in cystic fibrosis. This image is a derivative work, adapted from the following source, available under 😐. Courtesy of Dr. Yale Rosen. The image may have been modified by cropping, labeling, and/or captions. MedIQ Learning, LLC makes this image available under 😐.

657 **Restrictive lung diseases: Image A.** Pulmonary fibrosis. This image is a derivative work, adapted from the following source, available under 😐: Walsh SLF, Wells AU, Sverzellati N, et al. Relationship between fibroblastic foci profusion and high resolution CT morphology in fibrotic lung disease. *BMC Med.* 2015;13:241. DOI: 10.1186/s12916-015-0479-0.

658 **Sarcoidosis: Images B (X-ray of the chest) and C (CT of the chest).** This image is a derivative work, adapted from the following source, available under 😐: Lønborg J, Ward M, Gill A, et al. Utility of cardiac magnetic resonance in assessing right-sided heart failure in sarcoidosis. *BMC Med Imaging.* 2013;13:2. DOI: 10.1186/1471-2342-13-2.

658 **Inhalational injury and sequelae: Images A** (18 hours after inhalation injury) and **B** (11 days after injury). This image is a derivative work, adapted from the following source, available under 😐: Bai C, Huang H, Yao X, et al. Application of flexible bronchoscopy in inhalation lung injury. *Diagn Pathol.* 2013;8:174. DOI: 10.1186/1746-1596-8-174.

659 **Pneumoconioses: Image A.** Pleural plaques in asbestosis. This image is a derivative work, adapted from the following source, available under ⊚⊚⊚. Courtesy of Dr. Yale Rosen. The image may have been modified by cropping, labeling, and/or captions. MedIQ Learning, LLC makes this image available under ⊚⊚⊚.

659 **Pneumoconioses: Image B.** CT scan of asbestosis. This image is a derivative work, adapted from the following source, available under ⊚⊚⊚: Miles SE, Sandrini A, Johnson AR, et al. Clinical consequences of asbestos-related diffuse pleural thickening: a review. *J Occup Med Toxicol.* 2008;3:20. DOI: 10.1186/1745-6673-3-20.

659 **Pneumoconioses: Image C.** Ferruginous bodies in asbestosis. This image is a derivative work, adapted from the following source, available under ⊚⊚⊚. Courtesy of Dr, Michael Bonert. The image may have been modified by cropping, labeling, and/or captions. MedIQ Learning, LLC makes this image available under ⊚⊚⊚.

660 **Mesothelioma.** This image is a derivative work, adapted from the following source, available under ⊚⊚: Weiner SJ, Neragi-Miandoab S. Pathogenesis of malignant pleural mesothelioma and the role of environmental and genetic factors. *J Carcinog.* 2008;7:3. DOI: 10.1186/1477-3163-7-3.

660 **Acute respiratory distress syndrome: Image B.** Bilateral lung opacities. This image is a derivative work, adapted from the following source, available under ⊚⊚: Imanaka H, Takahara B, Yamaguchi H, et al. Chest computed tomography of a patient revealing severe hypoxia due to amniotic fluid embolism: a case report. *J Med Case Reports.* 2010;4:55. DOI: 10.1186/1752-1947-4-55.

662 **Pleural effusions: Images A** (before treatment) and **B** (after treatment). This image is a derivative work, adapted from the following source, available under ⊚⊚: Toshikazu A, Takeoka H, Nishioka K, et al. Successful management of refractory pleural effusion due to systemic immunoglobulin light chain amyloidosis by vincristine adriamycin dexamethasone chemotherapy: a case report. *Med Case Rep.* 2010;4:322. DOI: 10.1186/1752-1947-4-322.

664 **Pneumonia: Image B.** Lobar pneumonia, gross specimen. This image is a derivative work, adapted from the following source, available under ⊚⊚⊚. Courtesy of Dr. Yale Rosen. The image may have been modified by cropping, labeling, and/or captions. MedIQ Learning, LLC makes this image available under ⊚⊚⊚.

664 **Pneumonia: Image C.** Acute inflammatory infiltrates in bronchopneumonia. This image is a derivative work, adapted from the following source, available under ⊚⊚⊚. Courtesy of Dr. Yale Rosen. The image may have been modified by cropping, labeling, and/or captions. MedIQ Learning, LLC makes this image available under ⊚⊚⊚.

664 **Pneumonia: Image D.** Bronchopneumonia, gross specimen. This image is a derivative work, adapted from the following source, available under ⊚⊚⊚. Courtesy of Dr. Yale Rosen. The image may have been modified by cropping, labeling, and/or captions. MedIQ Learning, LLC makes this image available under ⊚⊚⊚.

665 **Lung cancer: Image B.** Adenocarcinoma histology. ⊚⊚⊚ Courtesy of the US Department of Health and Human Services and the Armed Forces Institute of Pathology.

665 **Lung cancer: Image C.** Squamous cell carcinoma. This image is a derivative work, adapted from the following source, available under ⊚⊚⊚. Courtesy of Dr. James Heilman. The image may have been modified by cropping, labeling, and/or captions. MedIQ Learning, LLC makes this image available under ⊚⊚⊚.

665 **Lung cancer: Image E.** Large cell lung cancer. This image is a derivative work, adapted from the following source, available under ⊚⊚⊚: Jala VR, Radde BN, Haribabu B, et al. Enhanced expression of G-protein coupled estrogen receptor (GPER/GPR30) in lung cancer. *BMC Cancer.* 2012;12:624. DOI: 10.1186/1471-2407-12-624.

666 **Lung abscess: Image A.** Gross specimen. This image is a derivative work, adapted from the following source, available under ⊚⊚⊚. Courtesy of Dr. Yale Rosen. The image may have been modified by cropping, labeling, and/or captions. MedIQ Learning, LLC makes this image available under ⊚⊚⊚.

666 **Lung abscess: Image B.** X-ray. This image is a derivative work, adapted from the following source, available under ⊚⊚: Courtesy of Dr. Yale Rosen.

666 **Pancoast tumor.** This image is a derivative work, adapted from the following source, available under ⊚⊚⊚: Manenti G, Raguso M, D'Onofrio S, et al. Pancoast tumor: the role of magnetic resonance imaging. *Case Rep Radiol.* 2013;2013:479120. DOI: 10.1155/2013/479120.

666 **Superior vena cava syndrome: Images A** (blanching of skin with pressure) and **B** (CT of chest). This image is a derivative work, adapted from the following source, available under ⊚⊚⊚: Shaikh I, Berg K, Kman N. Thrombogenic catheter-associated superior vena cava syndrome. *Case Rep Emerg Med.* 2013;2013:793054. DOI: 10.1155/2013/793054.

▶ NOTES

Index

About the Editors

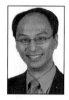

Tao Le, MD, MHS

Tao developed a passion for medical education as a medical student. He currently edits more than 15 titles in the *First Aid* series. In addition, he is Founder and Chief Education Officer of USMLE-Rx for exam preparation and ScholarRx for undergraduate medical education. As a medical student, he was editor-in-chief of the University of California, San Francisco (UCSF) *Synapse*, a university newspaper with a weekly circulation of 9000. Tao earned his medical degree from UCSF in 1996 and completed his residency training in internal medicine at Yale University and fellowship training at Johns Hopkins University. Tao subsequently went on to cofound Medsn, a medical education technology venture, and served as its chief medical officer. He is currently chief of adult allergy and immunology at the University of Louisville.

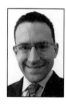

Matthew Sochat, MD

Matthew is a first-year hematology/oncology fellow at St. Louis University in St. Louis, Missouri. He completed his internal medicine residency training at Temple University Hospital in Philadelphia. He completed medical school in 2013 at Brown University and is a 2008 graduate of the University of Massachusetts, Amherst, where he studied biochemistry and the classics. Pastimes include skiing, cooking/baking, traveling, the company of friends/loved ones (especially his wonderful wife), the Spanish language, and computer/video gaming. Be warned: Matt also loves to come up with corny jokes at (in)opportune moments.

Mehboob Kalani, MD

Mehboob is a third-year internal medicine resident at Allegheny Health Network Medical Education Consortium in Pittsburgh. He was born in Karachi, Pakistan, grew up in Toronto, Canada, and pursued medicine upon completing high school. He earned his bachelor's and medical degrees at American University of Integrative Sciences in 2015. After residency, his interests lie in pulmonary critical care medicine, and he is researching COPD exacerbation treatment and readmission rates. In his limited leisure time, Mehboob enjoys playing or watching soccer, long drives, and family gatherings.

Andrew Zureick

Andrew is a fourth-year medical student at the University of Michigan who hopes to pursue residency training in radiation oncology. He earned his bachelor's degree at Dartmouth College in 2013, graduating Phi Beta Kappa and summa cum laude with high honors in Chemistry. He is a coauthor of *What Every Science Student Should Know*, a guidebook for undergraduate STEM majors published in 2016 by the University of Chicago Press. His interests include medical education and health policy. In his spare time, he enjoys playing the piano, golf, tennis, and creative writing.

Vikas Bhushan, MD

Vikas is a writer, editor, entrepreneur, and teleradiologist on extended sabbatical. In 1990 he conceived and authored the original *First Aid for the USMLE Step 1*. His entrepreneurial endeavors include a student-focused medical publisher (S2S), an e-learning company, and an ER teleradiology practice (24/7 Radiology). Trained on the Left Coast, Vikas completed a bachelor's degree at the University of California Berkeley; an MD with thesis at UCSF; and a diagnostic radiology residency at UCLA. His eclectic interests include technology, information design, photography, South Asian diasporic culture, and avoiding a day job. Always finding the long shortcut, Vikas is an adventurer, knowledge seeker, and occasional innovator. He enjoys novice status as a kiteboarder and single father, and strives to raise his children as global citizens.

Yash Chavda, DO

Yash is an emergency medicine resident at St. Barnabas Hospital in the Bronx. He earned his medical degree from NYIT College of Osteopathic Medicine, and completed his undergraduate degrees in biology and psychology at CUNY Baruch College in 2010. Yash has many interests outside of medicine and enjoys spending time with his loved ones. He is a developing photographer, former web/graphic designer (who still dabbles), video gamer, foodie, and avid explorer who wants to travel the world (whenever he actually gets a chance). He hopes to always keep improving at everything he does.

Kimberly Kallianos, MD

Originally from Atlanta, Kimberly graduated from the University of North Carolina at Chapel Hill in 2006 and from Harvard Medical School in 2011. She completed her radiology residency at the University of California, San Francisco (UCSF) in 2016 and is currently an Assistant Professor of Clinical Radiology at UCSF.